Food Engineering: Concepts and Applications

Food Engineering: Concepts and Applications

Edited by Lisa Jordan

SYRAWOOD
PUBLISHING HOUSE
New York

Published by Syrawood Publishing House,
750 Third Avenue, 9th Floor,
New York, NY 10017, USA
www.syrawoodpublishinghouse.com

Food Engineering: Concepts and Applications
Edited by Lisa Jordan

International Standard Book Number: 978-1-68286-620-7 (Hardback)

Cataloging-in-Publication Data

Food engineering : concepts and applications / edited by Lisa Jordan.
p. cm.
Includes bibliographical references and index.
ISBN 978-1-68286-620-7
1. Food industry and trade. 2. Food industry and trade--Technological innovations.
3. Food. 4. Food--Biotechnology. I. Jordan, Lisa.

TP370 .F66 2018
664--dc23

Printed in China.

TABLE OF CONTENTS

PREFACE

Food engineering studies the nature of food and processes related to the production of food. It helps in the development of new processed food products and new techniques of manufacturing these products. Some of the disciplines related to this subject are food technology, food preservation, food microbiology, food chemistry, etc. This book outlines the processes and applications of food science in detail. It is a vital tool for all those who are researching or studying food engineering as it gives incredible insights into emerging trends and concepts.

After months of intensive research and writing, this book is the end result of all who devoted their time and efforts in the initiation and progress of this book. It will surely be a source of reference in enhancing the required knowledge of the new developments in the area. During the course of developing this book, certain measures such as accuracy, authenticity and research focused analytical studies were given preference in order to produce a comprehensive book in the area of study.

This book would not have been possible without the efforts of the authors and the publisher. I extend my sincere thanks to them. Secondly, I express my gratitude to my family and well-wishers. And most importantly, I thank my students for constantly expressing their willingness and curiosity in enhancing their knowledge in the field, which encourages me to take up further research projects for the advancement of the area.

Editor

Rapid Molecular Identification of Human Taeniid Cestodes by Pyrosequencing Approach

Tongjit Thanchomnang[1,2], Chairat Tantrawatpan[1,3], Pewpan M. Intapan[1,4], Oranuch Sanpool[1,4], Penchom Janwan[1,5], Viraphong Lulitanond[1,6], Somjintana Tourtip[2], Hiroshi Yamasaki[7], Wanchai Maleewong[1,4]*

1 Research and Diagnostic Center for Emerging Infectious Diseases, Khon Kaen University, Khon Kaen, Thailand, **2** Faculty of Medicine, Mahasarakham University, Mahasarakham, Thailand, **3** Division of Cell Biology, Department of Preclinical Sciences, Faculty of Medicine, Thammasat University, Rangsit Campus, Pathum Thani, Thailand, **4** Department of Parasitology, Faculty of Medicine, Khon Kaen University, Khon Kaen, Thailand, **5** Department of Medical Technology, School of Allied Health Sciences and Public Health, Walailak University, Thasala, Nakhon Si Thammarat, Thailand, **6** Department of Microbiology, Faculty of Medicine, Khon Kaen University, Khon Kaen, Thailand, **7** Department of Parasitology, National Institute of Infectious Diseases, Tokyo, Japan

Abstract

Taenia saginata, T. solium, and *T. asiatica* are causative agents of taeniasis in humans. The difficulty of morphological identification of human taeniids can lead to misdiagnosis or confusion. To overcome this problem, several molecular methods have been developed, but use of these tends to be time-consuming. Here, a rapid and high-throughput pyrosequencing approach was developed for the identification of three human taeniids originating from various countries. Primers targeting the mitochondrial cytochrome *c* oxidase subunit 1 (*cox1*) gene of the three *Taenia* species were designed. Variations in a 26-nucleotide target region were used for identification. The reproducibility and accuracy of the pyrosequencing technology was confirmed by Sanger sequencing. This technique will be a valuable tool to distinguish between sympatric human taeniids that occur in Thailand, Asia and Pacific countries. This method could potentially be used for the molecular identification of the taeniid species that might be associated with suspicious cysts and lesions, or cyst residues in humans or livestock at the slaughterhouse.

Editor: Emmanuel Dias-Neto, AC Camargo Cancer Hospital, Brazil

Funding: This research was supported by grants from the National Science and Technology Development Agency (Discovery Based Development Grant), the Higher Education Research Promotion and National Research University Project of Thailand, the Office of the Higher Education Commission through the Health Cluster (SHep-GMS) and Khon Kaen University, Thailand. TT PMI WM are supported by TRF Senior Research Scholar Grant, Thailand Research Fund grant number RTA5580004. This work also was supported in part by a Grant-in Aid for Scientific Research from the Ministry of Health, Labour and Welfare, Japan (H24-25-Shinko-Ippan-014) to HY. The funders had no role in study design, data collection and analysis, decision to publish, or preparation of the manuscript.

Competing Interests: The authors have declared that no competing interests exist.

* Email: wanch_ma@kku.ac.th

Introduction

Human taeniasis is a disease caused by several *Taenia* spp., including *Taenia saginata, T. solium*, and *T. asiatica* [1–3]. Taeniids have a worldwide distribution [4]. Their definitive hosts are carnivores that become infected after eating larvae (cysticerci) contained in meat from herbivorous intermediate hosts. The larvae develop to adulthood in the small intestine and shed gravid proglottids, which pass to the outside in feces and disintegrate to release the eggs contained within. Eggs ingested by grazing herbivores develop to cysticerci in muscles and elsewhere. Human taeniasis is acquired from inadequately cooked infected pork (*T. solium* and *T. asiatica*) or beef (*T. saginata*). For many years there was debate about the status of *T. asiatica*, with many scientists considering it to be a variant of the beef tapeworm because of similarities in the adult worms [5]. It was named as a new species in 1993 [2]. Amongst the features distinguishing it from the beef tapeworm are morphological details of the cysticerci and the site where these are found (mostly the liver of pigs, whereas cysticerci of *T. saginata* are found mostly in muscles of bovids).

In the case of *T. solium*, if humans ingest eggs, these can develop into cysticerci in organs such as the brain, causing cysticercosis [1]. Cysticercosis, especially neurocysticercosis, due to *T. solium* can be fatal in humans [1]. *Taenia saginata* and probably *T. asiatica* are relatively harmless in humans: the adult worms occur in the small intestine and cause only a few specific symptoms, such as abdominal pain and nausea [6]. While *T. solium* and *T. saginata* have worldwide distributions, *T. asiatica* [5] is found mostly in Asian countries, including Korea, China, Taiwan, Thailand, Indonesia, Vietnam, Philippines, and Japan [7,8]. The early detection and adequate treatment of taeniasis is important for the prevention of *T. solium* infection and/or cysticercosis [9]. Necessary epidemiological tools for effective control of taeniasis or cysticercosis include accurate methods for parasite identification. At present, the morphological identification of proglottids and scolices expelled from tapeworm carriers, or of cysticerci collected from intermediate hosts, are the routine approaches that are employed.

In areas where these cestodes are sympatric, distinguishing between proglottids of *T. saginata* and *T. asiatica* is impeded by their strong morphological similarities. The diagnosis of taeniasis by micrococoscopy using fecal samples from patients is unreliable because the eggs of these species are very similar. The only reliable and completely accurate approach for the differentiation of taeniid eggs, cysticerci and proglottids is the use of DNA-based methods. Several PCR tests/assays targeting various genomic regions are available for differentiating human *Taenia* infections. These include PCR-restriction fragment length polymorphism (RFLP) methods [10–11], loop-mediated isothermal amplification (LAMP) [12], the use of species-specific DNA probes [13], the BESS T-base method [14], PCR for the differentiation of *T. saginata* and *T. solium* [15], multiplex PCR for the detection of *T. saginata* and *T. asiatica* and of the American/African and Asian genotypes of *T. solium* using primers from the *cox1* gene [16], a high-resolution multiplex PCR assay [17] and a nested PCR system [18]. Analyzing the results from these methods requires gel electrophoresis, which is slow, has a limited throughput, and is prone to carry-over contamination and subjective results.

A rapid DNA sequencing method, pyrosequencing, is a promising tool for yielding diagnostic data. The method relies on determining the sequence of addition of nucleotides to a primer complementary to a single stranded template. As a nucleotide is incorporated into the growing complementary strand by a polymerase, pyrophosphate is released which is converted to ATP by ATP sulphurylase. The ATP in turn is an energy source for luciferase, allowing it to oxidise luciferin and generate a detectable quantity of light [19]. Light is only generated when a newly added nucleotide is complementary to the next unpaired base in the template strand. The intensity of light is proportional to the number of sequential identical bases in homopolymers, but determining the exact length of a homopolymer can be a problem for this technique [19]. Pyrosequencing has been used in a broad range of applications, such as SNP genotyping, *de novo* mutation detection, gene identification and microbial genotyping [20]. It has recently been developed for the species-level identification of *Entamoeba* species [21] and has been applied to several parasite taxa, such as *Plasmodium* [22], *Paragonimus* [23] and *Trichinella* species [24]. The use of pyrosequencing for the identification of human taeniids has not yet been reported. The present study aimed to develop a pyrosequencing method for sequencing amplicons from *cox1* for the identification of *Taenia* species that are parasites of humans and intermediate hosts.

Materials and Methods

Parasite and DNA Materials

Forty-seven specimens of expelled proglottids were collected from patients who visited hospitals in Thailand, Japan, and China for medical treatment (Table 1). One cysticercus specimen was collected from a dead pig in the Kathmandu market, Kathmandu, Nepal; one cysticercus specimen was collected from a dead pig in the Cocal dos Alves market in Cocal dos Alves City, Piracuruca, Piaui State, northeastern Brazil; and one cysticercus specimen was from beef in the Saitama meat inspection center, Saitama City, Saitama Prefecture, Japan. All Thai samples of *T. saginata* (Table 1) were collected from patients who visited the Srinagarind Hospital, Faculty of Medicine, Khon Kaen University, Khon Kaen, Thailand. Additional *T. saginata* samples and two samples of *T. solium* proglottids were from patients of various nationalities treated in hospitals in Tokyo, Japan. A *Taenia asiatica* proglottid from China (case 8) was from a Chinese patient who was treated in a hospital in Dali, Yunnan province. In this case, the proglottid was expelled during mass treatment in the township. Three further *T. asiatica* samples were from Japanese patients who were treated in hospitals in the Tokyo area. The human cases diagnosed in Japan have been previously described [8]. In every case, each worm was analyzed individually.

All of the procedures used in this study were approved by the Human Ethics Committee of Khon Kaen University, based on the Ethics of Human Experimentation of the National Research Council of Thailand (Reference No. HE561396) and ethical approval (No. 177) of the Ethics Committee of the National Institute of Infectious Diseases, Tokyo, Japan. Because the parasites were recovered from diagnostic specimens acquired during routine laboratory investigations, and from fecal specimens from patients who visited the hospital for medical treatment, documented informed consent was not required by the Ethics Committees. Patient anonymity was maintained. The study was made up of research on pre-existing specimens. Specimens of cysticerci that were obtained from local markets and slaughter-houses do not correspond to the PLoS criteria for observational

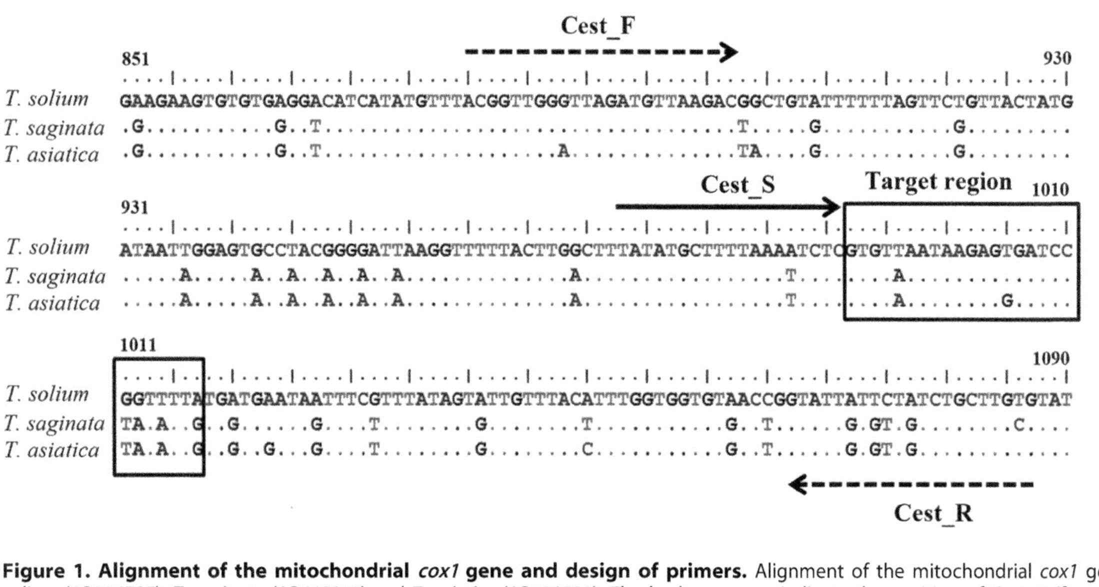

Figure 1. Alignment of the mitochondrial *cox1* gene and design of primers. Alignment of the mitochondrial *cox1* gene derived from *T. solium* (AB524785), *T. saginata* (AB645845) and *T. asiatica* (AB608739). The broken arrows indicate the position of Cest_F (forward primer) and the biotinylated Cest_R (reverse primer) for template amplification. The solid arrow indicates Cest_S (sequencing primer), and the rectangular box shows the position (992–1017) of the target region used for species level identification. The dots indicate identical nucleotides between the sequences.

Table 1. Characteristics and molecular identification of the 47 taeniasis cases examined in this study.

Patient				scolex/proglottids expelled	Locality	Sanger Sequencing	Pyrosequencing
Case No.	**Sex**	**Age, y**	**Year**				
1	M	30	2007	proglottid	Thailand	*T. saginata*	*T. saginata*
2	M	36	2007	proglottid	Thailand	*T. saginata*	*T. saginata*
3	M	65	2007	proglottid	Thailand	*T. saginata*	*T. saginata*
4	M	76	2007	proglottid	Thailand	*T. saginata*	*T. saginata*
5	M	48	2008	proglottid	Thailand	*T. saginata*	*T. saginata*
6	M	59	2008	proglottid	Thailand	*T. saginata*	*T. saginata*
7	F	61	2008	proglottid	Thailand	*T. saginata*	*T. saginata*
8	NR	NR	2008	proglottid	China	*T. asiatica*	*T. asiatica*
9	M	50	2009	proglottid	Thailand	*T. saginata*	*T. saginata*
10	M	56	2009	proglottid	Thailand	*T. saginata*	*T. saginata*
11	M	63	2009	proglottid	Thailand	*T. saginata*	*T. saginata*
12	M	76	2009	proglottid	Thailand	*T. saginata*	*T. saginata*
13	F	23	2009	proglottid	Thailand	*T. saginata*	*T. saginata*
14	F	67	2009	proglottid	Thailand	*T. saginata*	*T. saginata*
15	F	68	2009	proglottid	Thailand	*T. saginata*	*T. saginata*
16	F	NR	2009	proglottid	Thailand	*T. saginata*	*T. saginata*
17	NR	NR	2009	proglottid	Thailand	*T. saginata*	*T. saginata*
18	F	20	2009	proglottid	India*	*T. solium*	*T. solium*
19	M	19	2010	proglottid	Thailand	*T. saginata*	*T. saginata*
20	F	37	2010	proglottid	Thailand*	*T. saginata*	*T. saginata*
21	M	31	2010	proglottid	India*	*T. solium*	*T. solium*
22	M	58	2010	proglottid	Japan*	*T. asiatica*	*T. asiatica*
23	M	40	2010	proglottid	Japan*	*T. asiatica*	*T. asiatica*
24	F	39	2010	proglottid	Japan*	*T. asiatica*	*T. asiatica*
25	M	25	2011	proglottid	Thailand	*T. saginata*	*T. saginata*
26	M	28	2011	proglottid	Thailand	*T. saginata*	*T. saginata*
27	M	51	2011	proglottid	Thailand	*T. saginata*	*T. saginata*
28	M	88	2011	proglottid	Thailand	*T. saginata*	*T. saginata*
29	M	NR	2011	proglottid	Thailand	*T. saginata*	*T. saginata*
30	F	51	2011	proglottid	Thailand	*T. saginata*	*T. saginata*
31	F	70	2011	proglottid	Thailand	*T. saginata*	*T. saginata*
32	M	33	2011	proglottid	Sudan*	*T. saginata*	*T. saginata*
33	F	24	2011	proglottid	Ethiopia*	*T. saginata*	*T. saginata*
34	F	42	2011	proglottid	France*	*T. saginata*	*T. saginata*

Table 1. Cont.

Patient				scolex/proglottids expelled	Locality	Sanger Sequencing	Pyrosequencing
Case No.	Sex	Age, y	Year				
35	M	21	2012	proglottid	Thailand	*T. saginata*	*T. saginata*
36	M	28	2012	proglottid	Thailand	*T. saginata*	*T. saginata*
37	M	50	2012	scolex and proglottid	Thailand	*T. saginata*	*T. saginata*
38	M	50	2012	proglottid	Thailand	*T. saginata*	*T. saginata*
39	M	56	2012	proglottid	Laos	*T. saginata*	*T. saginata*
40	M	59	2012	proglottid	Thailand	*T. saginata*	*T. saginata*
41	M	62	2012	proglottid	Thailand	*T. saginata*	*T. saginata*
42	M	70	2012	proglottid	Thailand	*T. saginata*	*T. saginata*
43	M	75	2012	proglottid	Thailand	*T. saginata*	*T. saginata*
44	M	78	2012	proglottid	Thailand	*T. saginata*	*T. saginata*
45	M	60	2012	proglottid	Mali*	*T. saginata*	*T. saginata*
46	M	89	2013	proglottid	Thailand	*T. saginata*	*T. saginata*
47	F	51	2013	proglottid	Thailand	*T. saginata*	*T. saginata*

NR, no record.
*The samples were from patients who were treated in hospitals in Tokyo, Japan.

Table 2. Nucleotide patterns of the *cox1* gene to differentiate *Taenia solium, T. saginata* and *T. asiatica* using the pyrosequencing technique.

Species (Accession No.)	Nucleotide at positions					
	996	1005	1011	1012	1014	1017
T. solium (AB524785, AF360866)	T[a]	T	G/A[a]	G[a]	T[a]	A[a]
T. saginata (AB645845)	A	T	T	A	A	G
T. asiatica (AB608739)	A	G[b]	T	A	A	G

[a]Specific nucleotide to distinguish *T. solium* from *T. saginata* and *T. asiatica*.
[b]Specific nucleotide to distinguish *T. asiatica* from *T. solium* and *T. saginata*.

and field studies, and therefore separate ethics clearance was not required for these. No vertebrate specimens were used.

Primer Design

Sequences of the *cox1* gene (1,620 bp) of *T. solium* (GenBank accession no. AB524785), *T. saginata* (AB645845) and *T. asiatica* (AB608739) were used to guide primer design (Fig. 1). Based on these data, PCR primers (Cest_F; 5′-ACGGTTGGGTTA-GATGTTAAGAC -3′, corresponding to positions 880–902 and biotinylated Cest_R; biotin-5′- CGCAAGCAGACAACACAA-TAC - 3′, corresponding to positions 1087–1067) were designed. A sequencing primer, Cest_S (5′- TATATGCTTT-TAAATTCTC -3′, corresponding to positions 973–991), was also designed using pyrosequencing assay design software (Pyro-Mark Q96 ID software version 2.0; Biotage, Uppsala, Sweden) (Fig. 1). Sequences generated from this primer will differ between the three taeniid species (Fig. 1).

DNA Extraction and Plasmid Preparation

DNA was extracted from an individual proglottid of *T. saginata* obtained from each patient in Khon Kaen, Thailand, using the Nucleospin Tissue kit (Macherey-Nagel GmbH & Co, Duren, Germany). The DNA was eluted in 50 µl of distilled water, and 2 µl of the sample was used for each PCR reaction. The DNA samples were stored in a DNA bank at −70°C in the Department of Parasitology, Faculty of Medicine, Khon Kaen University until used. In all remaining cases, DNA was extracted from each sample using the DNeasy Blood & Tissue kit (Qiagen, Hilden, Germany).

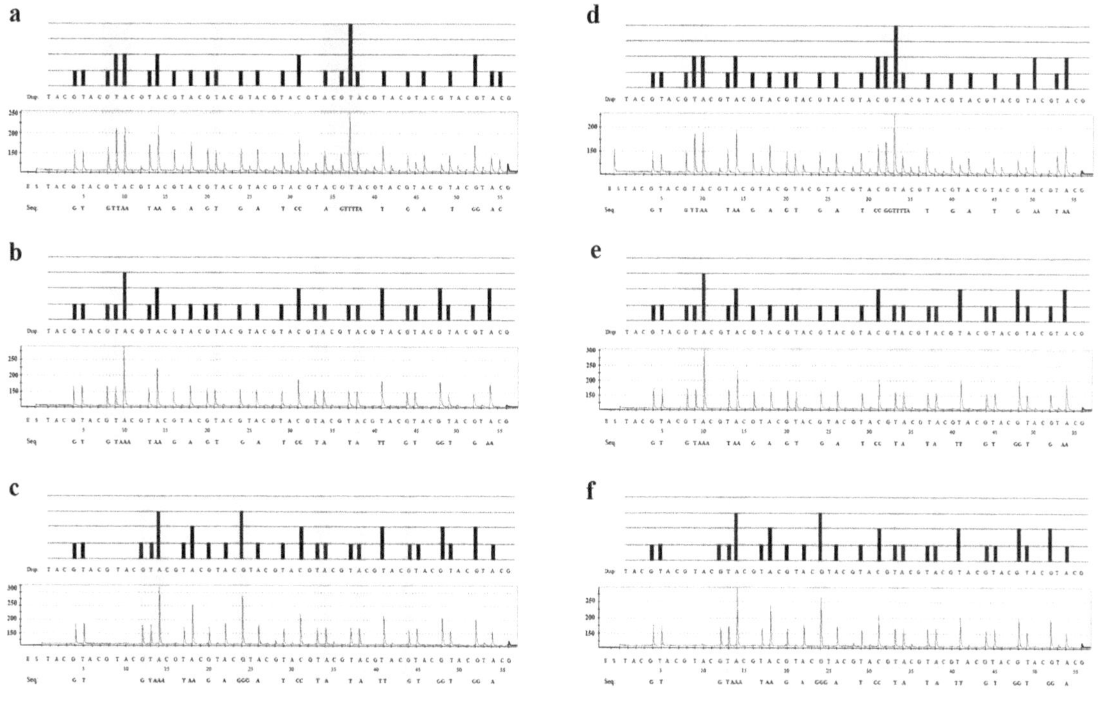

Figure 2. Sequence analysis pyrograms of *T. solium T. saginata* and *T. asiatica cox1* genes. Pyrograms showing the sequence analysis of 26-base fragments of the cox1 gene of T. solium (a, d) T. saginata (b, e) and T. asiatica (c, f) using pyrosequencing. The theoretical pyrogram patterns (top of each panel) and representative raw data from the control plasmids (a, b, c) and DNA extracted from taeniid proglottids (d, e, f) from pyrosequencing (bottom of each panel) are shown. The pyrosequencing was performed by the addition of enzyme (E), substrate (S), and four different nucleotides dispensed sequentially. The letters under the black bars show the dispensation (Disp:) order. The actual sequence detected by the pyrosequencing is indicated below the panels after "Seq:". The Y-axis represents the level of fluorescence emitted by the incorporation of a nucleotide base, and the X-axis represents the total number of bases added at that point in time; A, C, G, T, nucleotide bases. The light gray bars show the regions that can be used to distinguish between T. solium, T. saginata and T. asiatica.

For evaluation of the specificity, DNA samples from other parasites were used, including *Ascaris lumbricoides*, hookworm, *Trichuris trichiura*, *Capillaria philippinensis*, *Strongyloides stercoralis*, *Trichostrongylus* spp., *Schistosoma mekongi*, *Schistosoma japonicum*, *Opisthorchis viverrini*, *Haplorchis taichui*, *Clonorchis sinensis*, *Centrocestus* spp., *Stellantchasmus* spp., *Paragonimus heterotremus*, *Fasciola gigantica*, *Echinostoma malayanum*, intestinal lecithodendriid flukes, *Giardia duodenalis* and *Isospora belli*. Genomic DNA samples from human leukocytes (blood sample donated by W.M., approved by the Human Ethics Committee of Khon Kaen University) and beef and pork from dead animals (from the Khon Kaen market, Khon Kaen, Thailand) not infected with any taeniids were also analyzed.

Positive control plasmids of each of the *Taenia* species were constructed by ligation of each species-specific amplicon into a pGEM-T easy vector (Promega, WI), according to the manufacturer's instructions. Plasmids were propagated in *Escherichia coli* JM109 cells. Each inserted gene was sequenced in both directions using the Sanger method, and the resulting sequences were identical to the gene sequences from which the primers had been designed.

DNA Amplification by Polymerase Chain Reaction (PCR) and Pyrosequencing

The *cox1* gene fragments (208 bp) were amplified from *Taenia* DNA samples. Each PCR reaction had a final volume of 25 µl containing 1×PCR buffer (Invitrogen, Carlsbad, CA) with 0.2 mM of each dNTP, 2 mM $MgSO_4$, 0.2 µM of Cest_F primer, 0.2 µM of biotinylated Cest_R primer, 0.625 U of Platinum *Taq* DNA polymerase high fidelity (Invitrogen) and 2 µl of the DNA template. The amplification procedure was as follows: 5 min at 94°C for the initial denaturation, 35 cycles of denaturation for 30 s at 95°C, annealing for 30 s at 52°C, and extension for 30 s at 72°C, followed by a final extension for 10 min at 72°C. The molecular sizes of the amplicons were verified by electrophoresis on 1.5% agarose gels. After the PCR amplification, the biotinylated PCR products were placed in 96-well plates containing 0.4 µM Cest_S sequencing primer and processed by using the PyroMark Q96 ID instrument (Biotage) as previously described [22,23]. Following the completion of the pyrosequencing reaction, a pyrogram was produced and analyzed. The readouts were interpreted manually in case the target sequences contained homopolymers longer than four bases.

Results

The 26 nucleotides adjacent to the 3′ end of the sequencing primer were sufficient as a target region to distinguish between the three *Taenia* species using the pyrosequencing technique (Fig. 1, Fig. 2, Table 2). All of the results showed the expected sequence (Fig. 1, Table 2). *Taenia solium* could be discriminated from *T. saginata* and *T. asiatica* by nucleotides at 5 positions, and *T. asiatica* was distinct from *T. saginata* at one nucleotide position (Table 2). The reproducibility of the pyrosequencing approach was confirmed by Sanger sequencing of the amplicons, which yielded identical sequence data. The specificity of the PCR primer set was analyzed, and the results showed that no amplification product was detected with the DNA of other parasites or genomic DNA from human leukocytes or uninfected beef and pork (data not shown).

Discussion

Taenia solium, *T. saginata* and *T. asiatica* are sympatric in a number of Asian countries. Differentiating between *T. saginata* and *T. asiatica* proglottids is difficult because of their morphological similarities. It is hard to differentiate between the eggs of all three species using morphological features. A rapid, reliable and high-throughput molecular method to differentiate between these taeniid cestodes is therefore important for epidemiological and clinical reasons [7,8,16], as outlined in the introduction.

Previous molecular approaches to species identification/diagnosis i.e. the PCR-RFLP technique [10] the base excision sequence scanning thymine-base method [14], the multiplex PCR [16], the nested-PCR method [18], and the LAMP method [12,25,26], reviewed in the introduction, all have drawbacks. Most require many pairs and primers and gel or polyacrylamide electrophoresis; this electrophoresis is sluggish, has a limited throughput and is prone to carry-over contamination. The pyrosequencing technique is such a method. All of the steps, from the DNA extraction to pyrosequencing, can be completed within 4 h with the same degree of accuracy as Sanger sequencing, but without the need for labeled nucleotides, labeled primers and electrophoresis. Using pyrosequencing, a large number of samples can be analyzed in a short time, and at much lower cost for reagents [27]. Some limitations of this approach include the short read lengths (25–50 bp) and that long homopolymers, if present, create problems for the analysis. The latter problem can be resolved by manual evaluation of the pyrograms. In our experiments, pyrosequencing yielded exactly the same data as Sanger sequencing of PCR amplicons for the 26 nucleotides of the target region. The pyrosequencing technique can be used as an effective means for the identification of *T. saginata, T. asiatica* and *T. solium*. The primer set used in this present study was highly specific for *Taenia* species and did not amplify products from other parasites or genomic DNA from human leukocytes or uninfected beef and pork. A future application could be to use this technique for the species-specific identification of taeniid eggs or DNA in fecal samples, allowing for the identification of *T. solium*, *T. saginata* and *T. asiatica* without the need for proglottid samples. This identification application is important for the treatment and prevention of *T. solium,* which, being a causative agent of neurocysticercosis, is the most serious taeniid species for humans. More *T. asiatica* isolates should be investigated in future work to determine whether there is any intra-specific variation in the target region, especially in countries from which we did not have samples. Another potential use is the identification of tapeworm species suspected of producing cysts or other lesions in livestock at the slaughterhouse. The application of the technique needs to be further evaluated with those parasites/pathogens that might be misidentified by visual inspection.

We have presented here a rapid and reliable approach to distinguishing between the main species of *Taenia* that infect humans. This basic method can be modified to apply to other species of cestode, or indeed of any pathogens. The pyrosequencing method also lends itself to high-throughput analyses that might be required for broad-scale surveys.

Acknowledgments

We thank the Khon Kaen University Publication Clinic, Research and Technology Transfer Affairs, Khon Kaen University, for their assistance. The authors thank Drs. M.O. Sato (Universidade Federal do Tocantins, Palmas, Brazil), D. D. Joshi (National Zoonoses and Food Hygiene Research Centre, Kathmandu, Nepal) and M. Saito (Saitama Meat Inspection Center, Saitama, Japan) for proving cysticerci specimens of *T. solium* and *T. saginata.*

Author Contributions

Conceived and designed the experiments: TT PMI HY WM. Performed the experiments: CT OS PJ ST. Analyzed the data: TT VL WM. Contributed reagents/materials/analysis tools: PMI HY WM. Wrote the paper: TT HY WM. Critically reviewed the manuscript: TT PMI HY WM.

References

1. Ito A, Nakao M, Wandra T (2003) Human taeniasis and cysticercosis in Asia. Lancet 362: 1918–1920.
2. Jeon HK, Eom KS (2013) Molecular approaches to *Taenia asiatica*. Korean J Parasitol 51: 1–8.
3. Flisser A (2013) State of the art of *Taenia solium* as compared to *Taenia asiatica*. Korean J Parasitol 51: 43–49.
4. García HH, Gonzalez AE, Evans CA, Gilman RH (2003) Cysticercosis Working Group in Peru. *Taenia solium* cysticercosis. Lancet 362: 547–556.
5. Fan PC (1988) Taiwan *Taenia* and taeniasis. Parasitol Today 4: 86–88.
6. Pawlowski ZS, Murrell KD (2001) Taeniasis and cysticercosis. In: Hui YH, Sattar SA, Murrell KD, Nip W-K, Stanfield PS, editors. Foodborne Disease Handbook 2nd ed. New York: Marcel Dekker. 217–227.
7. Eom KS, Jeon HK, Rim HJ (2009) Geographical distribution of *Taenia asiatica* and related species. Korean J Parasitol 47: S115–S124.
8. Yamasaki H (2013) Current status and perspectives of cysticercosis and taeniasis in Japan. Korean J Parasitol 51: 19–29.
9. Gracey J, Collins DS, Huey RJ (1999) Cysticercosis. In: Collins DS, editor. Meat Hygiene 10th ed. London: W.B. Saunders. 669–674.
10. Bowles J, McManus DP (1994) Genetic characterization of the Asian *Taenia*, a newly described taeniid cestode of humans. Am J Trop Med Hyg 50: 33–44.
11. Gasser RB, Chilton NB (1995) Characterisation of taeniid cestode species by PCR-RFLP of ITS2 ribosomal DNA. Acta Trop 59: 31–40.
12. Nkouawa A, Sako Y, Li T, Chen X, Nakao M, et al. (2012) A loop-mediated isothermal amplification method for a differential identification of *Taenia* tapeworms from human: application to a field survey. Parasitol Int 61: 723–725.
13. Chapman A, Vallejo V, Mossie KG, Ortiz D, Agabian N, et al. (1995) Isolation and characterization of species-specific DNA probes from *Taenia solium* and *Taenia saginata* and their use in an egg detection assay. J Clin Microbiol 33: 1283–1288.
14. Yamasaki H, Nakao M, Sako Y, Nakaya K, Sato MO, et al. (2002) DNA differential diagnosis of human taeniid cestodes by base excision sequences canning thymine-base reader analysis with mitochondrial genes. J Clin Microbiol 40: 3818–3821.
15. González LM, Montero E, Morakote N, Puente S, Díaz de Tuesta JL, et al. (2004) Differential diagnosis of *Taenia saginata* and *Taenia saginata asiatica* taeniasis through PCR. Diagn Microbiol Infect Dis 49: 183–188.
16. Yamasaki H, Allan JC, Sato MO, Nakao M, Sako Y, et al. (2004) DNA differential diagnosis of taeniasis and cysticercosis by multiplex PCR. J Clin Microbiol 42: 548–553.
17. Jeon HK, Chai JY, Kong Y, Waikagul J, Insisiengmay B, et al. (2009) Differential diagnosis of *Taenia asiatica* using multiplex PCR. Exp Parasitol 121: 151–156.
18. Mayta H, Gilman RH, Prendergast E, Castillo JP, Tinoco YO, et al. (2008) Cysticercosis Working Group in Peru. Nested PCR for specific diagnosis of *Taenia solium* taeniasis. J Clin Microbiol 46: 286–289.
19. Ronaghi M (2001) Pyrosequencing sheds light on DNA sequencing. Genome Res 11: 3–11.
20. Ahmadian A, Ehn M, Hober S (2006) Pyrosequencing: history, biochemistry and future. Clin Chim Acta 363: 83–94.
21. Stensvold CR, Lebbad M, Verweij JJ, Jespersgaard C, von Samson-Himmelstjerna G, et al. (2010) Identification and delineation of members of the *Entamoeba* complex by pyrosequencing. Mol Cell Probes 24: 403–406.
22. Lulitanond V, Intapan PM, Tantrawatpan C, Sankuntaw N, Sanpool O, et al. (2012) Molecular markers for detection and differentiation of *Plasmodium falciparum* and *Plasmodium vivax* in human blood samples by pyrosequencing. J Clin Microbiol 50: 1455–1457.
23. Tantrawatpan C, Intapan PM, Janwan P, Sanpool O, Lulitanond V, et al. (2013) Molecular identification of *Paragonimus* species by DNA pyrosequencing technology. Parasitol Int 62: 341–345.
24. Sadaow L, Tantrawatpan C, Intapan PM, Lulitanond V, Boonmars T, et al. (2013) Molecular differentiation of *Trichinella spiralis*, *T. pseudospiralis*, *T. papuae* and *T. zimbabwensis* by pyrosequencing. J Helminthol 13: 1–6.
25. Nkouawa A, Sako Y, Li T, Chen X, Wandra T, et al. (2010) Evaluation of a loop-mediated isothermal amplification method using fecal specimens for differential detection of *Taenia* species from humans. J Clin Microbiol 48: 3350–3352.
26. Nkouawa A, Sako Y, Nakao M, Nakaya K, Ito A (2009) Loop-mediated isothermal amplification method for differentiation and rapid detection of *Taenia* species. J Clin Microbiol 47: 168–174.
27. Fakruddin M, Chowdhury A, Hossain MN, Mannan KS, Mazumda RM (2012) Pyrosequencing- principles and applications. Int J Life Sci Pharma Res 2: 65–76.

2

Subcutaneous Adipose Fatty Acid Profiles and Related Rumen Bacterial Populations of Steers Fed Red Clover or Grass Hay Diets Containing Flax or Sunflower-Seed

Renee M. Petri[1⁹], Cletos Mapiye[2,3⁹], Mike E. R. Dugan[2], Tim A. McAllister[1*]

1 Lethbridge Research Centre, Agriculture and Agri-Food Canada, Lethbridge, Alberta, Canada, **2** Lacombe Research Centre, Agriculture and Agri-Food Canada, Lacombe, Alberta, Canada, **3** Department of Animal Sciences, Faculty of AgriSciences, Stellenbosch University, Matieland, Western Cape, South Africa

Abstract

Steers were fed 70:30 forage:concentrate diets for 205 days, with either grass hay (GH) or red clover silage (RC), and either sunflower-seed (SS) or flaxseed (FS), providing 5.4% oil in the diets. Compared to diets containing SS, FS diets had elevated ($P<0.05$) subcutaneous *trans* (*t*)-18:1 isomers, conjugated linoleic acids and *n*-6 polyunsaturated fatty acid (PUFA). Forage and oilseed type influenced total *n*-3 PUFA, especially α-linolenic acid (ALA) and total non-conjugated diene biohydrogenation (BH) in subcutaneous fat with proportions being greater ($P<0.05$) for FS or GH as compared to SS or RC. Of the 25 bacterial genera impacted by diet, 19 correlated with fatty acids (FA) profile. *Clostridium* were most abundant when levels of conjugated linolenic acids, and *n*-3 PUFA's were found to be the lowest in subcutaneous fat, suggestive of their role in BH. *Anerophaga, Fibrobacter, Guggenheimella, Paludibacter and Pseudozobellia* were more abundant in the rumen when the levels of VA in subcutaneous fat were low. This study clearly shows the impact of oilseeds and forage source on the deposition of subcutaneous FA in beef cattle. Significant correlations between rumen bacterial genera and the levels of specific FA in subcutaneous fat maybe indicative of their role in determining the FA profile of adipose tissue. However, despite numerous correlations, the dynamics of rumen bacteria in the BH of unsaturated fatty acid and synthesis of PUFA and FA tissue profiles require further experimentation to determine if these correlations are consistent over a range of diets of differing composition. Present results demonstrate that in order to achieve targeted FA profiles in beef, a multifactorial approach will be required that takes into consideration not only the PUFA profile of the diet, but also the non-oil fraction of the diet, type and level of feed processing, and the role of rumen microbes in the BH of unsaturated fatty acid.

Editor: Ayyalasomayajula Vajreswari, National Institute of Nutrition, India

Funding: This work was financed by the Alberta Meat and Livestock Agency (ALMA). Dr. C. Mapiye acknowledges the receipt of NSERC Fellowships funded through ALMA (alma.alberta.ca). The funders had no role in study design, data collection and analysis, decision to publish, or preparation of the manuscript.

Competing Interests: The authors have declared that no competing interests exist.

* Email: tim.mcallister@agr.gc.ca

⁹ These authors contributed equally to this work.

Introduction

The healthfulness of beef has been challenged because of its relatively high concentrations of saturated fatty acids (SFA [1]), including myristic (14:0) and palmitic (16:0) acids which have been shown to raise serum levels of low-density lipoproteins, a risk factor for cardiovascular disease in humans [2]. However, meat also contains essential fatty acids (EFA) such as α-linolenic acid (18:3*n*-3, ALA) and its elongation and desaturation products including eicosapentaenoic acid (20:5*n*-3, EPA), docosapentenoic acid (22:5*n*-3) and docosahexaenoic acid (22:6*n*-3; DHA) and rumen biohydrogenation (BH) products including rumenic acid (*c*9,*t*11-18:2, RA) and its precursor vaccenic acid (*t*11-18:1, VA) which have purported human health-promoting properties [3–6]. In this context, current research efforts have been directed at finding dietary strategies that facilitate higher fore-stomach bypass of *n*-3 polyunsaturated fatty acids (PUFA) and specific PUFA BH products (*i.e*, VA and RA) for absorption and incorporation into adipose tissue.

Our previous studies have evaluated the effects of feeding 10 to 15% flaxseed (FS, a rich source of ALA) in the diet on ALA and its BH products in beef [7–9]. In an initial examination, feeding steers FS in a barley grain-based (73% of dry matter [DM]) diet resulted in limited absolute increases *n*-3 PUFA and their BH products in beef. In this research, the BH pathway promoted tissue accumulation of *t*13-/*t*14-18:1 rather than VA, and non-conjugated diene BH products (*i.e.*, atypical dienes, AD) in place of conjugated linoleic acids (CLA) [8]. In a second investigation, we fed cull cows grass hay (GH) or barley silage-based (50% of DM) diets supplemented with FS for 20 weeks and found that cows fed GH had a greater concentration of *n*-3 PUFA and BH products, with VA as the main *t*-18:1 isomer, as well as greater levels of AD instead of CLA in adipose tissue as compared to those fed barley silage [7,9].

Recent research in our laboratory has shown that supplementing a red clover silage (RC, 70% of DM) diet with FS for 215 days resulted in greater levels of *n*-3 PUFA and its BH products as a proportion of total fatty acids (FA) when compared to feeding other silages. As much as 2.9% of RA was found in the subcutaneous fat of cattle fed a RC diet supplemented with FS [10]. In this research, the increased amounts of PUFA BH products were in part associated with the amount and duration of FS feeding and the presence of relatively increased levels of polyphenol oxidase (PPO) activity which can produce quinones in RC, reducing the rate of PUFA lipolysis and BH in the rumen [11]. Consequently, adipose deposition of PUFA and their BH products was increased [12]. To our knowledge, no studies have directly compared RC with other forages for its effect on the concentrations of PUFA and BH intermediaries in beef adipose tissue [7].

Results from comparisons of different oilseeds suggest that those rich in linoleic acid (LA, 18:2*n*-6) such as sunflower-seed (SS) may be more effective at increasing VA and CLA in beef [13–15], while those rich in ALA increase ALA and its specific BH products. In this regard, it may be important to investigate how the deposition of VA, CLA and *n*-3 PUFA in beef differs when feeding RC as opposed to GH supplemented with SS or FS as PUFA sources.

Previously we have observed large coefficients of variation in concentrations of PUFA BH products among cattle, especially for VA, when feeding FS in high-forage diets [7,16], but the source of this inter-animal variation remains uncertain. Overall, differences in FA composition have been reported to originate from inter-animal variation in the rumen environment, including the kinds and numbers of rumen microbes present as well as other factors [17]. In this respect, determining an individual animal's rumen microbial profile with current metagenomic technologies could be useful in minimizing FA variation amongst animals consuming the same diet by designing management strategies that enhance the levels of beneficial FA in beef through microbial manipulation. It may also help to identify those microbial populations involved in BH that are inhibited by plant secondary compounds such as the quinones in RC, an outcome that results in a more favorable FA profile in beef. The objectives of the current research were to compare the effects on rumen bacterial populations and related subcutaneous FA profiles when steers were fed GH or RC diets supplemented with FS or SS. Subcutaneous fat was chosen as a representative tissue as it is used to make hamburger, which is the most consumed beef product in North America, and it is considered a more representative indicator of rumen FA metabolism than muscle [18].

Materials and Methods

Animals and diets

Animal management and diets were previously described by Mapiye et al. [19] with ethical experimental practices reviewed and approved (Protocol #201102) by Lacombe Research Centre Animal Care Committee using guidelines which are accredited by the national Canadian Council of Animal Care [20]. Briefly, 64 British × Continental crossbred steers were stratified by weight to four experimental diets, with two pens of eight steers per diet. The four diets were GH-FS, GH-SS, RC-FS and RC-SS. On a dry matter (DM) basis, diets contained 70% forage and 30% concentrate with sunflower-seed (SS) or flaxseed (FS) at a level that resulted in the addition of 5.4% oil to the diets (Table 1). In an attempt to equalize the digestible energy of the diets, additional ground-barley grain was also included in diets containing SS, and additional barley straw was added to diets containing FS. Flaxseed was triple rolled, while SS was fed whole. Nutrient and FA composition of the experimental diets are also shown in Table 1.

Sample collection procedures

Subcutaneous fat thickness was measured monthly by a certified ultrasound technician using an Aloka 500V diagnostic real-time ultrasound with a 17 cm 3.5 Mhz linear array transducer (Overseas Monitor Corporation Ltd., Richmond, B.C., Canada) following procedures of Brethour, [21]. Steers were slaughtered at the Lacombe Research Centre abattoir over four slaughter dates in November 2011 (two steers/pen/diet/slaughter day) at an average of 205 d on feed corresponding to subcutaneous fat depths of 6–8 mm between the 12th and 13th rib over the right *longissimus thoracis* muscle of each animal.

On the morning of slaughter, steers were transported 2 km to the Lacombe Research Centre abbatoir for immediate slaughter. At slaughter, final live weights were recorded and steers were stunned, exsanguinated and dressed in a commercial manner. At approximately 20 min *post-mortem*, samples of subcutaneous fat adjacent to the 12th rib were collected and stored at −80°C until analysed for FA. About 30 min *post-mortem*, the rumen was opened and the ruminal contents collected and thoroughly mixed. Thereafter, samples of ruminal contents (solids and fluid) were taken from mid-ventral region of the rumen (250 g) by the same researcher throughout the trial and placed into an open 2 L plastic container. Samples were then hand-mixed, subsampled and put in 2×50 ml plastic culture tubes. The tubes were immediately flash-frozen in liquid nitrogen and stored in a −80 freezer until DNA was extracted.

Bacterial DNA extraction, sequencing and quantification

From the 64 steers, 24 were selected for rumen bacterial analysis, based on which six animals in each dietary treatment had the lowest (n = 3) or the highest (n = 3) vaccenic acid in their subcutaneous fat. Subsamples of ruminal contents (25–40 ml) were lyophilized in a VirTis Freezemobile 25 freeze dryer (SP Industries Warminste, PA, USA), and 2–4 g of dried material was ground for 5 minutes at a frequency of 30 cycles/s in 10 ml grinding jars with a 20 mm stainless steel ball using a Qiagen TissueLyser II (Qiagen, Toronto, ON). Total DNA was extracted from dried, ground samples (30 mg) in two parallel procedures: one from the initial lysis supernatant, and the other from the initial lysis pelleted fraction of the QIAamp DNA Stool Kit as described by Narvaez et al. [22]. Final DNA elution volume was 150 µl for the supernatant fraction, and 100 µl for the pelleted fraction. Concentrations of DNA were determined spectrophotometrically using a NanoDrop 2000 (ThermoScientific, Wilmington, DE, USA), and supernatant and pellet elutions were pooled 1:1 (v/v).

Bacterial tag-encoded FLX-Titanium amplicon pyrosequencing (bTEFAP) of the pooled DNA, [23], was performed at MR DNA (Shallowater, TX, USA). Bacterial 16S primers 530F 5′–GTGCCAGCMGCNGCGG-3′ and 1100R 5′-GGGTTNCG-NTCGTTG-3′ were used in PCR amplification of the V4–V6 hyper-variable regions of 16S rRNA gene. Sequencing primers and barcodes were trimmed from the DNA sequences and quality control measures using Mothur [24] were used to exclude sequences <200 bp or those containing homopolymers longer than 8 base pairs. Pyrosequencing errors were minimized in the dataset, using the pre-cluster algorithm in Mothur [25], whereby rare sequences highly similar to abundant sequences were re-classified as their abundant homologue. Chimeras were removed from the samples, using the sequence collection as its own reference database [24]. Clean reads were submitted to EBI European Nucleotide Archive (ENA) database (http://www.ebi.ac.uk/ena, accession number PRJEB6402). Calculation of treatment based rarefaction curves, using the Mothur pipeline provided a way of comparing the phylogenetic richness among samples and determining the extent of sequencing relative to sampling needed to accurately describe the microbial community. While the total number of sequences obtained was decreased in the RC-FS

Table 1. Ingredient, nutrient and fatty acid composition of the experimental diets.

	Diet[1]			
Variable	**GH-FS**	**GH-SS**	**RC-FS**	**RC-SS**
Ingredient (% DM basis)				
Red clover silage	0.0	0.0	70.0	70.0
Grass hay	70.0	70.0	0.0	0.0
Barley straw	11.5	0.0	11.5	0.0
Sunflower-seed	0.0	18.4	0.0	18.4
Flaxseed	14.3	0.0	14.3	0.0
Vitamin/mineral supplement[2]	4.2	4.2	4.2	4.2
Barley grain	0.0	7.4	0.0	7.4
Nutrient (DM basis)				
Dry matter (%)	93.1	93.0	46.9	46.9
Crude protein (%)	13.3	13.4	14.2	14.0
Crude fat (%)	6.4	6.6	8.2	8.4
Calcium (%)	1.1	1.1	1.1	1.2
Phosphorus (%)	0.3	0.3	0.3	0.2
ADF (%)	44.3	45.4	43.0	44.0
NDF (%)	53.2	57.6	55.5	61.6
Digestible Energy[3] (Mcal/kg)	2.08	2.02	2.16	2.10
Fatty acid (% of total fatty acids)				
14:0	0.2	0.2	0.1	0.1
16:0	8.6	10.2	7.5	8.4
18:0	3.0	4.1	2.9	4.2
20:0	0.4	0.5	0.3	0.4
22:0	0.7	0.9	0.4	0.8
24:0	0.6	0.5	0.4	0.4
*c*9-18:1	11.6	11.3	11.6	11.7
*c*11-18:1	0.8	0.9	0.8	0.7
18:2*n*-6	23.4	66.0	21.4	70.4
18:3*n*-3	50.7	5.3	54.6	2.8

[1]GH-FS, grass hay + flaxseed; GH-SS, grass hay + sunflower-seed, RC-FS, red clover silage + flaxseed; RC-SS, red clover silage + sunflower-seed.
[2]Vitamin/mineral supplement per kg DM contained 1.86% calcium, 0.93% phosphorous, 0.56% potassium, 0.21% sulphur, 0.33% magnesium 0.92% sodium, 265 ppm iron, 314 ppm manganese, 156 ppm copper, 517 ppm zinc, 10.05 ppm iodine, 5.04 ppm cobalt, 2.98 ppm selenium, 49722 IU/kg vitamin A, 9944 IU/kg vitamin D3, and 3222 IU/kg vitamin E.
[3]Digestible energy was calculated according to Bull, [72].

compared to the other diets, the degree of coverage was similar across diets (Fig. S1). However, none of the curves reached a plateau, indicating that the observed level of richness (unique operational taxonomic unit), as determined by the unique sequences and overall sampling intensity was insufficient to fully describe the richness of rumen bacterial communities.

Sequences were then grouped according to diet in order to determine the effect of forage, oilseed and the forage by oilseed interaction and to account for low sequence abundance in some individual samples. A distance matrix was constructed using the average neighbour algorithm at 0.05 (genus) and 0.25 (phylum) phylogenetic distances to determine the most accurate phylogenetic tree structure. Pairwise distances between aligned sequences were calculated at a 0.97% similarity cut off and then clustered into unique OTUs (operational taxonomic unit). Any sequences aligning for more than 97% of the sequence were considered to be from the same bacterial species (OTU). In total, there were 64,396 quality reads with an average of 16,099±6731 reads and an average of 364 unique OTUs per diet. Mothur was also used to calculate the coverage for each treatment (Fig. S1), and to create a dendrogram based on treatment differences using OTU dissimilarity between the structures of two communities [26]. Calculations of percentage of sequences within taxonomic classifications at the genus level were performed using a custom summation script [27].

Subcutaneous fatty acid analysis

Subcutaneous fat samples (50 mg) were freeze-dried and directly methylated with sodium methoxide [28]. As an internal standard, 1 ml of 1 mg *c*10-17:1 methyl ester/ml toluene (standard no. U-42M form Nu-Check Prep Inc., Elysian, MN, USA) was added prior to addition of methylating reagents. Fatty acid methyl esters (FAME) were analysed by gas chromatography using a CP-Sil88 column (100 m, 25 μm ID, 0.2 μm film thickness) in a CP-3800 gas chromatograph equipped with an 8600-series autosampler (Varian Inc., Walnut Creek, CA, USA).

Table 2. Effect of forage type and oilseed interaction on fatty acid profiles of subcutaneous fat from beef steers.

	Grass hay		Red clover			P-value		
Variable	**Flax**	**Sunflower**	**Flax**	**Sunflower**	**SEM**	**Oilseed**	**Forage**	**O*F[1]**
∑ PUFA	1.97	2.10	1.80	2.11	0.07	0.001	0.25	0.19
∑ *n*-6	1.40	1.75	1.29	1.82	0.06	<0.001	0.78	0.15
18:2*n*-6	1.30	1.63	1.20	1.70	0.06	<0.001	0.81	0.17
20:2*n*-6	0.03	0.03	0.03	0.03	0.00	0.10	0.18	0.50
20:3*n*-6	0.04	0.05	0.03	0.05	0.00	<0.001	0.26	0.27
20:4*n*-6	0.03	0.04	0.03	0.05	0.00	<0.001	0.65	0.18
∑ *n*-3	0.58	0.35	0.51	0.29	0.02	<0.001	0.001	0.90
18:3*n*-3	0.50	0.30	0.44	0.24	0.02	<0.001	0.001	0.88
20:3*n*-3	0.02	0.01	0.02	0.01	0.00	<0.001	0.25	0.72
22:5*n*-3	0.06	0.04	0.05	0.04	0.00	<0.001	0.03	0.81
∑ CLNA	0.29[a]	0.08[b]	0.32[a]	0.05[b]	0.01	<0.001	0.90	0.03
*c*9,*t*11,*t*15-18:3	0.10	0.03	0.11	0.02	0.01	<0.001	0.66	0.16
*c*9,*t*11,*c*15-18:3	0.19[a]	0.05[b]	0.21[a]	0.03[b]	0.01	<0.001	0.71	0.04
∑ AD	2.61	1.68	2.35	1.17	0.09	<0.001	<0.001	0.17
∑ CLA	2.10	2.47	2.07	2.34	0.18	0.02	0.55	0.72
∑ *c*,*t*-CLA	1.91	2.37	1.90	2.26	0.18	0.001	0.65	0.73
∑ *t*,*t*-CLA	0.19	0.10	0.17	0.09	0.01	<0.001	0.06	0.95
∑ *t*-18:1	6.14	8.20	5.51	7.66	0.38	<0.001	0.09	0.90
∑ *c*-MUFA	45.2	44.7	46.0	43.5	1.09	0.16	0.85	0.35
*c*9-14:1	1.47	1.55	1.75	1.34	0.14	0.25	0.79	0.09
*c*7-16:1	0.20	0.19	0.22	0.22	0.01	0.42	0.001	0.74
*c*9-16:1	5.12	4.77	5.95	4.68	0.32	0.02	0.26	0.16
*c*9-17:1	0.78	0.68	0.83	0.71	0.03	0.001	0.27	0.76
*c*9-18:1	34.3	34.0	34.3	33.7	0.73	0.45	0.80	0.82
*c*11-18:1	1.33	1.11	1.32	1.12	0.09	0.02	0.97	0.88
*c*12-18:1	0.62[c]	1.38[a]	0.36[d]	0.81[b]	0.05	<0.001	<0.001	0.001
*c*13-18:1	0.44	0.38	0.47	0.34	0.03	0.01	0.90	0.29
*c*14-18:1	0.09	0.09	0.08	0.07	0.00	0.54	<0.001	0.43
*c*15-18:1	0.49	0.23	0.39	0.18	0.02	<0.001	<0.001	0.16
*c*16-18:1	0.08	0.08	0.07	0.07	0.00	0.10	0.06	0.70
*c*10-19:1	0.08	0.04	0.08	0.04	0.00	<0.001	0.19	0.53
*c*9-20:1	0.12	0.11	0.12	0.11	0.00	0.01	0.70	0.47
*c*11-20:1	0.15	0.13	0.15	0.14	0.01	0.23	0.67	0.40
∑ BCFA	2.01	1.83	1.93	1.90	0.04	0.01	0.86	0.07

Table 2. Cont.

Variable	Grass hay		Red clover			P-value		
	Flax	Sunflower	Flax	Sunflower	SEM	Oilseed	Forage	O*F[1]
iso-14:0	0.07	0.06	0.07	0.07	0.001	0.75	0.45	0.38
iso-15:0	0.24	0.22	0.22	0.22	0.01	0.07	0.16	0.07
anteiso-15:0	0.28	0.27	0.28	0.29	0.01	0.83	0.79	0.28
iso-16:0	0.29	0.27	0.29	0.30	0.01	0.80	0.16	0.24
iso-17:0	0.34	0.31	0.32	0.31	0.01	0.01	0.05	0.12
anteiso-17:0	0.64	0.57	0.61	0.59	0.01	0.001	0.88	0.07
iso-18:0	0.15	0.12	0.15	0.13	0.00	<0.001	0.89	0.32
∑ SFA	38.6	37.9	38.9	40.3	1.07	0.75	0.19	0.28
14:0	3.45	3.24	3.51	3.36	0.14	0.17	0.47	0.83
15:0	0.59	0.55	0.63	0.61	0.02	0.06	0.001	0.61
16:0	22.8	22.1	23.8	23.1	0.50	0.06	0.02	0.97
17:0	0.75[a]	0.68[c]	0.70[b]	0.75[a]	0.03	0.72	0.60	0.03
18:0	10.8	11.1	10.1	12.4	0.71	0.08	0.74	0.17
19:0	0.05	0.05	0.04	0.05	0.00	0.68	0.42	0.39
20:0	0.08	0.09	0.08	0.10	0.01	0.12	0.28	0.38
22:0	0.02	0.02	0.02	0.02	0.00	0.10	0.54	0.08

[a,b,c,d]Means with different superscripts for a particular fatty acid profile have a significant oilseed × forage interaction($P<0.05$); SEM, standard error of mean;

[1]Oilseed type × forage type interaction; *c*, *cis*; *t*, *trans*;

∑ PUFA, sum of polyunsaturated fatty acids = ∑ *n*-6 + ∑ *n*-3; ∑ *n*-6 = sum of 18:2*n*-6, 20:2*n*-6, 20:3*n*-6, 20:4*n*-6; ∑ *n*-3 sum of 18:3*n*-3, 20:3*n*-3, 22:5*n*-3; ∑CLNA, sum of conjugated α-linolenic acid = *c*9,*t*11,*t*15-, *c*9,*t*11,*c*15-; ∑AD, total atypical dienes = sum of *t*11,*t*15-, *c*9,*t*13-/*t*8,*c*12-, *t*8,*c*13-, *c*9,*t*12-/*c*16-18:1, *t*9,*c*12-, *t*11,*c*15-, *c*9,*c*15-, *c*12,*c*15-; ∑ CLA, conjugated linoleic acid = sum of *t*,*t*-CLA + sum of *c*,*t*-CLA; ∑ *trans*-*trans*-CLA = sum of *t*12,*t*14-, *t*11,*t*13-, *t*10,*t*12-, *t*9,*t*11-, *t*8,*t*10-, *t*7,*t*9- *t*6,*t*8-; ∑ *cis*-/*trans*-CLA = sum of *c*9,*t*11-, *t*7,*c*9-, *t*11,*c*13-, *t*12,*c*14-, *c*11,*t*13-, *t*10,*c*12-, *t*8,*c*10-, *t*9,*c*11-; ∑ *t*-18:1, sum of *trans*-18:1 isomers = *t*6,*t*7,*t*8-, *t*9-, *t*10-, *t*11-, *t*12-, *t*13,*t*14-, *t*15-, *t*16-; ∑ *c*-MUFA = sum of *c*9-14:1, *c*7-16:1, *c*9-16:1, *c*11-16:1, *c*9-17:1, *c*9-18:1, *c*11-18:1, *c*12-18:1, *c*13-18:1, *c*14-18:1, *c*15-18:1, *c*9-20:1, *c*11-20:1; ∑ BCFA, branched chain fatty acids = sum of *iso*-15:0, *anteiso*15:0, *so*16, *iso*17:0, *anteiso*17:0, *iso*18:0; ∑ SFA = sum of 14:0, 15:0, 16:0, 17:0, 18:0, 19:0, 20:0, 22:0.

Two gas chromatography (GC) analyses were conducted per sample using complementary temperature programs with 150°C and 175°C plateaus according to Kramer, et al. [29]. CLA isomers not separated by GC were further analysed using Ag^{+}-HPLC as described by Cruz-Hernandez et al. [30].

For the identification of FAME by GC, the reference standard no. 601 from Nu-Check Prep Inc, Elysian, MN, USA was used. Branched-chain FAME were identified using a GC reference standard BC-Mix1 purchased previously from Applied Science (State College, PA, USA). For CLA isomers, the UC-59M standard from Nu-Chek Prep Inc. was used which contains all four positional CLA isomers. *Trans*-18:1, CLA isomers and other BH products not included in the standard mixtures were identified by their retention times and elution orders as reported in literature [29–31]. The FAME were quantified, using chromatographic peak area and internal standard based calculations. Only FAME representing more than 0.01% of total FAME were included in tables and figures with the exception of BH products, where all the quantified isomers were reported.

Statistical analysis

All data were analysed, using the PROC MIXED procedure of SAS [32]. The statistical model for FA profiles and genus percent abundance included the fixed effects of oilseed, forage and oilseed × forage interaction,with slaughter date and pen considered as random effects and animal as the experimental unit. Since the random effect of pen nested within the oilseed × forage interaction was not significant, it was removed from the model. Treatment means were generated and separated, using the LSMEANS and PDIFF options respectively [32].

For the comparison of high and low levels of VA within diet to bacterial abundance using 2×2×2 factorial analysis, there was a significant FA level by oilseed type interaction. Therefore, data were reanalyzed as 2×4 factorial ANOVA comparing forage to high and low levels of a FA for each oilseed. For the analysis, treatment means were generated and separated, using Tukey-Kramer and PDIFF options [32]. To relate rumen bacterial profiles to FA profiles, percent abundance of genus level taxa were additionally analyzed in pairwise Pearson correlation to FA data, using the PROC CORR procedure of SAS [32]. The significance threshold for all statistical analyses was set at $P<0.05$.

Results

Animal performance

Data on animal performance are detailed in a companion paper by Mapiye et al [19]. In summary, steers fed SS diets (13.2±0.37) had higher ($P<0.05$) DM intake than those fed FS (12.1±0.37), and steers fed GH consumed more (13.3±0.37; $P<0.05$) feed than those fed RC (12.1±0.37). As a result, average daily gain and final live weights were higher ($P<0.05$) in steers fed SS (0.7 kg/d±0.08 and 550 kg±9.55) compared to FS (0.51 kg/d±0.08 and 503 kg±9.55) and final live weights were also higher ($P<0.05$) in steers fed GH (551 kg±9.55), as compared to those fed RC (517 kg±9.55). Steers fed SS diets (7.66±0.38 mm) had a tendency to have thicker (P=0.08) final subcutaneous fat depth than steers fed FS diets (6.69±0.38 mm), but forage type and its interaction with oilseed had no effect ($P>0.05$) on final subcutaneous fat thickness.

Subcutaneous fatty acid profiles

The proportions of total PUFA in subcutaneous fat were affected by oilseed type with steers fed SS diets having greater ($P<0.05$) proportions than those fed FS (Table 2). Oilseed type also influenced the proportions of total and individual *n*-6 PUFA (18:2*n*-6, 20:3*n*-6, 20:4*n*-6), with steers fed SS having greater ($P<0.05$) proportions in subcutaneous fat than steers fed FS. For all diets, LA was the most prominent *n*-6 PUFA, accounting for more than 90% of total *n*-6 PUFA.

For *n*-3 PUFA, diets containing FS as opposed to SS, and GH as opposed to RC exhibited elevated ($P<0.05$) proportions of total *n*-3 PUFA, 18:3*n*-3 (ALA) and 22:5*n*-3 (Table 2), but in general, increases were influenced more by oilseed than forage type. Alpha-linolenic acid was the most abundant *n*-3 PUFA, making up over 80% of total *n*-3 PUFA in all diets.

An oilseed × forage type interaction was detected for total conjugated linolenic acids (CLNA) and *c*9,*t*11,*c*15-18:3, but upon means separation only an effect of oilseed was detected with FS diets resulting in greater ($P<0.05$) proportions than SS diets (Table 2). The proportions of *c*9,*t*11,*t*15-18:3 were also only influenced by oilseed type, with steers fed FS having greater ($P<0.05$) proportions than those fed SS.

Based on the type of oilseed and forage fed, two AD isomer patterns were observed (Fig. 1A). The proportions of AD isomers likely largely derived from ALA (*t*8,*c*13-; *t*9,*t*12-/*c*9,*t*13-; *t*11,*c*15-; *t*11,*t*15-; *c*12,*c*15-18:2) were increased by FS (P<0.05). Of the isomers in this group, minor forage effects were found for *t*8,*c*13- and *t*9,*t*12-/*c*9,*t*13-18:2 ($P<0.05$), with diets containing GH resulting in slightly increased ($P<0.05$) proportions than diets containing RC. A small but significant forage × oilseed type interaction (P<0.05) was found for *c*12,*c*15-18:2 with the GH-FS diet resulting in the greatest proportions followed by RC-FS, GH-SS and RC-SS diets, respectively. For AD likely largely derived from LA (*t*8, *c*12-; *c*9,*t*12-; *t*9,*c*12-18:2), forage × oilseed type interactions were found ($P<0.05$) with amounts being greatest for the GH-SS diet. The dominant AD isomer irrespective of diet was *t*11, *c*15-18:2 accounting for up to 25% and 35% of total AD in steers fed SS and FS, respectively.

For CLA, two clear isomer patterns were found based on the type of oilseed fed (Fig. 1B). The proportions of CLA isomers with the first double bond at carbon 10 or closer to the carboxyl end (*t*7,*c*9-; *t*8,*c*10-; *c*9,*t*11- (RA); *t*9,*c*11-; *t*10,*c*12-; *t*10,*t*12-18:2) were more elevated ($P<0.05$) when feeding SS as compared to FS. Some minor forage effects were also found for *t*7,*c*9-; *t*8,*c*10-; *t*10,*c*12- and *t*10,*t*12-18:2 with diets containing GH *vs.* RC yielding slightly greater proportions. The proportions of CLA isomers with the first double bond at carbon 11 or further from the carboxyl end (*c*11,*t*13-; *t*11,*c*13-; *t*11,*t*13-; *c*12,*t*14-; *t*12,*t*14-; *t*12,*c*14-18:2) were mostly increased ($P<0.05$) by inclusion of FS. Minor forage effects were also noted for *c*12, *t*14-18:2 ($P<0.05$) while forage × oilseed type interactions were noted for *t*11,*c*13- and *t*12, *c*14-18:2 ($P<0.05$). For all diets, RA accounted for over 70% of total CLA (Fig. 1B).

For *t*-18:1, an isomer pattern was found based on the type of oilseed and forage fed (Fig. 1C). The proportions of *t*-18:1 isomers with double bonds from carbon 6 to 12 were primarily greater ($P<0.05$) with SS than FS, and for the majority of these isomers, feeding GH *vs.* RC diets also led to increases ($P<0.05$), but at a reduced magnitude as compared to oilseeds. For *t*-18:1 isomers with double bonds from carbon 13 to 16, the pattern of differences was less strongly linked to forage or oilseed effects (Fig. 1C). Feeding diets containing FS as opposed to SS increased ($P<0.05$) the proportions *t*15- and *t*16-18:1 (Fig. 1C). The proportions of *t*13-/*t*14- and *t*16-18:1 were elevated ($P<0.05$) by diets containing GH as opposed to RC. Vaccenic acid was the predominant *t*-18:1 isomer and accounted for 45% and 50% of total *t*-18:1 isomers in the subcutaneous fat of steers fed FS and SS diets, respectively (Fig. 1C).

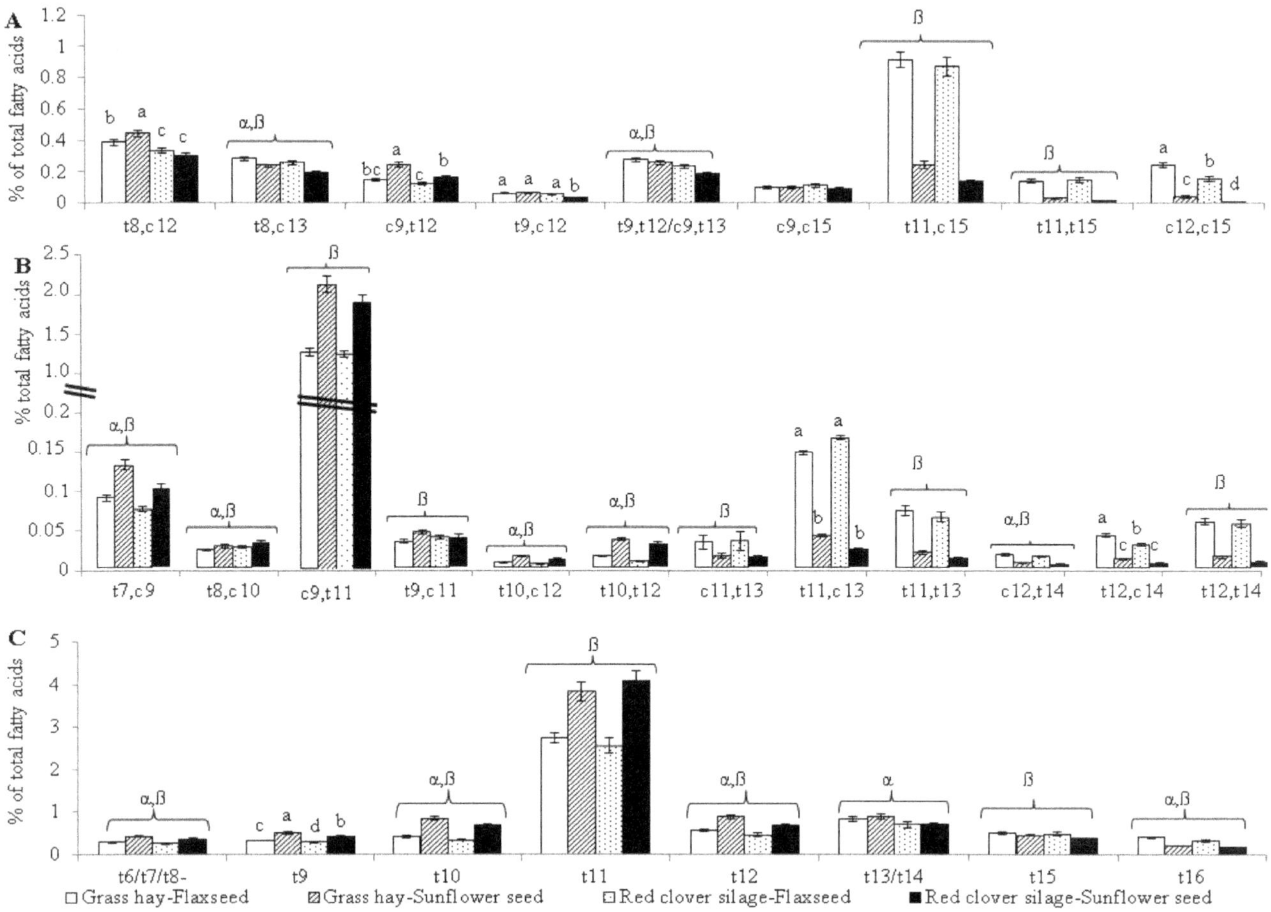

Figure 1. Effect of forage type and oilseed supplementation on atypical dienes (A), conjugated linoleic acid (B) and *trans*-18:1 isomers (C) in subcutaneous fat of beef steers. [a,b,c,d] Means (± standard error) with different superscripts for a particular fatty acid profiles are significantly different ($P<0.05$). α: Significant forage effect ($P<0.05$); β: Significant oilseed effect ($P<0.05$).

Overall, feeding diets containing FS as opposed to SS elevated ($P<0.\ 05$) the proportions of several individual *c*-monounsaturated fatty acids (MUFA) isomers (*c*9-16:1, *c*9-17:1, *c*11-18:1, *c*13-18:1, *c*15-18:1, *c*10-19:1, *c*9-20:1). An oilseed type × forage type interaction influenced the proportions of *c*12-18:1, with steers fed GH-SS having the largest proportions followed by those fed RC-SS, GH-FS and RC-FS, respectively ($P<0.05$; Table 2). Relative to feeding RC, GH reduced ($P<0.05$) the proportions of *c*7-16:1 and increased ($P<0.05$) the proportions of *c*14- and *c*15-18:1 (Table 2). Oleic acid (*c*9-18:1) was the dominant MUFA isomer, accounting for over 75% of total *c*-MUFA in all diets (Table 2).

Feeding diets containing FS compared to SS increased total branched-chain fatty acids (BCFA; $P<0.05$) as a result of increases in the proportions of *iso*-17:0, *anteiso*-17:0 and *iso*-18:0 ($P<0.05$) (Table 2). Neither oilseed nor forage type had any effect on total SFA ($P<0.05$), but proportions of 15:0, 16:0 and *iso*-17:0 were influenced by forage type, with steers fed RC having higher ($P<0.05$), 15:0, 16:0 and lower ($P<0.05$) *iso*-17:0 proportions than those fed GH. An oilseed type × forage type interaction was observed for steers fed GH-FS and RC-SS,,with steers fed RC-FS having intermediate and steers fed GH-SS having the lowest proportions of 17:0 ($P<0.05$). Palmitic acid (16:0) was the most abundant saturated FA (SFA), constituting about 60% of the total SFA in subcutaneous fat of steers across all diets.

Rumen bacterial profiles

The Yue and Clayton [26] measure of dissimilarity among communities was used to create a dendrogram showing the separation of OTU in samples from individual diets (Fig. 2). Despite clustering of diets based on type of forage, diets were not found to differ ($P = 1.0$). The OTU's calculated for each diet were used to construct a Venn diagram (Fig. 3), which identified a total of 558 OTU's across the 4 diets. The number of OTU's that were associated with each diet ranged from 326 to 427. Of these OTU's, 217 were shared by all 4 diets. Using non-parametric estimators in Mothur, it was predicted that the core microbiome was composed of 256 OTU's.

Using a summation script, the percent abundance of each of the 87 classified genera were determined and those which differed ($P<0.05$) by forage or oilseed type are listed in Table 3. Of these genera, 12 were impacted by forage type, 9 were impacted by oilseed type and 5 exhibited a forage × oilseed interaction. The taxa *Butyrivibrio*, and *Syntrophococcus* were higher ($P<0.05$) in the GH diets, whereas *Fibrobacter was* higher ($P<0.01$) in RC diets. *Blautia*, *Eubacterium*, and *Olsenella* were higher in the GH-FS diet and *Anaerophaga* was lowest in GH fed cattle. *Johnsonella* was highest with GH-SS, whereas *Mogibacterium* and *Wandonia* were highest in cattle fed RC-FS. When comparing oilseed supplementation, *Acidaminobacter* was the only taxon that was consistently higher in cattle fed FS. *Barnesiella* was abundant

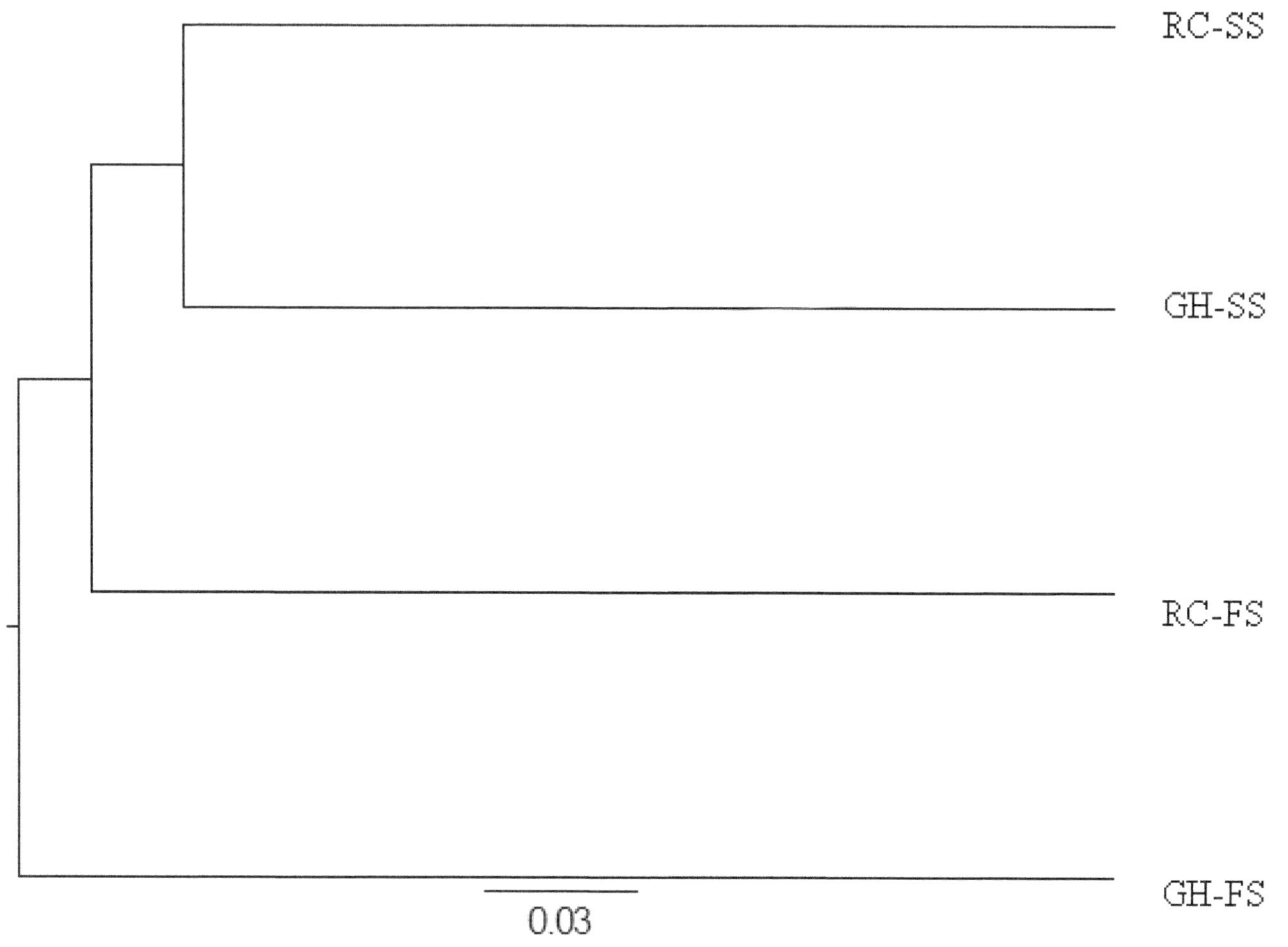

Figure 2. Dendrogram showing distances between dietary treatments based on similarity of sequences using Jaccard analysis (GH-SS: hay-sunflower seed, GH-FS: hay-flax seed, RC-SS: red clover-sunflower seed, RC-FS: red clover-flax seed).

across all diets, but it was higher ($P<0.05$) in the GH-FS diet and lowest with GH-SS. *Marvinbryantia* exhibited the opposite response being more abundant ($P<0.02$) with GH-SS than with GH-FS. *Bellilinea*, *Blautia*, *Guggenheimella*, *Nubsella* and *Sporobacter* were all influenced by an oilseed × forage interaction. Of these, *Bellilnea*, *Guggenheimella*, and *Nubsella* were present in greater abundance ($P<0.05$) in the RC-FS fed cattle.

Additionally, Pearson correlation was used to relate the percent abundance of measured bacterial taxa to measured subcutaneous FA. The highest correlation ($P<0.004$) between percent abundance and FA profile was for the genus *Clostridium IV* (Table 4). *Clostridium IV* was highly correlated to total n-3 PUFA ($P<0.004$; $R^2=0.32$), total CLNA ($P<0.001$; $R^2=0.38$) and total atypical dienes ($P<0.001$; $R^2=0.40$). The only other genera, which was highly correlated with specific FA profiles, was *Fibrobacter*, which correlated to total CLA ($P<0.001$; $R^2=0.40$) and *Marvinbryantia*, which correlated to total *t*MUFA ($P<0.002$; $R^2=0.36$). Additionally, two bacterial genera, *Acidaminobacter* and *Asteroleplasma* were highly ($P<0.001$) correlated to specific individual FA. *Acidaminobacter* was correlated to FA *iso*-18:0 with a $R^2=0.39$ and *Asteroleplasma* was correlated to *c*12-18:1 with a $R^2=0.44$.

This difference in VA levels coincided with changes in the percent abundance of several genera including *Anaerophaga*, *Asaccharobacter*, *Fibrobacter*, *Guggenheimella*, *Marvinbryantia*, *Paludibacter*, *Pseudosphingobacterium*, *Pseudozobellia* and *Syntrophococcus* (Table 5).

Discussion

Animal performance

The finding that steers fed diets containing FS grew slightly slower and had lower final live weight than steers fed diets containing SS may be related to palatability issues resulting from the addition of FS [33] and/or the inclusion of ground straw [34] in FS diets to balance for digestible energy across oilseed diets. The explanations for the lower final live weight observed, when feeding RC as opposed to GH are less clear, but the quality of silage fed and higher crude fat content of RC diets may have been partially responsible. Silage quality (dry matter content and fermentation quality) was not assessed in this experiment, but fat levels greater than 5% have been reported to inhibit ruminal fiber digestion, increasing rumen fill and reducing DM intake [35].

Subcutaneous fatty acid profiles

The elevated levels of total PUFA in the subcutaneous fat of steers fed diets containing SS was related to the increase in n-6 PUFA, especially LA. This resulted from the large proportion of LA in diets containing SS. In most diets, the extent of LA BH is lower than that of ALA [36] because greater levels of LA in the

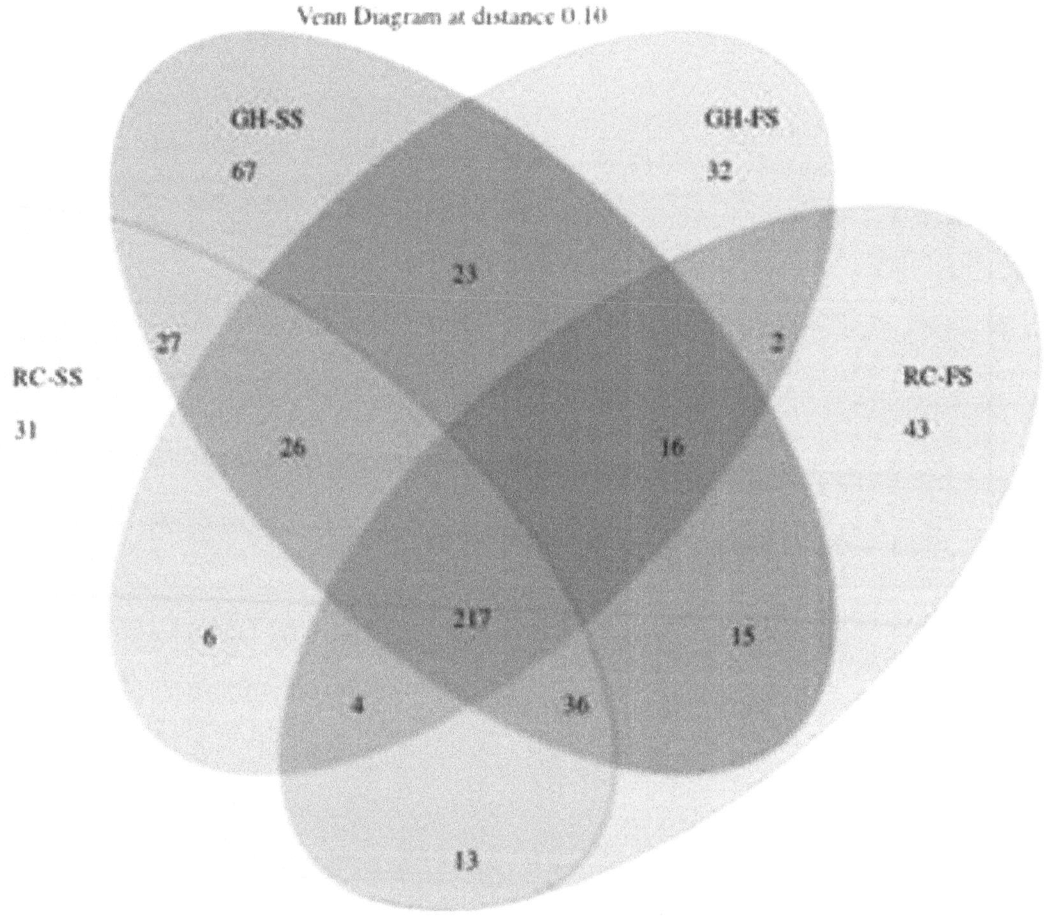

Figure 3. Venn diagram showing OTU's unique to and shared by each of the dietary treatments (GH-SS: hay-sunflower seed, GH-FS: hay-flax seed, RC-SS: red clover-sunflower seed, RC-FS: red clover-flax seed).

rumen inhibits the growth of many of the bacterial species involved in BH [37]. This inhibitory effect results in increased tissue deposition of LA and its long chain *n*-6 PUFA derivatives when compared to ALA and its long chain *n*-3 PUFA derivatives [38]. Additionally, the physical form of the oilseed fed (whole SS *vs.* triple rolled FS) might have also influenced BH in the rumen. Rolling has been reported to enhance the availability of PUFA in the rumen, thereby increasing the degree to which they are BH [39]. The increase in surface area as a result of rolling would have increased microbial attachment and therefore potentially increased the rate of lipolysis and BH. The effect of forage on FA profiles was confounded by the physical form of the feed. The lack of accumulation of PUFA in cattle fed RC diets was unexpected as it is well known that RC has increased levels of poly-phenol oxidase (PPO) which increases PUFA levels in meat and milk [11]. It is possible that the activity of PPO was reduced during ensiling.

As anticipated, feeding diets containing FS, a rich source of ALA, increased the deposition of ALA and its long chain derivatives, 20:3*n*-3 and 20:5*n*-3 in subcutaneous fat. This is likely due to part of dietary ALA escaping ruminal BH and therefore being available for direct deposition in the tissue. The reason for the increased *n*-3 PUFA proportions observed in steers fed diets containing GH diets remains uncertain, but may be partly associated with the higher feed intake previously reported for this diet [19] or the preservation method of the forage (i.e., hay *vs.* silage). It has been reported that ALA content in tissues is often higher, when hay as opposed to silage is fed due to a higher efficiency of transfer from the rumen to the tissue [40]. This could be related to changes in forage lipids, during preservation and/or ruminal lipid metabolism [41]. The process of ensiling has been shown to increase the levels of PUFA that are BH in the rumen due to lipolysis in the silo, which occurs as a result of increased moisture content during fermentation [42]. Biohydrogenation of PUFA's in the rumen has been shown to be lower in hay compared to ensiled forages, and therefore with hay a greater percentage of PUFA bypass the rumen and are available for uptake in the duodenum [40,43]. This may be a result of differences in physical properties of the forage impacting microbial attachment [43] or shifts in microbial communities that result in differences in lipid metabolism and outflow of FA [44]. In this investigation, the mean percentage concentration of ALA in subcutaneous fat (0.44–0.50% of total FA) of steers fed diets containing FS was higher than the mean percentage concentration of ALA in the subcutaneous fat of animals fed FS in high-grain diets (0.09–0.12%, [33]), but lower than those found, when feeding FS in 50:50 forage:grain (0.73–0.79%, [7]) or high-forage diets (0.8 7%, [13]; 1.1%, [9]). However, the differences in ALA across these trials could be related to a number of factors within these experiments including feeding management, forage type and quality or animal variability.

The finding that CLNA proportions in the subcutaneous fat were accentuated by feeding diets containing FS, as opposed to

Table 3. Percent abundance of genera impacted by forage type (F), oilseed type included in the diet (O), level of vaccenic acid (VA) in backfat or any interaction of these factors.

	Hay				Red Clover											
	Flax		Sunflower		Flax		Sunflower			*P*-value for indicated factor						
Bacterial Genera	High VA[1]	Low VA	High VA	Low VA	High VA	Low VA	High VA	Low VA	SEM	F	O	VA	F × O	F × VA	O × VA	F × O × VA
Acidaminobacter	0.00	0.37	0.00	0.00	0.17	0.17	0.00	0.00	0.11	0.93	0.03	0.24	0.93	0.24	0.24	0.24
Anaerophaga	0.76	1.86	0.92	1.82	1.99	2.21	1.90	2.66	0.40	0.01	0.68	0.02	0.85	0.38	0.77	0.52
Anaerosporobacter	0.61	0.42	0.61	0.71	0.20	0.54	0.37	0.00	0.19	0.04	0.91	0.83	0.24	0.90	0.47	0.09
Anaerostipes	0.18	0.22	0.18	0.00	0.47	0.73	0.00	0.23	0.17	0.10	0.03	0.49	0.15	0.21	0.63	0.70
Asaccharobacter	0.46	0.00	0.17	0.00	0.00	0.00	0.00	0.00	0.10	0.05	0.35	0.05	0.35	0.05	0.35	0.35
Asteroleplasma	0.00^{b}	0.00^{b}	0.83^{a}	0.21^{ab}	0.20^{ab}	0.00^{b}	0.00^{b}	0.43^{ab}	0.15	0.34	0.01	0.37	0.07	0.06	0.98	0.01
Blautia	1.48	1.31	1.19	0.99	0.47	0.66	1.34	0.89	0.23	0.02	0.45	0.35	0.02	0.87	0.31	0.36
Butyrivibrio	2.75	2.64	2.56	2.20	1.26	1.54	1.68	1.46	0.29	0.00	0.73	0.62	0.25	0.54	0.38	0.77
Clostridium_IV	0.88	0.70	1.09	1.13	0.77	0.83	1.47	1.50	0.25	0.30	0.01	0.96	0.33	0.76	0.79	0.73
Eubacterium	1.02	0.76	0.56	0.61	0.23	0.40	0.28	0.23	0.21	0.01	0.25	0.88	0.42	0.59	0.89	0.39
Faecalibacterium	0.00^{b}	0.26^{ab}	0.47^{ab}	0.00^{b}	0.68^{a}	0.23^{ab}	0.35^{ab}	0.60^{a}	0.23	0.10	0.70	0.55	0.82	0.99	0.96	0.04
Fibrobacter	0.59	1.89	0.37	0.98	2.06	2.18	1.48	2.85	0.38	0.00	0.36	0.01	0.28	0.70	0.62	0.09
Galbibacter	0.4^{c}	2.55^{c}	2.6^{c}	2.8^{bc}	3.41^{a}	3.71^{bc}	1.99^{c}	3.74^{ab}	0.11	0.00	0.52	0.44	0.10	0.77	0.00	0.00
Guggenheimella	0.40	2.55	2.60	2.63	2.61	3.49	1.99	3.09	0.50	0.05	0.38	0.01	0.03	0.89	0.20	0.12
Hallella	2.18^{a}	1.47^{ab}	1.19^{ab}	1.22^{ab}	1.54^{ab}	2.25^{a}	1.39^{ab}	1.08^{b}	0.30	0.82	0.01	0.73	0.93	0.22	0.73	0.05
Johnsonella	0.83	0.37	0.98	0.72	0.37	0.00	0.33	0.23	0.30	0.02	0.37	0.13	0.69	0.74	0.53	0.92
Marvinbryantia	1.43	0.55	1.88	1.30	1.38	1.12	1.66	1.21	0.24	0.78	0.03	0.01	0.24	0.28	0.88	0.49
Mogibacterium	0.17	0.18	0.40	0.00	0.88	0.71	0.70	0.50	0.17	0.00	0.48	0.13	0.35	0.95	0.37	0.43
Nubsella	0.27^{b}	1.45^{ab}	1.25^{ab}	1.13^{ab}	2.16^{a}	1.45^{ab}	0.85^{ab}	1.50^{ab}	0.28	0.03	0.44	0.22	0.03	0.17	0.93	0.00
Olsenella	0.48	0.20	0.18	0.00	0.00	0.00	0.00	0.00	0.10	0.03	0.19	0.22	0.19	0.22	0.77	0.77
Oscillibacter	0.00	0.61	0.60	0.76	0.54	0.53	0.80	0.79	0.19	0.21	0.03	0.18	0.68	0.16	0.43	0.42
Paludibacter	0.00	0.79	0.24	0.75	1.04	0.79	0.56	1.12	0.20	0.01	0.94	0.01	0.55	0.10	0.36	0.08
Phocaeicola	2.33^{a}	1.23^{ab}	1.06^{ab}	1.57^{ab}	1.05^{ab}	1.88^{ab}	1.39^{ab}	0.62^{b}	0.31	0.17	0.05	0.55	0.99	0.46	0.99	0.00
Pseudo-sphingobacterium	1.69^{b}	5.94^{a}	1.99^{b}	4.38^{ab}	6.7^{a}	5.64^{a}	4.52^{ab}	6.14^{a}	0.70	0.00	0.16	0.00	0.84	0.01	0.68	0.04
Pseudozobellia	0.18	0.54	0.00	0.00	0.00	0.41	0.00	0.19	0.15	0.80	0.05	0.04	0.26	0.57	0.21	0.76
Sporobacter	1.21	0.76	1.12	1.49	1.16	1.30	0.97	0.90	0.86	0.42	0.66	0.57	0.05	0.51	0.49	0.12
Syntrophococcus	2.31	1.50	2.28	1.55	1.36	1.35	1.61	1.08	0.23	0.00	0.99	0.01	0.94	0.14	0.51	0.37
Treponema	1.95^{b}	2.62^{ab}	2.56^{ab}	2.11^{ab}	2.52^{ab}	2.14^{ab}	2.06^{ab}	2.77^{a}	0.23	0.82	0.79	0.60	0.95	0.92	0.98	0.05
Wandonia	0.00	0.29	0.19	0.00	0.32	0.70	0.34	0.51	0.23	0.05	0.70	0.33	0.92	0.49	0.30	0.67

[a,b,c]Means with different superscripts within a row are significantly different ($P<0.05$) based on the three-way interaction.
[1]VA, Vaccenic acid; F, Forage; O, Oilseed; SEM, standard error of the mean.

Table 4. Correlation of bacterial genera to subcutaneous fatty acid groupings.

		Fatty Acid Group						
Genera Taxa		**Total n-6 and n-3**	**Total n-6**	**Total n-3**	**Total CLNA**	**Total AD**	**Total CLA**	**Total trans MUFA**
Acidaminobacter	P-value	0.75	0.31	0.05	0.07	0.26	0.33	0.03
	R^2	0.00	0.05	0.17	0.14	0.06	0.04	0.19
	Corr.[1]			+				−
Anaerostipes	P-value	0.03	0.02	0.57	0.16	0.56	0.36	0.03
	R^2	0.20	0.22	0.01	0.09	0.02	0.04	0.19
	Corr.	−	−					−
Asteroleplasma	P-value	0.20	0.11	0.32	0.17	0.53	0.14	0.05
	R^2	0.07	0.11	0.04	0.08	0.02	0.09	0.17
	Corr.							+
Clostridium_IV	P-value	0.39	0.06	0.004	0.001	0.001	1.00	0.38
	R^2	0.03	0.15	0.32	0.38	0.40	0.00	0.04
	Corr.			−	−	−		
Ethanoligenens	P-value	0.97	0.43	0.03	0.04	0.09	0.48	0.33
	R^2	0.00	0.03	0.19	0.19	0.12	0.02	0.04
	Corr.			−	−			
Fibrobacter	P-value	0.37	0.54	0.50	0.87	0.33	0.001	0.06
	R^2	0.04	0.02	0.02	0.00	0.04	0.40	0.15
	Corr.						−	
Galbibacter	P-value	0.20	0.25	0.83	0.52	0.66	0.01	0.31
	R^2	0.07	0.06	0.00	0.02	0.01	0.25	0.05
	Corr.						−	
Marvinbryantia	P-value	0.30	0.18	0.39	0.30	0.45	0.08	0.002
	R^2	0.05	0.08	0.03	0.05	0.03	0.13	0.36
	Corr.							+
Olsenella	P-value	0.54	0.28	0.17	0.26	0.04	0.26	0.49
	R^2	0.02	0.05	0.08	0.06	0.18	0.06	0.02
	Corr.					+		
Pseudo-butyrivibrio	P-value	0.42	0.43	0.97	0.74	0.64	0.03	0.38
	R^2	0.03	0.03	0.00	0.01	0.01	0.20	0.03
	Corr.						+	

[1]Positive (+) or negative (−) correlation (Corr.) for P<0.05.

Table 5. Changes in composition of bacterial abundance in animals with high *vs.*low vaccenic acid in the backfat.

	Vaccenic Acid within Treatment			
	High (n = 12)	Low (n = 12)-	SEM	P-value
Vaccenic Acid (% of total FAME)[1]	4.44	2.44	0.09	
Bacterial Abundance (% of total)				
Anaerophaga	1.39[b]	2.14[a]	0.02	0.02
Asaccharobacter[2]	0.02	0.00	0.01	0.05
Fibrobacter	1.13[b]	1.97[a]	0.02	0.01
Guggenheimella	1.90[b]	2.94[a]	0.02	0.01
Marvinbryantia	1.59[a]	1.04[b]	0.01	0.01
Paludibacter	0.46[b]	0.87[a]	0.01	0.01
Pseudosphingobacterium[2,3]	3.73	5.53	0.04	<0.01
Pseudozobellia	0.05[b]	0.28[a]	0.01	0.04
Syntrophococcus	1.89[a]	1.37[b]	0.01	0.01

[1]Significant two-way interaction of vaccenic acid level × oilseed ($P<0.05$).
[2]Significant two-way interaction of vaccenic acid level × forage ($P<0.05$).
[3]Significant three-way interaction of vaccenic acid level × oilseed × forage ($P<0.05$).
[a,b]Means with different superscripts within a row are significantly different ($P<0.05$).

feeding SS, was anticipated as ALA is known to initially get isomerised to CLNA as it undergoes BH in the rumen [45]. Current findings agree with our earlier results, when feeding GH or barley silage diets containing FS [7] and FS combined with RC [10]. Previous cell culture and animal model studies have demonstrated that plant-derived CLNA can improve biomarkers of cardiovascular health and has anti-inflammatory, immune-modulatory, anti-obesity and anti-carcinogenic properties [46]. Therefore, addition of FS to high-forage diets to achieve greater levels of CLNA in beef fat may be perceived as a positive outcome from a human health perspective.

The increase in AD isomers largely derived from ALA, including *t*11,*c*15-18:2 the major AD isomer in steers fed diets containing FS was expected as ALA is isomerised to CLNA, before BH [45]. These findings agree with previous reports with diets containing FS [7,10,47]. Some AD isomers (*t*8,*c*12-; *c*9,*t*12-; *c*9,*c*15-18:2) reported by Mapiye et al. [10] and Nassu et al. [7] were increased by FS, but in the present study these isomers were preferentially enriched by diets containing SS as reported by Bessa et al. [47]. This could imply that these isomers are found in common with BH pathways for both LA and ALA. The inconsistencies in AD proportions seen between steers fed GH *vs.* RC, may also reflect changes in the physical state of the RC as a result of ensiling increasing the degree of BH of PUFAs in the rumen [40,41], as enhanced microbial attachment to silage may have decreased the rumen bypass of PUFAs [43]. The observation that the proportions of AD likely largely derived from ALA were higher, when feeding diets containing FS as opposed to SS supports previous observations by Jenkins et al. [48] and Doreau et al. [49]. It was found that BH of ALA proceeds mostly through pathways incorporating AD *vs.* CLA, whereas BH of LA proceeds mostly through CLA. Definitive experiments on the impact of AD isomers on human health are required before recommendations can be made about including SS or FS in ruminant diets.

As found previously in ruminants [13,47,50], supplementing high-forage diets with SS as opposed to FS enhanced the proportions of CLA isomers with the first double bond from carbon 7 to 10 and *t*-18:1 isomers with double bonds between carbons 6 and 12. This is because of the common precursor LA, which is abundant in SS containing diets. Feeding cattle, a blend of oils or oilseeds rich in ALA and LA has previously been shown to result in a synergistic accumulation of VA [51] and CLA in the tissue [52]. Therefore, further investigations regarding whether blending SS and FS in high-forage diets would simultaneously enhance concentrations of VA, RA and *n*-3 PUFA in beef tissues are necessary. Furthermore, the blending of ALA and LA with long chain PUFA such as EPA and DHA, which are known inhibitors of BH of 18:1 to 18:0 in the rumen [53,54] merits investigation.

In this investigation, proportions of RA and VA in subcutaneous fat (2.1% and 2.6%, respectively) of steers fed diets containing SS were greater than those previously reported, when high-forage diets were supplemented with oils or oilseeds [7,55,56]. Conversely, mean percentage concentrations of RA and VA in subcutaneous fat was determined to be less than that observed, when grass pastures were grazed by cattle supplemented with FS or sunflower oil (2.7–3.9% and 7.5–9.7%, respectively; [13,56]) or RC with FS (2.9% and 5.9%; [10]). Variation in mean percentage concentrations of RA and VA across studies could be due to the effects of non-oil components of the diet on rumen BH. In the current study, the sunflower seeds were relatively low in oil (29.5%) compared to normal values of ≈1 40% [57]. As a result, the amount of SS that had to be added to the diet to get 5.4% oil was relatively high (18.4%), necessitating the addition of hulls that have a low energy value. Consequently, to balance the digestible energy content across diets, straw had to be added to flaxseed diets, leading to a diminished overall quality of forage in these diets. Therefore, the present findings strongly emphasize the importance of the non-oil components of the diet when trying to enrich for BH intermediates, particularly RA and VA, in beef. Overall, direct comparisons among studies are often difficult due to RA commonly being combined with other CLA isomers such as *t*7,*c*9-18:2, and VA containing more than one *t*-18:1 isomer.

The observation that feeding diets containing SS as compared to FS increased *t*10-18:1 confirms earlier reports by AbuGhazaleh and Jacobson [58] and Martínez Marín [59] that the BH of ALA as opposed to LA is less prone to promote *t*10-18:1 formation. The relative amounts of *t*10- and *t*13/*t*14-18:1 in the current study, are lower than those found by Juárez, et al., [8], whereas the relative amounts of *t*15- and *t*16-18:1 are less than those obtained by Nassu, et al., [7] and Mapiye et al [10]. These inconsistences could be attributed to differences in time on feed or levels, types and forms of forage fed in these experiments.

The increase in the proportions of minor CLA and *t*-18:1 isomers observed when feeding GH as opposed to RC may be partly associated with changes in the composition of ruminal microbes [60] or differences in ruminal and duodenal flow rates between these two forages [61]. For CLA and *t*-18:1 isomers, effects of oilseed type on these FA were greater than that of forage type.

This experiment showed that measured concentrations of *c*-MUFA isomers in subcutaneous fat were decreased when feeding SS as opposed to FS, which concurs with previous findings [62,63] when feeding LA- and ALA-rich diets to dairy cows and goats, respectively. Overall, the levels of *c*-MUFA in subcutaneous fat when feeding PUFA are indicative of their dietary levels, the level of PUFA BH to *c*-MUFA in the rumen and the capacity of PUFA/ or its BH products to inhibit stearoyl-CoA desaturase (SCD) activity, which converts 18:0 to *c*9-18:1 (oleic acid) in subcutaneous fat [64]. This further suggests that either LA has a slower BH rate and extent of ruminal BH in the rumen than ALA [36] or is more effective in down-regulating SCD activity than ALA [62]. In the present study, reductions in the proportions of total and individual *c*-MUFA isomers in steers fed SS diets could also relate to displacement of *c*-MUFA due to increased formation of *t*-18:1 during BH of PUFA in the rumen, as reflected by the elevated levels of total and individual *t*-18:1 isomers in subcutaneous fat.

Steers fed diets containing FS had a greater percentage of total BCFA as well as individual BCFA and odd-chain FA in subcutaneous fat than steers fed SS. This suggests that ALA did not inhibit rumen microbial FA synthesis as much as LA. In general, the decrease in BCFA and odd-chain FA in ruminant products is related to a direct inhibition of PUFA on microbial FA synthesis [65]. Given that BCFA have the potential to reduce necrotizing enterocolitis [66] and cancer [67,68] in humans, diets that increase levels of BCFA in beef are desirable from a human health perspective.

Rumen bacterial profiles

The fatty acid results of the present experiment demonstrate that feeding oilseeds in combination with diets containing a greater proportion of forage directly effects the mean percentage concentration of PUFA and their BH products in beef fat. However, there are many factors that simultaneously affect the amount and variation of PUFA and their BH products, making ad hoc estimation of fatty acid profiles extremely challenging. In order to perform such calculations a multifactorial approach is required, and among the potential variables, the bacterial ecosystem of the rumen will undoubtedly have an overriding influence. Where historically others have been able to culture isolated bacterial species which metabolize dietary FA [53,69], the global perspective of how the entire population may be changing in response to diet and correlate with differences in FA profiles is lacking. This prompted our study taking advantage of current technologies to more fully characterize differences in rumen bacterial populations and their relationship to diet and FA deposited in beef. Previous research has cultured individual bacteria to examine their role in BH [69,70]. However, the sensitivity of rumen bacteria to temperature, pH, osmolality, and the bacterial competition, quorum sensing, nutrient limitations and syntrophism within the rumen, makes it difficult to replicate this ecosystem in the laboratory [71,72]. The use of pyrosequencing of the rumen ecosystem creates the opportunity to gain an overview of rumen bacterial populations simultaneously at any one point in time and compare it to other points in time. By looking at changes in the overall ecosystem within a variety of diets and animal hosts, one may be able to predict which bacterial populations are involved in rumen BH. This approach has been previously used to document the role of rumen bacteria in acidosis [73]. Although the ability of pyrosequencing to identify individual species is limited, the data generated could be used as a guideline for further research and when combined with culture techniques provide insight into the manipulation of individual rumen species involved in BH.

While overall sequence data was unable to fully describe the rumen bacterial ecosystem in cattle fed each diet due to limited coverage (Fig. S1), it was able to show that there were a large number of OTU's shared regardless of forage or oilseed type (Fig. 3). Therefore, despite dietary differences, there was a core group of microbes that was similar among all diets. However, changes in both ingredient and nutrient composition can impact the prevalence and density of specific groups or species without impacting the overall bacterial community structure [74]. While a number of genera were clearly impacted by diet (Table 3), variations in diet quality (*i.e.*, ADF, NDF) and composition (*i.e.*, inclusion of barley straw *vs.* barley grain) confounded the impact of oilseed or forage source on bacterial abundance. Regardless of diet, more than half the genera in Table 3 were members of the phylum Firmicutes, class Clostridia, order Clostridiales. This order is known to be Gram-negative, obligate anaerobes with a large representation in the rumen ecosystem [75]. However, despite the extensive diversity of this genus, previous research has indicated a possible link between some of these species and rumen BH [76].

When the 25 bacterial genera impacted by diet where compared in a correlation analysis to individual and groups of FA, 19 showed a significant correlation to one or more of the FA's (Table 4). Of these 19, five genera including *Acidaminobacter*, *Clostrium IV*, *Fibrobacter*, *Marvinbryantia* and *Olsenella* showed correlation to 4 or more individual FA's. *Clostridium IV* were highly negatively correlated to levels of CLNAisomers *c*9,*t*11,*t*15-18:3 and *c*9,*t*11,*c*15-18:3, as well as ALA. Increased levels of ALA and its long chain derivatives were found in the subcutaneous fat of cattle fed diets containing FS. Therefore, the increased percent abundance of *Clostridium IV* and *Ethanoligenens* in diets containing SS and not FS indicates that these two genera may be negatively associated with ALA and other n-3 PUFA in the rumen. However, several other genera including *Barnesiella*, *Butyrivibrio*, *Eubacterium* and *Olsenella* all showed increased abundance in diets with increased levels of at least one *n*-3 PUFA. Since ALA is considered a beneficial FA for human consumption [3–6], further research into the role of these organisms in rumen BH of ALA could elucidate how to increase ruminal bypass of ALA to adipose tissue.

Anaerostipes was the only genus that was found to be negatively correlated ($P<0.001$) to *n*-6 PUFA, which is known to inhibit BH in the rumen. Interestingly, *n*-6 PUFA were found to be highest in diets containing SS and *Anaerostipes* was also most abundant in RC-FS diets. This bacterial group may be also be involved in the rumen BH process and could be an indicator of inhibition of BH.

Post hoc analysis comparing cattle with high *vs.* low levels of VA in subcutaneous fat showed a significant separation of means ($P< 0.001$; Table 5). Individuals with the lowest levels of VA in subcutaneous fat were found to have rumen populations with a greater abundance of *Anaerophaga*, *Fibrobacter*, *Guggenheimella*,

Paludibacter and *Pseudozobellia*. Increasing amounts of VA in adipose tissue has been a target for ongoing research as it is a precursor for RA and may have beneficial health effects on its own [77]. However, some rumen bacteria are able to hydrogenate VA to steric acid [48,69]. Therefore, bacteria found at significantly increased levels in cattle with low as compared to high VA in tissue may have greater VA BH activity in the rumen.

The main bacterial species within the rumen which is known to impact FA metabolism is *Butyrivibrio proteoclasticus* [69]. Similar to previous research, a relation between FA metabolism and *Butyrivibrio* was noted in the current experiment. However, increased levels of *Butyrivibrio* were related to increased levels of *n*-3 PUFA in the tissue and not increased levels of SFA as has been previously noted [69]. However, the current study was unable to identify changes in percent abundance of bacterial groups at a species level and therefore other *Butyrivibrio* spp may also be involved in rumen BH. Previous research has also indicated that *Propionibacteria acnes*, *Selenomonas ruminantium*, *Enterococcus faecium*, *Staphylococcus sp.*, *Flavobacterium sp.* and *Streptococcus bovis* may also play a role in the hydrogenation of *trans* FA to SFA [69]. While none of these bacterial groups were noted as being significantly different in this study, a number of previously unreported bacterial genera were identified as being correlated, either positively or negatively, to the levels of various FA in subcutaneous fat. These additional bacterial genera may also play a role in ruminal BH that has not yet been elucidated using traditional microbial culturing techniques. Further research is required to clarify the role of not only these bacterial groups but also of ciliate protozoa in relation to dietary changes impacting the FA profiles of adipose tissue in ruminants.

Conclusions

The present study showed that cattle fed high-forage diets supplemented with SS had increased proportions of VA, RA and LA in subcutaneous fat, whereas supplementing with FS increased *n*-3 PUFA, CLNA, and AD. Present results demonstrate that dietary changes have the potential to produce beef with enhanced levels of PUFA BH products. However, in order to produce beef with consistently increased levels of PUFAs, further knowledge regarding how the type of PUFA, composition of the non-oil fraction of the diet and the type and level of feed processing impact PUFA deposition in the subcutaneous fat is required. Optimizing ruminal outflows of BH products will also require a better understanding of the precise role of rumen microbes and how the individual animal's genetics contribute to inter-animal variation. While some bacterial genera in this experiment were found to be correlated to specific FAs, the effect of diet on lipolytic rumen microrganisms and preferential pathways for BH requires greater insight by combining molecular techniques with classical culture techniques. Bacterial genera positively correlated to increasing BH intermediates in the present experiment need to be further researched in order to confirm whether these correlations are consistent over a range of diet types.

Acknowledgments

Special thanks are extended to staff at the Lacombe Research Centre (LRC) Beef Unit of AAFC for animal care, animal management and sample collection. The slaughter and processing of the cattle by the LRC abattoir staff is gratefully acknowledged. Contributions of the meat grading and quality staff at the LRC to the result are appreciated. Ms. I.L. Larsen and Dr. D. Petri are acknowledged for their valuable assistance in statistical analysis.

Author Contributions

Conceived and designed the experiments: MERD TAM. Performed the experiments: RMP CM. Analyzed the data: RMO CM MERD. Contributed reagents/materials/analysis tools: MERD TAM. Wrote the paper: RMP CM MERD TAM.

References

1. Raes K, De Smet S, Demeyer D (2004) Effect of dietary fatty acids on incorporation of long chain polyunsaturated fatty acids and conjugated linoleic acid in lamb, beef and pork meat: a review. Animal Feed Science and Technology 113: 199–221.
2. Salter AM (2014) Dietary fatty acids and cardiovascular disease. Animal doi:10.1017/S1751731111002023. In press.
3. Dilzer A, Park Y (2012) Implication of conjugated linoleic acid (CLA) in human health. Critical Reviews in Food Science and Nutrition 52: 488–513.
4. Jaudszus A, Jahreis G, Schlörmann W, Fischer J, Kramer R, et al. (2012) Vaccenic acid-mediated reduction in cytokine production is independent of c9,t11-CLA in human peripheral blood mononuclear cells. Biochimica et Biophysica Acta - Molecular and Cell Biology of Lipids 1821: 1316–1322.
5. McNeill S, Van Elswyk ME (2012) Red meat in global nutrition. Meat Science 92: 166–173.
6. Sofi F, Buccioni A, Cesari F, Gori AM, Minieri S, et al. (2010) Effects of a dairy product (pecorino cheese) naturally rich in cis-9, trans-11 conjugated linoleic acid on lipid, inflammatory and haemorheological variables: A dietary intervention study. Nutrition, Metabolism and Cardiovascular Diseases 20: 117–124.
7. Nassu RT, Dugan MER, He ML, McAllister TA, Aalhus JL, et al. (2011) The effects of feeding flaxseed to beef cows given forage based diets on fatty acids of longissimus thoracis muscle and backfat. Meat Science 89: 469–477.
8. Juárez M, Dugan MER, Aalhus JL, Aldai N, Basarab JA, et al. (2011) Effects of vitamin E and flaxseed on rumen-derived fatty acid intermediates in beef intramuscular fat. Meat Science 88: 434–440.
9. He ML, McAllister TA, Kastelic JP, Mir PS, Aalhus JL, et al. (2012) Feeding flaxseed in grass hay and barley silage diets to beef cows increases alpha-linolenic acid and its biohydrogenation intermediates in subcutaneous fat. Journal of Animal Science 90: 592–604.
10. Mapiye C, Turner TD, Rolland DC, Basarab JA, Baron VS, et al. (2013) Adipose tissue and muscle fatty acid profiles of steers fed red clover silage with and without flaxseed. Livestock Science 151: 11–20.
11. Van Ranst G, Lee MRF, Fievez V (2011) Red clover polyphenol oxidase and lipid metabolism. Animal 5: 512–521.
12. Lee MRF, Evans PR, Nute GR, Richardson RI, Scollan ND (2009) A comparison between red clover silage and grass silage feeding on fatty acid composition, meat stability and sensory quality of the M. Longissimus muscle of dairy cull cows. Meat Science 81: 738–744.
13. Noci F, French P, Monahan FJ, Moloney AP (2007) The fatty acid composition of muscle fat and subcutaneous adipose tissue of grazing heifers supplemented with plant oil-enriched concentrates. Journal of Animal Science 85: 1062–1073.
14. Schmid A, Collomb M, Sieber R, Bee G (2006) Conjugated linoleic acid in meat and meat products: A review. Meat Science 73: 29–41.
15. Crumb DJ (2011) Conjugated linoleic acid (CLA)-An overview. International Journal of Applied Research in Natural Products 4: 12–15.
16. Mapiye C, Dugan MER, Turner TD, Rolland DC, Basarab JA, et al. (2013) Erythrocytes assayed early ante-mortem can predict adipose tissue and muscle trans-18:1 isomeric profiles of steers fed red clover silage with and without flaxseed. Canadian Journal of Animal Science 93: 1–5.
17. Hegarty RS (2004) Genotype differences and their impact on digestive tract function of ruminants: A review. Australian Journal of Experimental Agriculture 44: 459–467
18. Dugan MER, Rolland DC, Aalhus JL, Aldai N, Kramer JKG (2008) Subcutaneous fat composition of youthful and mature Canadian beef: emphasis

on individual conjugated linoleic acid and trans-18:1 isomers. Canadian Journal of Animal Science 88: 591–599.
19. Mapiye C, Turner TD, Rolland DC, Basarab JA, Baron VS, et al. (2013) Effects of feeding flaxseed or sunflower-seed in high-forage diets on beef production, quality and fatty acid composition Meat Science 95: 98–109.
20. Candian Council of Animal Care (CCAC) (1993) In Olfert ED, Cross BM, McWilliams AA, (Eds). (2nd ed.) Guide to the care and use of experimental animals, vol. 1, Ottawa, Ontario.
21. Brethour JR (1992) The repeatability and accuracy of ultrasound in measuring backfat of cattle. Journal of Animal Science 70: 1039–1044.
22. Narvaez N, Wang Y, Xu Z, Alexander T, Garden S, et al. (2013). Effects of hop varieties on ruminal fermentation and bacterial community in an artificial rumen (rusitec). Journal of the Science of Food and Agriculture 93: 45–52.
23. Dowd SE, Callaway TR, Wolcott RD, Sun Y, McKeehan T, et al. (2008). Evaluation of the bacterial diversity in the feces of cattle using 16S rDNA bacterial tag-encoded FLX amplicon pyrosequencing (bTEFAP). BMC Microbiology 8: 125.
24. Schloss PD, Westcott SL, Ryabin T, Hall JR, Hartmann M, et al. (2009). Introducing mothur: open-source, platform-independent, community-supported software for describing and comparing microbial communities. Applied and Environmental Microbiology 75: 7537–7541.
25. Schloss PD, Gevers D, Westcott SL (2011). Reducing the effects of PCR amplification and sequencing artifacts on 16S rRNA-based studies. PLOS ONE 6:e27310.
26. Huse SM, Welch DM, Morrison HG, Sogin ML (2010). Ironing out the wrinkles in the rare biosphere through improved OTU clustering. Environmental Microbiology 12: 1889–1898.
27. Petri RM, Schwaiger T, Penner GB, Beauchemin KA, Forster RJ, et al. (2013). Changes in the rumen epimural bacterial diversity of beef cattle as affected by diet and induced ruminal acidosis. Applied and Environmental Microbiology 79: 3744–3755.
28. Aldai N, Dugan MER, Rolland DC, Kramer JKG (2009) Survey of the fatty acid composition of Canadian beef: Backfat and longissimus lumborum muscle. Canadian Journal of Animal Science 89: 315–329
29. Kramer JKG, Hernandez M, Cruz-Hernandez C, Kraft J, Dugan MER (2008) Combining results of two GC separations partly achieves determination of all cis and trans 16:1, 18:1, 18:2 and 18:3 except CLA isomers of milk fat as demonstrated using ag-ion SPE fractionation. Lipids 43: 259–273
30. Cruz-Hernandez C, Deng Z, Zhou J, Hill AR, Yurawecz MP, et al. (2004) Methods for analysis of conjugated linoleic acids and trans-18:1 isomers in dairy fats by using a combination of gas chromatography, silver-ion thin-layer chromatography/gas chromatography, silver-ion liquid chrmatography. Journal of AOAC International 87: 545–562.
31. Gómez-Cortés P, Bach A, Luna P, Juárez M, de la Fuente MA (2009) Effects of extruded linseed supplementation on n-3 fatty acids and conjugated linoleic acid in milk and cheese from ewes. Journal of Dairy Science 92: 4122–4134.
32. SAS (2009) SAS user's guide: Statistics. SAS for windows. Release 9.2. Cary NC: SAS Institute Inc.
33. Kim CM, Kim JH, Oh YK, Park EK, Ahn GC, et al. (2009) Effects of flaxseed diets on performance, carcass characteristics and fatty acid composition of Hanwoo steers. Asian-Australasian Journal of Animal Sciences 22: 1151–1159.
34. Sarnklong C, Coneja JW, Pellikaan W, Hendriks WH (2010) Utilization of rice straw and different treatments to improve its feed value for ruminants: A review. Asian-Australasian Journal of Animal Sciences 23: 680–692.
35. Jenkins TC (1993) Lipid metabolism in the rumen. Journal of Dairy Science 76: 3851–3863.
36. Doreau M, Ferlay A (1994) Digestion and utilisation of fatty acids by ruminants. Animal Feed Science and Technology 45: 379–396.
37. Harfoot CG, Noble RC, Moore JH (1973) Factors influencing the extent of biohydrogenation of linoleic acid by Rumen micro-organisms in vitro. Journal of the Science of Food and Agriculture 24: 961–970.
38. Geay Y, Bauchart D, Hocquette JF, Culioli J (2001) Effect of nutritional factors on biochemical, structural and metabolic characteristics of muscles in ruminants, consequences on dietetic value and sensorial qualities of meat. Reproduction Nutrtion and Development 41: 1–26.
39. Doreau M, Aurousseau E, Martin C (2009) Effects of linseed lipids fed as rolled seeds, extruded seeds or oil on organic matter and crude protein digestion in cows. Animal Feed Science and Technology 150: 187–196.
40. Shingfield KJ, Salo-Väänänen P, Pahkala E, Toivonen V, Jaakkola S, et al. (2005) Effect of forage conservation method, concentrate level and propylene glycol on the fatty acid composition and vitamin content of cows' milk. Journal of Dairy Research 72: 349–361.
41. Shingfield KJ, Chilliard Y, Toivonen V, Kairenius P, Givens DI (2008) Fatty acids and bioactive lipids in ruminant milk in: Bioactive components of milk, Advances in experimental medicine and biology. In: Bösze Z (ed), Springer New York.
42. Khan NA, Cone JW, Hendriks WH (2009) Stability of fatty acids in grass and maize silages after exposure to air during the feed out period. Animal Feed Science and Technology 154: 183–192.
43. Scollan ND, Richardson I, De Smet S, Moloney AP, Doreau M, et al. (2005) Enhancing the content of beneficial fatty acids in beef and consequences for meat quality. Indicators of milk and beef quality, EAAP Publications: 151–162.
44. Halmemies-Beauchet-Filleau A, Kairenius P, Ahvenjarvi S, Crosley LK, Muetzel S, et al. (2013) Effect of forage conservation method on ruminal lipid metabolism and microbial ecology in lactating cows fed diets containing a 60:40 forage-to-concentrate ratio. Journal of Dairy Science, 96: 2428–2447.
45. Lee YJ, Jenkins TC (2011) Biohydrogenation of linolenic acid to stearic acid by the rumen microbial population yields multiple intermediate conjugated diene isomers. Journal of Nutrition 141: 1445–1450.
46. Hennessy AA, Ross RP, Devery R, Stanton C (2011) The health promoting properties of the conjugated isomers of α-linolenic acid. Lipids 46: 105–119.
47. Bessa RJB, Alves SP, Jerónimo E, Alfaia CM, Prates JAM, et al. (2007) Effect of lipid supplements on ruminal biohydrogenation intermediates and muscle fatty acids in lambs. European Journal of Lipid Science and Technology 109: 868–878.
48. Jenkins TC, Wallace RJ, Moate PJ, Mosley EE (2008) Board-Invited Review: Recent advances in biohydrogenation of unsaturated fatty acids within the rumen microbial ecosystem. Journal of Animal Science 86: 397–412.
49. Doreau M, Laverroux S, Normand J, Chesneau G, Glasser F (2009) Effect of linseed fed as rolled seeds, extruded seeds or oil on fatty acid rumen metabolism and intestinal digestibility in cows. Lipids 44: 53–62.
50. Jerónimo E, Alves SP, Alfaia CM, Prates JAM, Santos-Silva J, et al. (2011) Biohydrogenation intermediates are differentially deposited between polar and neutral intramuscular lipids of lambs. European Journal of Lipid Science and Technology 113: 924–934
51. AbuGhazaleh AA, Schingoethe DJ, Hippen AR, Kalscheur KF, Whitlock LA (2002) Fatty Acid profiles of milk and rumen digesta from cows fed fish oil, extruded soybeans or their blend. Journal of Dairy Science 85: 2266–2276.
52. Lock AL, Garnsworthy PC (2002) Independent effects of dietary linoleic and linolenic fatty acids on the conjugated linoleic acid content of cows' milk. Animal Science 74: 163–176
53. Maia MRG, Chaudhary LC, Figueres L, Wallace RJ (2007) Metabolism of polyunsaturated fatty acids and their toxicity to the microflora of the rumen. Antonie van Leeuwenhoek 91: 303–314.
54. Chow TT, Fievez V, Moloney AP, Raes K, Demeyer D, et al. (2004) Effect of fish oil on in vitro rumen lipolysis, apparent biohydrogenation of linoleic and linolenic acid and accumulation of biohydrogenation intermediates. Animal Feed Science and Technology 117: 1–12.
55. Basarab JA, Mir PS, Aalhus JL, Shah MA, Baron VS, et al. (2007) Effect of sunflower seed supplementation on the fatty acid composition of muscle and adipose tissue of pasture-fed and feedlot finished beef. Canadian Journal of Animal Science 87: 71–86.
56. Raes K, De Smet S, Balcaen A, Claeys E, Demeyer D (2003) Effect of diets rich in N-3 polyunsaturated fatty acids on muscle lipids and fatty acids in Belgian Blue double-muscled young bulls. Reproduction Nutrition Development 43: 331–345.
57. Gunstone FD, Harwood JL (1994) Occurrence and characterization of oils and fats. In Gunstone, F. D., Harwood, J. L., Padley, F. B., (Eds.), The Lipid Handbook (pp 101). New York: Chapman & Hall.
58. AbuGhazaleh AA, Jacobson BN (2007) The effect of pH and polyunsaturated C18 fatty acid source on the production of vaccenic acid and conjugated linoleic acids in ruminal cultures incubated with docosahexaenoic acid. Animal Feed Science and Technology 136: 11–22.
59. Martínez Marín AL, Gómez-Cortés P, Gómez Castro G, Juárez M, Pérez Alba L, et al. (2012) Effects of feeding increasing dietary levels of high oleic or regular sunflower or linseed oil on fatty acid profile of goat milk. Journal of Dairy Science 95: 1942–1955.
60. Kong Y, He M, McAlister T, Seviour R, Forster R (2010) Quantitative fluorescence in situ hybridization of microbial communities in the rumens of cattle fed different diets. Applied and Environmental Microbiology 76: 6933–6938.
61. Lee MRF, Harris LJ, Dewhurst RJ, Merry RJ, Scollan ND (2003) The effect of clover silages on long chain fatty acid rumen transformations and digestion in beef steers. Animal Science 76: 491–501.
62. Jacobs AAA, van Baal J, Smits MA, Taweel HZH, Hendriks WH, et al. (2011) Effects of feeding rapeseed oil, soybean oil, or linseed oil on stearoyl-CoA desaturase expression in the mammary gland of dairy cows. Journal of Dairy Science 94: 874–887.
63. Bernard L, Bonnet M, Leroux C, Shingfield KJ, Chilliard Y (2009) Effect of sunflower-seed oil and linseed oil on tissue lipid metabolism, gene expression, milk fatty acid secretion in Alpine goats fed maize silage–based diets. Journal of Dairy Science 92: 6083–6094.
64. Nakamura MT, Nara TY, (2004) Structure, function, dietary regulation of Δ6, Δ5, Δ9 desaturases, 2004. p. 345–376.
65. Vlaeminck B, Fievez V, Cabrita ARJ, Fonseca AJM, Dewhurst RJ (2006) Factors affecting odd- and branched-chain fatty acids in milk: A review. Animal Feed Science and Technology 131: 389–417.
66. Ran-Ressler RR, Khailova L, Arganbright KM, Adkins-Rieck CK, Jouni ZE, et al. (2011) Branched chain fatty acids reduce the incidence of necrotizing enterocolitis and alter gastrointestinal microbial ecology in a neonatal rat model. PLOS ONE 6: e29032
67. Wongtangtintharn S, Oku H, Iwasaki H, Toda T (2004) Effect of branched-chain fatty acids on fatty acid biosynthesis of human breast cancer cells. Journal of Nutritional Science and Vitaminology 50: 137–143.
68. Yang Z, Liu S, Chen X, Chen H, Huang M, et al. (2000) Induction of apoptotic cell death and in vivo growth inhibition of human cancer cells by a saturated branched-chain fatty acid, 13-methyltetradecanoic acid. Cancer Research 60: 505–509.

69. McKain N, Shingfield KJ, Wallace RJ (2010) Metabolism of conjugated linoleic acids and 18: 1 fatty acids by ruminal bacteria: products and mechanisms. Microbiology 156: 579–588.
70. Maia MR, Chaudhary LC, Figueres L, Wallace RJ (2007) Metabolism of polyunsaturated fatty acids and their toxicity to the microflora of the rumen. Antonie van Leeuwenhoek 91: 303–314.
71. Hobson PN (1965) Continuous Culture of some anaerobic and facultatively anaerobic rumen bacteria. Journal of General Microbiology 38: 167–180.
72. Russell JB, Baldwin RL (1979) Comparison of substrate affinities among several rumen bacteria: a possible determinant of rumen bacterial competition. Applied and Environmental Microbiology 37: 531–536.
73. Petri RM, Schwaiger T, Penner GB, Beauchemin KA, Forster RJ, et al. (2013) Characterization of the core rumen microbiome in cattle during transition from forage to concentrate as well as during and after an acidotic challenge. PLOS ONE 8: e83424.
74. Petri RM, Forster RJ, Yang W, McKinnon JJ, McAllister TA (2012) Characterization of rumen bacterial diversity and fermentation parameters in concentrate fed cattle with and without forage. Journal of Applied Microbiology 112: 1152–1162.
75. Yutin N, Galperin MY (2013) A genomic update on clostridial phylogeny: Gram-negative spore formers and other misplaced clostridia. Environmental Microbiology 15: 2631–2641.
76. Huws SA, Kim EJ, Lee MR, Scott MB, Tweed JK, et al. (2011) As yet uncultured bacteria phylogenetically classified as Prevotella, Lachnospiraceae incertae sedis and unclassified Bacteroidales, Clostridiales and Ruminococcaceae may play a predominant role in ruminal biohydrogenation. Environmental Microbiology 13: 1500–1512.
77. Field CJ, Blewett HH, Proctor S, Vine D (2009) Human health benefits of vaccenic acid. Applied Physiology, Nutrition, Metabolism 34: 979–991.

3

Modelling Size Structured Food Webs Using a Modified Niche Model with Two Predator Traits

Jan Klecka[1,2,3]*

1 Departmemt of Fish Ecology and Evolution, Eawag: Swiss Federal Institute of Aquatic Science and Technology, Kastanienbaum, Switzerland, **2** Laboratory of Theoretical Ecology, Institute of Entomology, Biology Centre of the Academy of Sciences of the Czech Republic, České Budějovice, Czech Republic, **3** Department of Ecosystems Biology, Faculty of Science, University of South Bohemia, České Budějovice, Czech Republic

Abstract

The structure of food webs is frequently described using phenomenological stochastic models. A prominent example, the niche model, was found to produce artificial food webs resembling real food webs according to a range of summary statistics. However, the size structure of food webs generated by the niche model and real food webs has not yet been rigorously compared. To fill this void, I use a body mass based version of the niche model and compare prey-predator body mass allometry and predator-prey body mass ratios predicted by the model to empirical data. The results show that the model predicts weaker size structure than observed in many real food webs. I introduce a modified version of the niche model which allows to control the strength of size-dependence of predator-prey links. In this model, optimal prey body mass depends allometrically on predator body mass and on a second trait, such as foraging mode. These empirically motivated extensions of the model allow to represent size structure of real food webs realistically and can be used to generate artificial food webs varying in several aspects of size structure in a controlled way. Hence, by explicitly including the role of species traits, this model provides new opportunities for simulating the consequences of size structure for food web dynamics and stability.

Editor: Luís A. Nunes Amaral, Northwestern University, United States of America

Funding: The study was supported by ERASMUS scholarship and the Grant Agency of the University of South Bohemia (grant no. GAJU 145/2010/P). The funders had no role in study design, data collection and analysis, decision to publish, or preparation of the manuscript.

Competing Interests: This author has declared that no competing interests exist.

* Email: jan.klecka@eawag.ch

Introduction

Animal communities form complex networks of interspecific interactions; the most traditionally studied type of such networks is the food web [1]. It is widely recognized that stability of food webs is driven by non-random features of food web structure [2–4]. Trophic links typically depend on the size of predators and prey [5–12] and it has been shown that predator-prey body mass ratios can affect food web stability [13,14]. Hence, we need to develop models that faithfully represent the empirically observed dependence of predation links on body masses of predators and prey to gain better insights into the structure and stability of food webs.

The lack of mechanistic models using body mass to explain or predict food web structure [15,16] is surprising given that the role of body mass for structuring food webs has been recognized already at least by Elton almost a century ago [1]. On the other hand, a family of phenomenological stochastic food web models has been developed with the intention to mimic the structure of real food webs using a set of simple rules which do not invoke any specific mechanisms. A prominent example is the niche model [17] which assumes that predators feed on a contiguous range of prey sorted along a single niche axis. The assumption of intervality has been relaxed in recent extensions of the model [18–20]; however empirical food webs are close to intervality [18,21,22], so the assumption of intervality is a reasonable simplification. It has been speculated that body mass is the key trait defining the position of species on the niche axis [7,17] and a body mass based version of the niche model, which makes this assumption explicit was published recently [20,23]. The original niche model and its modifications have been found to describe the structure of real food webs faithfully [17,18,20,23,24]. However, this conclusion was based almost exclusively on comparison of several summary statistics of food web structure between model generated and real food webs. The relationship between predator and prey body mass was not among them because the original niche model and most of its modifications [17,18] do not include any information on species body masses (but see [20,23]). However, it is widely recognized that predator and prey masses are strongly correlated in real food webs [8–11]. Testing whether this correlation is reproduced by theoretical food web models is of utmost importance.

There is also mounting evidence that other traits than body mass can modify the probability or strength of predator-prey links [25], such as foraging mode of the predator [26,27]. Models relating multiple species traits to the probability of feeding interactions [25] and interaction strength [28] have already been developed. These statistical models can be directly fitted to empirical data and used to test the importance of different species traits for feeding interactions [27]. However, the focus of this paper is on stochastic models, such as the niche model and its extensions. These models have usually been compared to empirical data indirectly by various metrics of food webs structure [17,29], although methods allowing to calculate model likelihood for directly comparing predicted and observed links have been recently developed [19,20,23]. These models are also prominently used in simulation studies of food web dynamics. They can be used to generate artificial food webs with specified properties; these model food webs can be used to explore the consequences of food web structure for dynamics, for example to test the effects of predator-prey mass ratios [13,14] or connectance [30,31] on food web stability.

Here I test whether a body mass based modification of the niche model represents size structure of feeding interactions in food webs realistically. Moreover, I introduce a novel extension of the niche model which directly includes empirically observed prey-predator body mass allometry [8–11]. Finally, I include a second trait modifying prey size selectivity of predators [26,27]. The aim of these empirically motivated modifications of the niche model is to develop a simple stochastic food web model capturing the size structure of a wide range of food webs. Such a model will be valuable for exploring the consequences of size structure for food web dynamics and stability in future simulation studies.

Materials and Methods

The original niche model

The niche model [17], referred to as "the original niche model" here, predicts the occurrence of feeding links in a food web with S species. Each potential link is an element a_{ij} of an $S \times S$ adjacency matrix A, where j is a potential consumer of species i. A link a_{ij} is either present ($a_{ij}=1$) or absent ($a_{ij}=0$). Key characteristics of the original niche model are that species can be sorted along a single niche axis, which defines a feeding hierarchy, and that the diets of consumers contain species distributed along a contiguous section of the niche axis [19]. Using only two parameters, species richness (S) and connectance (C), the original niche model generates a food web matrix using a simple set of instructions. Each species is assigned a position on a one-dimensional niche axis by drawing a random number n_j from a uniform distribution on an interval (0,1), diet breadth r_j and the centre of the feeding niche c_j from the interval $(\frac{r_j}{2}, n_j)$. Then, feeding links are assigned to all predator-prey combinations where a prey i has n_i within the range of $(c_j - \frac{r_j}{2}, c_j + \frac{r_j}{2})$ for predator j. The original niche model produces interval food webs, i.e. webs where each predator feeds on a contiguous range of prey along the niche axis. Another characteristic is that constraints on possible prey a predator can eat are weak and consequently there is only a small set of forbidden links (sensu [32,33]). A predator j can potentially feed on any prey i with $n_i < n_j$ and also on many prey with $n_i > n_j$; up to 50% of a predator's diet can have higher n_i than the predator's n_j.

Although it has been shown that body mass can be used as a basis for sorting species in food webs [5–7,20,23,24], the original niche model does not assume that predator-prey interactions depend on body mass. The niche value is an abstract value, which limits the applicability of the niche model to address specific biologically relevant questions about the role of body mass for food web stability. To circumvent this problem, it has been proposed that one can transform the niche value to body mass of species i as $w_i = 10^{x n_i}$, where x is a parameter fixing maximal predator-prey mass ratio, which is 10^x [14]. However, a direct way to incorporate body mass into the niche model was recently developed [20,23] (see below).

The body mass based niche model

A body mass based modification of the niche model uses body mass to calculate species niche values [20,23]. Several body mass based versions of the niche model developed by Williams et al. [20] also include other changes to the niche model. However, in its simplest form used here, the only difference compared to the original niche model is that the niche value is a function of body mass:

$$n_j = \frac{\ln(w_j) - \ln(w_{min})}{\ln(w_{max}) - \ln(w_{min})} \qquad \text{(eq.1)}$$

where w_j is body mass of species j, w_{min} and w_{max} is the mass of the smallest and the largest species in the food web, respectively. I will refer to this model as the "body mass based niche model". Stouffer et al. [18], Allesina et al. [19] and Williams et al [20] introduced further modifications of the niche model allowing for non-contiguous diets but I do not consider this aspect here because diets in real food webs have usually high degree of intervality [18,21,22]. Hence, the body mass based niche model explicitly assumes that body mass controls trophic position of individual species but otherwise the structure of the food webs generated by this model is identical to the original niche model. Code to generate food web structure (written in R) is avalaible as Supporting Information (Script S1).

Introducing the two traits allometric model

Here I propose further extensions of the body mass based niche model to incorporate predator-prey body mass allometry well known from empirical data and include a second predator trait to move from a simple body mass dependence of predator-prey interactions to multiple-trait based approach [25,27,28]. The centre of the feeding range c_j of a predator j is constrained to be a function of predator's body mass w_j. Empirical data show that predator's optimal prey mass w_{opt} is allometrically related to its body mass w_j:

$$\ln(w_{opt}) = \alpha + \beta \ln(w_j) \qquad \text{(eq.2)}$$

for a predator j [8–11]. This empirically derived predator-prey mass allometry is explicitly included in the model: the centre of the predator's feeding range c_j equals to the niche value n_i of a prey i with mass $w_i = w_{opt}$; i.e., predator's feeding range r_j is centred on a prey with the optimal mass for a given predator:

$$c_j = \frac{\ln(w_{opt}) - \ln(w_{min})}{\ln(w_{max}) - \ln(w_{min})} \qquad \text{(eq.3)}$$

where c_j is the centre of predator's feeding niche and w_{opt} is the optimal prey mass for predator j. The second modification I propose is an inclusion of a second predator trait k_j which modifies the optimal prey mass w_{opt} for a predator j. It models a situation when equally sized predators differing in foraging mode or another trait prefer prey of different sizes [26,27]. An illustrative example is shown in Figure 1. Specifically, I modify the allometry of predator mass and optimal prey mass (eq. 2):

$$\ln(w_{opt}) = \alpha + \beta \ln(w_j) + k_j \qquad \text{(eq.4)}$$

$$k_j \sim N(\mu, \sigma^2) \text{ and } (c_j - \frac{r_j}{2}) < k_j < (n_j - c_j)$$

where k_j denotes the effect of a second trait on the optimal prey mass for a predator j. I will refer to this model as the "two traits allometric model". I treat k_j as an unknown, or latent, trait [25] in the simulations. Because it is related to foraging behaviour of predators, I call it here a "foraging trait". I include the effect of the foraging trait k_j on optimal prey mass w_{opt} of each predator by drawing a random value from a truncated normal distribution and inserting it into the formula above (eq. 4). I used mean $\mu = 0$, various values of standard deviation σ; lower bound and upper bound was set to ensure that predator's c_j, which is a function of $\ln(w_{opt})$ (see eq. 3), lies within the range set by the basic constraints of the niche model; i.e. in the interval $(0, n_j)$. The effect of the second trait is independent of predator body mass (k_j and w_j are uncorrelated). The strength of the effect of the second trait k_j relative to body mass w_j can be manipulated by the choice of σ of the truncated normal distribution used to generate the values of k_j. Thanks to this feature, the two traits model covers the whole range of possibilities from the strictly size-dependent predation when $k_j = 0$ (eq. 2) to the very weak size constraints of the body mass based niche model (σ very large). For sufficiently large values of σ the two traits model converges to the body mass based niche model described above [20,23], where the centre of the feeding niche c_j is drawn uniformly from the interval $(\frac{r_j}{2}, n_j)$. Intermediate cases can be easily achieved by an appropriate choice of the standard deviation σ. A function rtruncnorm in the truncnorm package for R was used to sample from the truncated normal distribution [34]. Code to generate food web structure (written in R) is avalaible in Script S1.

Analysis of the structure of model food webs

I carried out extensive simulations in R 2.15.1 [35] to analyse the structure of model food webs generated by the body mass based niche model and its modifications described above. I also compared the results to those based on the original niche model where body mass is calculated post hoc from niche values as $w_i = 10^{x n_i}$ for species i, where x is a parameter fixing maximal predator-prey mass ratio, as described by Heckmann et al. [14]. To generate food webs with predator-prey interactions depending on species body mass using the body mass based niche and two traits models, I first set the number of species ($S = 100$ in the main results) and their body masses. Since the distribution of body masses is known to follow approximately a log-normal distribution, I assigned body masses to all species by randomly generating numbers from a log-normal distribution with $\mu = \ln(1)$ and $\sigma = 5$; the value of $\sigma = 5$ corresponds to total size range in the food web on average 10 orders of magnitude, which may represent, for example, a freshwater food web with species ranging from small zooplankton ($\sim 10\mu g$) to large fish ($\sim 100kg$). The effect of total mass range on the resulting food web structure was further explored by changing the value of σ of the log-normal distribution of body masses. In all results reported here, I set connectance $C = 0.1$ (C effectively controls the mean diet breadth of consumers) and excluded food webs with C differing from the target value by more than 3%, which is a standard procedure (e.g. [17,31]). In the case of the two traits allometric model, I also fixed the values of parameters describing the allometry of predator and prey masses (eq. 4). I set $\alpha = -3.63$ to get a predator-prey mass ratio of 37.7 for a predator of body mass $w_j = 1g$ and $\beta = 0.83$; these values are based on published analyses of a large database of predator-prey interactions [8–11]. I set the standard deviation σ of

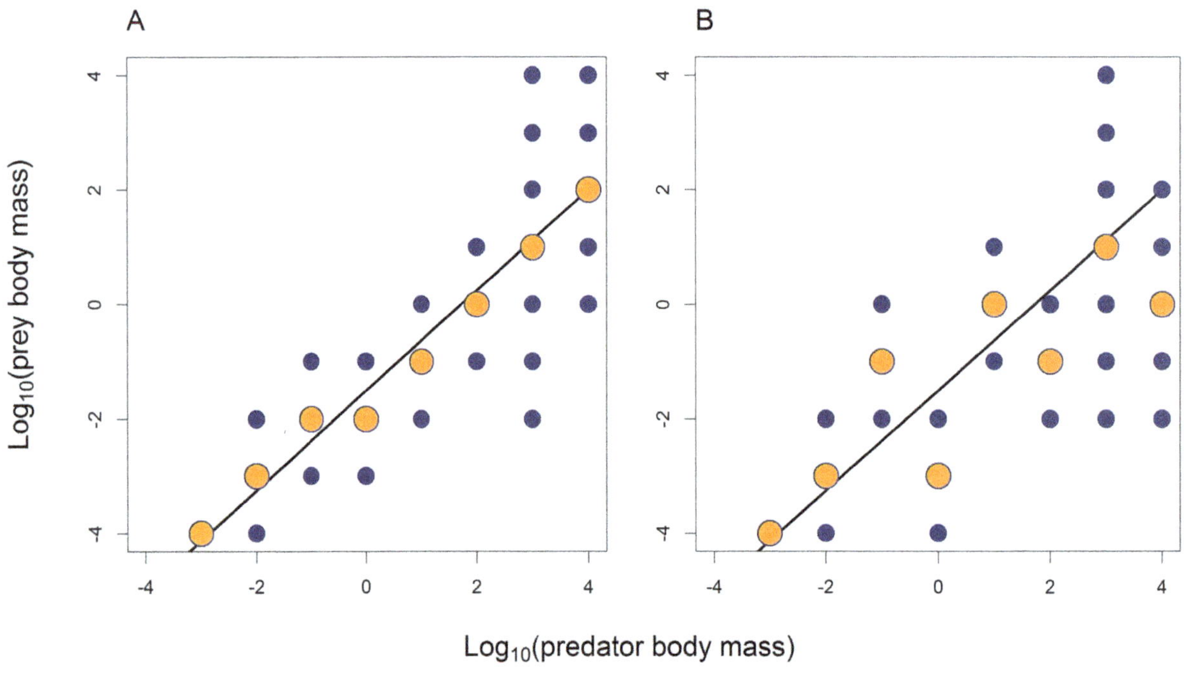

Figure 1. Comparison of two food webs with different importance of body mass for predator-prey interactions. An illustrative example of a small food web (9 species); each species is displayed on the x-axis as a predator and on the y-axis as a prey (the smallest species is a non-predatory basal species). The black line shows an allometric relationship between predator mass and optimal prey mass, large orange circles show the prey closest to the optimal prey mass for individual predators and smaller blue circles show other predator-prey links present in the network. In (A) optimal prey mass depends allometrically only on predator mass. In (B) optimal prey mass depends also on a second trait of a predator (a foraging trait), which causes deviations from the prey-predator body mass allometry depicted by the black line. Many real food webs are characterized by such a blurred relationship between prey and predator body masses.

k_j to several different values, which leads to a range of situations differing in the strength of the size dependence of feeding links. I also included the special case of $k_j = 0$, where the effect of the second trait is absent and optimal prey mass depends only on predator mass (eq. 2).

In the case of the original niche model, a different approach had to be used. I set the number of species and connectance as above and generated food web structure. Then, I calculated body masses form the niche values (instead of calculating niche values from body masses) using a method proposed by Heckmann et al. [14]. Here, $w_i = 10^{x n_i}$ for species i, where x is a parameter fixing maximal predator-prey mass ratio, which is 10^x. I set the value of x to match the mean value of total body mass range in the other models. This leads to a close correspondence between the original and body mass based niche models. Comparison of the results between these two models thus shows the consequences of the choice to (1) either generate niche values first and then use them to calculate body masses or (2) to use the opposite, arguably more natural, procedure of specifying species body masses first and then using them to calculate niche values. Distribution of body masses differs in these two cases because in the original niche model I calculated body masses as $w_i = 10^{x n_i}$ [14] and n_i is uniformly distributed on the interval (0,1). Hence, $\ln(w_i)$ is uniformly distributed, while in the body mass based niche and two trait models, body masses were generated from a log-normal distribution.

Food webs generated by the models were compared using several measures of network structure. I analysed the prey-predator body mass allometry using standardized major axis regression (SMA regression), which is frequently used to estimate allometries because it treats errors in both the explanatory and response variable equally [36]; the package smatr for R was used [37]. The analysis of size structure of model food webs was complemented by a comparison of twelve summary statistics commonly used to describe food web topology (e.g. [16,17,29]). The metrics used were: the proportion of basal, intermediate and top species, the proportion of herbivores, mean and maximum trophic level, mean omnivory level, clustering coefficient, standard deviation of generalism and vulnerability, maximum diet similarity and mean path length (the definitions follow [16]). I refrained from comparing these metrics directly to real data because improving the, already good, fit of the niche model was not an objective of this paper and because the utility of such comparisons for evaluating food web models is limited [38]. I instead focused on comparing the different models among themselves to test whether the changes in size structure in these models lead to changes in other structural properties.

Species richness and connectance were kept constant, although these parameters are important for addressing other questions, such as stability and robustness of food webs [13,39]. In the simulations reported here, species richness had no effect on the results and connectance only controlled mean diet breadth of predators, which slightly changed the quantitative output of the simulations but had no effect on comparing the models. Values of $S = 50$, 200 and $C = 0.05$, 0.2 were tested in additional simulations (results not shown) to verify that the results and conclusions presented here are robust.

Results

Body mass structure of model food webs

Both the original niche model and the two traits model produce food webs with the distribution of predator-prey body mass ratios (PPMR) comparable to empirical data from different habitats (Figure 2). Food webs generated by the original niche model have median PPMR = 253.8, while food webs produced by the two traits allometric model with no, weak and strong effect of the foraging trait have median PPMR = 191.4, 122.4 and 79.1, respectively. The empirical data have median PPMR = 87.1, 5.3 and 62.6 for freshwater, terrestrial and marine data, respectively. With increasing importance of the role of the foraging trait, the constraints set by the allometric dependence of optimal prey mass on predator mass are getting weaker, which leads to broader range of PPMR values (Figure 2). A notable difference from the empirical data is that all the models predict smaller numbers of interactions where predator is smaller than its prey than observed in empirical food webs (negative values of $\log_{10}$(PPMR) in Figure 2).

Individual models differ in the strength of the effects of predator and prey mass on the probability of occurrence of individual feeding links; also the set of "forbidden" links (i.e. links that never

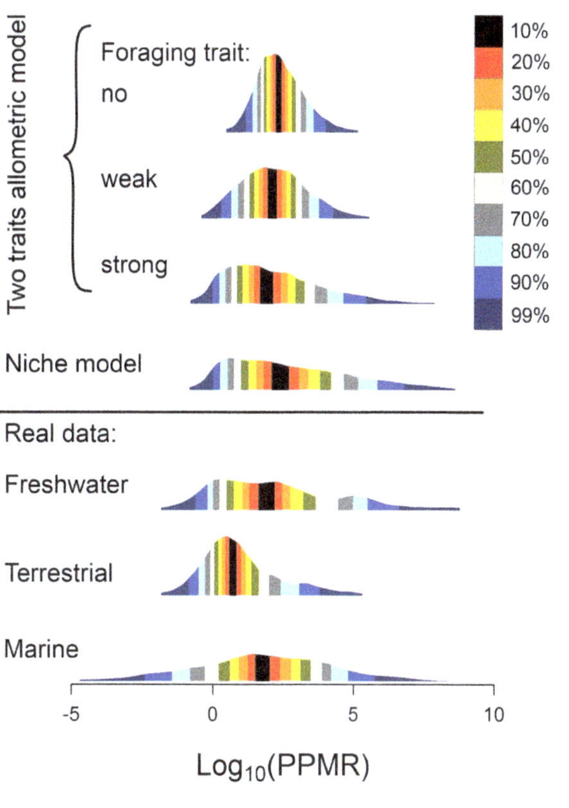

Figure 2. Predator-prey body mass ratios in model food webs and real data. The distributions of predator-prey body mass ratios produced by different models and real data from freshwater, marine and terrestrial predatory interactions (data from [8]). In the case of model data, results of 200 simulations of food web matrices with $S = 100$ species and $C = 0.1$ are presented for each model. In the case of the two traits allometric model, body masses were drawn from a lognormal distribution ($\mu = \ln(1)$ and $\sigma = 5$); this setting leads to the total body mass range in individual food webs ca. 10 orders of magnitude). Optimal prey mass is given as $\ln(w_{opt}) = -3.83 + 0.83 \cdot \ln(w_j) + k_j$, where w_j is predator mass and k_j denotes the effect of a predator's foraging trait on the optimal prey mass. Settings of the foraging trait are $k_j = 0$ (no effect), $k_j \sim N(\mu = 0, \sigma = 0.1)$ and $(c_j - \frac{r_j}{2}) < k_j < (n_j - c_j)$ (weak effect), and $k_j \sim N(\mu = 0, \sigma = 10)$ and $(c_j - \frac{r_j}{2}) < k_j < (n_j - c_j)$ (strong effect). See the methods section for more details. Plot shows estimated probability density functions with colours representing intervals with a given percentage of observations around the median (see the legend).

occur) varies (Figure 3). In the case of the two traits allometrical model with no effect of predator foraging trait, all interactions are constrained to a narrow band around the allometry of optimal prey and predator mass, and probability of the occurrence of feeding links decreases sharply with increasing difference from the allometry (Figure 3 A). With increasing importance of the predator foraging trait (and hence decreasing role of body mass constraints), the set of forbidden links decreases (Figure 3 B and C). In the original niche model, predators can feed on a wide range of prey and consequently, all links have a low probability of occurrence (<0.26) (Figure 3 D), as in the two traits allometric model with strong effect of predator foraging trait (Figure 3 C). The dependence of link probability on predator and prey masses holds independently on the total body mass range of species in a food web (not shown).

The prey-predator body mass allometry in model food webs with total body mass range of 10 orders of magnitude (Figure 2 and Figure 3) was similar in different models. The intercept estimated by SMA regression was -2.1, -1.9, and -2.1 in the two traits allometric model with no, weak and strong effect of predator foraging trait and -2.6 in the original niche model. The slope of the allometry was 0.91, 0.92, and 0.94 in the two traits allometric model with no, weak and strong effect of predator foraging trait and 0.98 in the original niche model. However, as already clear by the inspection of Figure 3, the amount of variance of prey body masses explained by predator body mass varied considerably: 82.7%, 58.8%, and 26.5% in the two traits allometric model with no, weak and strong effect of predator foraging trait and 35.1% in the original niche model.

Total body mass range of the food webs ($\frac{w_{max}}{w_{min}}$) affected the estimated intercept of the prey-predator body mass allometry in the original niche model (Figure 4 D). There was a sharp decrease in the intercept with increasing size range of the food webs; the same holds for the two traits allometric model with strong effect of the foraging trait (Figure 4 C). On the other hand, the intercept was almost independent of the total mass range of the food webs generated by the two traits allometric model with no or weak effect of the foraging trait (Figure 4 A and B). The slope of the prey-predator body mass allometry and the amount of explained variance were not or only weakly dependent on the total size range of the food webs (Figure 4).

Mean PPMR and the range of PPMR values increased considerably when the total body mass range was increased from 10^5 to 10^{20} in the original niche model and the two traits allometric model with strong effect of the foraging trait (Figure 5 C and D). On the other hand, mean PPMR was independent of the total mass range and the range of PPMR values changed less in the two traits allometric model with no or weak effect of the foraging trait (Figure 5 A and B).

Summary statistics of food web structure

Most summary statistics of food web structure varied systematically from the two traits allometric model with no effect of the foraging trait to the model with strong effect of the foraging trait (Figure 6). However, the distributions of all summary statistics overlapped (99% intervals overlapped in all metrics; in most cases the overlap was much larger), so the difference between model settings was not significant. The largest difference between the model with no and strong effect of the foraging trait was found in the case of maximum similarity (Figure 6 H), which reflects the fact that similarly sized predators have very similar diets when predator-prey links are driven only by body mass. The comparison of the two traits allometric model with strong effect of the foraging trait and the original niche model revealed no significant differences (Figure 6). However, it is noteworthy that the original niche model tends to produce slightly less basal, herbivorous and top species (median number of top species is zero) and more intermediate species (Figure 6 A, B, C and I). This pattern is connected to slightly higher level of omnivory in the original niche model food webs (Figure 6 J).

Summary statistics of food web structure varied with the total body mass range in the case of the two traits allometric model with no or weak effect of the foraging trait, while they were independent of the total body mass range in the original niche model and in the two traits allometric model with strong effect of the foraging trait (Figure 7). The observed sensitivity of the food web metrics to changes in the total body mass range results from the fact that prey mass depends allometrically on predator mass with a slope <1.0 in the case of the two traits allometric model with no or weak effect of the foraging trait. As the total body mass

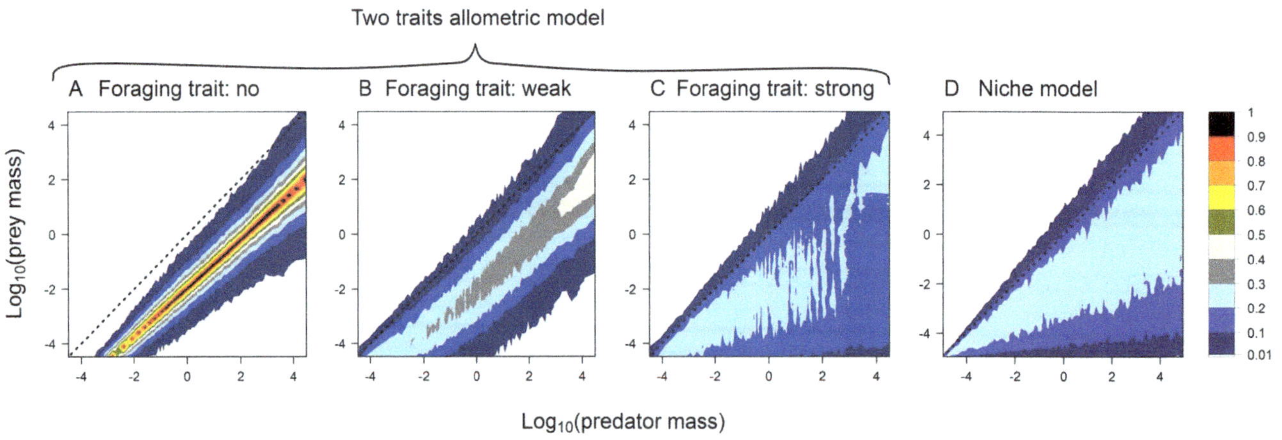

Figure 3. The two traits allometric model produces food webs with varying size structure. Results of 1000 simulations of food web matrices with $S=100$ species and $C=0.1$ using the same models as in Figure 2. The dotted diagonal line denotes situations when prey is of the same size as its predator; values above this line mean that predator is smaller than its prey. The colours show the probability of occurrence of feeding interactions between predator and prey of a given size in the simulated food webs (see the legend). The difference of values in (C) and (D) is small; for 82% of corresponding predator-prey pairs the difference in link probability is less than 0.05.

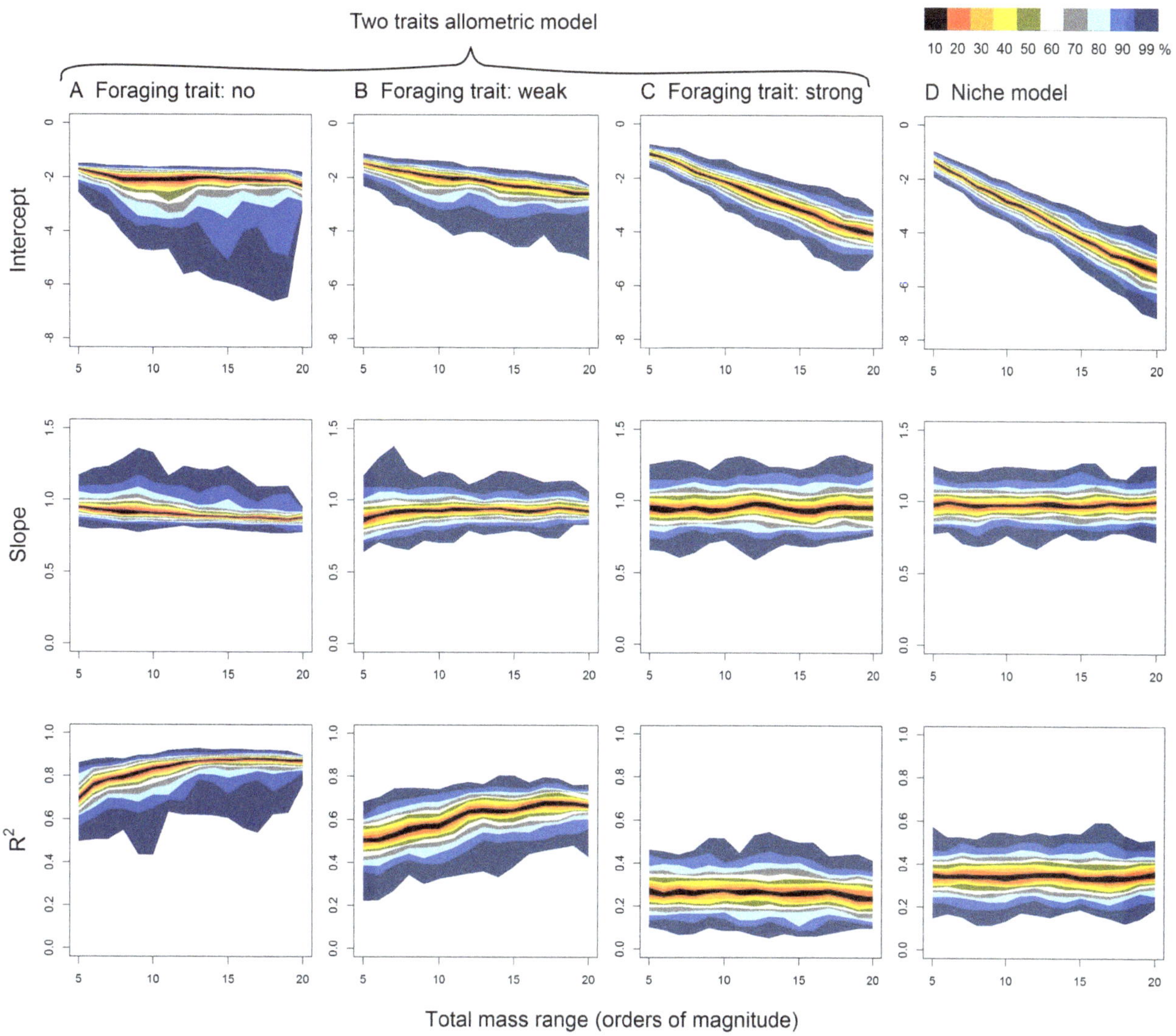

Figure 4. The dependence of the parameters of prey-predator body mass allometry on the total mass range of the food webs. The intercept, slope and explained variance of the dependence of $\log_{10}$ (prey mass) on $\log_{10}$ (predator mass) are plotted against the total mass range of the food webs. Parameters were estimated by standardized major axis regression. The same set of model food webs as in Figure 2 was used. Colours represent intervals with a given percentage of observations around the median (see the legend).

range increases, small predators become more similar in body mass to their prey and large predators become less similar to their prey (Figure 8). This alteration of the size structure of the food webs results in changes in summary statistics of food web structure (Figure 7).

Discussion

A plethora of different types of models seeking to explain food web structure has been developed in last several decades. Although truly mechanistic models attempting to predict food web structure based on optimal foraging have been developed recently [15,16], most of the models published so far are stochastic phenomenological models which generate more or less random food webs using a simple set of instructions. A prominent example is the niche model [17] which produces model food webs successfully mimicking real food webs according to comparisons of summary statistics, such as the proportion of top, intermediate and basal species to real data [17,29]. A pitfall of this approach is that a model may reproduce chosen metrics faithfully but still may fail to capture other untested aspects of food web structure; one of these is the relationship between predator and prey body mass. This paper aimed to evaluate the performance of the original niche model and its new empirically driven extensions in describing size structure of real food webs.

How well do the models capture real-world predator-prey body mass relationships?

The most apparent difference between real data and predator-prey mass ratios (PPMRs) in model generated food webs is that real food webs seem to contain a large proportion of predators feeding on prey larger than themselves (Figure 2). This could be partly an artifact caused by aggregating data on the species level instead of analysing them on the individual level, because many species, such as fish, grow in size over many orders of magnitude during ontogeny. When adults of a small species feed on juveniles

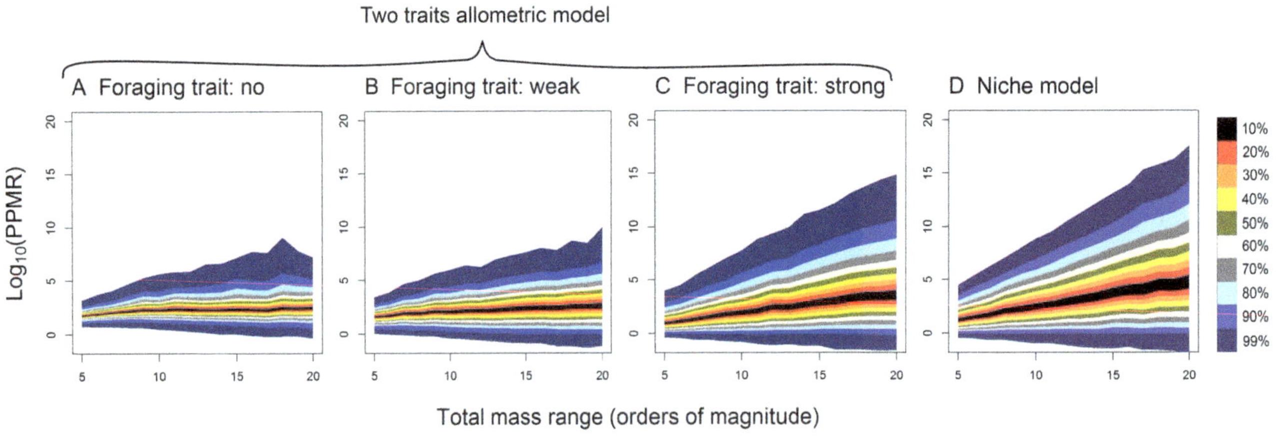

Figure 5. Predator-prey body mass ratios depend on the total mass range of the food webs. Plots show the values of predator-prey body mass ratios plotted against the total mass range of the food webs ($\frac{W_{max}}{W_{min}} = [10^5, 10^{20}]$). The total mass range was manipulated by changing the value of σ of the log-normal distribution of body masses in the case of the two traits allometric model and by changing the values of the parameter x in the case of the niche model (see methods for details). Colours represent intervals with a given percentage of observations around the median (see the legend).

of larger species, but the food web is analysed using species average or asymptotic body masses, we may draw a link where a predator is smaller than its prey. However, at the individual level, the predator may actually be larger than its prey [40,41]. Moving towards individual-based approaches in food webs is highly desirable for gaining novel insights [42], but most currently available data and current food web models use the species level.

The original niche model does not capture the relationship between predator and prey masses faithfully compared to empirical data. When the total mass range is set to 10 orders of magnitude, mean PPMR and the slope of the prey-predator mass allometry estimated by SMA regression correspond well to real data (Figure 2, [8–11]), although there is a lot of variation among individual simulations. However, the variance of prey body mass explained by predator body mass was only ca. 35% in the original niche model, compared to 86% in the analysis of empirical data by Brose et al. [8], which means that real food webs have much tighter prey-predator body mass allometry. Moreover, the intercept of the allometry and the range of PPMR values strongly depended on total range of body masses in the food web. This result stems from the fact that the niche model imposes only very weak constraints on predation – a predator can feed on any prey which is smaller than the predator and also on many larger prey species. Hence, maximum predator-prey mass ratio increases linearly with increasing total range of body masses in the food web (Figure 4). Cases when a large predator feeds on very small prey, such as whales feeding on krill are recognized as exceptions from general size-dependence of predatory interactions [8–12]. High sensitivity of the niche model predictions of the prey-predator body mass allometry to changes in the total mass range (Figure 5) limits the utility of the niche model to study the effect of predator and prey masses on food web stability [13,14].

The two traits allometric model generates food webs that capture predator-prey body mass relationships in real food webs well. When the effect of predator foraging trait is absent and predation is governed exclusively by prey-predator body mass allometry, predator mass explains on average 82% of prey mass variance, which corresponds to empirical data analyses by Brose et al. [8] ($R^2 = 86\%$). The proportion of variance in prey mass explained by predator mass decreases as the effect of the predator foraging trait increases. Importantly, the prey-predator mass allometry and mean PPMR do not depend on the total mass range unlike in the original niche model. However, with increasing total mass range, the range of PPMR values increases (Figure 5) as a natural consequence of the fact that because connectance remains fixed in the simulations (i.e. the mean number of prey species consumed by a predator does not change with body mass range), predators feed on prey of body masses deviating more strongly from the optimal prey mass. However, this effect is much weaker than the increase of the range of PPMR values in the body mass based niche model (Figure 5). This effect would be moreover counteracted if total body mass range increases in food webs with increasing species richness and decreasing connectance, which has been empirically observed [43–45]. By changing the value of the standard deviation of the truncated normal distribution used to assign the values of the foraging trait k_j, the model can cover the whole spectrum of food web size structure from that typical for the original niche model (σ very large) to that observed when the effect of foraging trait is absent and interactions are driven exclusively by body mass (σ close to 0). The role of body mass also varies among real food webs from different habitats and with different types of consumers [8,9,11,12,23]. In some food webs, the role of other traits may be even more important that the role of body mass [12]. The two traits allometric model captures a large part of this natural spectrum of food web structures depending on its parameter values.

Are there differences in food web structure among the models?

The comparison of twelve standard descriptors of food web structure (Figure 6) shows that although the three models differ in the size structure, most summary statistics of food web structure have similar values. These results suggest that many of these metrics are not tightly coupled with the size structure of food webs. This allows a model that makes not entirely realistic assumptions about the role of body mass in structuring food webs (i.e. the body mass based niche model) to provide very good fit to empirical food webs when the fit is judged by comparing values of summary statistics of food web structure [17,29]. There are other means of comparing food web models to empirical data, such as comparing the proportion of correctly predicted links or calculating model

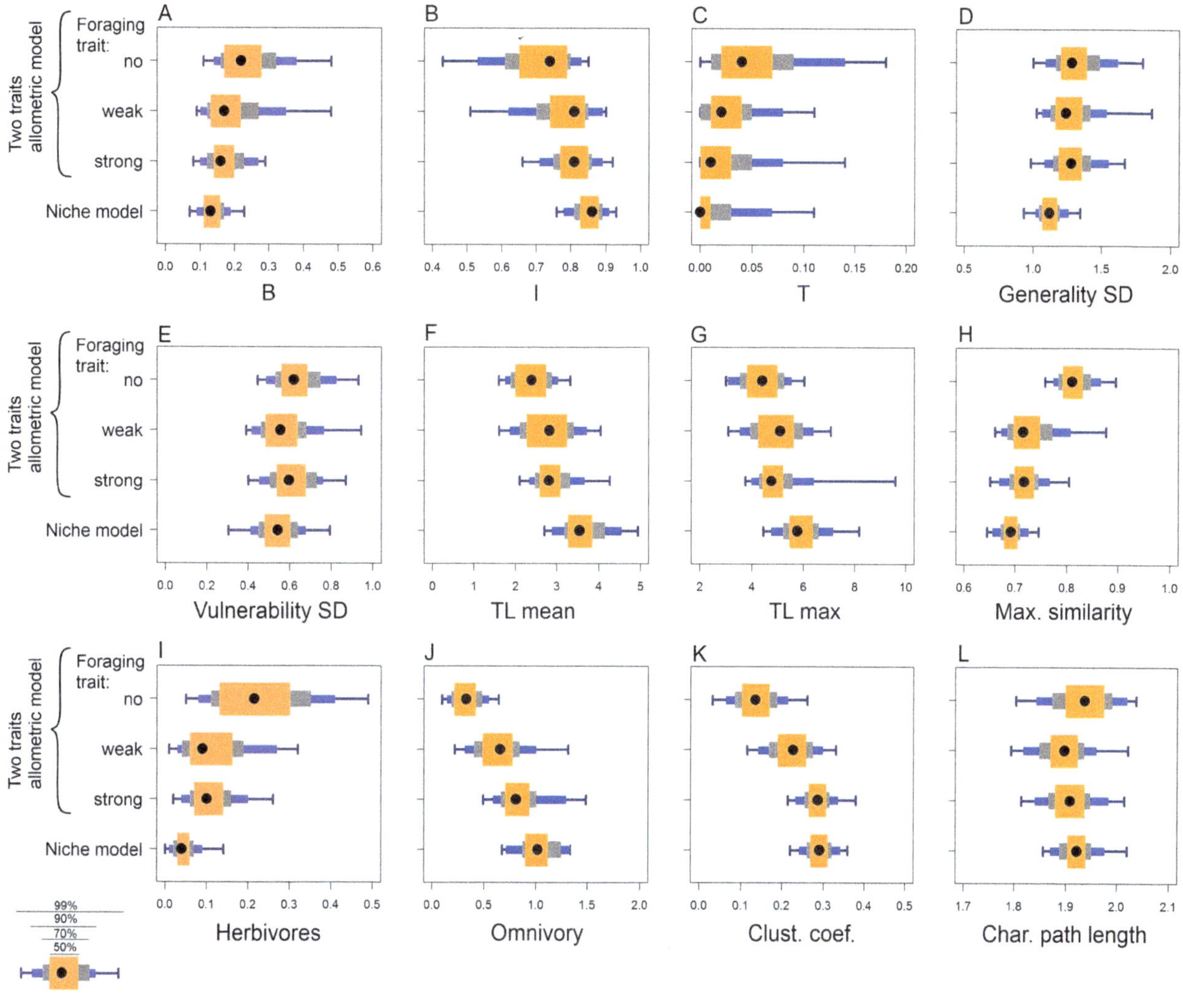

Figure 6. Comparison of metrics of food web structure among different models. Box-plots show the values of twelve metrics of food web structure calculated for a set of 200 food webs generated by each of the three settings of the two traits allometric model and the niche model with $S=100$ species and $C=0.1$. The same set of model food webs as in Figure 2 was used. The metrics shown are: proportion of basal (A), intermediate (B) and top (C) species, standard deviation of generality (D) and vulnerability (E), mean (F) and maximum (G) trophic level, maximum diet similarity (H), proportion of herbivores - i.e. consumers of basal species (I), mean omnivory level (J), clustering coefficient (K) and mean characteristic path length (L). Box-plot shows estimated intervals around the median (black circle) where a given percentage of observations lies: see the legend in the lower left corner.

likelihood [16,19,38,46]. However, fitting models to real data on food webs remains a tricky task [38] which may suffer from limitations beyond the choice of the appropriate metrics. Sampling effects may bias empirical descriptions of food web structure [47,48], which is certainly true also in the case of size structure because many common sampling methods are size selective and provide a distorted view of community composition in aquatic (e.g. [49–52]) as well as terrestrial (e.g. [53–55]) habitats. Moreover, I argue that stochastic structural food web models are better suited for studies simulating food web dynamics than for fitting to real data because they only describe food web structure without providing mechanistic explanations [38]. For the purpose of simulation studies, it is important that manipulating the size structure of food webs using the two traits allometric model has only minor consequences for other structural properties of food webs.

The original niche model [17] produces webs that are interval and species with similar niche value share predators but can still feed on different prey. Diet contiguity is retained in the two traits allometric model for the sake of simplicity because real food webs usually have high degree of intervality [18,21,22]. The two traits model allows species with similar body masses to feed on different prey because the second trait affects prey size preference of the predators. The inclusion of such a predator trait was motivated and is supported by empirical studies showing that foraging mode affects prey size selectivity of some predators. For example, filter-feeding zoopklanton prefers smaller prey than equally sized raptorial zooplankton [26] and suctorial predatory aquatic insects feed on larger prey than chewing predators of equal mass [27].

Using these models to understand real food webs

The two traits allometric model could be used to fit empirical data by specifying masses of individual species based on measurements and by choosing the parameters of the allometry of optimal prey mass and predator mass corresponding to a real

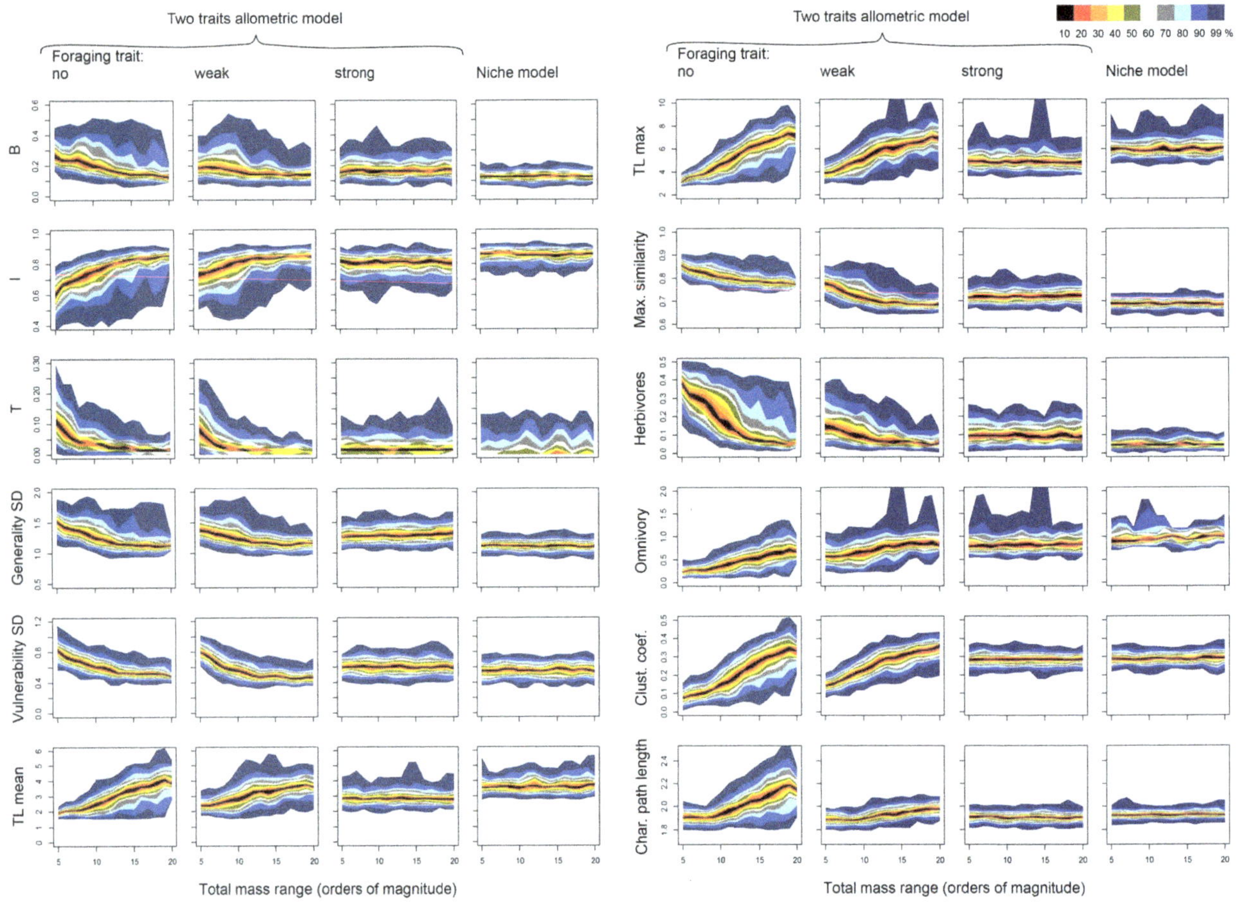

Figure 7. The dependence of metrics of food web structure on total body mass range in the food webs. The values of the same 12 metrics as in Figure 6 are plotted against the total body mass range in the food web (orders of magnitude) for individual models. Colours represent intervals with a given percentage of observations around the median (see the legend in the upper right corner).

food web in question or by optimizing parameter values to obtain the best possible fit. Stochastic food web models have been fitted to empirical data in this fashion [19,20,23,46], but the value of such comparisons is limited because the models are purely phenomenological and do not provide mechanistic insights [38]. It has been shown that any model obeying a few simple constraints will fit real food web data similarly well [56]. However, fitting models such as the body mass based niche model and the two traits allometric model can help to identify predators that deviate from predator-prey allometry obeyed by the rest of the species in the food web,

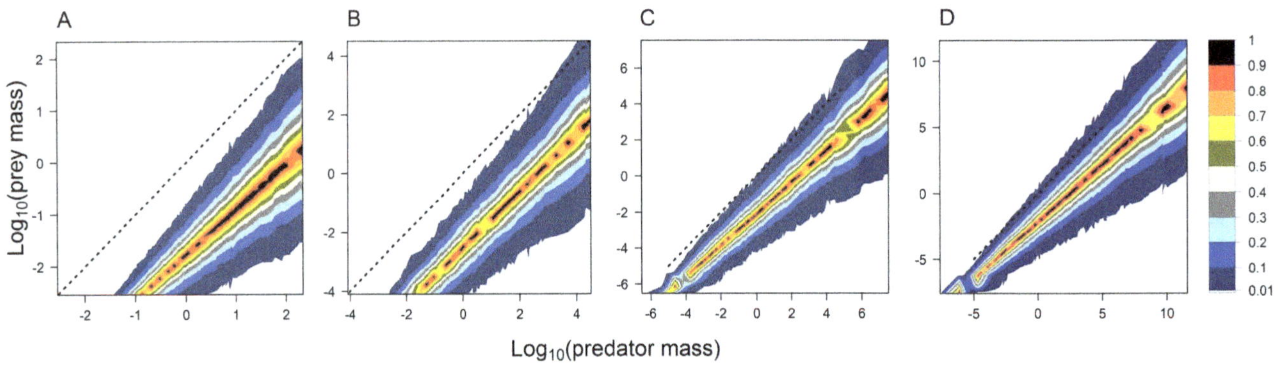

Figure 8. The dependence of size structure of the two traits allometric model with zero effect of the foraging trait on total body mass range in the food web. Results of 1000 simulations of food web matrices with $S=100$ species and $C=0.1$ for four different values of the total body mass range: 10^5 (A), 10^{10} (B), 10^{15} (C), and 10^{20} (D). The dotted line denotes situations when prey is of the same size as its predator; values above this line mean that predator is smaller than its prey. The colours show the probability of occurrence of feeding interactions between predator and prey of a given size in the simulated food webs (see the legend).

have unusual diet breadth, etc. [20,23]. Such explorations might pinpoint species worth studying in more detail to explain why are they different. This may be a fruitful way of connecting phenomenological food web models with real-world data to gain novel biological insights.

The explicit inclusion of species body mass to the niche model [20,23] and the possibility to manipulate size structure of food webs by directly including prey-predator mass allometry and other modifying traits into the model, as demonstrated in this paper, makes these models an increasingly flexible tool. The importance of body mass for structuring real food webs varies [8–12], so understanding the dynamical consequences of size structure is a key question of food web research [13,14]. The two traits model allows us to generate artificial food webs varying in size structure, which can be used in simulation studies of food web stability. Hence, this and similar models hold a significant promise for addressing the role of size structure of food webs for their dynamics and stability in a more detailed and direct way then was possible in previous studies.

I did not include prey traits other than body mass in the modifications of the niche model discussed in this paper for the sake of simplicity. However, recent results suggest that closely related prey are consumed by similar sets of predators but closely related predators have less similar diets; this asymmetry of the role of species similarity may be a consequence of differences in the roles of predator and prey traits [12]. New approaches in food web modelling based on multiple species traits [25,28,57] clearly hold a significant promise in moving towards more realistic descriptions of food web structure as they enable us to predict interaction strength based on biological traits of interacting species [27]. Different types of food web models can complement one another to address a broad range of questions using appropriate tools; such as trait-based models to predict individual feeding links and interaction strengths and stochastic structural models to study the links between structure and dynamics by simulation studies.

Supporting Information

Script S1 R script containing the code for the models used in the paper. The script contains a function niche.model which generates a food web using the original niche model and calculates species body masses from the niche values, a function niche.replicated which produces a list of n webs based on the original niche model, a function two.traits.model which generates a food web using the two traits allometric model and a function two.traits.replicated which produces a list of n webs based on the two traits allometric model.

Acknowledgments

I would like to thank Andrew P. Beckerman, Ludek Berec and David S. Boukal for stimulating discussions about food webs. Computation of summary statistics of food web structure was carried out partly using Owen L. Petchey's code freely available on his website (http://www.thetrophiclink.org/resources/food-web/).

Author Contributions

Conceived and designed the experiments: JK. Performed the experiments: JK. Analyzed the data: JK. Contributed reagents/materials/analysis tools: JK. Wrote the paper: JK.

References

1. Elton CS (1927) Animal Ecology. New York, 397 USA: Macmillan Co.
2. de Ruiter PC, Neutel AM, Moore JC (1995) Energetics, patterns of interaction strengths, and stability in real ecosystems. Science 269: 1257–1260.
3. McCann K, Hastings A, Huxel GR (1998) Weak trophic interactions and the balance of nature. Nature 395: 794–798.
4. Neutel AM, Heesterbeek JAP, de Ruiter PC (2002) Stability in real food webs: weak links in long loops. Science 296: 1120–1123.
5. Warren PH, Lawton JH (1987) Invertebrate predator-prey body size relationships: an explanation for upper triangular food webs and patterns in food web structure? Oecologia 74: 231–235.
6. Cohen JE, Pimm SL, Yodzis P, Saldana J (1993) Body sizes of animal predators and animal prey in food webs. Journal of Animal Ecology 62: 67–78.
7. Woodward G, Ebenman B, Emmerson M, Montoya JM, Olesen JM, et al. (2005) Body size in ecological networks. Trends in Ecology and Evolution 20: 402–409.
8. Brose U, Jonsson T, Berlow EL, Warren P, Banasek-Richter C, et al. (2006) Consumer-resource body-size relationships in natural food webs. Ecology 87: 2411–2417.
9. Bersier LF, Kehrli P (2008) The signature of phylogenetic constraints on food-web structure. Ecological Complexity 5: 132–139.
10. Naisbit RE, Kehrli P, Rohr RP, Bersier LF (2011) Phylogenetic signal in predator-prey body-size relationships. Ecology 92: 2183–2189.
11. Riede JO, Brose U, Ebenman B, Jacob U, Thompson R, et al. (2011) Stepping in Elton's footprints: A general scaling model for body masses and trophic levels across ecosystems. Ecology Letters 14: 169–178.
12. Naisbit RE, Rohr RP, Rossberg AG, Kehrli P, Bersier LF (2012) Phylogeny versus body size as determinants of food web structure. Proceedings of the Royal Society B: Biological Sciences 279: 3291–3297.
13. Brose U, Williams RJ, Martinez ND (2006) Allometric scaling enhances stability in complex food webs. Ecology Letters 9: 1228–1236.
14. Heckmann L, Drossel B, Brose U, Guill C (2012) Interactive effects of body-size structure and adaptive foraging on food-web stability. Ecology Letters 15: 243–250.
15. Beckerman AP, Petchey OL, Warren PH (2006) Foraging biology predicts food web complexity. Proceedings of the National Academy of Sciences 103: 13745–13749.
16. Petchey OL, Beckerman AP, Riede JO, Warren PH (2008) Size, foraging, and food web structure. Proceedings of the National Academy of Sciences 105: 4191–4196.
17. Williams RJ, Martinez ND (2000) Simple rules yield complex food webs. Nature 404: 180–183.
18. Stouffer DB, Camacho J, Amaral LAN (2006) A robust measure of food web intervality. Proceedings of the National Academy of Sciences 103: 19015–19020.
19. Allesina S, Alonso D, Pascual M (2008) A general model for food web structure. Science 320: 658–661.
20. Williams RJ, Anandanadesan A, Purves D (2010) The probabilistic niche model reveals the niche structure and role of body size in a complex food web. PLoS ONE 5: e12092.
21. Stouffer DB, Rezende EL, Amaral LAN (2011) The role of body mass in diet contiguity and food-web structure. Journal of Animal Ecology 80: 632–639.
22. Zook AE, Eklof A, Jacob U, Allesina S (2011) Food webs: Ordering species according to body size yields high degree of intervality. Journal of Theoretical Biology 271: 106–113.
23. Williams RJ, Purves DW (2011) The probabilistic niche model reveals substantial variation in the niche structure of empirical food webs. Ecology 92: 1849–1857.
24. Stouffer DB, Camacho J, Jiang W, Amaral LAN (2007) Evidence for the existence of a robust pattern of prey selection in food webs. Proceedings of the Royal Society B: Biological Sciences 274: 1931–1940.
25. Rohr RP, Scherer H, Kehrli P, Mazza C, Bersier LF (2010) Modeling food webs: exploring unexplained structure using latent traits. American Naturalist 176: 170–177.
26. Wirtz KW (2012) Who is eating whom? morphology and feeding type determine the size relation between planktonic predators and their ideal prey. Marine Ecology Progress Series 445: 1–12.
27. Klecka J, Boukal DS (2013) Foraging and vulnerability traits modify predator-prey body mass allometry: freshwater macroinvertebrates as a case study. Journal of Animal Ecology 82: 1031–1041.
28. Rossberg AG, Brännström Å, Dieckmann U (2010) How trophic interaction strength depends on traits. Theoretical Ecology 3: 13–24.
29. Williams RJ, Martinez ND (2008) Success and its limits among structural models of complex food webs. Journal of Animal Ecology 77: 512–519.
30. Kondoh M (2003) Foraging adaptation and the relationship between food-web complexity and stability. Science 299: 1388–1391.
31. Berec L, Eisner J, Křivan V (2010) Adaptive foraging does not always lead to more complex food webs. Journal of Theoretical Biology 266: 211–218.
32. Jordano P, Bascompte J, Olesen JM (2003) Invariant properties in coevolutionary networks of plant-animal interactions. Ecology Letters 6: 69–81.

33. Olesen JM, Bascompte J, Dupont YL, Elberling H, Rasmussen C, et al. (2011) Missing and forbidden links in mutualistic networks. Proceedings of the Royal Society B: Biological Sciences 278: 725–732.
34. Trautmann H, Steuer D, Mersmann O, Bornkamp B (2012) truncnorm: Truncated normal distribution.
35. R Core Team (2012) R: A Language and Environment for Statistical Computing. R Foundation for Statistical Computing, Vienna, Austria.
36. Warton DI, Wright IJ, Falster DS, Westoby M (2006) Bivariate line-fitting methods for allometry. Biological Reviews of the Cambridge Philosophical Society 81: 259–291.
37. Warton DI, Duursma RA, Falster DS, Taskinen S (2012) smatr 3 - an r package for estimation and inference about allometric lines. Methods in Ecology and Evolution 3: 257–259.
38. Petchey OL, Beckerman AP, Riede JO, Warren PH (2011) Fit, efficiency, and biology: Some thoughts on judging food web models. Journal of Theoretical Biology 279: 169–171.
39. Dunne JA, Williams RJ, Martinez ND (2002) Network structure and biodiversity loss in food webs: Robustness increases with connectance. Ecology Letters 5: 558–567.
40. Woodward G, Warren PH (2007) Body size and predatory interactions in freshwaters: Scaling from individuals to communities. Body Size: The Structure and Function of Aquatic Ecosystems: 98–117.
41. Woodward G, Blanchard J, Lauridsen RB, Edwards FK, Jones JI, et al. (2010) Individual-based food webs: Species identity, body size and sampling effects. Advances in Ecological Research 43: 211–266.
42. Melián CJ, Vilas C, Baldó F, González-Ortegón E, Drake P, et al. (2011) Eco-evolutionary dynamics of individual-based food webs. Advances in Ecological Research 45: 225–268.
43. Schmid-Araya JM, Schmid PE, Robertson A, Winterbottom J, Gjerløv C, et al. (2002) Connectance in stream food webs. Journal of Animal Ecology 71: 1056–1062.
44. Montoya JM, Solé RV (2003) Topological properties of food webs: from real data to community assembly models. Oikos 102: 614–622.
45. Riede JO, Rall BC, Banasek-Richter C, Navarrete SA, Wieters EA, et al. (2010) Scaling of food-web properties with diversity and complexity across ecosystems. Advances in Ecological Research 42: 139–170.
46. Allesina S (2011) Predicting trophic relations in ecological networks: a test of the allometric diet breadth model. Journal of Theoretical Biology 279: 161–168.
47. Goldwasser L, Roughgarden J (1993) Construction and analysis of a large caribbean food web. Ecology 74: 1216–1233.
48. Bersier LF, Dixon P, Sugihara G (1999) Scale-invariant or scale-dependent behavior of the link density property in food webs: A matter of sampling effort? American Naturalist 153: 676–682.
49. Klecka J, Boukal DS (2011) Lazy ecologist's guide to water beetle diversity: Which sampling methods are the best? Ecological Indicators 11: 500–508.
50. Hamley JM (1975) Review of gillnet selectivity. Journal of the Fisheries Board of Canada 32: 1943–1969.
51. Harley SJ, Myers RA (2001) Hierarchical bayesian models of length-specific catchability of research trawl surveys. Canadian Journal of Fisheries and Aquatic Sciences 58: 1569–1584.
52. Jennings S, Dulvy NK (2005) Reference points and reference directions for size-based indicators of community structure. ICES Journal of Marine Science: Journal du Conseil 62: 397–404.
53. Mommertz S, Schauer C, Kosters N, Lang A, Filser J (1996) A comparison of d-vac suction, fenced and unfenced pitfall trap sampling of epigeal arthropods in agro-ecosystems. Annales Zoologici Fennici 33: 117–124.
54. Lang A (2000) The pitfalls of pitfalls: a comparison of pitfall trap catches and absolute density estimates of epigeal invertebrate predators in arable land. Journal of Pest Science 73: 99–106.
55. Sanders D, Entling MH (2011) Large variation of suction sampling efficiency depending on arthro-pod groups, species traits, and habitat properties. Entomologia Experimentalis et Applicata 138: 234–243.
56. Stouffer DB, Camacho J, Guimera R, Ng CA, Amaral LAN (2005) Quantitative patterns in the structure of model and empirical food webs. Ecology 86: 1301–1311.
57. Rossberg AG, Matsuda H, Amemiya T, Itoh K (2006) Food webs: Experts consuming families of experts. Journal of Theoretical Biology 241: 552–563.

4

Modifications to the Aesop's Fable Paradigm Change New Caledonian Crow Performances

Corina J. Logan[1]*, Sarah A. Jelbert[2], Alexis J. Breen[3], Russell D. Gray[2], Alex H. Taylor[2]

1 SAGE Center for the Study of the Mind, Department of Psychological and Brain Sciences, University of California Santa Barbara, Santa Barbara, California, United States of America, **2** School of Psychology, University of Auckland, Auckland, New Zealand, **3** School of Psychology and Neuroscience, University of St Andrews, St Andrews, United Kingdom

Abstract

While humans are able to understand much about causality, it is unclear to what extent non-human animals can do the same. The Aesop's Fable paradigm requires an animal to drop stones into a water-filled tube to bring a floating food reward within reach. Rook, Eurasian jay, and New Caledonian crow performances are similar to those of children under seven years of age when solving this task. However, we know very little about the cognition underpinning these birds' performances. Here, we address several limitations of previous Aesop's Fable studies to gain insight into the causal cognition of New Caledonian crows. Our results provide the first evidence that any non-human animal can solve the U-tube task and can discriminate between water-filled tubes of different volumes. However, our results do not provide support for the hypothesis that these crows can infer the presence of a hidden causal mechanism. They also call into question previous object-discrimination performances. The methodologies outlined here should allow for more powerful comparisons between humans and other animal species and thus help us to determine which aspects of causal cognition are distinct to humans.

Editor: Thomas Boraud, Centre national de la recherche scientifique, France

Funding: CJL was supported by a SAGE Junior Research Fellowship at the SAGE Center for the Study of the Mind at the University of California Santa Barbara, and received a National Geographic Society/Waitt Grant (number 252-12) to conduct field work. RDG and AHT were supported by the Marsden Fund. The funders had no role in study design, data collection and analysis, decision to publish, or preparation of the manuscript. Publication costs were provided by the University of California Santa Barbara Open Access Pilot Fund Program.

Competing Interests: The authors have declared that no competing interests exist.

* Email: corina.logan@psych.ucsb.edu

Introduction

Humans have an excellent understanding of the relationships between cause and effect [1-3]. Currently, little is known about which aspects of this understanding are unique to our species or how such understanding evolves, despite a number of recent claims for human uniqueness [2,4]. One reason for the slow progress in this area is that, until recently, the predominant test of causal cognition was the trap-tube task, where food has to be moved out of a horizontal tube while avoiding a hole [5–11]. There are a number of issues with this paradigm [12–13], including the failure of critical controls by adult humans [14], the large effect that small modifications to the paradigm have on problem-solving capabilities [7], and the inability of large numbers of individuals from each species tested to learn any strategy to solve the task [5–6,11].

The Aesop's Fable paradigm has recently emerged as an alternative test of causal cognition [15]. This paradigm is useful because it requires a novel form of tool use (stone dropping into water-filled tubes), which is not seen in the wild and thus allows cross-species comparisons of causal cognition [16]. In this paradigm, subjects are presented with a water-filled tube that contains an out-of-reach floating food reward. To solve this problem, subjects must drop objects into the tube to raise the water level, thus bringing the food within reach. Rooks (*Corvus frugilegus*), Eurasian jays (*Garrulus glandarius*), New Caledonian crows (*Corvus moneduloides*) and children (*Homo sapiens*) can discriminate between functional and non-functional substrates (water vs. sand/sawdust/air) and objects (large vs. small, sinking vs. floating, hollow vs. solid) when presented with choices [13,15–18]. However, these species differ in their reactions to the U-tube task, a variant of the Aesop's Fable paradigm. This task examines how subjects respond to an unexpected effect after dropping a stone into a tube, namely that the stone causes water to rise in a seemingly unconnected adjacent tube.

Eurasian jays were the first species presented with the U-tube task, in an attempt to determine whether a confusing cause and effect relationship would inhibit their learning of a simple rule [18]. In the task, two large tubes were positioned adjacent to a small middle tube containing food. Since the small tube was too small to drop stones into, subjects had to drop stones into one of the large tubes. Only one of the large tubes was connected to the small tube under the table, thus making this tube the functional option, though because the base was covered, the causal mechanism was hidden. Each large tube was marked with a distinct color cue. To solve the task, subjects had to notice that dropping a stone into a tube marked with one color resulted in the rise of the floating food in the middle tube. None of the jays solved this task, indicating that a confusing causal relationship appears to inhibit the learning of a simple associative rule: 'drop the stone in the red tube'. All New Caledonian crows [13] and all 5-year-old children also fail this task, though all children 7 years and older solve it [16]. One explanation for the bird's failure is that the distance between the two large tubes was smaller than in the other tasks, which might have interfered with successful discrimination [19]. In other water tube discrimination experiments that involve two tubes, such as the sand vs. water experiment, the tubes are positioned 30 cm apart [13,15–18]. In the U-tube experiment, the two large tubes are only 15 cm apart [13,16,18]. It could be that this reduction in distance made it more difficult for the birds to inhibit switching between tubes and so prevented discrimination. A further issue with the current U-tube methodology is that, even if subjects succeed, such as children 7 to 10 years of age, there are two competing hypotheses for their performance. One possibility is that they have inferred the presence of a hidden causal mechanism, namely the connection between the two tubes. Another possibility is that the subjects are highly sensitive to perceptual feedback [16,18,20–21], and thus notice the effect stone dropping has on the adjacent small tube.

An additional limitation of previous studies concerns the ability of crows to make functional object discriminations. While current results suggest the crows make discriminations based on the causal properties of the objects involved, an alternate possibility is that they discriminate simply because they prefer to handle one object type over another. In particular, preferences could be driven by familiarity. For example, crows could prefer to handle solid rather than hollow objects simply because solid objects look more similar to the stones they have previously dropped in the tube and encountered in the wild. While simple preferences for approaching previously rewarded objects were controlled for in one study [17], no study has so far examined if subjects have a preference for handling certain objects.

Given the history of the trap-tube task, where small modifications to the procedure such as letting subjects pull rather than push the food leads to large behavioral differences [7], it is critical that the effect of modifications to the Aesop's Fable task be explored. Here, we use the Aesop's Fable paradigm to test causal cognition in New Caledonian crows. This species may have sophisticated causal cognition in the wild since it makes and uses tools to extract hidden food [22] and appears to make inferences about hidden causal agents [23]. We addressed the limitations of the U-tube and object preference tasks outlined above. First, we replicated the object and substrate experiments in Jelbert and colleagues [13] to ensure that our results were consistent with results from previous studies on New Caledonian crows. We also replicated Jelbert and colleagues' [13] volume discrimination experiment. However, instead of providing the crows with 12 objects, which allowed individuals to obtain food from either tube if they persisted long enough, we provided the crows with only enough objects (four) to correctly solve the task by choosing the more efficient tube. We then addressed the methodological limitation of the U-tube experiment by increasing the distance between large tubes, such that it was identical to the distance used in standard tube discrimination experiments. Additionally, we gave each wide tube its own narrow tube to make the distinction between the two sets of tubes clear. To investigate whether object preferences are actually related to the functionality of the task, we presented crows with hollow and solid objects of the same weight when the task required an object with a particular weight, rather than a particular displaceable volume. Finally, to test whether New Caledonian crows make inferences about a hidden causal mechanism, we designed a novel uncovered U-tube task to be given after subjects had attempted to solve the original U-tube task. We removed all arbitrary cues and exposed the hidden mechanism, the connecting pipe between two of the tubes. If subjects successfully solved the original covered U-tube task by inferring that the large and small tube were connected, we expected them to subsequently choose the visibly connected large tube rather than the unconnected one. However, if they had simply learned the association between the arbitrary color cue and the movement of the food, then their learning should be disrupted by the removal of this cue.

Methods

Ethics Statement

This research was carried out in accordance with the University of Auckland's Animal Ethics Committee (permit number R602). All aspects of the study protocols were approved as part of this permit.

Subjects

Eight wild-caught New Caledonian crows (2 adults, 6 juveniles; 3 females, 5 males) were studied from May to July 2013 in an aviary on Grand Terre, New Caledonia. Crows were housed in 2×3×3 m aviaries, had *ad libitum* access to water, and were fed dog food, papaya, eggs, and meat daily. Sex was estimated from body weight [24] and age was determined from mouth coloring. Birds were tested individually and in visual isolation of others. If a bird was not participating in a trial, bait was placed on the table to encourage participation. In experiments where two tubes were involved, the bait was located halfway between the tubes and birds were given up to 30 seconds to inspect the tubes before the objects were placed on the table. Birds had access to four stones, weighing 14–17 g and displacing 4–5 mm of water, in each experiment except sinking vs. floating, solid vs. hollow, and wide vs. narrow. The object discrimination and wide vs. narrow experiments followed the methodology of Jelbert and colleagues [13]. Twenty trials were conducted for each experiment. Experiments 1 through 7 were carried out in sequential order on all of the birds, with some of the birds experiencing experiment 8 before experiment 1 as noted in the section for experiment 8.

Stone Dropping

Before participating in this experiment, birds were trained to drop stones onto a platform, which collapsed to release a food reward. The apparatus was a clear cast acrylic box (180×110×85 mm) with a 90 mm tube (outer diameter = 51 mm, inner diameter = 40 mm) on top and a platform inside held up by a magnet. When a stone was dropped through the tube and onto the platform, the platform collapsed and the meat sitting on top of the platform fell out (Figure 1). Four stones were provided for this task. Once birds began stone dropping, they were given a further 24 trials on this task before proceeding to multi-stone training.

Multi-stone Training

After having successfully conducted the single stone dropping trials, each bird carried out 10 multi-stone dropping trials where they had to drop several stones in each trial onto a platform to receive the food. The apparatus consisted of a platform balanced on a stick inside a clear cast acrylic box (200×180×150 mm) with a 50 mm tube (outer diameter = 50 mm, inner diameter = 44 mm) on top of the box (Figure 2). The platform tipped and the food fell out when 2–4 stones were dropped down the tube because there were counterweights on the opposite side of the platform. This apparatus trained the crows to drop multiple stones to gain meat. Seven birds passed the multi-stone training and one (Kitty) skipped this training due to experimenter error and went straight to water vs. sand. Six birds completed 10 trials proficiently and one bird (Buster) required 32 trials to become proficient at this task.

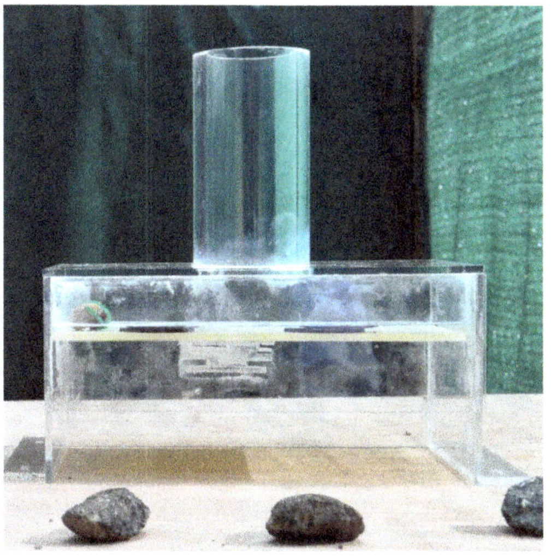

Figure 1. Single stone dropping apparatus.

Reachable Distance

The reachable distance is defined as the water level at which the bird can reach the floating food (meat cube attached to cork) with its bill and was measured from the base of the cast acrylic tube to the top of the floating food inside the tube. We determined the reachable distance by presenting the bird with a tube filled with usually 120 mm of water. If the bird could reach the food, the water level was lowered until their reachable distance was known. During the experiment, 12 mm was subtracted from their reachable distance such that the food would be out of reach enough to require dropping 2–4 stones to bring the food within reach. Reachable distances were calculated for each bird for the standard tube and small tube (in the U-tube experiments), and the average reachable distance (128 mm) as found by Jelbert and colleagues [13] was used for the wide and narrow tubes.

Experiment 1: Water vs. Sand

Each tube was clear cast acrylic with an outer diameter of 51 mm, inner diameter of 40 mm, and height of 170 mm, and was glued to a 300×300×12 mm clear cast acrylic base. Birds were given 10 habituation trials for the sand (non-functional) and water (functional) tubes by presenting the tubes in a pseudorandomized order (alternating sides for the first two trials, presenting the same tube on the same side up to two times consecutively). The tube openings were taped shut and meat cubes were placed on top and at the base of each tube. The first tube from which a bird ate food was noted to evaluate whether the bird showed a preference. If an obvious preference developed as habituation trials progressed, more meat was placed on the least preferred tube to reduce the preference, to ensure the bird attended to the functional properties of the task when the experiment began. If a bird did not confidently approach the tubes within 10 trials, the taped tubes were placed in their home aviary, meat was periodically placed on the tubes until the bird habituated, and then another 10 habituation trials ensued. After habituation, the experiment began and the sand and water tubes were pseudorandomized for side. Four stones were placed between the tubes with two sitting on the left tube's base and two sitting on the right tube's base (Figures 3 and 4).

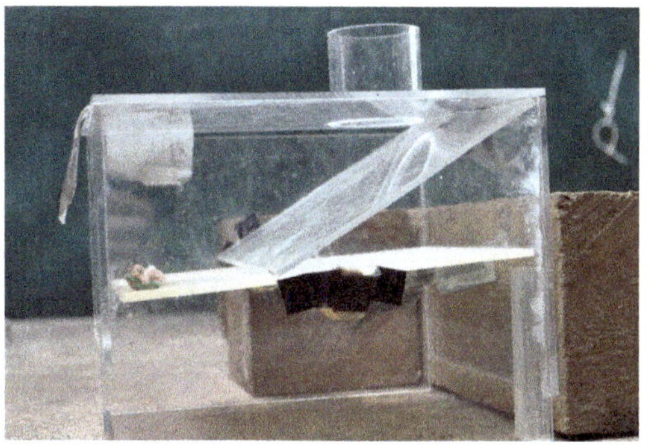

Figure 2. Multi-stone dropping apparatus.

Experiment 2: Sinking vs. Floating

The functional sinking objects were erasers (9 g, 20×20×10 mm) that displaced 3.5 mm of water in the standard tube and the non-functional floating objects were polystyrene blocks (0 g, 20×20×10 mm) that displaced 0.3 mm of water. Birds were habituated to the objects by giving them three trials where one sinking and one floating object were placed on the table and meat was put on top and below the objects so the bird had to interact with them to get the food. The first object touched during a habituation trial was noted to document preferences. In the experiment, we gave birds four erasers and four polystyrene objects placed in pseudorandomized pairs in front of the tube (Figure 5).

Experiment 3: Solid vs. Hollow

The more functional solid objects were metal cubes that were empty inside (9 g, 20×20×20 mm) and displaced 6 mm of water and the less functional hollow objects were metal cube frames that lacked sides (9 g, 20×20×20 mm) and displaced 1 mm of water. Birds were habituated to the objects using the same method as in the sinking vs. floating experiment. We gave birds four solid and four hollow objects arranged as in the sinking vs. floating experiment.

Experiment 4: Wide vs. Narrow Equal Water Levels

In this experiment, the narrow tube was the functional tube because the water levels in both tubes were set to the narrow tube's reachable distance. Since the wide tube required more objects to make the water rise the same distance, the food would not come within reaching distance even if all four objects were dropped in. The narrow (24×24×174 mm, volume = 100,224 mm^3) and wide

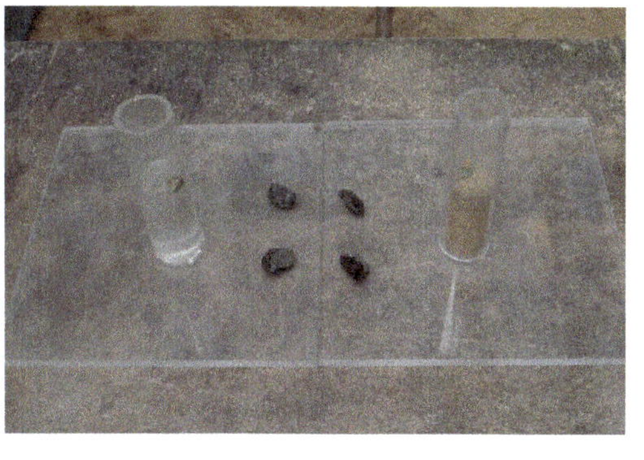

Figure 3. Water vs. sand experimental set up.

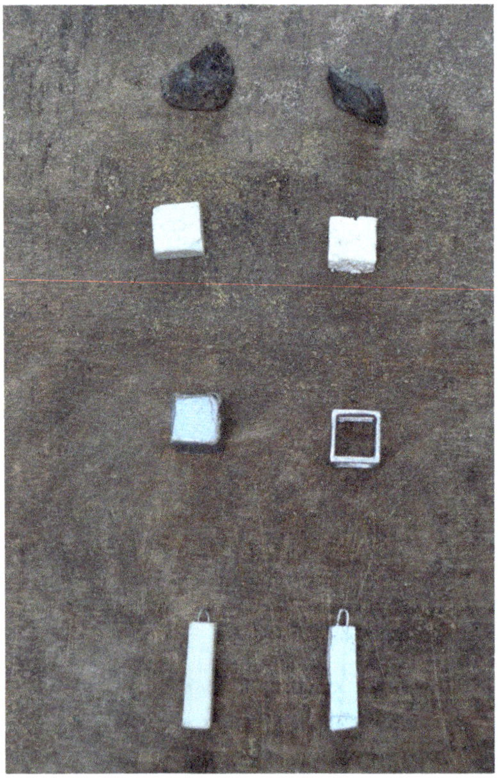

Figure 4. Objects used: top pair = stones, second pair = eraser/polystyrene for sinking vs. floating, third pair = solid/hollow, bottom pair = eraser/fimo clay for wide vs. narrow.

(44×44×174 mm, volume = 336,864 mm^3) tubes were made out of clear cast acrylic sheets and glued to 300×300 mm bases (Figure 6). Both tubes had clear cast acrylic lids with holes of the same diameter (25 mm) to equalize how far the bill could reach through the hole into the tube. The relative differences in volume between the standard cylindrical water tube (213,628 mm^3) and the wide and narrow tubes were roughly equivalent (wide tube = 123,236 mm^3 larger than standard tube and narrow tube = 113,404 mm^3 smaller than standard tube). Birds had access to four objects of the same type (8–10 g erasers that displaced 9 mm in narrow or 1 mm in wide tube, or 5–7 g fimo clay cuboids that displaced 9 mm in narrow or 3 mm in wide tube; both objects were 40×10×10 mm) with metal handles on one end. We

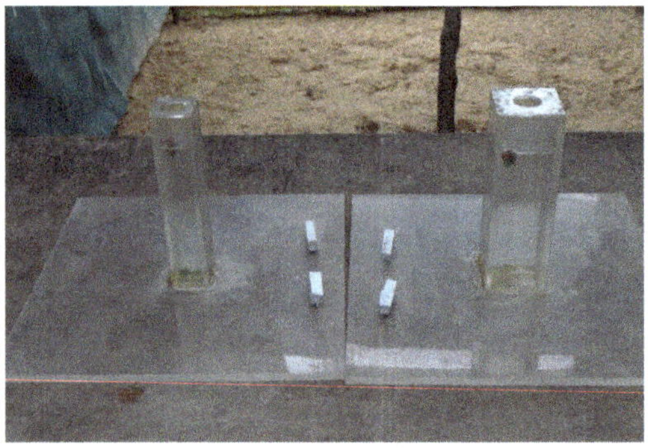

Figure 6. Narrow and wide tubes with equal water levels.

switched from erasers to clay objects because Damien began eating the erasers. Therefore, Q, 007, Kitty, and Lady had erasers for objects, while Damien and Buster had clay objects. Objects were placed between the tubes as in the sand vs. water experiment.

Experiment 5: Wide vs. Narrow Unequal Water Levels

The water level in the narrow tube was completely unreachable at 50 mm, regardless of how many objects were dropped in, while the water level in the wide tube was set to a distance such that dropping the objects in would raise the food within reach (Figure 7). Birds that passed the wide vs. narrow equal water level experiment were given this experiment to determine whether they were able to switch their preference when the opposite tube becomes more functional.

Experiment 6: Colored U-tube

This experiment consisted of two apparatuses, each containing a standard tube and a small tube (small tube: outer diameter = 25.4 mm, inner diameter = 19 mm) 25 mm apart, with 170 mm sticking out and 80 mm below a clear cast acrylic lid (300×400×12 mm) on a wooden box (Figure 8). The lid was covered with paper to prevent subjects from observing the tubes underneath. The small tubes contained food. Stones were too large to drop into the small tubes; they could only be dropped into the standard tubes. Under the lid, one apparatus had a tube (outer diameter = 25.4 mm, inner diameter = 19 mm) that connected the standard and small tubes such that when stones were dropped into the standard tube, the water in the small tube would also be displaced, raising the food reward. The other apparatus did not have a connector tube, thus it was non-functional. Each apparatus,

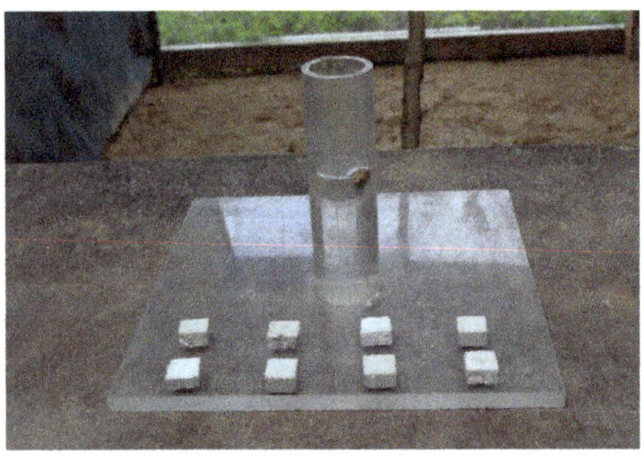

Figure 5. Sinking vs. floating experimental set up.

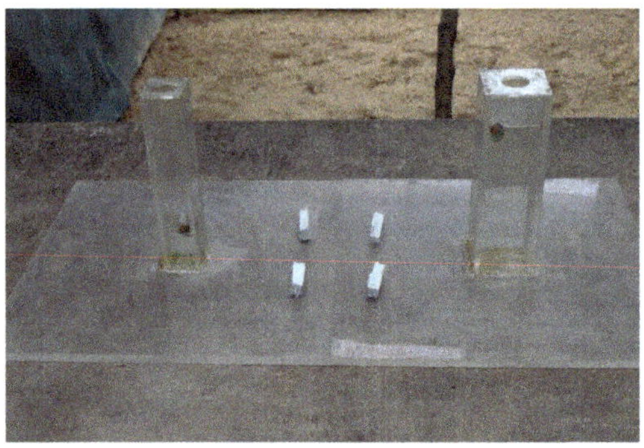

Figure 7. Narrow and wide tubes with unequal water levels.

the connected or non-connected, was marked with red or blue tape at the top and base (red triangle or blue square on the paper cover over the lid) of the standard tube to indicate which apparatus was connected. The apparatuses were oriented with the small tubes nearest each other, making the distance between them 300 mm, and the connected and non-connected apparatuses were pseudorandomized for which side they were placed on. Birds were habituated to the two apparatuses in the same way as in the sand vs. water experiment (all tubes were taped over the top and had equal water levels), and their reachable distances for the small tube were carried out with the standard tube water level matching that of the small tube. We gave birds access to four stones lined up between the apparatuses as in the sand vs. water experiment.

Experiment 7: Uncovered U-tube

This experiment was the same as the colored U-tube experiment, except that we removed the colored tape, the paper cover over the lid, and the front and back of the wooden box so the bird could see which apparatus was connected (Figure 9).

Experiment 8: Solid vs. Hollow on the Multi-stone Platform

This was the same as the solid vs. hollow experiment with the water tube, except that instead of a water tube, the multi-stone platform was used. Since both object types weighed the same, they were equally functional on the platform, whereas the solid was the functional object in the water tube since it displaces more water. Half of the birds were given this experiment before having experience with water tubes and half after the solid vs. hollow experiment with the water tube to determine whether they attended to the functional properties of the objects.

Side Bias

If, during the experiments involving two tubes, a bird showed a side bias, the trials were paused and 5–20 trials of color choice were given, after which the experiment was restarted. The color choice test draws their attention to color rather than space and can break their pattern of always choosing one side without attending to the details of the task. In the color choice test, birds were presented with two PVC tubes (diameter = 32.5 mm, length = 45 mm glued to two 45×45 mm pieces of plywood): one gold tube that always contained meat and one silver tube that never contained meat. The tubes were placed, left side first, in a pseudorandomized order on the table and oriented such that the bird could not see into the tube without approaching it. The first tube approached and looked into was considered the chosen tube and once the bird left that tube, the trial was stopped. All birds were trained on the color choice test to an accuracy of at least 17 successful trials out of 20 before beginning the water tube experiment.

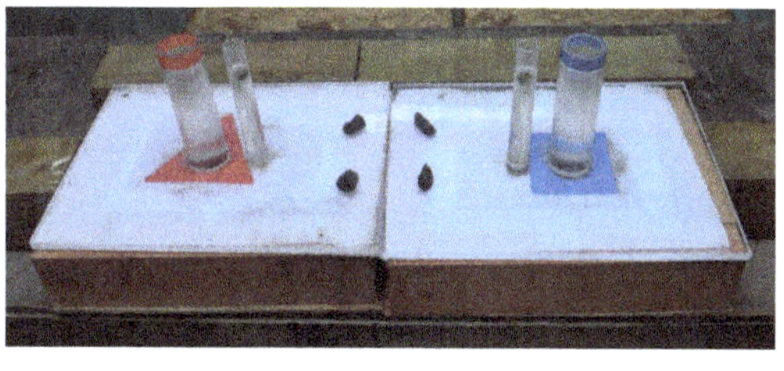

Figure 8. Colored U-tube experimental set up.

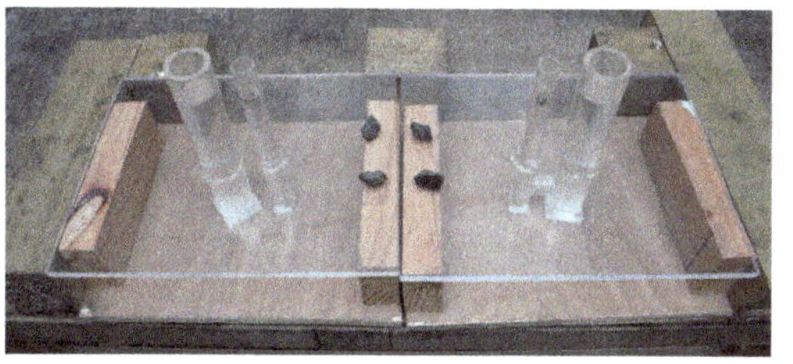

Figure 9. Uncovered U-tube experimental set up.

Analysis

The exact binomial test was applied to the first choice in first trials for all birds in experiments 1–3, 4–5, and 6–7, and to all correct choices for each bird in each experiment at the 20-trial level to determine whether there were significantly more successes than predicted by chance (probability of 0.5) using the statistical software R [25]. P-values within each hypothesis were adjusted to correct for type 1 errors from conducting multiple tests using the Holm-Bonferroni method (R package: stats, function: p.adjust, method: Holm). A Generalized Linear Mixed Model (GLMM) was used to determine whether performance, the percentage of correct choices per bird per trial (response variable), changed across the 20 trials (trials grouped to determine where learning occurred: 1–5, 6–10, 11–15, and 16–20) in any given experiment (explanatory variables; see Table S1.1 in File S1). The GLMM had a Poisson distribution and log link (R package: lme4 [26]), and bird was included as a random factor to account for repeated tests on each subject. The response variable was categorical, thus did not need to adhere to a normal distribution. The top model was selected by comparing all possible model combinations according to their Akaike weight (scale: 0–1, all models sum to 1) using the dredge function in the R package MuMIN [27]. The top model was only considered reliable if its Akaike weight was 0.90 or higher [28].

Results

See (Tables S2.1–2.8 in File S2) to see the order in which each choice was made for all trials in all experiments.

Experiment 1: Water vs. Sand

Three birds passed this experiment by dropping stones into the water-filled tube significantly more than the sand-filled tube (see Holm-Bonferroni corrected binomial test p-values per bird in Table 1). Q made only three errors, which occurred in his first six trials. Two birds failed and three did not complete it. Of those that did not complete it, two were removed from the experiment because they would not drop stones into water. Of all of the stones that were dropped by the five birds that participated in this experiment, 74% were dropped into the water-filled tube. No birds showed a preference for either tube during the habituation trials (Holm-Bonferroni corrected binomial test: $p = 1.00$ for every bird, $n = 8$ birds).

Experiment 2: Sinking vs. Floating

Six out of six birds passed this test by choosing the sinking objects significantly more (85% of the time across all birds) than the floating objects (Table 1). Damien and Buster made no mistakes and Lady made only four errors, which occurred in her first three trials. Across all birds, there were no preferences for

Table 1. Summary of which birds passed which 20-trial experiments according to the Holm-Bonferroni corrected binomial test (p values listed in each cell).

Bird (color bands)	Age	Water vs. Sand	Sink vs. Float	Solid vs. Hollow	Wide vs. Narrow Equal	Wide vs. Narrow Unequal	Colored U-tube	Uncovered U-tube
Q (YG)	Juvenile	<0.001	0.004	<0.001	0.02	0.02	0.74	0.2
007 (Y)	Juvenile	<0.001	0.004	<0.001	1.00	–	0.08	1.00
Trooper (BO)	Juvenile	X	–	–	–	–	–	–
Kitty (WR)	Juvenile	0.08	<0.001	<0.001	0.03	0.3	0.04	1.00
Candy (WO)	Juvenile	X	–	–	–	–	–	–
Lady (YR)	Adult	<0.001	<0.001	<0.001	0.02	<0.001	0.74	1.00
Buster (OO)	Adult	X	<0.001	<0.001	<0.001	<0.001	X	–
Damien (WLB)	Juvenile	1.00	<0.001	<0.001	1.00	–	0.15	1.00
		n = 5	n = 6	n = 6	n = 6	n = 4	n = 5	n = 5

X = did not complete this experiment, – = did not participate in this experiment.

either object during habituation trials (uncorrected binomial test: p = 0.81, n = 6 birds).

Experiment 3: Solid vs. Hollow

Six out of six birds passed by choosing the solid objects significantly more (95% of the time across all birds) than the hollow objects (Table 1). 007, Kitty, Lady, and Buster made no mistakes and Damien made only two errors, however no bird made an error until trial eight. Across all birds, there were no preferences for either object during habituation trials (uncorrected binomial test: p = 0.39, n = 7 birds).

Experiment 4: Wide vs. Narrow Equal Water Levels

Four birds passed this test by dropping objects into the narrow tube significantly more (64% of the time across all six birds) than in the wide tube, and two birds failed (Table 1, Video S1). There were no preferences for either tube during habituation trials (uncorrected binomial test: p = 1.00, n = 2 birds).

Experiment 5: Wide vs. Narrow Unequal Water Levels

Of the four birds that passed experiment 4, three of them also passed the unequal water level experiment by dropping significantly more objects into the wide tube (79% of the time across all birds), and one bird failed (Table 1). Buster was error-free and Lady made only four mistakes.

Experiment 6: Colored U-tube

One bird, Kitty, passed this test by dropping stones significantly more into the connected apparatus, while four birds failed and one stopped participating (the connected tube was chosen 47% of the time across all birds; Table 1, Video S2). No birds showed a preference for either the red or blue tube during the habituation trials (Holm-Bonferroni corrected binomial test: p = 1.00 for each bird, n = 6 birds).

Experiment 7: Uncovered U-tube

Five out of five birds failed this test by dropping stones randomly into either the connected or the non-connected apparatus (the connected tube was chosen 44% of the time across all birds; Table 1). Birds rarely bent over to inspect the part of the apparatus that was newly exposed, which included the connector tube.

Experiment 8: Solid vs. Hollow on the Multi-stone Platform

Three birds (Trooper, Lady, and Damien) experienced the platform experiment before the water tube experiment, two birds (007 and Kitty) experienced the platform experiment after the water tube experiment, and one (Buster) experienced only the platform experiment. All birds in both experiments dropped significantly more solid objects than hollow objects into water tubes and platforms regardless of their prior experience (20-trial Holm-Bonferroni corrected binomial test p-values for the platform experiment: Trooper<0.001, Lady<0.001, Damien<0.001, 007<0.001, Kitty<0.001; 95% of objects dropped across all birds were solid).

First choices in first trials

Birds chose the correct substrate (water) and object (sinking and solid) as their first choice in their first trial significantly more than expected by chance when combining data from experiments 1–3 (uncorrected binomial test: p = 0.002, 15 correct choices out of 17 total choices, n = 5 birds in experiment 1, n = 6 birds in experiments 2 and 3). Experiments 1–3 tested similar types of preferences and were combined to increase the sample size for the binomial test. Regarding volume discriminations, the correct volume was not chosen significantly more than chance when combining results from experiments 4 and 5 (uncorrected binomial test: $p = 1.00$, 5 correct choices out of 10 total choices, $n = 6$ birds in experiment 4, $n = 4$ birds in experiment 5). The correct tube in the U-tube experiments was not chosen significantly above chance when combining data from experiments 6 and 7 (uncorrected binomial test: $p = 1.00$, 5 correct choices out of 10 total choices, $n = 5$ birds in experiments 6 and 7).

Did performance increase with an increasing number of trials?

Performance was influenced by experiment and trial and by an interaction between experiment and trial as evidenced by the fact that the best model of all possible model combinations was the full model (performance ~ experiment * trial + (1|bird), Akaike weight = 1). Performance increased with an increasing number of trials in all experiments, except in solid vs. hollow, where the best performances were in the first five trials, and the uncovered U-tube where performance decreased as trials increased, potentially due to their lack of motivation to complete this difficult and unrewarding experiment (Table 2). Performance increased for trials 11–20 in water vs. sand, sinking vs. floating, and both wide vs. narrow experiments, indicating that birds learned about the task primarily during the first 10 trials. While learning occurred during the first five trials and trials 11–15 of the U-tube experiment, it was not sufficient for most birds to pass this test.

Discussion

As in past studies, New Caledonian crows preferred to drop stones into water-filled, rather than sand-filled tubes, and they preferred to drop objects that sank or were solid, rather than floating or hollow objects [13,17]. However, while past work suggested that New Caledonian crows cannot discriminate between water-filled tubes of different volumes [13], here three of the six birds tested not only preferred to drop stones into a narrow tube, but then switched their preference to a wide tube when the water level in this tube was significantly higher. This switch from the narrow to the wide tube shows that the success in the equal water level condition is not simply due to these three crows having a preference for narrow tubes. While previous work has suggested that New Caledonian crows [13], like Eurasian jays [18], and children under 7 years of age [16], cannot solve the U-tube task, here one crow, Kitty, was able to do so by learning the connection between the arbitrary color cue and the movement of the food. However, all crows, including Kitty, subsequently failed our novel U-tube task with the exposed connection, which suggests that Kitty's success on the colored U-tube was due to the color cue association and not to the inference of a hidden causal mechanism or attention to the movement of the food. Crows also showed a preference for solid, rather than hollow, objects of the same weight when presented with a task not involving water, which suggests that they may have a bias for solid objects independent of the task at hand.

In first trials, significantly more correct choices were made in the substrate and object discrimination experiments, but not in the narrow vs. wide equal water levels, colored U-tube, and uncovered U-tube experiments. The crows' lack of an initial preference for particular tubes or objects during habituation suggests that first trial performance was not based on a bias to approach specific objects. In the experiments where first choices on first trials were correct, aside from the solid vs hollow condition, crows showed a learning effect in the first 10 trials, with performance improving in trials 11-20. This suggests that, while they had high overall levels of success across 20 trials, the crows needed experience with the objects, substrates, and tubes to settle on the functional option. These results are consistent with previous water tube experiments where rooks, Eurasian jays, and other New Caledonian crows showed some learning effects across the first five trials [13,15,17–18].

While our results show that the crows did not have a bias to approach objects to gain food, they may have had a bias towards the type of objects they preferred to pick up, given that all three birds without water tube experience chose solid rather than hollow objects of the same weight when presented with a platform apparatus. This finding calls into question the previous object discrimination choices of children [16], jays [18], and New Caledonian crows [13,21]. The possibility that, irrespective of the task at hand, subjects have preferences for particular objects (*i.e.*, solid and sinking objects), particularly those that look more like objects they have previous experience with (*i.e.*, stones), has not been sufficiently well controlled for in past studies. Interestingly, it was only in the solid vs. hollow condition that no learning effect was shown, which suggests that the crows may have had a specific bias for solid objects, rather than a more general bias for the functional objects in our experiments. However, further work is required to test this hypothesis. It is also important to note that a handling preference has not yet been controlled for in children [16], and it may explain children's performances to date.

Our results differ from previous findings where no crows passed the wide vs. narrow equal water level experiment [13]. It appears that providing enough objects (four rather than twelve) for the bird to succeed only in the narrow tube, but not in both of the tubes, provided the motivation to choose the more efficient tube. That three birds then preferred a wide tube when the water level was unequal shows that these crows made discriminations based on water volume because they switched their preference from the narrow to the wide tube, indicating that they did not simply prefer to drop objects into the narrow tube. This finding raises two possibilities. The first is that crows are able to imagine changes in the magnitude of a causal relation. The crows only had prior experience dropping stones into a tube of one volume to raise its water level. They could have used their knowledge of the relationship between this tube size, the object, and the water level to mentally model the effect on the water level of dropping the same object into a bigger or smaller tube. This would have led them to choose the narrow tube. In contrast to this high level explanation, an alternate possibility is that the crows attended to differences in the feedback generated by dropping objects into the narrow tube (the floating reward moved significantly closer to the top of the tube) and the wide tube (minimal movement occurred). Further testing is required, using a tube where visual feedback is not available, to distinguish between these causal relation and feedback explanations

The performance of Kitty in solving our modified U-tube apparatus raises the possibility that past failures by corvids [13,18] may be due to problems with tube discrimination when the stone dropping tubes are close together. Kitty's successful solution of this problem suggests two hypotheses. Like 42% of children between ages 4 and 10 [16], Kitty may have inferred the presence of a hidden causal mechanism linking the two tubes of the U-tube task. Alternatively, consistent with the most likely explanation for children's success on this task, she may have paid more attention to feedback than the other crows: by carefully watching the effect of a stone drop into each tube she may have noticed which tube caused the water level in the small tube to rise. However, these

Table 2. The best fitting generalized linear mixed model (GLMM) examining the effect of experiment and trial on performance (percent correct choices per bird per trial) with bird as a random factor (variance and standard deviation for the random factor are reported in the estimate and SE columns respectively).

Factor	Trials	Estimate	SE
Intercept (U-tube)	1–5	3.90	0.04
U-tube	6–10	0.27	0.04
	11–15	0.06	0.04
	16–20	0.18	0.04
Water vs Sand	1–5	0.46	0.04
	6–10	−0.26	0.05
	11–15	−0.08	0.05
	16–20	−0.07	0.05
Sinking vs Floating	1–5	0.53	0.04
	6–10	−0.26	0.05
	11–15	0.06	0.05
	16–20	−0.04	0.05
Solid vs Hollow	1–5	0.71	0.03
	6–10	−0.30	0.05
	11–15	−0.11	0.05
	16–20	−0.22	0.05
Wide vs Narrow Equal	1–5	0.25	0.04
	6–10	−0.27	0.05
	11–15	0.19	0.05
	16–20	0.02	0.05
Wide vs Narrow Unequal	1–5	0.36	0.04
	6–10	−0.26	0.05
	11–15	0.14	0.05
	16–20	0.01	0.05
Uncovered U-tube	1–5	0.19	0.04
	6–10	−0.27	0.05
	11–15	−0.23	0.06
	16–20	−0.58	0.06
Random effect: Bird		0.005	0.07

SE = Standard Error.

hypotheses both predict that Kitty should have passed both U-tube experiments. Though Kitty chose the correct tube on the first trial of the uncovered U-tube experiment, she did not consistently choose the connected tube. Thus, rather than inferring the presence of a hidden causal mechanism or attending to feedback, Kitty may have instead associated the color cue with the eventual receipt of the food. Further testing is required, given that children have not yet been tested on the novel uncovered U-tube task used here. Past research has shown the pitfalls of assuming how humans will react when faced with causal problems [29].

Despite the last 20 years of work on what animals understand about their physical world, we still have a rudimentary understanding of the cognition behind how animals solve problems. One of the key issues in the past has been the lack of rigorous testing of the experimental methodologies themselves, particularly the relation between small changes in procedure and animals' performance, which has resulted in the formation of strong conclusions about issues, such as human uniqueness, before the hypotheses under examination have been thoroughly tested [2,6–7,10]. The results here highlight a number of methodological limitations in the Aesop's Fable paradigm. With appropriate modifications to this paradigm, it should be possible to overcome these issues in future studies and so produce useful results for comparative cognition research. Comparisons will be particularly interesting between corvids and apes as they will provide insights into how the very differently structured bird and mammalian brains understand the causality of the world.

Acknowledgments

We thank Joe Jablonski for machining the acrylic tubes, Gavin Hunt for field support, and three anonymous reviewers for helpful feedback on the manuscript.

Author Contributions

Conceived and designed the experiments: CJL SAJ RDG AHT. Performed the experiments: CJL AJB. Analyzed the data: CJL. Contributed reagents/materials/analysis tools: CJL SAJ RDG AHT. Wrote the paper: CJL AHT. Edited the manuscript: SAJ AJB RDG.

References

1. Gopnik A, Wellman HM (1994) The theory theory. In: Lawrence A, editor,. Mapping the mind: Domain specificity in cognition and culture. New York, NY US: Cambridge University Press. pp. 257–293.
2. Penn D, Povinelli D (2007) Causal cognition in human and nonhuman animals: A comparative, critical review. Annu Rev Psychol 58: 97–118.
3. Bonawitz EB, Ferranti D, Saxe R, Gopnik A, Meltzoff AN, et al. (2010) Just do it? Investigating the gap between prediction and action in toddlers' causal inferences. Cognition 115: 104–117.
4. Penn DC, Holyoak KJ, Povinelli DJ (2008) Darwin's mistake: Explaining the discontinuity between human and nonhuman minds. Behav Brain Sci 31: 109–129.
5. Visalberghi E, Limongelli L (1994) Lack of comprehension of cause effect relations in tool-using capuchin monkeys (*Cebus apella*). J Comp Psychol 108: 15–22.
6. Povinelli DJ, Reaux JE, Theall LA, Giambrone S, Humphrey N (2000) Folk physics for apes: The chimpanzee's theory of how the world works. Oxford: Oxford University Press.
7. Mulcahy NJ, Call J (2006) How great apes perform on a modified trap-tube task. Anim Cogn 9:193–199.
8. Seed AM, Tebbich S, Emery NJ, Clayton NS (2006) Investigating Physical Cognition in Rooks, *Corvus frugilegus*. Curr Biol 16: 697–701.
9. Martin-Ordas G, Call J, Colmenares F (2008) Tubes, tables and traps: great apes solve two functionally equivalent trap tasks but show no evidence of transfer across tasks. Anim Cogn 11: 423–430.
10. Seed AM, Call J, Emery NJ, Clayton NS (2009) Chimpanzees solve the trap problem when the confound of tool-use is removed. J Exp Psychol Anim B, 35: 23–34.
11. Taylor AH, Hunt GR, Medina FS, Gray RD (2009) Do New Caledonian crows solve physical problems through causal reasoning? P Roy Soc B-Biol Sci 276: 247–254.
12. Taylor AH, Clayton NS (2012) Evidence from convergent evolution and causal reasoning suggests that conclusions on human uniqueness may be premature. Behav Brain Sci 35: 241–242.
13. Jelbert SA, Taylor AH, Cheke LG, Clayton NS, Gray RD (2014) Using the Aesop's Fable paradigm to investigate causal understanding of water displacement by New Caledonian crows. PLOS ONE 9: e92895.
14. Silva FJ, Page DM, Silva KM (2005) Methodological-conceptual problems in the study of chimpanzees' folk physics: how studies with adult humans can help. Anim Learn Behav 33: 47–58.
15. Bird CD, Emery NJ (2009) Rooks use stones to raise the water level to reach a floating worm. Curr Biol 19: 1410–1414.
16. Cheke LG, Loissel E, Clayton NS (2012) How do children solve Aesop's fable? PLOS ONE 7: e40574.
17. Taylor AH, Elliffe DM, Hunt GR, Emery NJ, Clayton NS, et al. (2011) New Caledonian crows learn the functional properties of novel tool types. PLOS ONE 6: e26887.
18. Cheke LG, Bird CD, Clayton NS (2011) Tool-use and instrumental learning in the Eurasian jay (*Garrulus glandarius*). Anim Cogn 14: 441-455.
19. Mulcahy NJ, Call J (2009) The Performance of Bonobos (Pan paniscus), Chimpanzees (Pan troglodytes), and Orangutans (Pongo pygmaeus) in two versions of an object-choice task. J Comp Psychol 123: 304–309.
20. Taylor AH, Gray RD (2009) Animal cognition: Aesop's fable flies from fiction to fact. Curr Biol 19: R731–R732.
21. Taylor AH, Medina FS, Holzhaider JC, Hearne LJ, Hunt GR, et al. (2010) An investigation into the cognition behind spontaneous string pulling in New Caledonian crows. PLOS ONE 5: e9345.
22. Hunt GR (1996) Manufacture and use of hook-tools by New Caledonian crows. Nature 379:249–251.
23. Taylor AH, Miller R, Gray RD (2012) New Caledonian crows reason about hidden causal agents. Proc Natl Acad Sci 109: 16389–16391.
24. Kenward B, Rutz C, Weir AAS, Chappell J, Kacelnik A (2004) Morphology and sexual dimorphism of the New Caledonian crow *Corvus moneduloides*, with notes on its behaviour and ecology. Ibis 146: 652–660.
25. R Core Team (2013) R: a language and environment for statistical computing. R Foundation for Statistical Computing, Vienna Austria. R Project website. Available: http://www.R-project.org Accessed 2013 Nov 2.
26. Bates D, Maechler M, Bolker B (2011) lme4: Linear mixed-effects models using S4 classes. R package version 0.999375-42. R Project website. Available: http://CRAN.R-project.org/package = lme4. Accessed 2013 November 2.
27. Barton K (2012) MuMIn: Multi-model inference. R package version 1.7.7. R Project website. Available: http://CRAN.R-project.org/package = MuMIn. Accessed 2013 November 2.
28. Burnham KP, Anderson DR (2002) Model selection and multimodel inference: a practical information- theoretic approach, 2nd edn. Springer, New York.
29. Silva FJ, Silva KM, Cover KR, Leslie AL, Rubalcaba MA (2008) Humans' folk physics is sensitive to physical connection and contact between a tool and reward. Behav Process, 77: 327–333.

5

A New Method to Monitor the Contribution of Fast Food Restaurants to the Diets of US Children

Colin D. Rehm[1]*, **Adam Drewnowski**[1,2]

1 Center for Public Health Nutrition, University of Washington, Seattle, Washington, United States of America, **2** Institute for Cardiometabolism and Nutrition, Groupe Hospitalier Pitié-Salpêtrière, Paris, France

Abstract

Background: American adults consume 11.3% of total daily calories from foods and beverages from fast food restaurants. The contribution of different types of fast food restaurants to the diets of US children is unknown.

Objective: To estimate the consumption of energy, sodium, added sugars, and solid fats among US children ages 4–19 y by fast food restaurant type.

Methods: Analyses used the first 24-h recall for 12,378 children in the 2003–2010 cycles of the nationally representative National Health and Nutrition Examination Survey (NHANES 2003–2010). NHANES data identify foods by location of origin, including stores and fast food restaurants (FFR). A novel custom algorithm divided FFRs into 8 segments and assigned meals and snacks to each. These included burger, pizza, sandwich, Mexican, Asian, fish, and coffee/snack restaurants. The contribution of each restaurant type to intakes of energy and other dietary constituents was then assessed by age group (4–11 y and 12–19 y) and by race/ethnicity.

Results: Store-bought foods and beverages provided 64.8% of energy, 61.9% of sodium, 68.9% of added sugars, and 60.1% of solid fats. FFRs provided 14.1% of energy, 15.9% of sodium, 10.4% of added sugars and 17.9% of solid fats. Among FFR segments, burger restaurants provided 6.2% of total energy, 5.8% of sodium, 6.2% of added sugars, and 7.6% of solid fats. Less energy was provided by pizza (3.3%), sandwich (1.4%), Mexican (1.3%), and chicken restaurants (1.2%). Non-Hispanic black children obtained a greater proportion of their total energy (7.4%), sodium (7.1%), and solid fats (9.5%) from burger restaurants as compared to non-Hispanic white children (6.0% of energy, 5.5% of sodium, and 7.3% of solid fat).

Conclusions: These novel analyses, based on consumption data by fast food market segment, allow public health stakeholders to better monitor the effectiveness of industry efforts to promote healthier menu options.

Editor: Harry Zhang, Old Dominion University, United States of America

Funding: This study was funded by a research grant from McDonald's Corp. to the University of Washington. The funders had no role in study design, data collection and analysis, decision to publish, or preparation of the manuscript.

Competing Interests: CR has no conflicts to report. AD advises McDonald's on nutrition issues and has also received grants, honoraria, and consulting fees from numerous food and beverage companies and other commercial and nonprofit entities with interests in nutrition. The University of Washington has received grants, donations, and contracts from both the public and the private sector.

* Email: crehm@uw.edu

Background

Consumption of foods away from home (FAFH) is thought to contribute to poor diet quality among children and adults [1–6]. FAFH represent a broad category that can include meals and snacks eaten at restaurants, schools, or at entertainment or sports events. The impact of fast foods on diet quality of children has received much research attention [7–11]. Nutritional analyses of fast food menu offerings have focused on the amount of energy, sodium, added sugars, and fats for fast food meals and menu items [12–14].

Since 2003, the National Health and Nutrition Examination Survey (NHANES), the primary source of dietary surveillance data in the US, has coded all foods and beverages consumed by their location of origin, which is reported by survey respondents. Among such locations were supermarkets and grocery stores, fast food restaurants/pizza (FFR), full-service restaurants (FSR), school cafeterias, and vending machines, among many others. The fast food industry generally segments fast food restaurants into 8 different types: burger, pizza, sandwich, chicken, Mexican, Asian, and fish restaurants, as well as coffee/snack shops [15]. However, the NHANES dataset does not distinguish among different FFRs by restaurant type [10,16].

The present study provides the first analysis of children's consumption patterns by the type of FFR. Custom algorithms, developed by the authors, subdivided the NHANES FFR/pizza category into 8 different types. Meals and snacks consumed at each type of restaurant were then analyzed for energy, sodium, added sugars, and solid fats. The present focus was on the relative contribution of different types of FFR to US children's diets.

Analysis of actual consumption data, instead of menu offerings, can provide an alternate picture of the contribution of the fast food

Table 1. Mean and % of total for energy and selected dietary factors (and standard errors) by location of origin.

	Energy (kcal)		Sodium (mg)		Added sugars (kcal)		Solid fats (kcal)	
	Mean	% of total	Mean	% of total	Mean	% of total	Mean	% of total
Overall (age 4–19 y)								
Store	1345 (13)	64.8 (0.6)	2005 (25)	61.9 (0.7)	238 (4)	68.9 (0.6)	252 (3)	60.1 (0.7)
Fast food restaurant	293 (9)	14.1 (0.4)	515 (16)	15.9 (0.5)	36 (1)	10.4 (0.4)	75 (2)	17.9 (0.5)
Full-service restaurant	116 (7)	5.6 (0.4)	226 (16)	7.0 (0.5)	16 (1)	4.5 (0.3)	26 (2)	6.2 (0.4)
School	150 (9)	7.2 (0.4)	247 (17)	7.6 (0.5)	17 (1)	4.9 (0.4)	34 (2)	8.1 (0.5)
Other	171 (5)	8.2 (0.3)	248 (9)	7.6 (0.3)	39 (2)	11.4 (0.5)	32 (1)	7.7 (0.4)
Age 4–11 y								
Store	1246 (16)	65.6 (0.8)	1854 (26)	63.9 (0.9)	204 (4)	66.9 (1.0)	245 (5)	62.3 (1.0)
Fast food restaurant	212 (11)	11.2 (0.6)	356 (20)	12.3 (0.7)	27 (2)	8.8 (0.5)	54 (3)	13.8 (0.8)
Full-service restaurant	84 (7)	4.5 (0.4)	158 (14)	5.5 (0.5)	12 (1)	4.1 (0.4)	18 (2)	4.7 (0.5)
School	173 (11)	9.1 (0.6)	277 (19)	9.5 (0.6)	19 (1)	6.3 (0.5)	39 (3)	10.0 (0.7)
Other	184 (8)	9.7 (0.4)	258 (12)	8.9 (3.9)	42 (3)	13.9 (0.8)	36 (2)	9.2 (0.5)
Age 12–19 y								
Store	1441 (19)	64.2 (0.7)	2150 (40)	60.3 (9.5)	271 (6)	70.3 (0.7)	258 (5)	58.2 (0.9)
Fast food restaurant	371 (12)	16.5 (0.5)	668 (24)	18.7 (0.7)	45 (2)	11.6 (0.4)	95 (3)	21.4 (0.7)
Full-service restaurant	147 (10)	6.5 (0.5)	291 (26)	8.2 (0.7)	19 (2)	4.9 (0.4)	33 (3)	7.5 (0.6)
School	127 (11)	5.6 (0.5)	219 (20)	6.1 (0.5)	15 (2)	3.8 (0.4)	29 (3)	6.5 (0.6)
Other	159 (7)	7.1 (0.4)	237 (14)	6.7 (0.4)	36 (2)	9.4 (0.5)	29 (2)	6.5 (0.4)

industry to the diets of US children and youth. Detailed analyses by FFR type will also allow for better monitoring of food industry trends by interested public health stakeholders. The present study is the first-ever analysis of children's diets by specific type of fast food restaurant. Rather than assess the caloric contribution of specific food items (e.g. burgers or pizza) [16,17], the present analyses provide the first estimate of calories, sodium, added sugars and solid fats from burger or pizza restaurants.

Methods

Dietary intake data sources

Data analyses were based on the first 24-h recall from 4 cycles of the nationally representative National Health and Nutrition Examination Survey (NHANES) for the years 2003–2010. The NHANES 24-h dietary recall utilizes a multi-pass method, where all foods and beverages consumed in the preceding 24-h, from midnight to midnight were reported. The name, time and place of consumption for each eating occasion were also measured. For children 4–5 y, a parent or guardian completed the dietary recall. For children 6–11 y, the child was the primary respondent, but the parent was present and able to assist. For children 12–19 y, the child was the primary respondent, but could be assisted by an adult [18].

Data from the MyPyramid Equivalents Database (MPED) were used to assess intakes of added sugars and solid fats [19]. The MPED 2.0 database was updated for use with more recent NHANES cycles by imputing the MPED equivalents for a limited number of foods (n = 291). Energy from solid fats was estimated as 9 kcal/g of solid fat. Since the MPED database provided added sugars in teaspoon equivalents, this value was converted to energy (1 tsp = 16 kcal) [20].

The 5 principal locations of origin for all foods and beverages were obtained from NHANES data. These were: grocery stores, fast food restaurants (FFR), full-service restaurants (FSR), school cafeterias, and other [21]. The "other" category included foods or beverages from someone else or as a gift, child-care centers, sports/recreational facilities, vending machines, and grown or caught among other categories [21]. Since no further data about the FFR category are provided in NHANES data, a multi-step algorithm was developed by the authors to assign FFR meals and snacks into one of 8 market segments as defined by the restaurant industry [15].

The FFR segmentation

The 8 FFR segments were burger restaurants (e.g., McDonald's or Burger King), pizza restaurants (e.g., Pizza Hut or Domino's), sandwich restaurants (e.g., Subway or Quiznos), chicken restaurants (e.g., KFC or Chick-fil-A), Mexican restaurants (e.g., Taco Bell), Asian restaurants (e.g., Panda Express), fish restaurants (e.g., Long John Silver's) and coffee/snack shops (e.g., Starbucks or Baskin-Robbins). The NHANES data included meals and snacks from national chains as well as regional or local restaurants: the specific brand names provided above are for reference only.

FFR meals were assigned to one of the eight pre-defined segments based on the foods and beverages consumed at that meal. First, unique meals were defined as eating occasions that occurred at the same time and at the same location (i.e., at-home or away from home). Both fast foods consumed at-home and away-from-home were included in the coding algorithm; the place of eating was simply used to define unique eating occasions. Second, an iterative algorithm scanned the 24-h recall individual foods file for "sentinel" foods that could be used to identify a specific market segment. Among the 26 sentinel foods were burgers, pizza, Mexican dishes (e.g., tacos or burritos), chicken strips/nuggets, fried chicken, submarine/deli sandwiches, and hot breakfast items as well as pretzels, hot dogs, side-dishes often served with fried chicken (e.g., baked beans, mashed potatoes and gravy, biscuits, potato salad, where no fried chicken was served), French fries alone, or soda alone.

Foods and food combinations (e.g., hamburger, fried chicken, or pizza) indicated the type of fast food restaurant. If a given meal occasion included only one of these sentinel main dishes, it was coded as such. Examples of meal components that were readily coded and assigned to a given FFR segment were burgers, pizza, Mexican dishes, fried chicken (but not chicken strips/nuggets), or Asian dishes (e.g., fried rice or General Tso's chicken). Meals that contained multiple potential main dishes were flagged for further refinement (described below). Most of the meal components could be unambiguously assigned to a single and identifiable FFR segment. The initial scan coded 77.3% of single items, while the remainder was assessed manually.

Table 2. Mean energy and % of total energy (and standard errors) by FFR segment and age group.

	Total (n = 12,378)		Age 4–11 y (n = 5,681)		Age 12–19 y (n = 6,697)	
	Mean	% of total	Mean	% of total	Mean	% of total
Burger	128 (6.1)	6.2 (0.3)	102 (8.1)†	5.4 (0.4)‡	154 (6.7)	6.8 (0.3)
Pizza	69 (4.8)	3.3 (0.2)	51 (5.9)†	2.7 (0.3)‡	87 (7.3)	3.9 (0.3)
Sandwich	29 (2.2)	1.4 (0.1)	15 (2)†	0.8 (0.1)†	42 (3.9)	1.9 (0.2)
Chicken	26 (2.3)	1.2 (0.1)	23 (3.3)	1.2 (0.2)	28 (3.6)	1.2 (0.2)
Mexican	27 (2.4)	1.3 (0.1)	12 (2.7)†	0.6 (0.1)†	41 (4)	1.8 (0.2)
Asian	9 (1.4)	0.4 (0.1)	4 (1.2)‡	0.2 (0.1)‡	13 (2.4)	0.6 (0.1)
Coffee/snack	3 (0.5)	0.2 (0.0)	3 (0.6)	0.2 (0.0)	4 (0.8)	0.2 (0.0)
Fish	3 (0.9)	0.1 (0.0)	1 (0.7)	0.1 (0.0)	4 (1.6)	0.2 (0.1)
Other sources	1782 (14.2)	85.9 (0.4)	1688 (13.8)‡	88.8 (0.6)†	1873 (21.7)	83.5 (0.5)
Total energy	2076 (13.7)	–	1900 (15.4)†	–	2244 (21.0)	–

†$p<0.001$; ‡$0.001<p<0.01$ for difference between two age groups. Significance testing conducted separately for mean and % of total energy. Value in parentheses is the standard error.

Table 3. Mean sodium and % of total sodium (and standard errors) by FFR segment and age group.

	Total (n = 12,378)		Age 4–11 y (n = 5,681)		Age 12–19 y (n = 6,697)	
	Mean	% of total	Mean	% of total	Mean	% of total
Burger	189 (9.8)	5.8 (0.3)	142 (12.1)†	4.9 (0.4)†	233 (12.3)	6.5 (0.4)
Pizza	142 (9.7)	4.4 (0.3)	102 (11.2)†	3.5 (0.4)‡	180 (15.4)	5.0 (0.4)
Sandwich	62 (4.8)	1.9 (0.2)	34 (4.4)†	1.2 (0.2)†	89 (8.8)	2.5 (0.2)
Chicken	42 (4.0)	1.3 (0.1)	37 (4.6)	1.3 (0.2)	48 (7.0)	1.3 (0.2)
Mexican	49 (4.9)	1.5 (0.1)	21 (5.1)†	0.7 (0.2)†	76 (8.0)	2.1 (0.2)
Asian	22 (3.5)	0.7 (0.1)	13 (3.5)‡	0.5 (0.1)¶	31 (5.7)	0.9 (0.2)
Coffee/snack	5 (1.1)	0.1 (0.0)	4 (1.5)	0.1 (0.1)	5 (1.5)	0.1 (0.0)
Fish	4 (1.4)	0.1 (0.0)	2 (0.8)	0.1 (0.0)	6 (2.5)	0.2 (0.1)
Other sources	2726 (33.9)	84.1 (0.5)	2548 (29.3)†	87.7 (0.7)†	2897 (51.7)	81.3 (0.7)
Total sodium	3242 (30.9)	–	2903 (26.7)†	–	3566 (49.8)	–

†$p<0.001$; ‡$0.001<p<0.01$; ¶$0.01<p<0.05$ for difference between two age groups. Significance testing conducted separately for mean and % of total sodium. Value in parentheses is the standard error.

For some meals, the assignment to a FFR segment was more complex. For example, chicken nuggets/strips are typically sold at both burger and chicken restaurants. Other examples include soda consumed alone, hot breakfast dishes, French fries alone, or ice cream. These meals were randomly assigned to each segment according to a deterministic probability based on weights from sales data for the 50 largest chains. For example, all chicken and burger establishments selling a chicken nugget/strip product were identified and assigned a weight to each segment that randomly divided such meals according to weighted sales. This approach assumes that the relative revenues from each product were similar across different brand segments. For the chicken strips/nugget meal component, 84.3% were assigned to the burger segment while 15.7% were applied to the chicken segment [15].

The reliability of the algorithm was evaluated by an independent coder who assigned 138 random meals (412 individual food items) into the 8 FFR segments. The chance-corrected concordance (Kappa) was estimated at 0.89, indicating a high level of agreement. Some refinements were made to the algorithm following the reliability sub-study. Specifically, sweet and sour sauce was originally coded as an indicator food for Asian-type dishes, but it became clear it was most often associated with eating chicken nuggets/strips.

Analytical approach

Analyses were conducted for all children (ages 4–19 y) and by age group (ages 4–11 and 12–19 y). Three race/ethnicity groups were examined: non-Hispanic whites, Mexican-Americans and non-Hispanic blacks. The race/ethnicity analysis excluded a subsample of the population for which presentation of race/ethnicity specific estimates is not recommended [22]. The three race/ethnicity groups examined constituted 89% of the population.

Dependent measures were dietary energy (kcal/d), sodium (mg/d), added sugars (kcal/d) and solid fats (kcal/d). These dietary constituents were most frequently cited in past analyses of foods away from home, and our important components of summary

Table 4. Mean energy from added sugars and % of total energy from added sugars (and standard errors) by FFR segment and age group.

	Total (n = 12,378)		Age 4–11 y (n = 5,681)		Age 12–19 y (n = 6,697)	
	Mean	% of total	Mean	% of total	Mean	% of total
Burger	21 (1.1)	6.2 (0.3)	17 (1.3)†	5.5 (0.4)¶	26 (1.3)	6.7 (0.3)
Pizza	3.4 (0.4)	1.0 (0.1)	3.0 (0.5)	1.0 (0.2)	3.9 (0.6)	1.0 (0.1)
Sandwich	3.3 (0.4)	1.0 (0.1)	1.7 (0.3)†	0.5 (0.1)†	4.9 (0.6)	1.3 (0.2)
Chicken	3.2 (0.4)	0.9 (0.1)	2.9 (0.6)	1.0 (0.2)	3.5 (0.6)	0.9 (0.2)
Mexican	3.0 (0.3)	0.9 (0.1)	1.3 (0.2)†	0.4 (0.1)†	4.6 (0.6)	1.2 (0.1)
Asian	0.5 (0.1)	0.2 (0.0)	0.2 (0.1)¶	0.1 (0.0)¶	0.8 (0.2)	0.2 (0.1)
Coffee/snack	0.8 (0.2)	0.2 (0.0)	0.8 (0.2)	0.3 (0.1)	0.8 (0.3)	0.2 (0.1)
Fish	0.3 (0.1)	0.1 (0.0)	0.2 (0.1)	0.1 (0.0)	0.4 (0.2)	0.1 (0.1)
Other sources	310 (4.0)	89.6 (0.4)	278 (4.8)†	91.2 (0.5)†	340 (5.8)	88.4 (0.4)
Total added sugars	346 (4.5)	–	305 (5.1)†	–	385 (6.4)	

†$p<0.001$; ¶$0.01<p<0.05$ for difference between two age groups. Significance testing conducted separately for mean and % of total added sugars. Value in parentheses is the standard error.

Table 5. Mean energy from solid fats and % of total energy from solid fats (and standard errors) by FFR segment and age group.

	Total (n = 12,378)		Age 4–11 y (n = 5,681)		Age 12–19 y (n = 6,697)	
	Mean	**% of total**	**Mean**	**% of total**	**Mean**	**% of total**
Burger	32 (1.7)	7.6 (0.4)	25 (2.1)†	6.4 (0.5)†	38 (1.9)	8.6 (0.5)
Pizza	20 (1.6)	4.8 (0.4)	15 (2.1)†	3.8 (0.5)‡	25 (2.3)	5.7 (0.5)
Sandwich	6.5 (0.5)	1.6 (0.1)	3.8 (0.5)†	1.0 (0.1)†	9.2 (0.8)	2.1 (0.2)
Chicken	6.1 (0.6)	1.5 (0.1)	5.7 (0.7)	1.4 (0.2)	6.6 (0.9)	1.5 (0.2)
Mexican	7.2 (0.7)	1.7 (0.2)	3.2 (0.8)†	0.8 (0.2)†	11.1 (1.2)	2.5 (0.3)
Asian	1.3 (0.3)	0.3 (0.1)	0.5 (0.1)‡	0.1 (0.0)¶	2.1 (0.6)	0.5 (0.1)
Coffee/snack	0.9 (0.2)	0.2 (0.0)	0.8 (0.2)	0.2 (0.1)	1.0 (0.2)	0.2 (0.1)
Fish	0.7 (0.3)	0.2 (0.1)	0.3 (0.1)	0.1 (0.0)	1.2 (0.5)	0.3 (0.1)
Other sources	344 (4.4)	82.1 (0.5)	339 (5.3)	86.2 (0.8)†	349 (6.5)	78.6 (0.7)
Total energy from solid fats	419 (4.0)	–	393 (5.3)†	–	443 (6.5)	–

†$p<0.001$; ‡$0.001<p<0.01$; ¶$0.01<p<0.05$ for difference between two age groups. Significance testing conducted separately for mean and % of total solid fats. Value in parentheses is the standard error.

measures of diet quality [12–14,23,24]. Two summary measures were assessed: the survey-weighted mean and the survey-weighted population proportion. The population proportion is the percent of each dietary constituent provided by FFR segment. This measure, interpreted as a ratio of the means, rather than a mean of the ratios, is best suited for examinations of population-level habits [25].

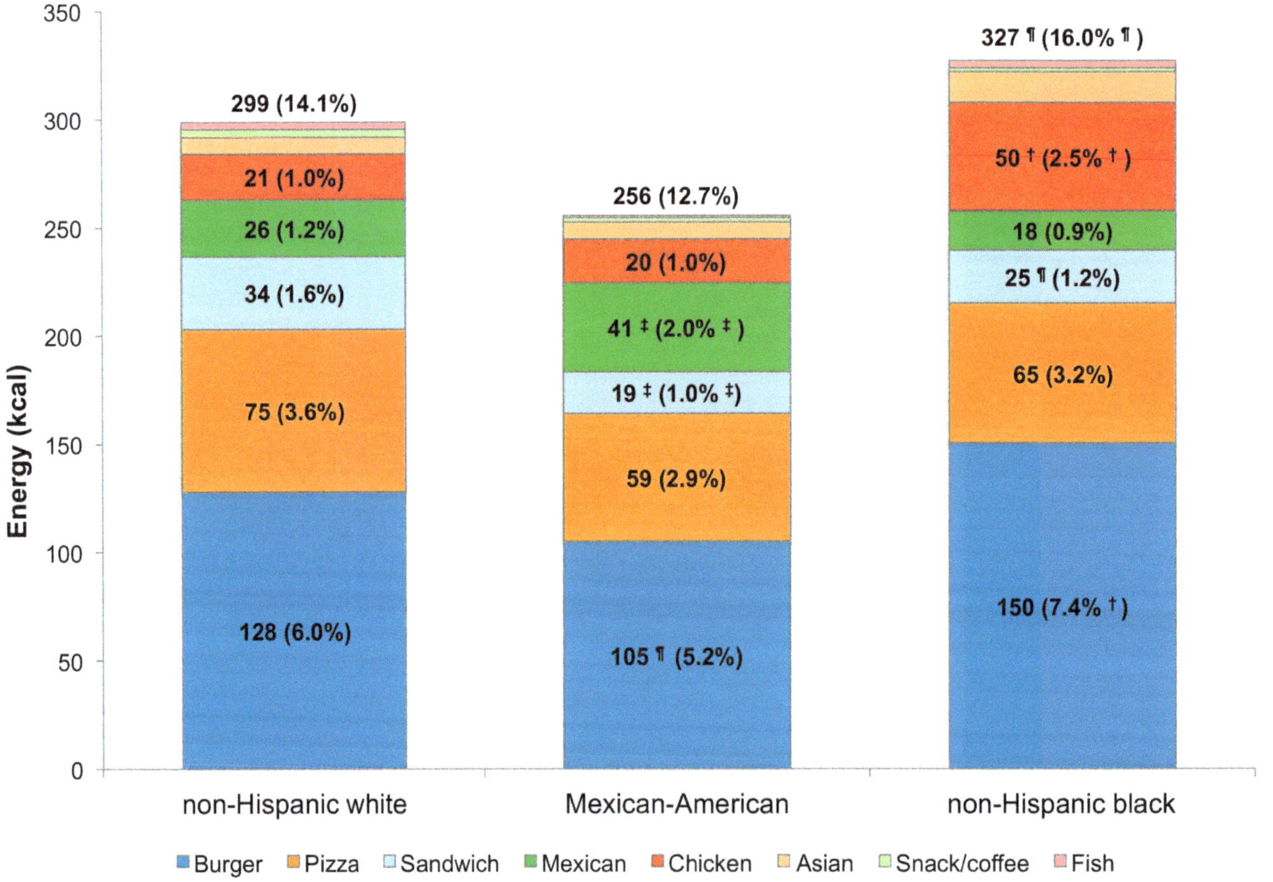

Figure 1. Estimated energy (kcal) intake and population proportion by FFR segment and race/ethnicity, age 4–19 y. †$p<0.001$; ‡$0.001<p<0.01$; ¶$0.01<p<0.05$ for difference, with non-Hispanic whites as the reference group. Significance testing conducted separately for population mean and population proportion (value in parentheses is the population proportion).

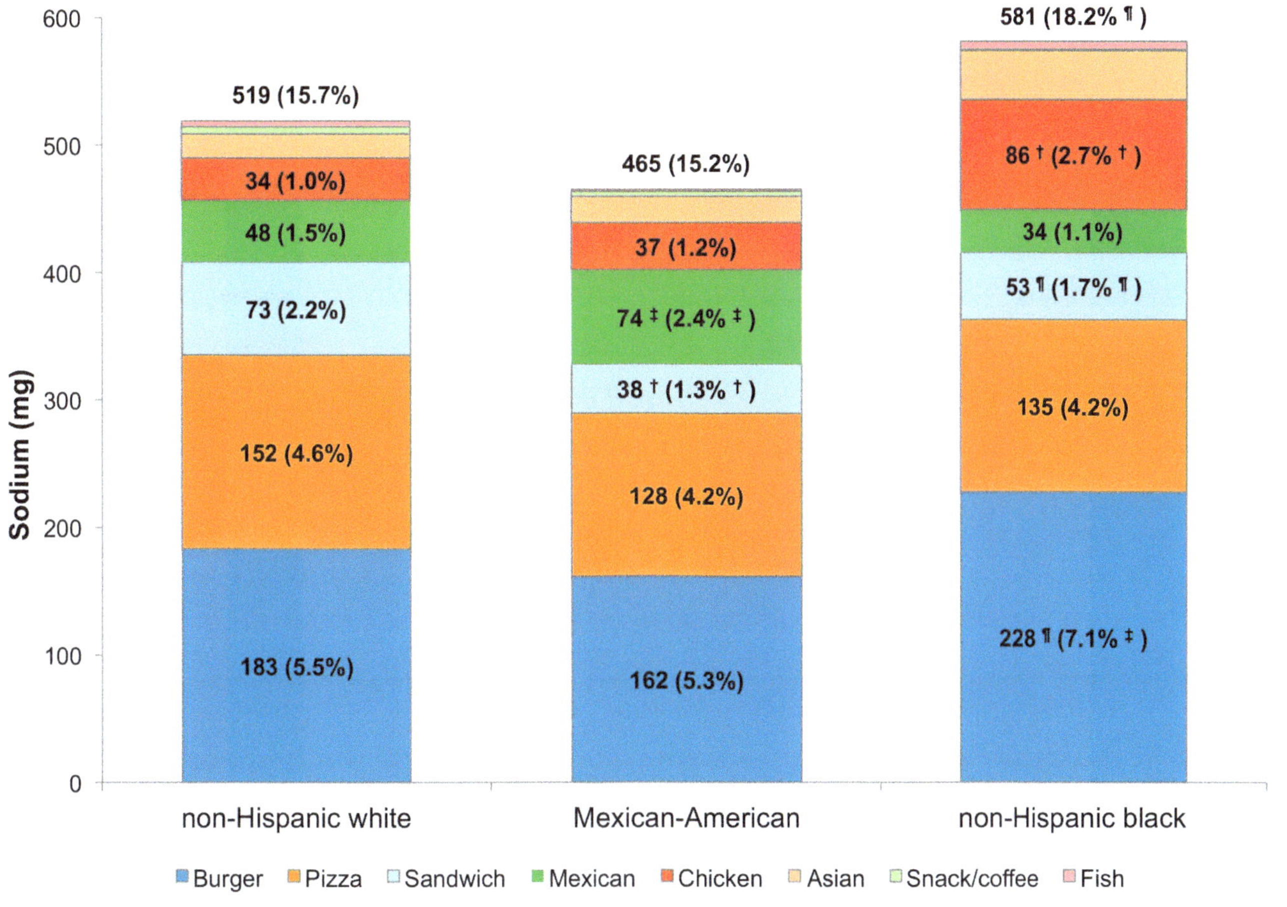

Figure 2. Estimated sodium (mg) intake and population proportion by FFR segment and race/ethnicity, age 4–19 y. †$p<0.001$; ‡$0.001<p<0.01$; ¶$0.01<p<0.05$ for difference, with non-Hispanic whites as the reference group. Significance testing conducted separately for population mean and population proportion (value in parentheses is the population proportion).

Additional analyses examined the energy-adjusted contribution of these dietary constituents by NHANES location of origin and FFR segment. Sodium was presented in mg/1000 kcal, and energy from added sugars and solid fats as a percentage of total energy from that segment.

A survey-weighted Wald test was used to determine the statistical significance of differences in means and proportions between sub-populations by age and race/ethnicity, with adolescents (12–19 y) and non-Hispanic adults as the reference groups. A total of 12,378 children and adolescents were included in all analyses, with the exception of those by race/ethnicity, which included 10,847. All analyses accounted for the complex NHANES stratified multistage sampling design and for over-sampling. The analysis also accounted for survey non-response and all results were representative of the US child population from 2003–2010. Analyses were conducted using Stata 12.1 (StataCorp, College Station, TX).

Data availability and ethical approval

The necessary IRB approval for NHANES had been obtained by the National Center for Health Statistics (NCHS) [26]. The study was exempt from human subjects review per University of Washington policies. All data used here are publicly available on the NCHS website [27].

Results

Consumption patterns by NHANES location

Table 1 shows the survey-weighted means and population proportion for energy, sodium, added sugars and solid fats by NHANES food location and age group. Overall, foods and beverages from supermarkets and grocery stores accounted for the bulk of dietary energy (65%), sodium (62%), added sugars (69%) and solid fats (60%). FFRs were the second most important source of these dietary factors, contributing 14% of total energy, 16% of sodium, 10% of added sugars, and 18% of solid fats. FFRs contributed more energy to the diets of 12–19 y olds (16.5%) than to the diets of 4–11 y olds (11.2%). Approximately 21% of total energy came from FSRs, schools, and other sources.

Consumption patterns by fast food restaurant type

Overall, 35.7% (95% CI 33.9–37.7%) of all children ages 4–19 y consumed fast food items on a given day. Seventeen percent (95% CI 16.1–18.8%) of all children consumed items from burger restaurants, whereas 9.0% (95% CI 8.0–10.1%) consumed items from pizza restaurants. About 4% of all children consumed any items from sandwich, chicken, and Mexican FFRs.

Table 2 provides the mean and population proportion of energy by fast food restaurant type and age group. Within the FFR category, burger restaurants provided the most energy (6.2% overall, 5.4% for 4–11 y olds and 6.8% for 12–19 y olds). Among

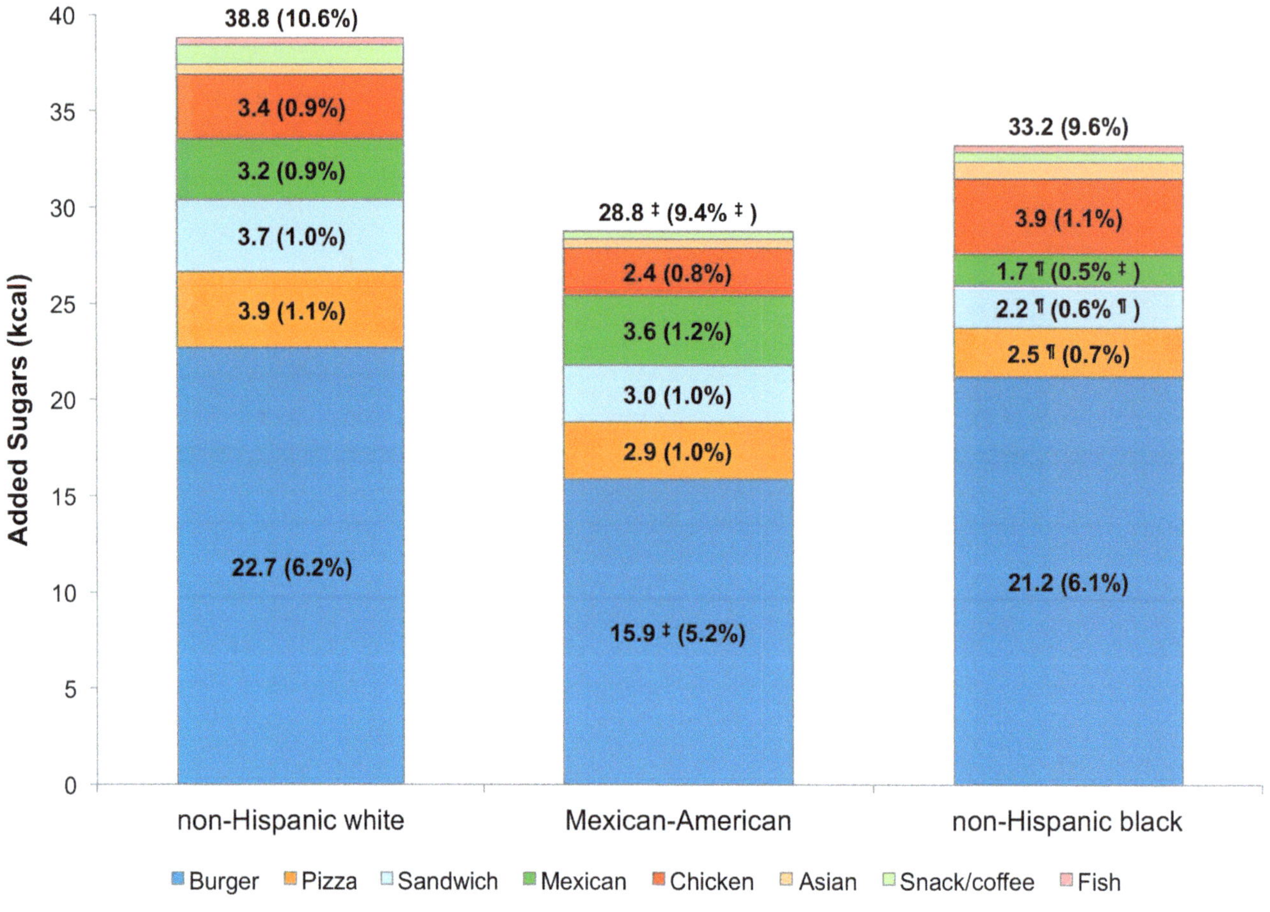

Figure 3. Estimated intake of energy from added sugars (kcal) and population proportion by FFR segment and race/ethnicity, age 4–19 y. †p<0.001; ‡0.001<p<0.01; ¶0.01<p<0.05 for difference, with non-Hispanic whites as the reference group. Significance testing conducted separately for population mean and population proportion (value in parentheses is the population proportion).

the FFR types, pizza restaurants provided the second most energy (3.3% overall, 2.7% for 4–11 y olds, and 3.9% for 12–19 y olds). Overall, sandwich, chicken and Mexican restaurants each provided less than 1.5% of total energy. The Asian, coffee/snack and fish segments each provided less than 0.5% of total energy. Given the strong correlation between energy and other dietary components, the contribution of each FFR segment to sodium (**Table 3**), added sugars (**Table 4**) and solid fats (**Table 5**) tracked the results for energy. Among the different FFR segments, burger restaurants provided the most sodium, added sugars and solid fats.

Figure 1 shows total energy intakes analyzed by fast food restaurant type and race/ethnicity. The distribution of energy intakes by FFR segment varied by race/ethnicity. Non-Hispanic black children derived more energy from fast food restaurants (327 kcal and 16.0% of total) than did non-Hispanic white children (299 kcal and 14.1% of total). Compared to non-Hispanic white children (6.0%), Mexican-American children derived significantly less energy from burger restaurants, whereas non-Hispanic black children derived significantly more (7.4%). By contrast, non-Hispanic white children derived significantly more energy from sandwich restaurants compared to the other race/ethnicity groups, while Mexican-American children derived more calories from Mexican restaurants when compared to non-Hispanic white children. Non-Hispanic black children derived significantly more energy from chicken restaurants than did non-Hispanic white children. From sandwich, Mexican, and chicken FFRs combined, there were no differences in energy by race/ethnicity (81 kcal for non-Hispanic white children, 80 kcal for Mexican-American children and 93 kcal for non-Hispanic black children). Comparable findings were obtained for the other dietary components (see **Figures 2–4** for sodium, energy from added sugars and energy from solid fats, respectively).

Energy-adjusted consumption of sodium, added sugars and solid fats by fast food restaurant type

Table 6 shows the energy-adjusted amounts of sodium and percent of total energy from added sugars and solid fats by FFR type. The data were expressed as a percent of total energy, for solid fats and added sugars, or as mg/1,000 kcal for sodium. Overall, fast food restaurants contributed significantly more sodium per 1,000 kcal and percent of energy from solid fats than stores, while stores contributed significantly more energy from added sugars than FFRs. Pizza, sandwich, Mexican and Asian FFRs contributed significantly more sodium per 1,000 kcal than the burger segment. By contrast, pizza, sandwich, chicken, Mexican and Asian FFRs accounted for a lower proportion of their total energy from added sugars, when compared to burger restaurants. For percent of energy from solid fats, pizza FFRs contributed a greater proportion of total energy from solid fats

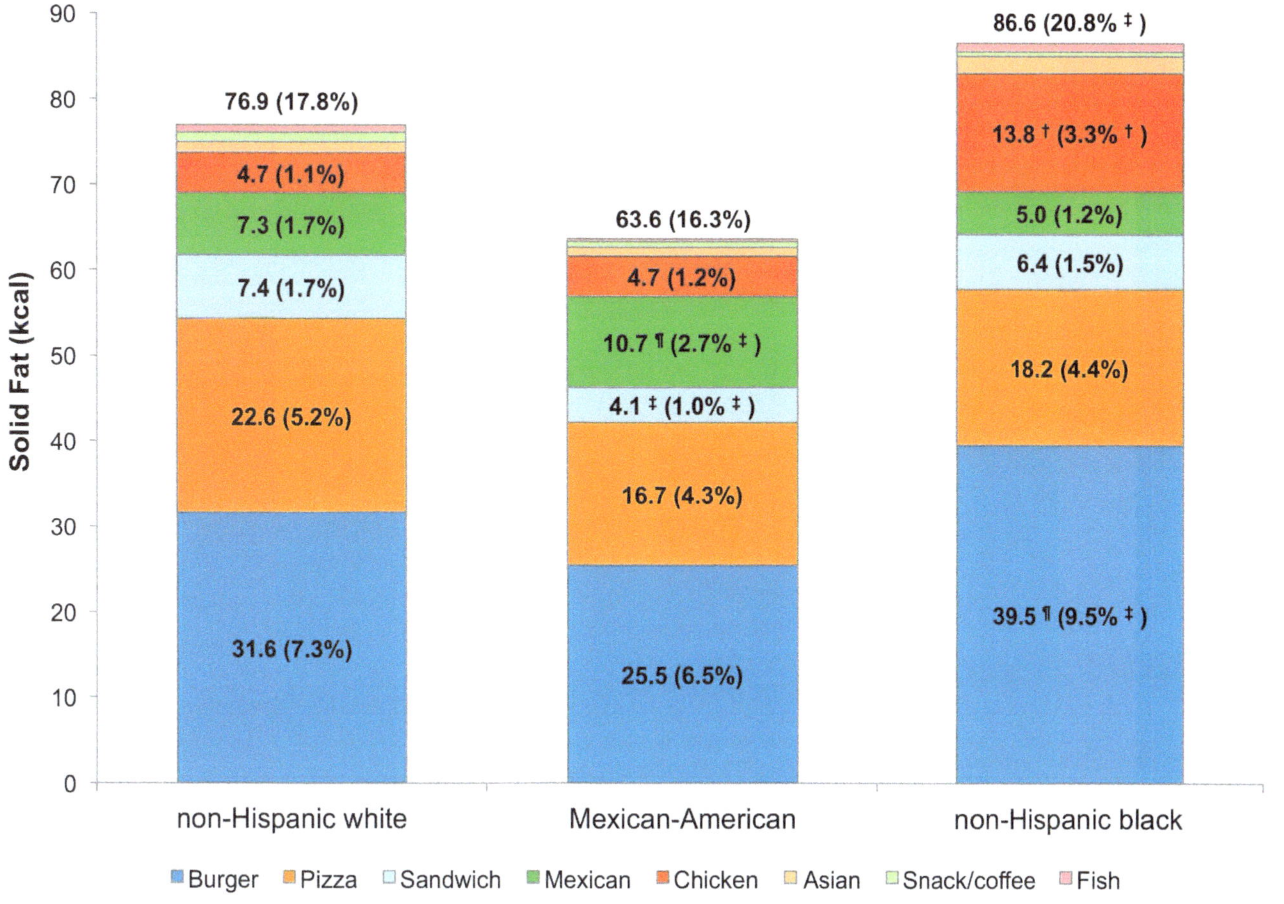

Figure 4. Estimated intake of energy from solid fats (kcal) and population proportion by FFR segment and race/ethnicity, age 4–19 y. †p<0.001; ‡0.001<p<0.01; ¶0.01<p<0.05 for difference, with non-Hispanic whites as the reference group. Significance testing conducted separately for population mean and population proportion (value in parentheses is the population proportion).

than did burger FFRs, while Asian FFRs contributed the lowest proportion of total energy from solid fats.

Discussion

The present analyses are the first example of stratifying consumption data for a nationally representative sample of US children by fast food restaurant type. First, analyses of consumption data are a useful supplement to the numerous prior analyses of fast food menu offerings [12–14]. Second, separating the FFR category into specific market segments as defined by the restaurant industry allows interested stakeholders to monitor the impact of public health policies and programs aimed at improving the quality of children's diets.

The present analyses complement published studies of US diets by NHANES location of origin, where foods were aggregated based on a National Cancer Institute coding scheme [16,17]. The present analyses are unique in that they accounted for all foods and beverages eaten at different types of fast food restaurants. Items consumed at burger restaurants may include burgers but may also include fries, chicken, salad, beverages, milkshakes, desserts, fruit and coffee. Thus, burgers alone contributed 1.2% of energy to the diets of the 6–11 y age group and 1.9% of energy to the 12–19 y age group, as reported previously [16]. By contrast, the total contribution of calories from burger restaurants was much higher: 6.2% overall, 5.4% for 4–11 y olds, and 6.8% for 12–19 y olds.

The present estimates, based on nationally representative federal datasets, were generally consistent with FFR segment sales, as published by industry sources [15]. Among FFRs, burger restaurants are the leading segment, as reflected in the consumption data. In 2009, total sales for burgers among leading national chains were $66 billion (or 47.7% of all FFR sales). The present estimate was that 43.5% (95% CI 40.2–47.4%) of FFR calories consumed by US children came from the burger segment. In this age group, pizza was far and away the second most important source of energy. Nationally, the sandwich, snack, chicken, pizza and Mexican segments were the 2nd–6th leading segments in terms of sales, respectively. The infrequent consumption of coffee among children/adolescents explains why the snack/coffee segment was not observed as an important source of energy in this study. The present approach allows publicly available federal data to be used for identifying the relative importance of different FFR segments for specific demographic groups of interest, a definite advantage over the use of menu offerings or sales data. This approach can also be used to monitor population-based trends in dietary intakes from different types of FFRs.

The present consumption-based analyses complement past studies on the nutrient density of foods/meals from FFRs that are generally based on menu offerings [12–14,28–31]. No nationally representative data on food consumption by FFR

Table 6. Mean sodium per 1,000 kcal and percent of energy from added sugars and solid fats (and standard errors) by FFR segment.

	Sodium		Added sugars		Solid fats	
	Sodium (mg) per 1,000 kcal	% of total sodium	% of total energy from added sugars[1]	% of total added sugars	% of total energy from solid fats[1]	% of total solid fats
FFR segment						
Burger (ref)	1458 (24)	5.8 (0.3)	16.5 (0.5)	6.2 (0.3)	25.3 (0.5)	7.6 (0.4)
Pizza	2028 (33)¶	4.4 (0.3)	4.5 (0.6)¶	1.0 (0.1)	30.6 (1.3)¶	4.8 (0.4)
Sandwich	2005 (76)¶	1.9 (0.2)	12.1 (0.9)¶	1.0 (0.1)	22.6 (0.9)	1.6 (0.1)
Chicken	1577 (67)	1.3 (0.1)	13.0 (1.1)¶	0.9 (0.1)	23.9 (0.8)	1.5 (0.1)
Mexican	1841 (36)¶	1.5 (0.1)	11.5 (0.9)¶	0.9 (0.1)	27.0 (0.8)	1.7 (0.2)
Asian	2590 (204)¶	0.7 (0.1)	6.2 (1.2)¶	0.2 (0.0)	16.6 (2.5)¶	0.3 (0.1)
Coffee/snack	1579 (267)	0.1 (0.0)	22.2 (4.4)	0.2 (0.0)	26.2 (1.8)	0.2 (0.0)
Fish	1420 (97)	0.1 (0.0)	14.3 (4.2)	0.1 (0.0)	28.8 (1.5)	0.2 (0.1)
Location of origin						
All FFR (ref)	1756 (20)	15.9 (0.5)	12.0 (0.4)	10.4 (0.4)	26.3 (0.4)	17.9 (0.5)
Store	1466 (11)¶	61.9 (0.7)	18.3 (0.3)¶	68.9 (0.6)	18.2 (0.1)¶	60.1 (0.7)
FSR	1892 (61)	7.0 (0.5)	13.8 (0.8)	4.5 (0.3)	23.1 (0.7)¶	6.2 (0.4)
School	1635 (78)	7.6 (0.5)	11.5 (0.5)	4.9 (0.4)	23.1 (0.5)¶	8.1 (0.5)
Other	1499 (40)¶	7.6 (0.3)	20.6 (0.9)¶	11.4 (0.5)	19.9 (0.7)¶	7.7 (0.4)

[1]Value can be interpreted as the proportion of energy from each segment that is from added sugars or solid fats. For example, of all energy from burger FFRs, 16.5% came from added sugars.
¶Indicates p-value <0.05. Reference group for segment analysis is burger. Reference group for location of origin is all FFR. Hypothesis testing only conducted for sodium (mg) per 1,000 kcal, and percent of total energy from added sugars and solid fats. Value in parentheses is the standard error.

segment has previously been published. Merging market segmentation and public health surveillance approaches, the present method has the potential to transform ways in which the contribution of different food sources to the total diet can be evaluated and monitored over time. In particular, given efforts by the food and restaurant industry to improve the composition of menus and food products, a surveillance system needs to be established. The approach used here can also be adapted for a large number of dietary outcomes, including fruit, vegetable, low-fat dairy, fiber, potassium or any other dietary constituent or food group of interest.

The present study had several limitations. First, the present analyses were based on a 24-hour recall, which may result in under-reporting of foods perceived to be less healthful [32,33]. This may result in a falsely minimized estimation of energy from both full-service and fast food restaurants or from food groups such as desserts, salty snacks, pizza or soda. However, such underreporting should not affect the relative rankings of consumption patterns by FFR segment. For younger children, dietary reporting by proxy respondent may result in under-reporting of foods consumed while the parent is not present. However, such a reporting error is less likely for restaurant foods, where parents are likely to be present, as opposed to school/childcare settings.

The NHANES food location of origin may also have some error. In particular, stores include supermarkets, grocery stores, convenience stores and pharmacies where people buy food. The FFR-segment coding algorithm also had some limitations; a small proportion of eating occasions could not be unambiguously assigned to a specific FFR category and were coded instead based on the relative market share of each segment.

Despite these limitations, the present work represents the only assessment of the contribution of different types of fast food restaurants to the diets of US children. The present analyses advance the field in two important ways. First, consumption data can supplement the ongoing analyses of menu offerings, while offering better insight into what is eaten. Second, intakes of energy and dietary constituents of public health concern can now be assigned to different types of fast food restaurants: burger, pizza, sandwich, chicken, Mexican, Asian, fish, and coffee/snack. The present approach can be usefully applied to monitor the effectiveness of industry and public health policies aimed at improving the dietary habits of American children.

Author Contributions

Conceived and designed the experiments: CDR AD. Analyzed the data: CDR. Wrote the paper: CDR AD.

References

1. Bauer KW, Larson NI, Nelson MC, Story M, Neumark-Sztainer D (2009) Fast food intake among adolescents: secular and longitudinal trends from 1999 to 2004. Prev Med 48: 284–287.
2. Mancino L, Todd J, Lin B-H (2009) Separating what we eat from where: Measuring the effect of food away from home on diet quality. Food Policy 34: 557–562.
3. U.S. Food and Drug Administration: Backgrounder - Keystone Forum on Away-From-Home Foods: Opportunities for Preventing Weight Gain and Obesity. Available at: http://www.fda.gov/Food/LabelingNutrition/ReportsResearch/ucm082064.htm.
4. Guthrie JF, Lin BH, Frazao E (2002) Role of food prepared away from home in the American diet, 1977–78 versus 1994–96: changes and consequences. J Nutr Educ Behav 34: 140–150.
5. Todd J, Mancino L, Lin BH (2010) The impact on food away from home on adult diet quality. Economic Research Report 2010.

6. Jeffery RW, French SA (1998) Epidemic obesity in the United States: are fast foods and television viewing contributing? Am J Public Health 88: 277–280.
7. Bowman SA, Gortmaker SL, Ebbeling CB, Pereira MA, Ludwig DS (2004) Effects of fast-food consumption on energy intake and diet quality among children in a national household survey. Pediatrics 113: 112–118.
8. Paeratakul S, Ferdinand DP, Champagne CM, Ryan DH, Bray GA (2003) Fast-food consumption among US adults and children: dietary and nutrient intake profile. J Am Diet Assoc 103: 1332–1338.
9. Taveras EM, Berkey CS, Rifas-Shiman SL, Ludwig DS, Rockett HR, et al. (2005) Association of consumption of fried food away from home with body mass index and diet quality in older children and adolescents. Pediatrics 116: e518–524.
10. Powell LM, Nguyen BT (2013) Fast-food and full-service restaurant consumption among children and adolescents: effect on energy, beverage, and nutrient intake. JAMA Pediatr 167: 14–20.
11. Schmidt M, Affenito SG, Striegel-Moore R, Khoury PR, Barton B, et al. (2005) Fast-food intake and diet quality in black and white girls: the National Heart, Lung, and Blood Institute Growth and Health Study. Arch Pediatr Adolesc Med 159: 626–631.
12. Hearst MO, Harnack LJ, Bauer KW, Earnest AA, French SA, et al. (2013) Nutritional quality at eight U.S. fast-food chains: 14-year trends. Am J Prev Med 44: 589–594.
13. Wu HW, Sturm R (2014) Changes in the Energy and Sodium Content of Main Entrees in US Chain Restaurants from 2010 to 2011. J Acad Nutr Diet 114: 209–219.
14. Wu HW, Sturm R (2013) What's on the menu? A review of the energy and nutritional content of US chain restaurant menus. Public Health Nutr 16: 87–96.
15. Oches S (2011) Top 50 breakdown by market segments. QSR Magazine online. Available at: http://www.qsrmagazine.com/reports/top-50-breakdown-market-segments.
16. Drewnowski A, Rehm CD (2013) Energy intakes of US children and adults by food purchase location and by specific food source. Nutr J 12: 59.
17. Drewnowski A, Rehm CD (2013) Sodium intakes of US children and adults from foods and beverages by location of origin and by specific food source. Nutrients 5: 1840–1855.
18. National Health and Nutrition Examination Survey: MEC In-Person Dietary Interviewers Procedure Manual. Available at: http://www.cdc.gov/nchs/data/nhanes/nhanes_09_10/DietaryInterviewers_Inperson.pdf.
19. Bowman SA, Friday JE, Moshfegh A (2008). MyPyramid Equivalents Database, 2.0 for USDA Survey Foods, 2003–2004 [Online] Food Surveys Research Group. Beltsville Human Nutrition Research Center, Agricultural Research Service, U.S. Department of Agriculture, Beltsville, MD.
20. Ervin RB, Ogden CL (2013) Consumption of added sugars among U.S. adults, 2005–2010. NCHS Data Brief: 1–8.
21. National Health and Nutrition Examination Survey. Dietary Interview: Individual Foods – First Day (DR1IFF_F) Codebook. Available at: http://www.cdc.gov/nchs/nhanes/nhanes2009-2010/DR1IFF_F.htm.
22. (2011) National Health and Nutrition Examination Survey. Analytic Note Regarding 2007–2010 Survey Design Changes and Combining Data Across other Survey Cycles. Available at: http://www.cdc.gov/nchs/data/nhanes/analyticnote_2007-2010.pdf.
23. Guenther PM, Casavale KO, Reedy J, Kirkpatrick SI, Hiza HA, et al. (2013) Update of the Healthy Eating Index: HEI-2010. J Acad Nutr Diet 113: 569–580.
24. Guenther PM, Reedy J, Krebs-Smith SM (2008) Development of the Healthy Eating Index-2005. J Am Diet Assoc 108: 1896–1901.
25. Krebs-Smith SM, Kott PS, Guenther PM (1989) Mean proportion and population proportion: two answers to the same question? J Am Diet Assoc 89: 671–676.
26. National Health and Nutrition Examination Survey. NCHS Research Ethics Review Board (ERB) Approval. Available at: http://www.cdc.gov/nchs/nhanes/irba98.htm.
27. (2014) National Center for Health Statistics, Centers for Disease Control and Prevention. National Health and Nutrition Examination Survey Questionnaires, Datasets and Related Documentation. Available at: http://www.cdc.gov/nchs/nhanes/nhanes_questionnaires.htm.
28. Kirkpatrick SI, Reedy J, Kahle LL, Harris JL, Ohri-Vachaspati P, et al. (2013) Fast-food menu offerings vary in dietary quality, but are consistently poor. Public Health Nutr: 1–8.
29. Namba A, Auchincloss A, Leonberg BL, Wootan MG (2013) Exploratory analysis of fast-food chain restaurant menus before and after implementation of local calorie-labeling policies, 2005–2011. Prev Chronic Dis 10: E101.
30. Bauer KW, Hearst MO, Earnest AA, French SA, Oakes JM, et al. (2012) Energy content of U.S. fast-food restaurant offerings: 14-year trends. Am J Prev Med 43: 490–497.
31. Bruemmer B, Krieger J, Saelens BE, Chan N (2012) Energy, saturated fat, and sodium were lower in entrees at chain restaurants at 18 months compared with 6 months following the implementation of mandatory menu labeling regulation in King County, Washington. J Acad Nutr Diet 112: 1169–1176.
32. Rasmussen LB, Matthiessen J, Biltoft-Jensen A, Tetens I (2007) Characteristics of misreporters of dietary intake and physical activity. Public Health Nutr 10: 230–237.
33. Lafay L, Mennen L, Basdevant A, Charles MA, Borys JM, et al. (2000) Does energy intake underreporting involve all kinds of food or only specific food items? Results from the Fleurbaix Laventie Ville Sante (FLVS) study. Int J Obes Relat Metab Disord 24: 1500–1506.

6

Effects of Low-Level Deuterium Enrichment on Bacterial Growth

Xueshu Xie, Roman A. Zubarev*

Division of Physiological Chemistry I, Department of Medical Biochemistry and Biophysics, Karolinska Institutet, Stockholm, Sweden

Abstract

Using very precise (±0.05%) measurements of the growth parameters for bacteria *E. coli* grown on minimal media, we aimed to determine the lowest deuterium concentration at which the adverse effects that are prominent at higher enrichments start to become noticeable. Such a threshold was found at 0.5% D, a surprisingly high value, while the ultralow deuterium concentrations (≤0.25% D) showed signs of the opposite trend. Bacterial adaptation for 400 generations in isotopically different environment confirmed preference for ultralow (≤0.25% D) enrichment. This effect appears to be similar to those described in sporadic but multiple earlier reports. Possible explanations include hormesis and isotopic resonance phenomena, with the latter explanation being favored.

Editor: Vipul Bansal, RMIT University, Australia

Funding: This work was supported by the Swedish Research Council (Grant # 2011-3726). The funder had no role in study design, data collection and analysis, decision to publish, or preparation of the manuscript.

Competing Interests: The authors have declared that no competing interests exist.

* Email: Roman.Zubarev@ki.se

Introduction

Since the discovery of D_20 (heavy water) in 1932 by Urey, Brickwede and Murphy [1], its biological effects have attracted a great deal of researchers' interest. Already early experiments have revealed that deuterium has profound effect on living organisms. Between 1934 and the beginning of the second World war in 1939, a total of 216 publications appeared dealing with biological effects of deuterium [2]. Excess of deuterium in water was found to cause reduction in synthesis of proteins and nucleic acids, disturbance in cell division mechanism, changes in enzymatic kinetic rates and cellular morphological changes [3,4]. Yet it is possible to grow microorganisms (e.g. some variants of *Escherichia coli*) in a highly substituted medium, and achieve almost complete deuterium substitution [5,6].

The biological effects of stable isotopes are usually observed shortly after the microorganism is placed in an isotopically different medium [7]. At first, prokaryotic cells experiences an "isotopic shock" manifested through the growth arrest and morphology changes. After a period of adaptation ("lag phase"), growth resumes, but the rate is usually slower than in normal isotopic environment [8]. The changes in the growth rate can be explained by the impact of isotopic substitutions on the kinetics of enzymes [9], pattern of hydrogen bonds and similar relatively subtle but cumulatively potentially important effects.

The Katz group who have studied multiple heavy-isotope (^{13}C, ^{15}N and ^{18}O) substitutions in *Chlorella vulgaris* grown in heavy water found that all additional isotopic substitutions resulted into abnormal effects in cell size, appearance, growth rate and division [10]. The effects were progressively stronger as the isotopic composition deviated from the normal. The authors concluded that "*organisms of different isotopic compositions are actually different organisms, to the degree that their isotopic compositions are removed from naturally occurring compositions*" [10].

The question is whether this conclusion made for heavy enrichments levels (>50%) remains true for low levels of enrichment (<10%). Since isotopic compositions of microorganisms grown in a slightly enriched environment showed deficit of heavy isotopes [11], one can reasonably assume that even low levels of deuterium enrichment may cause biological effects. Indeed, the earliest works on biological effect of deuterium reported in the 1930s were performed using low levels of deuterium, as high enrichment was still not available. Barnes *et al.* studied the physiological effect of low deuterium concentration on the growth of *Spirogyra*, flatworms and *Euglena*. They found an increased growth of these three organisms at 0.06% of D in water compared to ordinary water that contains 156 ppm D (0.0156%). More specifically, they observed increased cell division for *Euglena*, longer longevity for flatworms, and both less cell disjunction and greater longevity for *Spirogyra* [12–15]. Lockemann and Leunig's study on the effect of heavy water with less than 0.54% D upon *E. coli* and *Pseudomonasa* revealed that concentrations as low as 0.04% D favored growth [16]. Curry *et al.* observed ca. 10% faster growth for *Aspergillus* at 0.05% D, but the result was not statically significant due to large errors of measurements [17]. After the first half of 1930s, the research focus has shifted to the effects of highly enriched deuterium, which were more pronounced and largely negative. The interested to low deuterium enrichment has returned in the 1970s and 1980s, when Lobyshev *et al.* studied the Na, K-ATPase activity at different concentration of deuterium and found it to increase at low deuterium concentrations, with a maximum reached at 0.04–0.05% [18,19]. Lobyshev *et al.* then performed experiments with regeneration of hydrioid pohyps *Obelia geniculata* in a wide range of deuterium added to sea water and found faster regeneration at and below 0.1% D [20]. Somlyai *et al.* have shown that 0.06% D in tissue culture activated the growth of L_{929} fibroblast cell lines [21]. Nikitin *et al.* have studied growth of bacteria with different membrane lipid composition in liquid media in a range of deuterium concentration in water varied from 0.01% to 90% and observed pronounced activation in growth for *Methylobacterium organopholium* and *Hyphomonas jannaschiane* at around 0.01% enrichment [22]. Recent studies on the impact of D_2O on the life span of *Drosophila melanogaster* revealed the biggest positive effect of deuterium at the lowest D concentration tested in that work, 7.5% of enrichment [23].

In the current study, we probed enrichment levels starting from 0.03%, i.e. double the normal deuterium abundance of 156 ppm. Disregarding the earliest reports from 1930s on the biological effects of 0.06% deuterium in water which suffered from the lack of statistical analysis and proper controls, we expected the size of the biological effects to be commensurable with the enrichment levels, i.e. to be exquisitely small. To address the expected minute size of the phenomena, we developed a very sensitive method for detecting the biological effects of unspecific deuterium incorporation in the model organism. *E. coli* was chosen as such because of the ease of handling, robustness and speed of growth as well as the ability to thrive on minimal media with easily changeable isotopic composition.

The applied method utilizes robotized sample preparation, automated and massively parallel data acquisition (hundreds of individual experiments per concentration point) and measures three independent parameters per growth curve: maximum growth rate, the lag phase duration and maximum density (Figure 1). Massive parallel measurement approach is achieved using the BioScreen C automated fermentor that affords up to 200 experiments run at the same time. Every second experimental well in a 100-well plate was kept at standard isotopic conditions (Figure S1), and the data from each "test" well was normalized by that of the neighboring standard well, providing the accuracy of relative measurements close to those achieved with internal standard. Using massive statistics, we achieved the precision of relative measurements close to 0.05% (standard error).

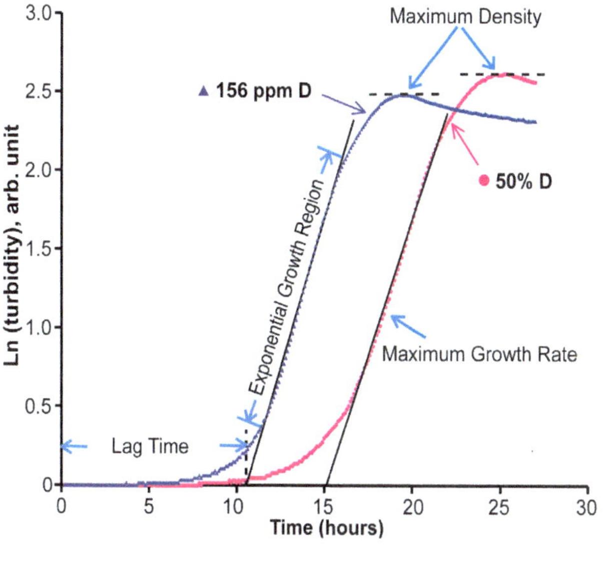

Figure 1. Typical growth curve and the three growth parameters derived from the curve.

Materials and Methods

Chemicals and Materials

Glycerol stock of *E. coli* BL 21 strain (stored at −80°C) was obtained from the microbiology lab of our department. The M9 minimal media [24] was prepared using D-glucose ($C_6H_{12}O_6$), disodium hydrogen phosphate ($Na_2HPO_4.2H_2O$), monopotassium phosphate (KH_2PO_4), sodium chloride (NaCl), magnesium sulfate ($MgSO_4$), calcium chloride ($CaCl_2$), ammonia chloride (NH_4Cl), heavy water (99.9% of ^2H), all purchased from Sigma-Aldrich (Schnelldorf, Germany), and distilled water prepared with a Milli-Q device from Millipore (Billerica, MA, USA). Heavy water (99.9% of ^2H) was also purchased from Sigma-Aldrich (Schnelldorf, Germany).

Vacuum filtration system with 0.2 µm polyethersulfone (PES) membrane for bacteria media sterilization was purchased from VWR (Stockholm, Sweden). Petri dishes (90×14 mm) and inoculating sterile loops were purchased from Sigma-Aldrich. Sterile plastic conical tubes (50 mL and 15 mL) for sample preparation were purchased from Sarstedt (Nümbrecht, Germany). The BioScreen C automatic fermentor was obtained from Oy Growth Curves AB Ltd (Helsinki, Finland).

M9 minimal media preparation

5-time concentrated M9 minimal salts stock solution was prepared by dissolving 42.5 g $Na_2HPO_4.2H_2O$, 15 g KH_2PO_4 and 2.5 g NaCl in Milli-Q water to a final volume of 1000 mL. The solution was then sterilized by autoclaving and stored at 4°C for further use. To prepare M9 minimal media, the salts stock solution was diluted five times in Milli-Q water.

M9 minimal media were prepared by mixing the following components: 800 mL Milli-Q water, 200 mL M9 concentrated salts stock solution, 2 mL of 1 M $MgSO_4$ solution, 0.1 mL of 1 M $CaCl_2$ solution, 5 g D-glucose ($C_6H_{12}O_6$) and 1 g NH_4Cl.

Preparation of streak agar plates

M9 minimal media agar plates were prepared by dissolving 3 g of agar powder in 200 mL M9 minimal media. The obtained mixture was sterilized by autoclaving, then cooled down to ca. 60°C and finally poured into Petri dishes (ca. 15 mL agar solution per plate). The agar plates were allowed to solidify at room temperature for ca. 10 min, sealed with parafilm and stored at 4°C till further use.

E. coli streak agar plates were prepared by streaking [25] *E. coli* from −80°C glycerol stock onto M9 minimal media agar plate followed by 40-hour incubation at 37°C to form visible isolated colonies. Streak agar plates were stored for experiments for maximum one week at 4°C.

Measurement of *E. coli* growth

From the *E. coli* agar plate, one isolated colony was picked with a sterile loop into 5 mL M9 minimal media and incubated at 37°C while shaking with 200 r.p.m for 5–6 hours until it reached its early exponential phase with optical density (OD_{590}) around 0.2, measured with Colorimeter WPA CO75 (York, UK).

Sample preparation workflow is shown in Figure 2. In each experiment, four stock solutions were used. Stock A for preparing sample S_A, and stock B for preparing sample S_B were obtained by mixing M9 minimal media with sterilized heavy water at a certain ratio (Table 1). For the preparation of stock solutions of standard A and standard B, M9 minimal media were mixed with sterile Milli-Q water at the same ratio as stock A and stock B. The final solutions were dispensed into the honeycomb well plates using

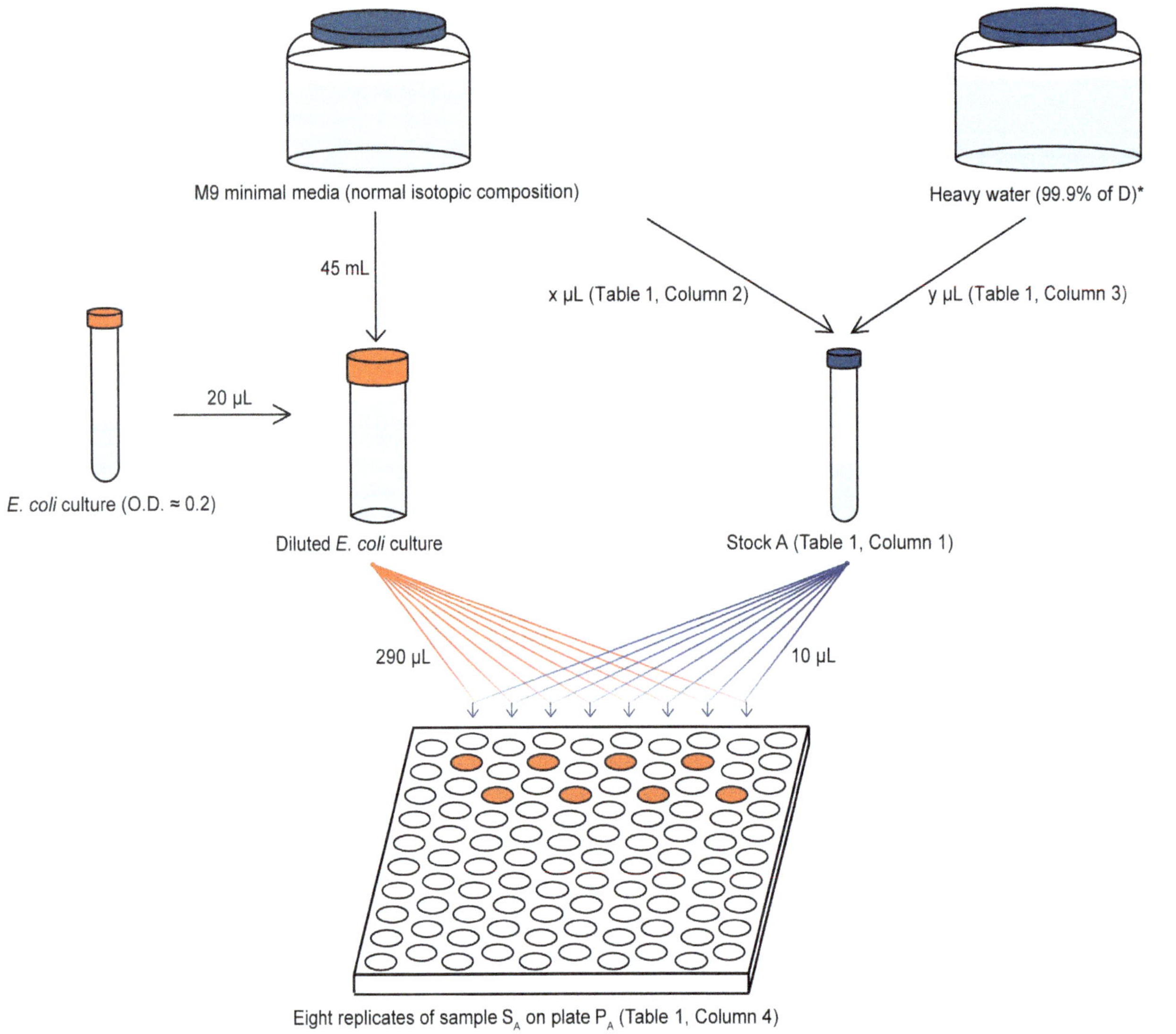

Figure 2. Experimental workflow. For each plate, 32 samples (S_A) and 32 standards were prepared. Stock A was used for preparing 32 samples on plate P_A. * Milli-Q water was used instead of heavy water to prepare stock solution for the preparation of standards.

programmed robotic system (Tecan, Genesis RSP 150, Männedorf, Switzerland).

A 20 μL aliquot of the incubated *E. coli* culture (O.D. ≈0.2) was diluted in 45 mL M9 minimal media for robotic sample preparation. First, 300 μL M9 minimal media without bacteria were introduced into each of the border wells ("edge cells") on both plates P_A and P_B (72 wells in total) to serve as blank samples (no color code in Figure S1). Second, 30 μL (10 μL for samples with <4% enrichment of deuterium) aliquot of stock A was dispensed into each "sample" well (marked with purple on plate P_A in Figure S1) to prepare 32 replicates of sample S_A. Third, 30 μL (10 μL for samples with <4% enrichment of deuterium) aliquot of stock solution of standard A was added into each "standard" well (marked with yellow on plate P_A in Figure S1) to prepare 32 reference standards on plate. In the same way, wells were filled on plate P_B. Finally, 270 μL (290 μL for <4% D) of the diluted *E. coli* culture was dispensed into each well except blank wells. In total, 32 replicate pairs of "sample" and "standard" wells were prepared on each plate. Sample configuration is shown in Figure S1.

Bioscreen C monitors *E. coli* concentration in each well by measuring turbidity (with wide band filter 420–580 nm) in it at 39°C with continuous bacterial agitation by shaking. In our experiments, turbidity was sampled every six minutes and was monitored for ca. 24 hours.

E. coli adaptation to different deuterium content

One *E. coli* colony was inoculated into 5 mL M9 minimal media (normal isotopic condition) from a fresh M9 minimal media agar plate, and cultured at 37°C until O.D. 1.0. For every deuterium concentration point (156 ppm, 0.03%, 0.25%, and 1%), 2 μL *E. coli* culture was diluted 2500 times into 5 mL M9 minimal media with the corresponding D content and cultured overnight at 37°C. After the culture reached its maximum density (O.D. ≈1.4), for each *E. coli* culture, 10 μL was then diluted 500 times into 5 mL media with the same D content, and culturing continued at 37°C. In this way, each *E. coli* culture was diluted 500 times twice a day, with nine generations grown between dilutions. The process continued until the 400th generation was obtained, after which the difference in the rate

Table 1. Stock solutions and their corresponding D content in the final samples.

D content in stock solution	M9 minimal media (μL)	Heavy water (μL)	D content in the final sample (honey comb well plate)
0.0156%	5948	28 (Milli-Q water)	0.0156%
0.48%	5948	28	0.03%
1.42%	5892	84	0.06%
3.29%	5957	202	0.12%
7.04%	5728	433	0.25%
14.52%	5620	955	0.5%
29.50%	4403	1844	1%
59.46%	2437	3581	2%
39.80%	3667	2427	4%
79.73%	1222	4830	8%

Stock solution (column one) was prepared by mixing M9 minimal media and heavy water at a certain ratio that resulted in the final D content in the sample (column four). For each sample, stock solution for its corresponding standards (below it is called stock solution of standard X) was prepared in the same way but using Milli-Q water instead of heavy water.

of growth of the adapted bacteria on the corresponding content of deuterium versus normal D content was measured using Bioscreen C.

Data Analysis

Using Microsoft Excel, the logarithm of turbidity was plotted against time (Figure 1). The slope for every 8-h interval was calculated, and the maximum value was determined. The extrapolation of the line with maximum slope to the background level of turbidity gave the lag time. The maximum turbidity for each replicate was taken as the maximum density. The obtained three values for each growth curve were treated in the same way as below.

For each "sample" A, the obtained value was normalized by that of the "standard" B. To minimize the influence of nonstatistical outliers that could arise due to gross errors in sample preparation and handling (e.g. robot or BioScreen C malfunction), the 32 replicates were divided into 4 groups according to their positions on the honey comb well plate (group 1: columns 1 and 2; …, group 4: columns 7 and 8). In each group, the median of the eight values was calculated and then the four medians were averaged to obtain the value for a given plate and its standard deviation.

Altogether, nine independent 32-replicate experiments were performed for each D content point and six experiments per each D point for adapted bacteria. To compensate for small systematic errors of measurement (e.g., differences in the geometry of the honeycomb wells, position-dependent sensitivity of the BioScreen C detector, etc.), the obtained average values of the maximum growth rate, lag time as well as the maximum density within each experiment were normalized to that of the sample with terrestrial D composition (156 ppm). The final result was obtained when the average of $9\times4=36$ ($6\times4=24$ for adapted bacteria) median values, and the corresponding standard error, were calculated. Since after normalization, the values for terrestrial composition were all unities, the p-values for non-terrestrial compositions were calculated using two-tailed, paired Student's t-test comparing the relative value R and its inverse 1/R.

Results and Discussion

High enrichment (50% D)

To learn the behavior of the growth parameters at high enrichment, bacteria were grown first at 50% D. The growth curve showed significant deviation from the normal (Figure 1), with the growth rate reduced by ca. 5%, maximum density increased by ca. 15% and the lag phase extended by almost 40% (Figure S2). While reduction in the growth rate and lag time extension were expected based on abundant previous research, the increase in maximum density was surprising: at adverse growth conditions, the maximum density usually follows the declining growth rate trend. The increase in maximum density at 50% D, or at least the magnitude of the increase, could be overestimated by the optical density measurements if the optical properties of the deuterated bacteria are different than that of bacteria with normal D content. Indeed, literature suggests that the size and shape of the bacteria may be quite distorted when grown in a highly deuterated media, especially in the beginning of growth [3,4,7]. If this is the case, and the maximum density at 50% D is overestimated, then the growth rate reduction at 50% D may be underestimated in our measurements. However, both these possible effects should be relatively small at <10% D, and especially at <1% D. Besides, our prime goal was to identify the lowest concentration of deuterium at which biological effects become detectable. Thus we did not make any corrections for these hypothetical effects in low-enrichment measurements.

Low enrichment (<10% D)

Growth behavior of *E. coli* in minimal media under ten different content of deuterium (including 156 ppm, 0.03%, 0.06%, 0.1%, 0.25%, 0.5%, 1%, 2%, 4%, 8%) were investigated, starting with 156 ppm of deuterium (terrestrial condition) and increasing the content of deuterium by a factor of 2 until ca. 10% D is reached. In each run of the BioScreen C instrument, *E. coli* was grown in minimal media on two honey comb well plates each containing wells with two different contents of deuterium, one always being the normal D content (156 ppm), giving 32 replicates for each plate (*vide infra*). This way, five runs were required to cover the entire range of deuterium content, which constituted one experiment.

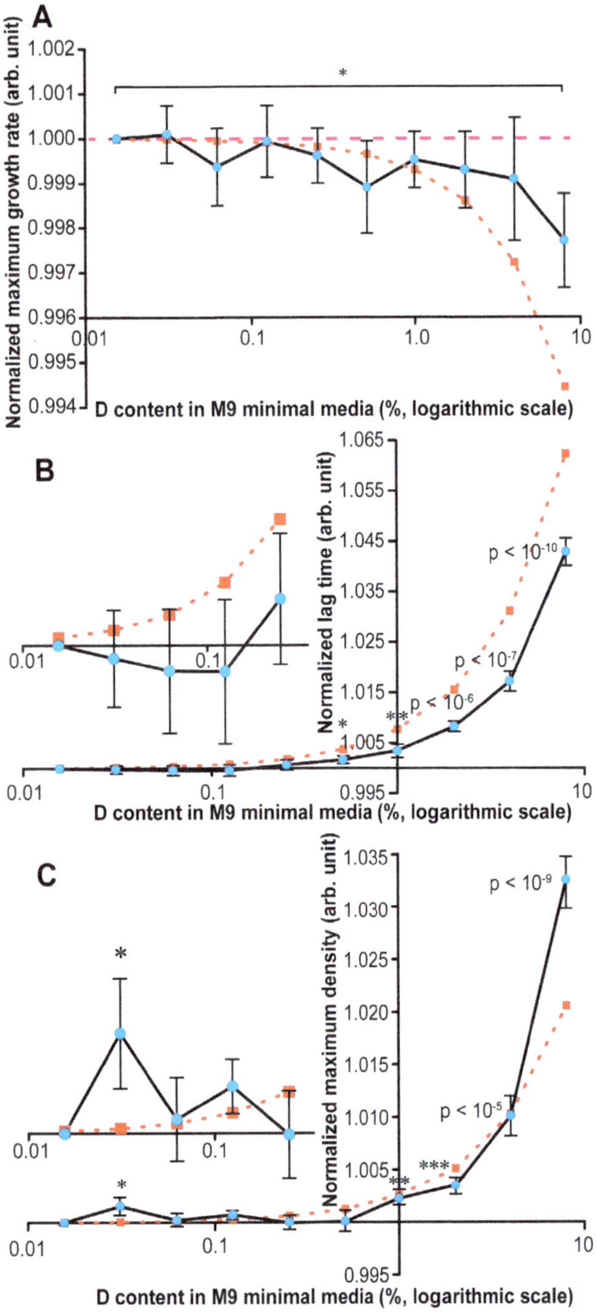

Figure 3. Maximum growth rate, lag time, maximum density of *E. coli* grown in minimal media. (**A**) Blue circles: maximum growth rate of *E. coli* grown in M9 minimal media normalized by that at normal deuterium content of 156 ppm. * denotes $p<0.05$, ** - $p<0.005$, etc. Brown squares: predicted maximum growth rate calculated according to the maximum growth rate of *E. coli* grown in 50% of deuterium. (**B**) Blue circles: lag time of *E. coli* grown in M9 minimal media normalized by that at terrestrial content of deuterium from 156 ppm (terrestrial value) to 8%. Inset shows a zoom-in of the ultralow enrichment region. Brown squares: predicted lag time calculated according to the lag time of *E. coli* grown in 50% of deuterium. (**C**) Blue circles: maximum density of *E. coli* grown in M9 minimal media normalized by that at terrestrial deuterium content from 156 ppm (terrestrial value) to 8%. Inset shows a zoom-in of the ultralow enrichment region. Brown squares: predicted maximum density calculated according to maximum density of *E. coli* grown in 50% of deuterium.

Figure 3A shows the normalized maximum growth rate. The curve is trending downwards, but only at the highest enrichment the statistical significance at $p<0.05$ is reached. The observed trend significantly (by a factor of 4) lags behind the linear extrapolation of the 50% D results to low-enrichment levels (i.e., a 5% slower growth at 50% D means growth rate ≈1–0.001*%D).

In contrast, the lag phase curve (Figure 3B) fluctuates at ultralow enrichment levels slightly below the normal level. But after 0.1% D, the lag time increases dramatically, reaching statistical significance at 0.5% D. The curve lags behind the linear prediction by a factor of two. Even if linear extrapolation is made based on 8% D results instead of 50% D, the actual trend remains below the predicted one.

The maximum density curve (Figure 3C) shows surprising behavior: at the lowest enrichment level of 0.03% D amounting to only twice the normal D content, there is a small but significant ($p<0.05$) peak corresponding to a ≈0.16% higher density. The increase in the maximum density continues at higher D content, and vanishes at 0.25% D, to increase again above the significance level at 1% D. For the interval 0.2%–4% D, the maximum density curves lags behind the linear extrapolation, but at 8% D it actually exceeds it, increasing by 3.2% compared to the predicted 2.4%.

Summarizing the above observations, the effects typical for high D enrichment (slower growth, longer lag and higher maximum density), start to be noticeable at 0.5% D. This is a surprisingly high threshold, given that the 0.05% precision of the measurements would allow us to detect with statistical significance as small changes in growth parameters as 0.1%. According to the 50% D results, if the effect of D content on *E. coli* growth was linear, the expected detection threshold for biological effects would be around 0.1–0.2% D. That no significant change was detected at 0.25% D indicates the presence of a previously unreported threshold for isotopic phenomena. Moreover, the results hint on the existence of an "inverted region" at ultralow enrichment levels with statistically significant fluctuations in the direction of higher comfort, rather than adverse reaction as at ≥0.5% D. The existence of such a region would be in agreement with previous studies, even though many of the actually found much bigger effects than were observed in our experiments [12–22].

Validity of ultralow enrichment effect

The biological effect at <0.25% D in our study does not result from one or two aberrantly high measurements: in six out of nine constituent experiments, the maximum density was enhanced compared to normal % D. Another way to test the validity is to investigate the variability of measurements: usually, stronger biological effect results in larger variability. Indeed, the standard error of the maximum density determination at normal D content was 0.05%, while for 8% D it was five times larger, 0.25%. At 0.03% D, the corresponding standard error was 0.08%, which is the highest value for all measurements below 1% D. Also for the other two growth parameters, the maximum growth rate and the lag phase, the standard error at 0.03% D was higher than at normal conditions. Curiously, of all the data points, only 0.03% D shows an increase (however slight and statistically insignificant) in the maximum growth rate on Figure 3A. Another supporting evidence in favor of the opposite trend at ultralow enrichment is the fact that, at such enrichment, all three growth parameters lag behind the trend extrapolated from 50% D measurements, and two out of three (lag phase and maximum density) – of the trend extrapolated from 8% D results. These results speak in favor of the validity of the biological effect at 0.03% D.

The effect at the ultralow enrichment levels, assuming it is real, in unlike that at high enrichments. While the growth rate does not change, the lag phase shortens (although insignificantly in statistical sense), and the maximum density increases above the expected trend. Overall, it's a signature of growth in a more comfortable environment. In contrast, at high enrichments the signature is definitely that of a more hostile environment, with a very long lag phase and slower growth. What is common for both regimes, though, is the increased maximum density, but the origins of this effect may differ (*vide supra*).

How to explain the presumed effect of ultralow deuterium enrichment on bacterial growth? The previous research has not produced any convincing explanation [12–22], which probably was one of the factors why this research has largely became forgotten. One of possible explanations is the effect of hormesis. The concept of hormesis suggests that, at low dosages, the effects of adverse agents (e.g. chemical toxins or radiation) can be stimulating for growth. Hormetic effect on *E. coli* growth has previously been detected at low concentrations of chemical toxins [26]. However, the size of the effect in our study (≈0.16% in maximum density) is disproportionally large compared to the enrichment degree (0.032% D, or +0.016% D compared to normal composition, Figure S3), which speaks against the role of hormesis in the studied situation.

Adaptation to ultralow enrichment conditions

Hormesis is usually explained by activation of protecting mechanisms that, in effect, boost the growth at low concentrations of adverse agents. But gradual adaptation of the organism to slightly adverse environment should increase the threshold for activation and thus reduce this effect. To test this hypothesis, we grew bacteria for ca. 400 generations at normal isotopic conditions, 0.03% D, 0.25% D and 1% D, changing the media every 12 hours (Figure S4). After that, the growth parameters in the same media were measured, using as control the same adapted bacteria growing at normal isotopic conditions. Adaptation has dramatically reduced the lag time from 10–11 h to 6–7 h, and increased the maximum growth rate as well as the maximum density by about 15–20% (Figure S5). The directions of the changes in growth parameters are consistent with bacteria feeling much more comfortable in the minimal media after adaptation.

In the isotopically different environment, the growth rate has increased by 0.10–0.15% at ultralow enrichment ($p<0.05$ at 0.25%, Figure 4A), while the lag time has increased insignificantly by the same amount (Figure 4B). The maximum density has shown most significant changes of ca. 0.2% ($p<0.05$, Figure 4C) at 0.25% D, but was elevated also at 0.03% D. Overall, two out of three parameters showed statistically significant changes characteristic for better adaptation in isotopically different environment compared to normal media. Note that at 1% D this effect disappeared.

Strictly speaking, deuterium is not toxic for *E. coli*, as this organism can grow at very high enrichment levels. Even at 50% D, the maximum growth rate is only slightly (5%) lower than at normal conditions. Therefore, deuterium enriched medium is more correctly characterized as an unusual, rather than toxic, environment. Thus the applicability of the hormetic explanation to ultralow deuterium enrichment is questionable.

An alternative to hermetic explanation could be provided by the isotopic resonance hypothesis [27]. Briefly, the hypothesis suggests that, at certain isotopic compositions of the elements C, H, N and O that together compose ≥96% of the living matter of prokaryotes and many eukaryotes, the rate of all chemical and biochemical reactions, including the bacterial growth, should increase. Normal terrestrial isotopic compositions are very close to one such resonance. The existing small deviation from the perfect

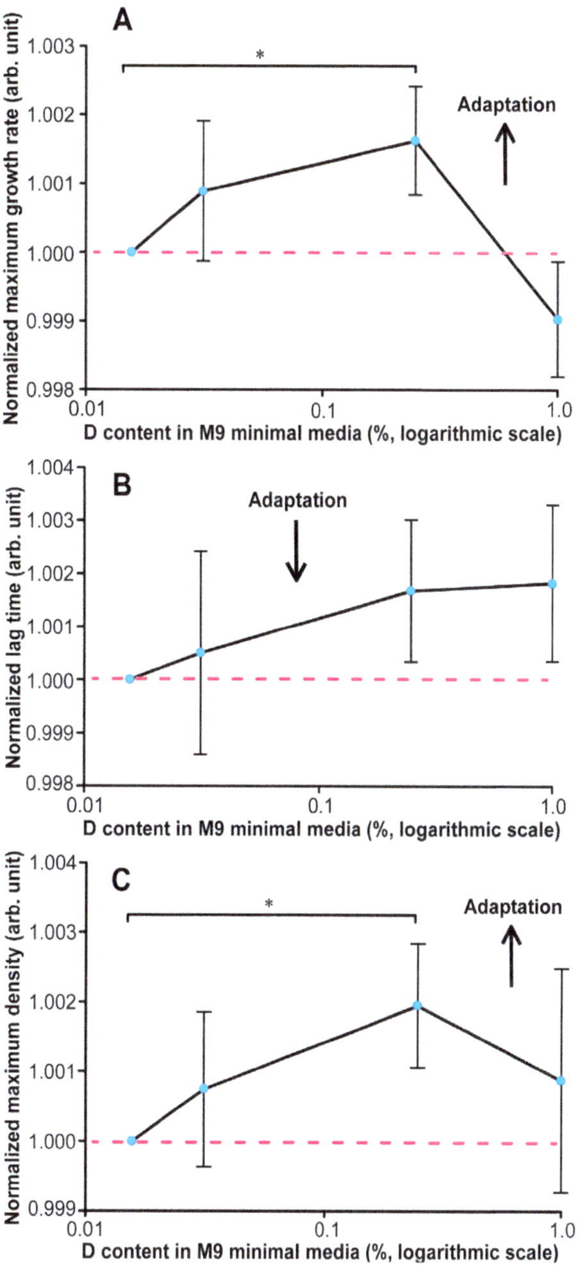

Figure 4. Maximum growth rate, lag time and maximum density of aged *E. coli*. (**A**) Maximum growth rate of aged *E. coli* grown in M9 minimal media with ultralow composition of deuterium. * denotes $p<0.05$. (**B**) Lag time of aged *E. coli* grown in M9 minimal media with ultralow composition of deuterium. (**C**) Maximum density of aged *E. coli* grown in M9 minimal media with ultralow composition of deuterium. * denotes $p<0.05$.

resonance, suggests the hypothesis, can be corrected by "tuning" the isotopic composition of any of the elements C, H, N and O. After such tuning the growth rate of all organisms should slightly increase. The size of the effect is not predicted, but the required value of the D content for the perfect "terrestrial" isotopic resonance is close to 0.03% [28]. Since the isotopic composition of water inside the *E. coli* bacteria has much lower deuterium enrichment compared to the growth media [29], the resonance conditions should occur in the region 0.03–0.06% of D. Such an agreement between the predictions of the hypothesis and the experiment could be spurious, but it receives strong support from earlier studies [12–22]. Taken together, these results suggest that the growth behavior of *E. coli* and other organisms at ultralow enrichment levels well worth exploring further, using even more precise measurements.

Conclusions

Here we studied the growth behavior of *E. coli* at low enrichment levels of deuterium, and found that the adverse effects characteristic for high enrichment levels become noticeable at 0.5% D, which is several times higher level than expected given the 0.05% precision of our measurements. This discrepancy highlights the "buffering capacity" of living organisms that can partially compensate the adverse nature of the isotopically altered growth medium by reduced incorporation levels of heavy isotopes [28]. On the other hand, there seems to be a small but significant fingerprint of more comfortable environment at an ultralow enrichment level of 0.03% D. This behavior, which begs for additional verification by more precise measurements, could be explained by both hormesis as well as the isotopic resonance hypothesis. The latter theory predicts the exact location of the "resonance" at ≈0.03%–0.06% D, which is in a broad agreement with sporadic but multiple earlier reports [12–22].

Supporting Information

Figure S1 Sample configuration on the honey comb well plates.

Figure S2 Maximum growth rate, maximum density and lag time of *E. coli* grown in M9 minimal media with deuterium content of 50% normalized by that at normal deuterium content of 156 ppm. ** is equivalent to $p<0.005$.

Figure S3 Change of maximum density per percentage of deuterium for *E. coli* grown in M9 minimal media with content of deuterium from 156 ppm (terrestrial value) to 8%. * is equivalent to $p<0.05$, ** is equivalent to $p<0.005$, etc.

Figure S4 Workflow of adapting the bacteria to growth media.

Figure S5 Growth curves of *E. coli* grown in minimal media with 156 ppm of D before and after adaptation.

Acknowledgments

The authors thank the Swedish Research Council for funding this work.

Author Contributions

Conceived and designed the experiments: RAZ XX. Performed the experiments: XX. Analyzed the data: XX. Contributed reagents/materials/analysis tools: XX. Wrote the paper: XX RAZ.

References

1. Urey HC, Brickwedde FG, Murphy GM (1932) A hydrogen isotope of mass 2. Phys Rev 39: 164–166.
2. Koletzko B, Sauerwald T, Demmelmair H (1997) Safety of stable isotope use. Eur J Pediatr 156: S12–S17.
3. Katz JJ, Crespi HL, Hasterlik RJ, Thomson JF, Finkel AJ (1957) Some observations on biological effects of deuterium, with special reference to effects on neoplastic processes. J Natl Cancer Inst 18: 641–658.
4. Katz JJ, Crespi HL (1971) Isotope effects in biological systems. In: Collins, C J, Bowman NS, editor. Isotope effects in chemical reactions. New York: Van Nostrand Reinhold Co. 286–363.
5. Rokop S, Gajda L, Parmerter S, Crespi HL, Katz JJ (1969) Purification and characterization of fully deuterated enzymes. Biochim Biophys Acta 191: 707–715.
6. Paliy O, Bloor D, Brockwell D, Gilbert P, Barber J (2003) Improved methods of cultivation and production of deuteriated proteins from E. coli strains grown on fully deuteriated minimal medium. J Appl Microbiol 94: 580–586.
7. Katz JJ, Crespi HL (1966) Deuterated organisms: Cultivation and uses. Science 151: 1187–1194.
8. Ernest B, Rittenberg D (1960) Anomalous growth of microorganisms produced by changes in isotopes in their environment. Proc Natl Acad Sci 46: 777–782.
9. Fowler EB, Adams WH, Christenson CW, Kollman VH, Buchholz JR (1972) Kinetic studies of C. pyrenoidosa using 94% 13C CO2. Biotechnol Bioeng 14: 819–829.
10. Uphaus RA, Flaumenhaft E, Katz JJ (1967) A living organism of unusual isotopic composition sequential and cumulative replacement of stable isotopes in Chlorella vulgaris. Biochim Biophys Acta 141: 625–632.
11. Kreuzer-Martin HW, Jarman KH (2007) Stable isotope ratios and forensic analysis of microorganisms. Appl Environ Microbiol 73: 3896–3908.
12. Barnes TC (1933) A possible physiological effect of the heavy isotope of H in water. J Am Chem Soc 55: 4332–4333.
13. Barnes TC (1933) Further experiments on the physiological effect of heavy water and of ice water. J Am Chem Soc 55: 5059–5060.
14. Barnes TC, Larson EJ (1935) The influence of heavy water of low concentration on Spirogyra, Planaria and enzyme action. Protoplasma 22: 431–443.
15. Barnes TC (1934) The effect of heavy water of low concentration on Euglena. Science 79: 370.
16. Lockemann G, Leunig H (1934) Über den Einfluβ des "schweren Wassers" auf die biologischen Vorgänge bei Bakterien. Berichte der Dtsch Chem Gesellschaft (A B Series) 67: 1299–1302.
17. Curry J, Partt R, Trelease SF (1935) Does dilute heavy water influence biological processes? Science 81: 275–277.
18. Lobyshev VI, Tverdislov VA, Vogel J, Iakovenko LV (1978) Activation of Na, K-ATPase by small concentrations of D_2O, inhibition by high concentrations. Biofizika 23: 390–391.
19. Lobyshev VI, Fogel' Iu, Iakovenko LV, Rezaeva MN, Tverdislov VA (1982) D_2O as a modifier of ionic specificity of Na, K-ATPase. Biofizika 27: 595–603.
20. Lobyshev VI (1983) Activating influence of heavy water of small concentration on the regeneration of hydroid polyp obelia geniculata. Biofizika 28: 666–668.
21. Somlyai G, Jancsó G, Jákli G, Vass K, Barna B, et al. (1993) Naturally occurring deuterium is essential for the normal growth rate of cells. FEBS Lett 317: 1–4.
22. Nikitin DI, Oranskaya MN, Lobyshev VI (2003) Specificity of bacterial response to variation of isotopic composition of water. Biofizika 48: 678–682.
23. Hammel SC, East K, Shaka AJ, Rose MR, Shahrestani P (2013) Brief early-life non-specific incorporation of deuterium extends mean life span in drosophila melanogaster without affecting fecundity. Rejuvenation Res 16: 98–104.
24. Sambrook J, Russell DW (2001) Molecular cloning: A laboratory manual. 3rd ed. New York: Cold Spring Harbor Laboratory Press.
25. Madigan M, Martinko J, Stahl D, Clark D (2012) Brock biology of microorganisms. 13th ed. San Francisco: Pearson.
26. Calabrese EJ, Hoffmann GR, Stanek EJ, Nascarella MA (2010) Hormesis in high-throughput screening of antibacterial compounds in E coli. Hum Exp Toxicol 29: 667–677.
27. Zubarev RA, Artemenko KA, Zubarev AR, Mayrhofer C, Yang H, et al. (2010) Early life relict feature in peptide mass distribution. Cent Eur J Biol 5: 190–196.
28. Zubarev RA (2011) Role of stable isotopes in life-testing isotopic resonance hypothesis. Genomics Proteomics Bioinformatics 9: 15–20.
29. Kreuzer-Martin HW, Lott MJ, Ehleringer JR, Hegg EL (2006) Metabolic processes account for the majority of the intracellular water in log-phase Escherichia coli cells as revealed by hydrogen isotopes. Biochemistry 45: 13622–13630.

7

Dancing Bees Improve Colony Foraging Success as Long-Term Benefits Outweigh Short-Term Costs

Roger Schürch[1]*, Christoph Grüter[2¤]

1 Laboratory of Apiculture and Social Insects, School of Life Sciences, University of Sussex, Falmer, United Kingdom, 2 Departamento de Biologia da Faculdade de Filosofia, Ciências e Letras de Ribeirão Preto, Universidade de São Paulo, Ribeirão Preto, São Paulo, Brazil

Abstract

Waggle dancing bees provide nestmates with spatial information about high quality resources. Surprisingly, attempts to quantify the benefits of this encoded spatial information have failed to find positive effects on colony foraging success under many ecological circumstances. Experimental designs have often involved measuring the foraging success of colonies that were repeatedly switched between oriented dances *versus* disoriented dances (i.e. communicating vectors *versus* not communicating vectors). However, if recruited bees continue to visit profitable food sources for more than one day, this procedure would lead to confounded results because of the long-term effects of successful recruitment events. Using agent-based simulations, we found that spatial information was beneficial in almost all ecological situations. Contrary to common belief, the benefits of recruitment increased with environmental stability because benefits can accumulate over time to outweigh the short-term costs of recruitment. Furthermore, we found that in simulations mimicking previous experiments, the benefits of communication were considerably underestimated (at low food density) or not detected at all (at medium and high densities). Our results suggest that the benefits of waggle dance communication are currently underestimated and that different experimental designs, which account for potential long-term benefits, are needed to measure empirically how spatial information affects colony foraging success.

Editor: Nicolas Chaline, Universidade de São Paulo, Brazil

Funding: RS was funded by the Swiss National Science Foundation (Grant PA00P3_139731). CG was funded by a Science without Borders fellowship from the Brazilian National Council for Scientific and Technological Development (CNPq, Process-number: 400664/2012-7) and an Ambizione fellowship from the Swiss National Science Foundation (PZ00P3_142628/1). The funders had no role in study design, data collection and analysis, decision to publish, or preparation of the manuscript.

Competing Interests: The authors have declared that no competing interests exist.

* Email: R.Schuerch@sussex.ac.uk

¤ Current address: Department of Ecology and Evolution, Biophore, University of Lausanne, Lausanne, Switzerland

Introduction

Colony success in social insects often depends on the colony's ability to mobilize workers and allocate them to where work is needed [1-4]. Accordingly, insects have evolved different ways to communicate in these situations, such as when nestmates must be recruited to valuable resources [1,2]. One of the most remarkable means of recruitment is the honeybee waggle dance. Foragers perform this dance-like behavior inside the nest after finding a profitable food source or on a swarm during nest-hunting to advertise suitable nest-sites [3,5-8]. Other foragers following a waggle dance learn the location and are subsequently able to fly to the area of the food source [8–12], where they use additional visual and olfactory information to localize the food [6,8,13,14].

Only recently have attempts been made to quantify empirically the colony level benefits of this spatial information [15–19]. Surprisingly, these studies found that colonies would often not benefit from spatial communication [16–19]. For example, Donaldson-Matasci and Dornhaus [17] tested the effect of spatial communication in five different habitats, but found a positive effect of communication only in one. Dornhaus & Chittka [18] found benefits only in a tropical habitat, but not in temperate European habitats. These findings suggest that the benefits of spatial information strongly depend on the spatiotemporal distribution of food sources, a conclusion that is in agreement with theoretical studies [20–22]. Recruitment by waggle dances is costly in terms of time and energy [21,23,24] and it is thus conceivable that these costs outweigh the benefits under certain conditions, for example when food sources are easy to find by independent search (scouting).

However, the apparent absence of benefits resulting from spatial information use in many habitats could also be the result of confounding effects caused by the experimental designs used to quantify these benefits. In previous studies, researchers took advantage of the fact that honeybees are unable to perform oriented dances on a horizontal comb with no or only diffuse light [16–19]. It is thus possible to create colonies with oriented (with spatial information; SI) or disoriented (no direction information; NI) dances and compare the foraging success of colonies in these two conditions. Importantly, in these studies, colonies were kept in one condition for relatively short time periods (2 or 3 days in [16–18]; a variable number of days with a mean of ~12 days in [19]) and repeatedly switched between the two experimental conditions (SI vs. NI), presumably to use paired statistical tests.

If a bee that was recruited on the last day of the SI treatment returns to that food source on the following day, the food she collects on that day will be added to the NI treatment, even though her success was a consequence of acquiring spatial information during the SI treatment. Thus, the continued availability of food sources combined with "site fidelity" (persistency) leads to confounded results and makes the interpretation of such data challenging. This seems particularly important since flower patches can remain in bloom for weeks or even months [25], and honeybees often return to the same foraging sites for days and up to 3 weeks [6,8,26–34].

Here we explored, using an agent-based simulation model, whether there is a benefit to the use of spatial information over longer periods of time than previously explored. We hypothesized that forager persistency causes long-term benefits of successful recruitment events, and therefore the benefits of spatial information might have been underestimated in experimental designs such as those used in empirical studies. Furthermore, we hypothesized that the degree to which results are confounded depends on various factors, including the duration of the experimental period, the longevity of food patches, the density of food sources, and the size of the colony.

Model Description

The present model is a spatially explicit agent-based simulation model (ABM) of two types of agents in a foraging context, scouts and recruits. We used NetLogo 4.1.3 to implement the model (Text S1), and we follow the "Overview, Design Concepts, and Details" (ODD) protocol in our description of it below [35,36].

Purpose

We explored how potential long-term effects of spatial communication by means of waggle dances affect honeybee colony success in different environments. We then tested how different experimental designs that were used previously to measure empirically the benefits of spatial communication [16–19] affect foraging success of our virtual colonies in different environments. Our model shared many parameters with previous models, but was different in two key aspects. First, rather than exploring the effects of spatial communication during a few hours [20] or days [22], we monitored colonies during 48 days, allowing us to explore long-term effects of spatial communication. Second, recruits had a high probability of returning to profitable food sources on subsequent days (Figure S1). This assumption is well established by empirical research [29,30,33] – bees can even persistently visit unrewarding food sources up to 7 days [37].

Entities, state variables and scale

Our agents were located on a two-dimensional square grid with 201×201 patches. The agents' nest was located on the center patch. Every other patch on the grid could either be void or contain suitable forage for our agents. Food patches were of variable quality (Table 1) and lasted for a limited number of days.

The population of agents ($N_{default}$ = 300) consisted of two groups, the scouts ($N_{default}$ = 30) and the recruits ($N_{default}$ = 270). We used a default colony size of 300 agents, but we also tested other colony sizes to explore if results are sensitive to colony size. Colony size had no effect on the benefits of communication in a previous model [22] and was chosen to be similar to colony size in [38]. Honeybee scouts usually represent 5–25% of all foragers [3]. They search for food source locations without following waggle dances and have a high probability to abandon even rewarding food sources and search for new ones [39]. Scouts could assume any of six states: idle in the colony, scouting for food sources, feeding at a food source, returning to the colony, recruiting of idle foragers to the newly discovered food source, returning to the nest without having discovered food. Recruits decoded waggle dances to find a food patch, but they could also scout (Table 1) if they were unable to find a dancing bee [40]. Recruits could adopt any of 8 states: idle in the nest, idly waiting to be recruited, flying to food source, feeding on food source, returning to colony after feeding, recruiting new idle foragers, scouting for forage, returning to the colony without having discovered food.

Simulations were run in discrete time steps (t). We choose the model parameters (Table 1) such that one time step in a simulation corresponded to approximately 10 s real time, so that each simulated day was t_{day} = 8640 time steps long, with days starting at 6:00 in the morning. The simulated world allowed foraging when the following condition was true: $\sin\left((2\cdot\pi\cdot\frac{t}{t_{day}})\cdot\frac{180}{\pi}\right) > 0.1$. Conditions were therefore suitable between 6:23 and 17:37 real time. There was no change of foraging time with the progression of a simulation run (no seasonal change), and all days were assumed to have weather suitable for the agents to forage all day long. Often plants offer nectar during the better part of the day, but in varying amounts and qualities [41]. With our parameters (Table 1), the width of a patch corresponded to ca. 100 m, e.g. a group of trees or a flower field, and the world expanded 10 km from the nest patch. No foraging occured on the central patch. This means that our agents could not exploit food sources that were closer than 50 m to the nest. The agents could occupy any specific location on the two-dimensional plane (i.e. they were not restricted to move on a lattice) at every point in time.

Process overview and scheduling

Each simulation experiment was preceded by a 3 day non-experimental phase where a colony of agents learned about the foraging patches surrounding the nest. Only then did the 48 days experimental phase start. Thus, in total each simulation run lasted 51 days, or 440,640 time steps.

At the beginning of each simulation run and every subsequent morning, idle scouts left the nest with a probability p_{Exit}, and idle recruits waiting for food locations to be communicated to them (dances) left the nest with a probability p_{RS} and started scouting. We chose p_{Exit} relatively high, so that scouts left the hive early in the morning [39]. Successful scouts or scouting recruits fed on patches that offered forage, and then returned to the nest. After unloading, they could communicate the location of the food source in a ritualized dance to N_{Dance} recruits, each of which had a probability of p_{Dance} to learn the food source. N_{Dance} = 1 and p_{Dance} = 0.25 were chosen so that each dance had a 25% probability to recruit a forager to the advertised food patch (empirically determined values usually range from 0.1 to 1.0; [22,23,42–44]). The probability to dance p_d depended on the quality of the visited foraging patch q_{Patch} and the distance to this patch (Figure S1), as well as on the current influx of returned foragers (scouts N_{rs} and recruits N_{rr}, see Figure S2). A higher influx of foragers decreased the probability to dance [3,45,46]. On days when dances were disoriented (NI), dances animated recruits to scout for themselves instead, with N_{Dance} = 1 and p_{Dance} = 1, i.e., one recruit per dance left the hive. Scouts and recruits became idle once finished with dancing, from which state they could then leave the nest again with p_{Exit}. Scouts consequently searched for new food sources, while recruits re-visited the previously visited food source for the rest of the day or until they died.

Every morning recruits with foraging experience decided whether to continue visiting the food source they had been visiting

Table 1. Overview of the model parameters and the values used in our simulations.

		Default values	Other values tested
N_{Scouts}	Number of scouts in the agent population	30	60, 120
$N_{Recruits}$	Number of recruits in the agent population	270	540, 1080
t_{Day}	Time steps per day	8640 time steps	
t_{Init}	Time before experimental switches start	3 days	
t_{Switch}	Duration of experimental switches	3 days	2, 12 days
p_{Exit}	Probability of a scout to leave the nest per time step [39]	0.815	0.01, 0.1, 0.5, 0.8
p_{RS}	Probability that idle recruits will leave the nest and scout per time step [22]	0.00009	
d_{Patch}	Density of patches	0.05	0.01, 0.1
a_{max}	Maximum age of patches	14 days	1, 7, 28
y_{Patch}	Yield of a foraging trip [82]	50 mg	
$t_{Patch} \pm \sigma_t$	Mean ± SD nectar handling time on patch [28,83]	180 ± 60 time steps	
t_{Nest}	Nectar handling time in the nest [84]	6 time steps	
$q_{Patch} \pm \sigma_q$	Mean ± SD nectar quality [51]	1 ± 0.2 mol/l	
v	Agent speed	0.7 patch width/time step	
$\mu_{Lévi}$	Lévi flight parameter [48]	2.4	1, 2, 3, 4
c_{Rest}	Energy costs per time step t when resting [85,86]	0.04861 J	
c_{Move}	Energy costs per time step t when moving [22,85]	$9 \times c_{Rest}$ J	
m	Mortality per time step t [86]	0.000007	
E_{mol}	Energy per mol sugar	5645000 J	
$c_{Recruit}$	Energy costs incurred by recruits [22]	325 J	0 J
N_{Dance}	Number of recruits following a dance of a scout	1	
p_{Dance}	Probability of dance success [43,44,87]	0.25	

on the previous day or became idle recruits. The probability to abandon the food source depended on the quality of the forage, as well as on the distance to the patch (Figure S1), as did the probability to dance. If they did not abandon the patch, they left the nest with the probability p_{Exit}. If the patch had vanished overnight, the recruits returned to the nest and became idle recruits.

Each time step, every agent had a probability of m to die. If an agent died, a completely equivalent new agent was born in the nest. This agent lacked foraging experience, and started out as an idle scout or recruit.

Each day forage patches with an age that exceeded a_{max} were replaced by empty patches. And empty patches could become forage patches with a probability d_{Patch} and quality q_{Patch}.

Experiments 1: benefits of SI with varying food density and experimental designs. In the first sets of experiments we tested the agents in an environment with high ($d_{Patch} = 0.1$), medium ($d_{Patch} = 0.05$) and low food density ($d_{Patch} = 0.01$). Analyzing the emergent foraging distances from model runs confirmed that these distributions led to naturally realistic median foraging distances between approx. 0.5–2 km [3,47]. In each of the food densities, we performed model runs with colonies having either no switches, or 2-day, 3-day or 12-day cycles. In the no switch case, after the initial 3 days of information gathering, the colonies were allocated to their respective state (NI or SI) and did not switch state for the remaining 48 days. In the treatments with switches, we ran equal amounts of simulation runs with SI or NI in the first cycle, and subsequently switched back and forth.

Experiments 2: benefits of SI with varying patch longevities and experimental designs. In the second set of experiments we fixed the food patches at the medium density $d_{Patch} = 0.05$. We ran simulations for patch longevity of a day ($a_{max} = 1$), a week ($a_{max} = 7$), 2 weeks ($a_{max} = 14$) and 4 weeks ($a_{max} = 28$). Like for the first set of experiments, we ran simulations with having either no switches between SI and NI states, or 2-day, 3-day or 12-day cycles.

Design concepts

The model mimicked a central place foraging situation. Honeybee workers collected their food from a variety of sources, and brought it back to the nest for storage. Our model implemented the core properties necessary to simulate central place foraging with spatial information about the food source. The energy a colony of agents could extract from the simulated world was an emergent property. This energy intake could be affected by other emergent properties, such as waiting times during interactions. The agents adapted to their environment in many ways. Agents could sense the environment for whether it was good to leave the nest, they could assess whether a food source wass good enough for dancing, and whether a food source was worth visiting the next day. The agents could learn about the spatial location of the food source they had visited, or they could learn such a location from a returned forager, that communicated the location *via* oriented dances. This communication was the only interaction between agents. Whether a patch became a foraging patch was stochastically determined, as was the quality of the forage on the patch. Stochasticity also played a role in agents to determine whether agents left the nest, whether they danced for a food source, whether they could learn the location of a food source, whether they abandoned a food source, or whether they died.

At the end of each day, the nest stores of energy were sampled, as well as the median distance at which foraging occurred.

Initialization

The patches, except the central nest patch, were randomly set to be foraging patches with a probability d_{Patch}, and with quality $q_{Patch} \pm \sigma_{qPatch}$. At initialization, the patch age was chosen to be uniformly distributed between 1 and $a_{\max}$. All scouts and recruits were initially set to be idle within the nest. The random number generator was initialized using the system's date-time.

Submodels

The Lévy flight. To mimic the random search of honeybees, the agents moved using an optimal Lévy flight routine [48]. The agents first turned uniform randomly into a direction before moving. If the length of a leg was 0, because the journey on that leg had not started yet, a new distance for that leg was calculated as $d_{Lévy} = e^{\ln a \cdot \frac{1}{1-\mu_{Lévy}}}$, where a was a uniform random variable drawn from the interval [0, 1) and a default $\mu_{Lévy} = 2.4$ [48]. For the next time steps, the agent would move on the randomly chosen trajectory, until it had flown $d_{Lévy}$.

The decision to dance or abandon food sources. Returned scouts and recruits could advertise the food source they had just visited with the dance, as long as the day still allowed for flying. For each time step, as long as the time spent unloading $t_{Unloading} < t_{Nest}$, the agent would decide whether to dance or not. We relied on Table 1 in [49] to determine the probability to dance for food sources of different energetic values at short foraging distances and on [50] to determine the relationship between the energetic value of a food source and the dancing probability at larger distances (up to several km, see Figure S1). Thus, the probability of dancing p_d was calculated to be depending on distance d and the quality of the food source q_{Patch}, $p_{qt} = \dfrac{0.956937}{1 + e^{\left(\frac{0.2721966 - \ln q_t}{0.2624014}\right)}}$, where $q_t = 1.02 + q_{Patch} - 0.04915919 - 2.851457 \cdot 10^{-5} \cdot d + 3.174098 \cdot 10^{-8} \cdot d^2$. The probabilifty of dancing further depended on the influx of other foragers, $p_{Influx} = \begin{cases} 1 - 0.035 \cdot N_{Influx} & N_{Influx} \leq 20 \\ 0.3 & N_{Influx} > 20 \end{cases}$, so that the final probability to dance was $p_d = p_{qt} \cdot p_{Influx}$ (see also Figure S2). Because recruits often need several excursions to find an advertised food source [23,24], they incurred a penalty in terms of energy consumption $c_{recruit} = 325\text{J}$ for locating the foraging patch in the field [22]. In case communication of the location was not allowed, recruits turned into scouting recruits without incurring the energy penalty.

Following Figure 6 in [51] we assumed that the shape of the curve of the relationship between food source profitability and dancing is the same as between food source profitability and abandonment of the food patch. The decision to abandon the patch was thus modelled analogously to the decision to dance or not. $p_a = 1 - \dfrac{0.956937}{1 + e^{\left(\frac{0.2721966 - \ln(q_t + 0.6687)}{0.2624014}\right)}}$, where q_t was calculated in exactly the same way as in the dance probability (Figure S1). The curve for the abandonment of the food source from one day to the next was approximated using data taken from [29], where a food source that led to a dance probability of 50% per foraging trip caused 80% of experienced foragers to return to this feeder the following day (Figure S1).

Sensitivity analyses

Due to stochasticity we performed $N = 12$ runs in each of our artificial experiments. We used standard errors (shown in Figures) to explore whether this number of runs was sufficient for interpretation without the need to perform additional statistical analysis.

To analyze how sensitive our model is to changes in parameters that were not under direct investigation, we chose default values presented in Table 1 for the duration of the experimental cycles t_{Switch}, the food density d_{Patch}, and the patch longevity $a_{\max}$. With these default values, we tested how the relative benefits of spatial information were influenced by colony size $N_{Scouts} + N_{Recruits}$, the scouts' probability to exit the hive p_{Exit}, the Lévi-flight parameter $\mu_{Lévi}$, and the energy costs of recruiting $c_{Recruit}$. None of these factors alter the main results presented in that paper.

Statistical methods

We used R to calculate means and standard errors per run or day [52]. In all cases, we ignored the 3 day acclimatization period when calculating means. To calculate means of the persistency of agents, we used the fitdistr function from the MASS package [53]. We assumed a Poisson distribution for the persistency.

Results

Experiments 1: switch durations, density and foraging success

When there is no switching between SI and NI, spatial information transfer improves colony foraging success at all food source densities. The benefits increase when food resources are at lower densities (Figure 1; +2.5% at high density and +21.6% at low density). For all densities, the lack of spatial information leads to smaller variance in the colony energy intake compared to the situation where spatial information is always available (Figure 1).

In contrast, when switching colonies back and forth between SI and NI states every 2 or 3 days, the benefit of the information transfer remain undetected in all situations except when food density is low (Figure 1). But even in this situation, the detected relative benefits of SI are substantially lower than in untreated colonies with SI (+4.4% and +5.4% vs. + 21.6%). Of the 3 experimental designs, the results most similar to the untreated condition come from colonies subjected to 12-day experimental periods. Here, colonies benefit almost as much when having SI (+ 6.6% compared to NI over all densities), as in untreated colonies (+ 8.8%). The explanation for the lower relative benefits in switch experiments can be seen in Figure 1: switching between experimental states causes considerable carry-over effects, so that the collected energy on the first day of a new cycle is strongly dominated by the previous cycle.

In our model, the difference between recruits and scouts in individually collected energy per day is higher at low food densities but diminishes at higher densities. At low food densities ($d_{Patch} = 0.01$) recruits have more than double the efficiency compared to scouts (236.1005 vs. 98.85329 $^{\text{J}}/_{\text{day}}$ per forager) when information transfer is allowed. The increased efficiency then diminishes at higher densities ($d_{Patch} = 0.05$, 243.8685 vs. 213.02885 $^{\text{J}}/_{\text{day}}$ per forager; $d_{Patch} = 0.1$, 250.1621 vs. 230.75986 $^{\text{J}}/_{\text{day}}$ per forager).

Experiments 2: switch durations, patch longevity and foraging success

Experiment 1 used the default patch longevity of 14 days. Experiment 2 explored the effect of environmental stability by

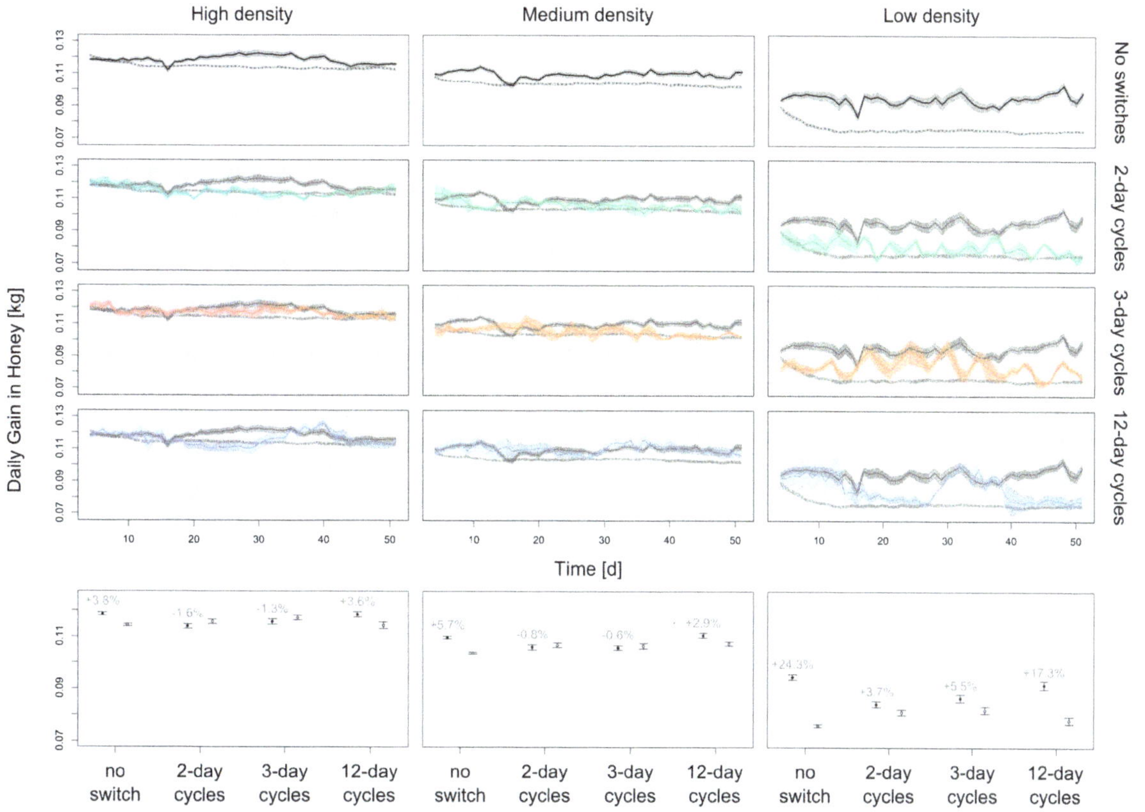

Figure 1. A comparison of foraging success measured as daily gain in honey under high, medium and low food densities, either with spatial information transfer (SI) or without spatial information transfer (NI). Model runs lasted 48 days after an initial period of 3 days SI (the 3 day acclimatization period is not shown). The first row shows the pure SI (solid black line) and NI (dotted black line) cases. These baselines are also shown for the model runs where switching between SI and NI occurred (rows 2–4, black solid and dotted lines). Rows 2–4 show the cases for SI (white background)/NI (grey background) cycles that last 2 days, 3 days or 12 days respectively. All the simulations shown here started with the SI treatment on day 4. The last row shows the aggregated simulation results (means ± s.e.) for the three food densities and SI/NI cycles (solid circles: SI, open circles: NI) including the second set of simulations that started with the NI treatment on day 4.

testing additional patch longevities at a medium food density. Surprisingly, the results show that the benefits of SI increase in untreated colonies as patch longevity increases. If patches only last 1 day, spatial dance information is even detrimental (−15.8%). But as patches last longer, colonies gain more from having spatial dance information (+11% for 28 days). Experiments with 2-day and 3-day experimental cycles provide very different results for all patch longevities, except for when patches last only for 1 day (Figure 2). If patches persist longer (≥ 7 days), colonies perform more or less equally well during SI and NI periods. Again, the best results are obtained using 12-day experimental cycles. But even in this situation the relative benefit of SI is less than half the benefit in the untreated colonies in a very stable environment (+11% vs. + 4.9%).

Recruitment success and, consequently, the energetic costs of recruitment are likely to be variable [22]. To test whether this affects our findings, we tested a situation with higher recruitment success ($p_{Dance} = 1$) and no recruitment costs ($c_{Recruit} = 0$) in a separate set of model runs. This could represent a situation in certain tropical habitats with many large and clustered food patches, where recruits locate advertised foraging sites quickly. The simulations show that SI is again beneficial and that the relative benefits of SI increase in a more stable environment (Figure 3; +5.8% when patches last for 7 days, +9.5% when patches last for 21 days), but the benefits of SI are again underestimated by a factor of 3.5 to 9.5 for 7 day patches and 21 day patches respectively when using 2-day experimental cycles.

The longevity of food patches also has an impact on the individual foragers. The longer patches last, the longer single agents can be persistent. The mean persistency of agents ranged from 1.008±0.004 day when patches lasted for a day to 2.842±0.0124 days when patches lasted for 28 days (Figure S3), but the maximum persistence was only limited by the patch longevities.

Sensitivity analyses

Qualitatively our main result, that switching hives between SI and NI treatments will obscure potential benefits of the dance, was robust under a wide range of parameters. The difference between SI and NI treatments were minimal for switching under a range of different colony sizes (Figure S4), differences in the random walk's Lévy parameter (Figure S5), or different probabilities for scouts to leave the hive (Figure S6).

Discussion

Spatial location information of waggle dancing bees increased colony foraging success under almost all simulated circumstances. Spatial information did not improve colony success when patches lasted just 1 day, which is unrealistic for most natural habitats [25,54–56]. The most surprising finding is that the relative benefits

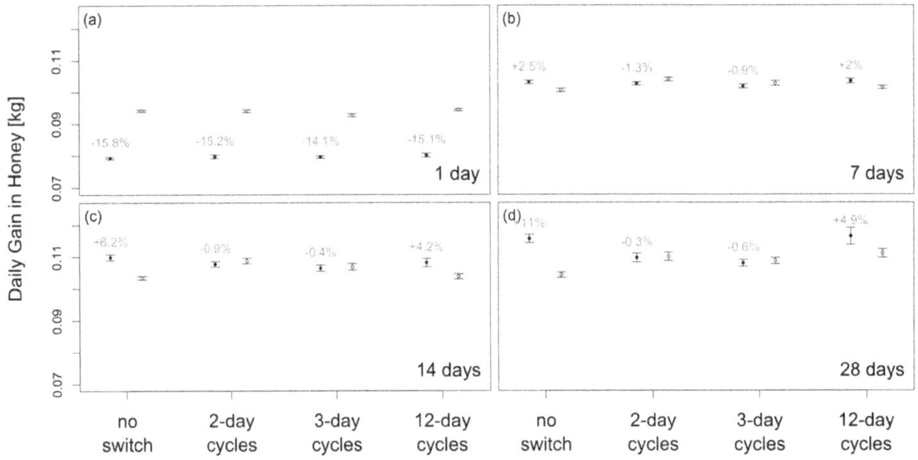

Figure 2. A comparison of foraging success measured as mean daily gain in honey (means ± s.e.) under varying patch longevities and with various intervals between experimental switches of spatial information transfer (SI) and no spatial information transfer (NI) treatments (no switches, 2-day cycles, 3-day cycles, 12-day cycles). The benefit of SI varies with patch longevity, with increasing benefits from one day (a), 7 days (b), 14 days (c), to 28 days (d). SI is more beneficial, if patches are relatively stable over time. Switching between SI and NI treatment hides the benefit of SI to a large degree (solid circle: SI, open circles: NI).

of spatial information increased as environmental stability increased (Figure 2). This contradicts the common assumption that dance information is most beneficial in an environment with ephemeral food sources [18,19,29,57].

A closer examination of our model and the existing literature suggests that our results of long term benefits of the dance are plausible. Recruitment in honeybees is costly [21,23,24]: recruits need to wait for a dancing bee [21], and they usually require several field excursions before locating the advertised food source after following a dance [23,58–60]. Thus, potential recruits incurred both energy and opportunity costs in our model. But after the advertised food source is located, the energetic returns are higher than for scouts. This result is consistent with empirical studies, which found that recruits tend to discover food sources of higher quality than scouts [23,24,60]. By dancing only for high quality food sources (see Figure S1 and [3,8]) foraging bees effectively filter information, which allows recruits to exploit selectively the best food sources known to the colony [3,61,62]. After successful recruitment, costs of continuing to visit the food patch are low as bees quickly locate the previously visited patches using route-memory [63,64], while benefits potentially remain high. The more stable the environment, the longer these benefits can accumulate. This is true even if there are short term fluctuations in a given patch's quality, such that it switches back and forth between profitable and non-profitable, because colonies with persistent individuals using private information can quickly decide which is the most profitable patch at a given time [65]. In contrast, if the environment completely changes (e.g., profitable patches become permanently unprofitable and vice versa), as in the case where patches only lasted for a day, recruits repeatedly have to pay the recruitment costs, while benefits remain short-lived.

One major difference between our model and previous models is our assumption that patches could last several days (and up to 4 weeks). Three lines of evidence suggest that this is a realistic assumption. First, it is known that flower patches in both tropical and temperate habitats often bloom for several days or even months [25,54–56,66]. Second, observations on naturally foraging honeybees show that foragers often return to the same patches for days and or even weeks [6,8,26,28–30,32–34]. Bees recruited by waggle dances are particularly likely to show site fidelity because food sources located by recruits are more profitable than those located by individually exploring bees [23,24] and profitability positively affects site fidelity [33,37]. In our model, foragers visited

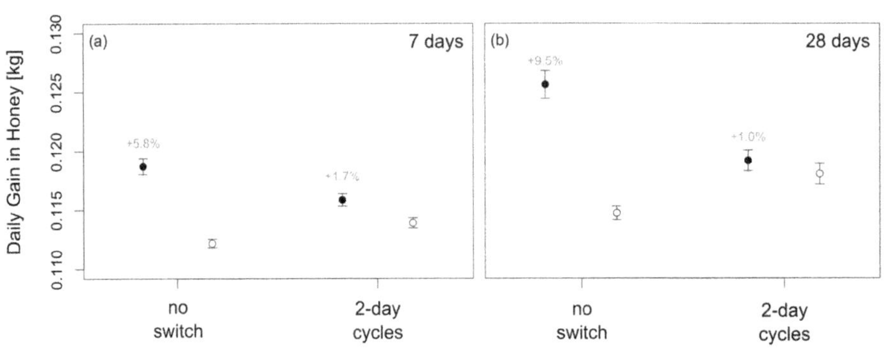

Figure 3. A comparison of foraging success measured as mean daily gain in honey (means ± s.e.) under the absence of costs to spatial information transfer (SI) and with SI, or no spatial information transfer (NI). The switching between SI and NI treatments masks the benefit of SI even if there are no costs to SI (solid circle: SI, open circles: NI).

the same food patch for an average of 1 to 2.8 days, depending on the longevity of food patches (Figure S3). Third, honeybees readily learn the time of day when food sources are most rewarding and return to feeding sites on subsequent days at the appropriate time of day [27,31,67,68]. This suggests that foragers are adapted to an environment where the spatiotemporal availability of the currently exploited food source is predictive for the next day. On the other hand, studies analyzing foraging locations by decoding waggle dances [3] show considerable daily changes in the locations that are advertised by dances. However, while such daily changes in dance maps inform us about the number of patches that receive increased exploitation (pp. 48 in [3]), they provide no information about how long individual foragers exploit patches. Clearly, the long-term foraging behavior of honeybee foragers in natural flower patches deserves further study.

Our findings help to explain the puzzling observation that experienced foragers following dances frequently ignore spatial waggle dance information [29,69–74]. Our results show that foragers should continue to visit familiar food sources if these remain profitable in order to avoid recruitment costs and the lower benefits of individual exploration [23,24,60]. Decoding the spatial information of dances that advertise alternative food patches would become more beneficial if the currently visited patch deteriorates and using memory no longer provides rewards [29,61,75]. Accordingly, a recent simulation study found that individuals do best if they rely on learned behaviors most of the time and tailor social information-use to circumstances when the environment changes [76]. It is not yet entirely clear why experienced foragers follow dances at all if they subsequently ignore the spatial information. It is possible that these foragers follow dances mainly to acquire up-to-date information about the time period a particular flower species produces rewards, rather than its location, and is therefore worth inspecting by other foragers at other locations [6,13,60,69,77].

We hypothesized that treating colonies by repeatedly switching between SI and NI states leads to confounded results and obscures the benefits of spatial information. Our simulations corroborate this hypothesis. When we used short treatment periods (2-day or 3-day cycles), as in previous empirical studies [16–18], we often found no improved collection performance during periods with spatial information (Figure 1 and 2), even in environments where colonies with continuous access to SI (no switch) outperformed those without SI. The best estimates of dance benefits were obtained with 12-day treatment periods (similar to [19]). However, even this experimental design lead to a considerable underestimation of the relative benefits of spatial information in some environmental situations (Figure 1 and 2). Our simulations suggest that the problems of repeatedly switching between SI and NI are caused by carry-over effects (Figure 1): the foraging success of colonies during the first days of a new treatment is affected by the foraging success during the last days of the previous treatment (Figure 1). It takes a few days before these carry-over effects are no longer apparent. Allowing for site-fidelity, foragers collecting at a good food source have a high probability to continue visiting this food sources irrespective of treatment changes. Hence, colonies newly switched to the NI state will initially perform well because foragers continue to visit the high quality food sources to which they were recruited by waggle dances during SI periods. If we prevented the agents from being true to a site, these carry-over effects disappeared (Figure S7).

An additional problem for the interpretation of data from switch-experiments is that the degree to which data is confounded depends on the spatiotemporal distribution of food sources (Figure 1). This makes it especially challenging to meaningfully compare the foraging success of colonies in switch-experiments in different environments or seasons. To solve the methodological problems, we propose the following changes to experimental designs: First, switch experiments should allow colonies to recover for several days between SI and NI periods. Second, SI and NI periods should not be shorter than the average patch-age to make sure the environment changes substantially. With such a design, differences in the gained weight (or energy) should be noticeable between treatments. Alternatively, if only a qualitative result needs to be obtained (whether SI or NI is better), researchers could look at the change in weight gain over time instead of the weight gain. In other words, instead of recording the weight of colonies and calculating the day to day weight gain or loss ((weight on day t + 1) – (weight on day t)), one would calculate the day to day change in the weight gain or loss ((weight change on day t + 1) – (weight change on day t)). This latter solution does not involve a different experimental protocol and should therefore be straightforward to implement, but because of carry-over effects it would still be impossible to gain quantitative data on the difference between pure SI and NI treatments.

So far, we have discussed our results in the context of honeybee recruitment by waggle dances. However, the main findings of the model – the beneficial effects of social information, particularly in more stable environments – are probably not restricted to honeybees alone. If acquiring social information is (i) more costly and (ii) subsequently associated with higher rewards than asocial information (e.g. individual exploration), then we would expect the relative payoff of social information to increase with increasing environmental stability. In support of the first assumption (i), Dechaume-Moncharmont and colleagues [21] show with a model that social information is often costlier than asocial information due to time costs (waiting for a demonstrator). The recent finding that social information is usually of high quality because demonstrators perform the most successful behavior they know of [62] supports the second assumption (ii). However, empirical research is needed to estimate costs and benefits of different types of information and test the role of environmental stability.

Communication about food source locations is common in the Apini and many Meliponini (as pheromone trails), but not in bumble bees. The specific circumstances that lowered the costs or increased the benefits to dancing in *Apis* bees so it could evolve in the first place are not known, and our model is not concerned with the initial evolution of the dance. Recent phylogenies suggest that dancing evolved only once (reviewed in [5]), suggesting some constraints to dance evolution even if simpler forms of recruitment seem to evolve readily [78]. Temperate bumble bees might be exposed to different resource distribution [78]. Additionally, even though the range of tested colony sizes did not affect our main result, a critical colony size for the dance to be beneficial is likely: if the waiting costs to recruits are too long, for example because only a small work force is collecting food, the benefit of finding high quality food might not outweigh these waiting costs [79–81].

In summary, our study and previous simulation studies suggest that dancing is most beneficial in environments where food sources vary greatly in quality [20], are hard to find [22,38] and persist for several days or weeks. In such an environment, spatial information helps a colony to allocate its foragers to highly profitable, but hard-to-find food sources and exploit those for extended time periods. We argue that dancing is beneficial in almost every natural environment, but new empirical studies using different experimental designs are needed to test this prediction.

Supporting Information

Figure S1 The probability that an agent will dance upon its return to the colony, and the probability that a recruit will continue to visit a given food source was modelled to be dependent on the quality of the food as well as the distance to the food source. Depicted are the probabilities to dance in relation to food quality after foraging at 0, 2.5, 5 and 10 km (solid black lines), and the probability that a recruit will continue to visit a given food source the next day at 10 km foraging distance (grey line). At all times, the probability to visit a food source the next day is 30% higher at the food quality that elicits a dance response 50% of the times. See the main text for more details on implementation.

Figure S2 The probability of an agent to dance after a foraging trip in response to the influx of returned foragers. When more foragers return they are less likely to dance. We modelled this as a linear decrease of the probability to dance up to 20 foragers, at which level the dance probability remained constant.

Figure S3 The effect of patch longevity on foragers' persistence to remain with a foraging patch. The longer patches yield energy, the longer a forager stays with a patch to which it is committed (except for the patch longevity all parameters were set to the default values given in table 1 of the main text).

Figure S4 The effect of population size on the foraging success measured as mean daily gain in honey (means ± s.e.) with spatial information transfer (SI) or no spatial information transfer (NI). At all population sizes (**a**) $N = 300$; **b**) $N = 600$; **c**) $N = 1200$) the switching between SI and NI treatments masks the benefit of SI (solid circle: SI, open circles: NI).

Figure S5 The effect of the Lévy flight parameter $\mu_{\text{Lévi}}$ on the foraging success measured as mean daily gain in honey (means ± s.e.) with spatial information transfer (SI) or no spatial information transfer (NI). At all levels for the Lévy flight parameter (**a**) $\mu_{\text{Lévi}} = 1$; **b**) $\mu_{\text{Lévi}} = 2$; **c**) $\mu_{\text{Lévi}} = 3$; **d**) $\mu_{\text{Lévi}} = 4$) the switching between SI and NI treatments masks the benefit of SI (solid circle: SI, open circles: NI).

Figure S6 The effect of the exit probability p_{Exit} on the foraging success measured as mean daily gain in honey (means ± s.e.) with spatial information transfer (SI) or no spatial information transfer (NI). At all exit probabilites (**a**) $p_{\text{Exit}} = 1$; **b**) $p_{\text{Exit}} = 2$; **c**) $p_{\text{Exit}} = 3$; **d**) $p_{\text{Exit}} = 4$) the switching between SI and NI treatments masks the benefit of SI (solid circle: SI, open circles: NI).

Figure S7 A comparison of foraging success measured as mean daily gain in honey (means ± s.e.) when recruits were switching food sources every day as opposed to visit food sources for multiple days (according to Fig. S1). Persistency allows the agents to gain long-term benefits from the spatial information transfer.

Text S1 The downloadable file, TextS1_BeeBenefitOfDance.nlogo, runs in NetLogo versions 4.1.3. NetLogo is freely available from the World Wide Web.

Acknowledgments

We are grateful to Margaret Jane Couvillon, Elli Leadbeater and Francisca Segers, Matina Donaldson-Matasci and Anna Dornhaus for comments on earlier drafts.

Author Contributions

Conceived and designed the experiments: RS CG. Performed the experiments: RS CG. Analyzed the data: RS CG. Contributed to the writing of the manuscript: RS CG. Programming and testing of the model: RS CG.

References

1. Hölldobler B, Wilson EO (2009) The Superorganism: the Beauty, Elegance, and Strangeness of Insect Societies. WW Norton & Company.
2. Jarau S, Hrncir M (2009) Food Exploitation by Social Insects: Ecological, Behavioral, and Theoretical Approaches. CRC Press.
3. Seeley T (1995) The Wisdom of the Hive: The Social Physiology of Honey Bee Colonies. Cambridge: Harvard University Press.
4. Wilson EO (1971) The Insect Societies. Belknap Press of Harvard University Press Cambridge.
5. Couvillon M (2012) The dance legacy of Karl von Frisch. Insect Soc 59: 297–306.
6. Grüter C, Farina WM (2009) The honeybee waggle dance: can we follow the steps? Trends Ecol Evol 24: 242–247.
7. von Frisch K (1946) Die Tänze der Bienen. Österr zool Z 1: 1–148.
8. von Frisch K (1967) The Dance Language and Orientation of Bees. Cambridge, MA: Harvard University Press.
9. Esch HE, Zhang S, Srinivasan MV, Tautz J (2001) Honeybee dances communicate distances measured by optic flow. Nature 411: 581–583.
10. Riley JR, Greggers U, Smith AD, Reynolds DR, Menzel R (2005) The flight paths of honeybees recruited by the waggle dance. Nature 435: 205–207.
11. Tanner D, Visscher P (2008) Do honey bees average directions in the waggle dance to determine a flight direction? Behav Ecol Sociobiol 62: 1891–1898.
12. Towne WF, Gould JL (1988) The spatial precision of the honey bees' dance communication. J Insect Behav 1: 129–155.
13. Farina WM, Grüter C, Arenas A (2012) Olfactory information transfer during recruitment in honey bees. In: Honeybee Neurobiology and Behavior, Springer. pp. 89–101.
14. Wenner AM, Wells PH (1990) Anatomy of a Controversy. New YorkColumbia University Press
15. Okada R, Ikeno H, Kimura T, Ohashi M, Aonuma H, et al. (2012) Mathematical analysis of the honeybee waggle dance. Acta Biol Hung 63 Suppl 2: 75–79.
16. Donaldson-Matasci MC, DeGrandi-Hoffman G, Dornhaus A (2013) Bigger is better: honeybee colonies as distributed information-gathering systems. Anim Behav 85: 585–592.
17. Donaldson-Matasci MC, Dornhaus A (2012) How habitat affects the benefits of communication in collectively foraging honey bees. Behav Ecol Sociobiol 66: 583–592.
18. Dornhaus A, Chittka L (2004) Why do honey bees dance? Behav Ecol Sociobiol 55: 395–401.
19. Sherman G, Visscher PK (2002) Honeybee colonies achieve fitness through dancing. Nature 419: 920–922.
20. Beekman M, Lew JB (2008) Foraging in honeybees–when does it pay to dance? Behav Ecol 19: 255–261.
21. Dechaume-Moncharmont FX, Dornhaus A, Houston A, McNamara J, Collins E, et al. (2005) The hidden cost of information in collective foraging. Proc R Soc B 272: 1689–1695.
22. Dornhaus A, Klügl F, Oechslein C, Puppe F, Chittka L (2006) Benefits of recruitment in honey bees: effects of ecology and colony size in an individual-based model. Behav Ecol 17: 336–344.
23. Seeley T, Visscher P (1988) Assessing the benefits of cooperation in honeybee foraging: search costs, forage quality, and competitive ability. Behav Ecol Soc 22: 229–237.
24. Seeley TD (1983) The ecology of temperate and tropical honeybee societies: Ecological studies complement physiological ones, offering a new perspective on patterns of honeybee adaptation. Amer Sci 71: 264–272.
25. Gentry AH (1974) Flowering phenology and diversity in tropical Bignoniaceae. Biotropica 6: 64–68.
26. Beekman M, Doyen L, Oldroyd B (2005) Increase in dance imprecision with decreasing foraging distance in the honey bee *Apis mellifera* L. is partly explained by physical constraints. J Comp Physiol A 191: 1107–1113.
27. Beling I (1929) Über das Zeitgedächtnis der Bienen. Z vergl Physiol 9: 259–338.
28. Butler C, Jeffree E, Kalmus H (1943) The behaviour of a population of honeybees on an artificial and on a natural crop. J Exp Biol 20: 65–73.

29. Grüter C, Ratnieks FL (2011) Honeybee foragers increase the use of waggle dance information when private information becomes unrewarding. Anim Behav 81: 949–954.
30. Moore D (2001) Honey bee circadian clocks: behavioral control from individual workers to whole-colony rhythms. J Insect Physiol 47: 843–857.
31. Moore D, Doherty P (2009) Acquisition of a time-memory in forager honey bees. J Comp Physiol A 195: 741–751.
32. Moore D, Van Nest BN, Seier E (2011) Diminishing returns: the influence of experience and environment on time-memory extinction in honey bee foragers. J Comp Physiol A 197: 641–651.
33. Ribbands CR (1949) The foraging method of individual honey-bees. J Anim Ecol : 47–66.
34. von Frisch K (1923) Über die "Sprache" der Bienen, Eine tierpsychologische Untersuchung, volume 40 of *Sonderabdruck aus "Zoologische Jahrbücher" Abteilung für allgem. Zoologie und Physiologie*. G. Fischer.1186
35. Grimm V, Berger U, Bastiansen F, Eliassen S, Ginot V, et al. (2006) A standard protocol for describing individual-based and agent-based models. Ecol Model 198: 115–126.
36. Grimm V, Berger U, DeAngelis DL, Polhill JG, Giske J, et al. (2010) The ODD protocol: A review and first update. Ecol Model 221: 2760–2768.
37. Al Toufailia H, Grüter C, Ratnieks FL (2013) Persistence to unrewarding feeding locations by honeybee foragers (*Apis mellifera*): the effects of experience, resource profitability and season. Ethology 119: 1096–1106.
38. Beekman M, Gloag R, Even N, Wattanachaiyingchareon W, Oldroyd B (2008) Dance precision of apis florea–clues to the evolution of the honeybee dance language? Behav Ecol Sociobiol 62: 1259–1265.
39. Liang ZS, Nguyen T, Mattila HR, Rodriguez-Zas SL, Seeley TD, et al. (2012) Molecular determinants of scouting behavior in honey bees. Science 335: 1225–1228.
40. Beekman M, Gilchrist AL, Duncan M, Sumpter DJ (2007) What makes a honeybee scout? Behav Ecol Sociobiol 61: 985–995.
41. Kleber E (1935) Hat das Zeitgedächtnis der Bienen biologische Bedeutung? Z vergl Physiol 22: 221–262.
42. Gould JL, Henerey M, MacLeod MC (1970) Communication of direction by the honey bee: Review of previous work leads to experiments limiting olfactory cues to test the dance language hypothesis. Science 169: 544–554.
43. Seeley TD, Towne WF (1992) Tactics of dance choice in honey bees: do foragers compare dances? Behav Ecol Sociobiol 30: 59–69.
44. Tautz (1996) Honeybee waggle dance: recruitment success depends on the dance floor. J Exp Biol 199: 1375–1381.
45. Lindauer M (1948) Über die Einwirkung von Duft- und Geschmacksstoffen sowie anderer Faktoren auf die Tänze der Bienen. Z vergl Physiol 31: 348–412.
46. Lindauer M (1952) Ein Beitrag zur Frage der Arbeitsteilung im Bienenstaat. Z vergl Physiol 34: 299–345.
47. Couvillon MJ, Schürch R, Ratnieks FL (2014) Dancing bees provide an integrated seasonal picture of foraging challenges. PloS ONE 9: e93495.
48. Reynolds AM, Swain JL, Smith AD, Martin AP, Osborne JL (2009) Honeybees use a Lévy flight search strategy and odour-mediated anemotaxis to relocate food sources. Behav Ecol Sociobiol 64: 115–123.
49. Seeley TD, Camazine S, Sneyd J (1991) Collective decision-making in honey bees: how colonies choose among nectar sources. Behav Ecol Sociobiol 28: 277–290.
50. Boch R (1956) Die Tänze der Bienen bei nahen und fernen Trachtquellen. Z vergl Physiol 38: 136–167.
51. Seeley TD (1986) Social foraging by honeybees: how colonies allocate foragers among patches of flowers. Behav Ecol Sociobiol 19: 343–354.
52. R Core Team (2013) R: A Language and Environment for Statistical Computing. R Foundation for Statistical Computing. Vienna, Austria. http://www.R-project.org/.
53. Venables WN, Ripley BD (2002) Modern Applied Statistics with S. New York: Springer, fourth edition. http://www.stats.ox.ac.uk/pub/MASS4. ISBN 0-387-95457-0.
54. Primack RB (1985) Longevity of individual flowers. Annu Rev Ecol Syst 16: 15–37.
55. Rathcke B, Lacey EP (1985) Phenological patterns of terrestrial plants. Annu Rev Ecol Syst 16: 179–214.
56. Vogel S (1983) Ecophysiology of zoophilic pollination. InLange O LNobel P SOsmond C BZiegier HeditorsPhysiological Plant Ecology IIIBerlin, Germany; New York, NY: Springer 559–624.
57. Seeley T (2012) Progress in understanding how the waggle dance improves the foraging efficiency of honey bee colonies. InGalizia CEisenhardt DGiurfa MeditorsThe Neurobiology and Behavior of Honeybeesa Tribute to Randolf Menzel, Heide lbergSpringer. pp. 77–88.
58. Esch H, Bastian JA (1970) How do newly recruited honey bees approach a food site? Z vergl Physiol 68: 175–181.
59. Mautz D (1971) Der Kommunikationseffekt der Schwänzeltänze bei *Apis mellifica carnica* (Pollm.). Z vergl Physiol 72: 197–220.
60. Seeley TD, Visscher PK, Schlegel T, Hogan PM, Franks NR, et al. (2012) Stop signals provide cross inhibition in collective decision-making by honeybee swarms. Science 335: 108–111.
61. Grüter C, Leadbeater E, Ratnieks FL (2010) Social learning: the importance of copying others. Curr Biol 20: R683–R685.
62. Rendell L, Boyd R, Cownden D, Enquist M, Eriksson K, et al. (2010) Why copy others? insights from the social learning strategies tournament. Science 328: 208–213.
63. Collett M (2009) Spatial memories in insects. Curr Biol 19: R1103–R1108.
64. Collett TS, Collett M (2002) Memory use in insect visual navigation. Nat Rev Neurosci 3: 542–552.
65. Granovskiy B, Latty T, Duncan M, Sumpter DJT, Beekman M (2012) How dancing honey bees keep track of changes: the role of inspector bees. Behav Ecol 23: 588–596.
66. Wilms W, Imperatriz-Fonseca VL, Engels W (1996) Resource partitioning between highly eusocial bees and possible impact of the introduced Africanized honey bee on native stingless bees in the Brazilian Atlantic rainforest. Stud Neotrop Fauna E 31: 137–151.
67. Bogdany F (1978) Linking of learning signals in honeybee orientation. Behav Ecol Soc 3: 323–336.
68. Naeger NL, Van Nest BN, Johnson JN, Boyd SD, Southey BR, et al. (2011) Neurogenomic signatures of spatiotemporal memories in time-trained forager honey bees. J Exp Biol 214: 979–987.
69. Biesmeijer J, Seeley T (2005) The use of waggle dance information by honey bees throughout their foraging careers. Behav Ecol Sociobiol 59: 133–142.
70. Grüter C, Balbuena MS, Farina WM (2008) Informational conflicts created by the waggle dance. Proc R Soc B 275: 1321–1327.
71. Grüter C, Segers FHD, Ratnieks FL (2013) Social learning strategies in honeybee foragers: do the costs of using private information affect the use of social information? Anim Behav 85: 1443–1449.
72. Johnson DL (1967) Communication among honey bees with field experience. Anim Behav 15: 487–492.
73. Menzel R, Kirbach A, Haass WD, Fischer B, Fuchs J, et al. (2011) A common frame of reference for learned and communicated vectors in honeybee navigation. Curr Biol 21: 645–650.
74. Wray MK, Klein BA, Seeley TD (2012) Honey bees use social information in waggle dances more fully when foraging errors are more costly. Behav Ecol 23: 125–131.
75. Grüter C, Leadbeater E (2014) Insights from insects about adaptive social information use. Trends Ecol Evol 29: 177–184.
76. Rendell L, Boyd R, Enquist M, Feldman MW, Fogarty L, et al. (2011) How copying affects the amount, evenness and persistence of cultural knowledge: insights from the social learning strategies tournament. Phil Trans R Soc B 366: 1118–1128.
77. Gilley D, Kuzora J, Thom C (2012) Hydrocarbons emitted by waggle-dancing honey bees stimulate colony foraging activity by causing experienced foragers to exploit known food sources. Apidologie 43: 85–94.
78. Dornhaus A, Chittka L (1999) Insect behaviour: Evolutionary origins of bee dances. Nature 401: 38–38.
79. Anderson C, Ratnieks F (1999) Task partitioning in foraging: general principles, efficiency and information reliability of queueing delays. InDetrain CDeneu-Deneubourg J LeditorsInformation Processing in Social InsectsBirkhäuser Verlag, Berlin 31–50.
80. Beekman M, Sumpter DJ, Ratnieks FL (2001) Phase transition between disordered and ordered foraging in pharaoh's ants. Proc Natl Acad Sci U S A 98: 9703–9706.
81. Anderson C, Ratnieks FLW (1999) Task partitioning in insect societies. I. effect of colony size on queueing delay and colony ergonomic efficiency. Am Nat154521–535.
82. Nuñez JA (1966) Quantitative Beziehungen zwischen den Eigenschaften von Futterquellen und dem Verhalten von Sammelbienen. Z vergl Physiol 53: 142–164.
83. Park (1926) Water-carriers versus nectar-carriers. J Econ Entomol 4: 656–664.
84. de Marco R, Farina W (2003) Trophallaxis in forager honeybees (*Apis mellifera*): resource uncertainty enhances begging contacts? J Comp Physiol A 189: 125–134.
85. Schmid-Hempel P, Kacelnik A, Houston A (1985) Honeybees maximize efficiency by not filling their crop. Behav Ecol Soc 17: 61–66.
86. Van Nest BN, Moore D (2012) Energetically optimal foraging strategy is emergent property of time-keeping behavior in honey bees. Behav Ecol 23: 649–658.
87. Gould JL (1976) The dance-language controversy. Quart Rev Biol 51: pp. 211–244.

8

Effects of Long-Term Feeding of the Polyphenols Resveratrol and Kaempferol in Obese Mice

Mayte Montero, Sergio de la Fuente, Rosalba I. Fonteriz, Alfredo Moreno, Javier Alvarez*

Instituto de Biología y Genética Molecular (IBGM), Departamento de Bioquímica y Biología Molecular y Fisiología, Facultad de Medicina, Universidad de Valladolid and Consejo Superior de Investigaciones Científicas (CSIC), Valladolid, Spain

Abstract

The effect of the intake of antioxidant polyphenols such as resveratrol and others on survival and different parameters of life quality has been a matter of debate in the last years. We have studied here the effects of the polyphenols resveratrol and kaempferol added to the diet in a murine model undergoing long-term hypercaloric diet. Using 50 mice for each condition, we have monitored weight, survival, biochemical parameters such as blood glucose, insulin, cholesterol, triglycerides and aspartate aminotransferase, neuromuscular coordination measured with the rotarod test and morphological aspect of stained sections of liver and heart histological samples. Our data show that mice fed since they are 3-months-old with hypercaloric diet supplemented with any of these polyphenols reduced their weight by about 5–7% with respect to the controls fed only with hypercaloric diet. We also observed that mice fed with any of the polyphenols had reduced levels of glucose, insulin and cholesterol, and better marks in the rotarod test, but only after 1 year of treatment, that is, during senescence. No effect was observed in the rest of the parameters studied. Furthermore, although treatment with hypercaloric diets induced large changes in the pattern of gene expression in liver, we found no significant changes in gene expression induced by the presence of any of the polyphenols. Thus, our data indicate that addition of resveratrol or kaempferol to mice food produces an initial decrease in weight in mice subjected to hypercaloric diet, but beneficial effects in other parameters such as blood glucose, insulin and cholesterol, and neuromuscular coordination, only appear after prolonged treatments.

Editor: Hemachandra Reddy, Texas Tech University Health Science Centers, United States of America

Funding: This work was supported by grants from Ministerio de Ciencia e Innovación [BFU2008-01871 and BFU 2011-25763; (http://www.idi.mineco.gob.es/portal/site/MICINN/)] and from Junta de Castilla y León [VA029A12-1 and GR105, (http://www.educa.jcyl.es/educacyl/cm/universidad)]. Sergio de la Fuente had an FPI (Formación de Personal Investigador) fellowship from the Spanish Government. The funders had no role in study design, data collection and analysis, decision to publish, or preparation of the manuscript.

Competing Interests: The authors have declared that no competing interests exist.

* Email: jalvarez@ibgm.uva.es

Introduction

The importance of the presence of vegetables in human food has been widely debated, and in the last years considerable scientific literature has been published in relation with the effects in health of diets rich in vegetables or in particular types of polyphenols. Most of these studies are epidemiological, and associate the amount of polyphenols present in the diet with a reduction in the risk for cardiovascular diseases and cancer [1–8]. Some studies have also described other positive effects in neurodegenerative diseases [9,10] or inflammatory diseases [11], and they have also been shown to activate lipolysis [12,13]. All these potentially beneficial effects have led to proposals for their addition in foods as a nutritional supplement.

Moreover, some studies have investigated the effects of some of these individual molecules in cellular or animal models. The more striking example is resveratrol, a polyphenol abundant in red wine, which has been shown to improve the survival and several plasmatic, neurological and genomic markers in mice fed with hypercaloric diets [14]. Previously, it had been shown that this compound was able to prolong considerably the lifespan in several species, including Saccharomyces cerevisiae, Caenorhabditis elegans, Drosophila melanogaster and a short-lived fish [15–19]. More recently, it has also been shown to protect pancreatic islets against oxidative stress in db/db mice [20]. These effects have been attributed not only to the antioxidant properties of this compound, but rather to the specific activation by resveratrol of sirtuins, a family of NAD^+-dependent deacetylases and mono ADP-rybosiltransferases that mediate the physiological effects of caloric restriction. From these data an entire industry has emerged to provide food supplements, cosmetics, and other products based on resveratrol. However, recent data has questioned the results obtained with resveratrol in C. elegans and D. melanogaster [21] and this point is now a matter of strong debate [22–24].

Although at a smaller scale, similar studies have also been carried out with other related polyphenols, but significant differences appear among the reported effects. We were particularly interested in the flavonoid kaempferol, as we showed several years ago that this compound was a potent stimulator of the mitochondrial Ca^{2+} uniporter, a Ca^{2+} channel essential to modulate mitochondrial energy production [25]. It has been shown that kaempferol increases oxygen consumption in cell cultures and isolated mitochondria, potently activates the synthesis of thyroid hormones and modulates a whole series of enzymes and proteins related to metabolism [26]. In addition, a 30 days administration of a kaempferol glucoside to Wistar rats feed with hypercaloric diet reduced the weight and the plasmatic levels of triglycerides [27]. Kaempferol, however, was much less effective as activator of sirtuins [15], and resveratrol, instead, was ineffective as stimulator of thyroid hormone synthesis [14] and little effective as activator of mitochondrial Ca^{2+} uptake [25].

Both compounds (resveratrol and kaempferol) thus seem to act through different signaling pathways, and we thought it would be very interesting to compare their effects on several biochemical, neurological and genomic parameters during a lifetime treatment with these compounds in mice. We have then decided to make a large and complete study of this point by using a very large number (250) 3-months old C57BL mice and carrying out the treatment for the entire life of the mice (24 months). As in previous reports [14,27], we have also studied the effects of these polyphenols in mice fed with hypercaloric diet, periodically monitoring parameters such as food intake, weight, blood glucose, insulin, triglycerides, cholesterol and transaminase activity. Motor coordination was estimated using the rotarod test [28,29], and we have also compared mortality rates, analyzed histological sections of liver and heart, and looked for changes in gene expression patterns in liver using Affymetrix gene expression arrays.

Methods and Materials

Ethics statement

The study was approved by the Ethical Committee for Animal Research of the School of Medicine of the University of Valladolid (Permit Number: 7-2007), and was carried out in strict accordance with the recommendations in the Guide for the Care and Use of Laboratory Animals of the National Institutes of Health.

Mice treatment and diets

250 C57BL male mice were obtained from Janvier (53947 Saint Berthevin Cedex, France) and fed with control diet (Diet D12450B from Research Diets Inc., New Brunswick, NJ 08901 USA) until they were 3-months old and at that moment the different diets were started. This diet contains 3.85 kcal/g. Mice were maintained in standard housing conditions at 22°C, with a 12 h light/dark cycle and with free access to tap water. They were distributed in 5 groups with 50 mice in each of them, and placed in cages containing 10 mice in each for all their life. Group Control (C) continued with the same control diet. Group Hypercaloric Control (HC) was fed with a standard hypercaloric diet (Diet D12492 from Research Diets Inc.), a diet containing a larger proportion of lard and providing 5.24 kcal/g. Control diet contains 1.9% lard, providing 4.44% of the total kcal, while hypercaloric diet contains 31.66% lard, providing 54.35% of the total kcal. Group Hypercaloric Resveratrol (HR) was fed with hypercaloric diet (D12492) supplemented with 250 mg/kg-diet (0,025%) of resveratrol. Group Hypercaloric low Kaempferol (Hk) was fed with hypercaloric diet (D12492) supplemented with 50 mg/kg-diet (0,005%) of kaempferol. Group Hypercaloric high Kaempferol (HK) was fed with hypercaloric diet (D12492) supplemented with 250 mg/kg-diet (0,025%) of kaempferol. Food was stored at 4°C, sealed and at dark. Both resveratrol and kaempferol were obtained from Apin Chemicals Limited, Abingdon, Oxon, OX14 4RU, U.K., and sent to Research Diets to prepare the different types of foods, which were identified by color codes.

The amount of food ingested was measured by putting known amounts of food in every cage and weighting the remaining food every two days. As shown in Fig. 1 and Table S1, the amount of food ingested kept quite constant along the whole study for all the conditions, although some small changes among the groups could be detected (see Results). The initial weight of the mice was around 25 g, and so the initial dose of the compounds was 25 $mg{\cdot}kg^{-1}{\cdot}day^{-1}$ in groups HR (as in ref. 14) and HK, and 5 $mg{\cdot}kg^{-1}{\cdot}day^{-1}$ in group Hk. Mice fed hypercaloric diets increased progressively weight along the study (Fig. 2a), reaching values of 55–60 g after 1 year of treatment.

Once the treatment was started, we monitored a series of parameters along the whole life of the mice: mice weight every 15 days, blood glucose, insulin, triglycerides, cholesterol and aspartate aminotransferase every three months, neurological performance with the rotarod test every 3 months, histological studies of liver and heart after 6 and 12 months of hypercaloric diet, and gene expression studies with Affymetrix arrays in liver extracts after 12 months.

Blood biochemistry

Glucose was measured using the Ascensia Breeze 2 Blood Glucose Meter (Bayer HealthCare AG, Wuppertal, Germany).

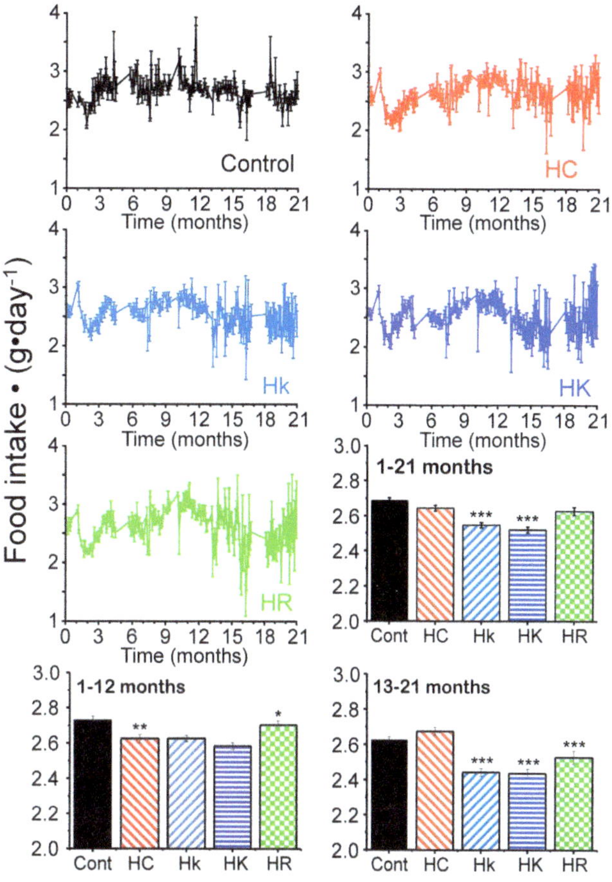

Figure 1. Variation of the mean amount of food ingested by each group of mice along their lifespan. Data are calculated as food intake per mice and per day. Each data was obtained as mean±s.e, n = 5 (5 mice cages containing 10 mice each). The bar diagrams shows the mean±s.e. of all the measurements obtained for each group of mice (n = 197 measurements for whole period, n = 112 for the first 12 months, n = 85 for 13–21 months) and the significance (*, $p<0.05$; **, $p<0.005$; ***, $p<0.001$) of the differences (HC group, compared with the control; Hk, HK and HR groups, compared with the HC group).

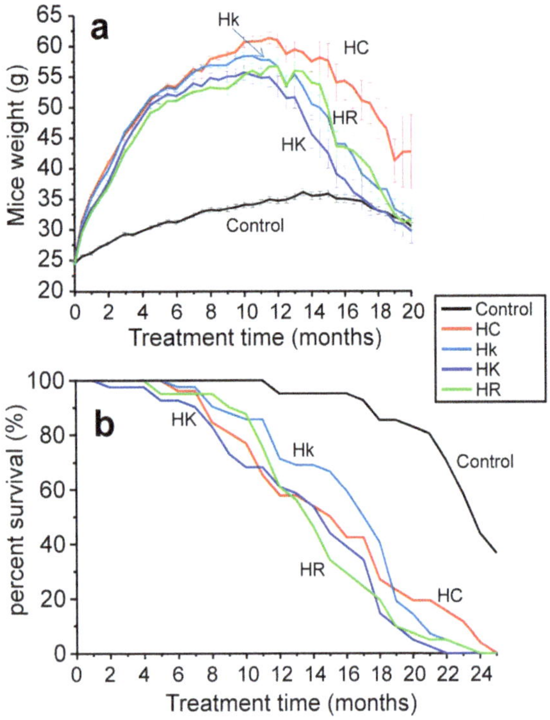

Figure 2. Evolution with time of mice weight and survival. Panel a. Evolution of mice weight along the study from the start of the hypercaloric diets (time 0 in the figure). Data are mean±s.e, n = 50 data for each value at the beginning, the number of data then decreasing with time according to the survival. **Panel b.** Evolution of mice survival with time in all the groups, expressed as percentage of the starting mice number.

Insulin was measured by ELISA using the kit for mouse insulin from DRG Diagnostics, Marburg, Germany (Ref. EIA-3439). Triglycerides, total cholesterol and alanine aminotransferase were measured using the corresponding kits from BioSystems, Barcelona, Spain (Refs. 11528, 11505 and 11533, respectively). All these measurements were made using blood taken from the tail after overnight fast.

Rotarod test

The Ugo Basile (Comerio, Italy) Mouse Rota Rod was used for the tests. Starting at 0 rpm, the rotarod was accelerated at constant rates of 4–40 rpm. All the mice in the same cage were first trained on the rotarod the day before at a constant rate of 4 rpm until they were able to stay on for one minute. The next day, 5 mice were randomly chosen in that cage and labeled. Then each mice was subjected to three rotarod trials, with 30 min intervals, consisting in a constant acceleration along 5 min from 4 rpm to 40 rpm. The final time to fall of each mouse was obtained as the mean±s.e. of all the measurements for that mouse. Rotarod tests were carried out every 3 months in all the mice groups.

Histological studies

Mice were sacrificed by cervical dislocation. The heart and liver were removed and washed several times in 4°C cold PBS. Tissues were cut in small pieces and fixed for 24 hours in 4% formalin at 4°C. After fixation, tissues were washed 3 times for 30 min in cold PBS, once in distilled water and finally once in 70% ethanol. The tissue sections were then embedded in paraffin in a carousel tissue processor cut in 4 μm sections and mounted on Superfrost slides. They were then let dry overnight at 37°C before they were finally stained with Haematoxyline and Eosin and imaged in a Nikon Eclipse 80i upright microscope at 20× and 40×.

Gene expression

Three mice of each group (3×5) were sacrificed and their livers were separately minced, immersed in RNAlater RNA stabilization Reagent (Quiagen) and frozen. For RNA extraction, liver chunks were homogenized using the Minibeadbeater-8, and RNA was then extracted using the RNeasy mini kit (Qiagen). RNA concentrations were measured using a NanoDrop spectrophotometer (NanoDrop Technologies, Wilmington, DE, USA), and samples were analyzed using 15 Mouse Gene 1.0 ST arrays, one for each mice, in the Genomic facility of the Cancer Research Center, Salamanca, Spain. Background correction, intra- and inter-microarray normalization, and expression signal calculation was made using a robust microarray analysis algorithm [30–32]. This algorithm calculates the absolute expression signal for each gene in each microarray. Then, a method known as significance analysis of microarray [33] was applied to calculate significant differential expression. This method provides an estimation of the error using the false discovery rate algorithm (FDR) [34]. A FDR of less than 0.1 (10% false positives) was used as standard for all the differential expression calculations, although in some cases it was increased to 0.15 (15% false positives), as indicated. All these methods were applied using R and Bioconductor packages.

Statistics

Data are expressed as mean±s.e. Significance analysis was made with the ANOVA test.

Results

Food ingestion

The mean amount ingested by the group treated with HC diet was significantly smaller in the first 12 months, although its caloric value was still much higher (see Fig. 1 and Table S1). Food intake was little modified in the groups treated with the drugs compared with the HC group in the first 12 months, but it was significantly decreased (by 5–9%) in the senescence period (13–21 months).

Mice weight

Control mice (C) started with a weight of about 25 g, which increased to stabilize at around 30–35 g at one year, and then slowly declined with senescence (see figure 2a). The weight of mice fed high-calorie diet (HC) increased rapidly, reaching around 60 g after one year of treatment with this diet. Then it started to decrease with senescence, tending to return to the original values after 2 years of treatment. Mice treated with HC diet with resveratrol (HR, 25 mg/kg body weight per day) increased weight 7.0±0.4% less (mean±s.e. obtained from the first 20 weight measurements, obtained every 15 days) than HC mice during the first year, and this effect was statistically significant for every measurement (see Table S2). Then, weight also began a rapid decline with senescence, in parallel with the weight loss observed in the HC mice, but starting about 3 months earlier. In the case of mice treated with kaempferol at low concentration (Hk, 5 mg/kg body weight per day), there were no significant differences in weight during most of the first year of treatment (Table S2), but the subsequent drop in weight associated with senescence also occurred about 3 months earlier than in the case of the controls with HC diet. In the case of mice treated with HC diet and kaempferol at high concentration (HK, 25 mg/kg body weight per day), there was also an initial decrease in weight of a 5.0±0.5% (mean±s.e. obtained from the first 20 weight measurements, obtained every 15 days), which was statistically significant for most of the measurements, but not all of them (Table S2). Then, the subsequent decline in weight associated with senescence began even earlier, around 4 months earlier than in control mice treated with HC diet, so that the differences in weight with the HC group remained highly significant for most of the senescence period (Table S2). In summary, kaempferol and resveratrol treatments produced significant decreases (5–7%) in weight in mice fed with HC diet during the first year of treatment, and induced an early start of the decrease in weight associated with senescence.

Survival study

In control mice, mortality was very small before they were 18 months old. Feeding with HC diet significantly reduced survival (Fig. 2b), so that 50% mortality was already reached by 15 months of life (compared with only 5% mortality in controls of the same age). The administration of dietary kaempferol or resveratrol at high concentrations did not significantly change the mortality curve with respect to that of the HC mice. In the case of kaempferol at low concentration, 50% mortality was obtained 2 months later, at 17 months, but the subsequent decrease of the survival curve was faster, equaling with the group of mice with HC diet at 19 months. In summary, our data show that treatment with kaempferol or resveratrol did not modify survival in mice fed with hypercaloric diet.

Glucose

Blood glucose levels in control mice were stable around 80–120 mg/dl throughout all the study. In all the other conditions having HC diet, there was a rapid increase in the blood glucose levels, which doubled the previous glucose levels immediately after establishment of the HC diet treatment (Fig. 3a). These high levels were not significantly modified by any of the polyphenols used throughout the first year of treatment. Then, during senescence, there was a slight decrease in the glucose levels, which was more rapid and pronounced in mice treated with polyphenols. In particular, kaempferol at high doses produced a significant decrease with respect to the HC mice ($p<0.005$, ANOVA test) in blood glucose levels at 15 months of treatment (see red arrows), and both kaempferol and resveratrol produced a decrease ($p<0.05$) in these values at 18 months. Therefore, significant effects of the polyphenols were only observed after more than 1 year of treatment.

Insulin

Insulin levels in control mice remained around 0.2 to 0.3 µg/l throughout the study. In contrast, in all conditions of HC diet-fed mice there was a large increase in blood insulin levels to values 10–15 times higher (Fig. 3b). Treatment with polyphenols did not modify this increase in the initial measurements. However, there was a statistically significant decrease in the insulin values obtained in mice treated with the high dose of kaempferol between 9 and 15 months (see red arrows, $p<0.05$ at 9 months, $p<0.005$ at 15 months). Resveratrol and the low dose of kaempferol also produced statistically significant decreases in insulin levels at 15 months of treatment ($p<0.05$ and $p<0.005$, respectively). Thus, as in the case of the glucose levels, a reduction in insulin levels was only apparent after about 1 year of treatment with the polyphenols.

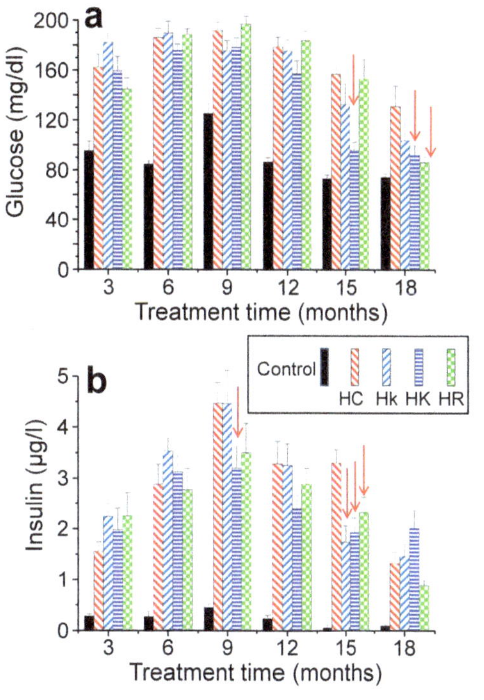

Figure 3. Mean blood glucose (panel a) and insulin (panel b) values obtained every 3 months along the study, from the start of the hypercaloric diet. Arrows indicate the presence of differences statistically significant when the HC condition is compared to the Hk, HK and HR ones (see the text). Data are mean±s.e, n = 10 data for each value.

Cholesterol

Cholesterol levels in blood were maintained at around 80–100 mg/dl in control mice throughout the study. The administration of HC diet increased these values to levels around 200 mg/dl, which were insensitive to treatment with polyphenols during the first year of treatment (Fig. 4a). In the second year there was a decrease in cholesterol levels in all the conditions. However, this decrease occurred earlier in mice treated with polyphenols. Thus, we observed a significant decrease in cholesterol levels at 15 months of treatment in mice treated with the high dose of kaempferol ($p<0.005$) or resveratrol ($p<0.05$) with respect to HC mice. Then, after 18 months of treatment, cholesterol levels were also reduced in the HC mice and the differences disappeared. In the case of mice treated with the high dose of kaempferol, there was also a significant decrease in cholesterol values ($p<0.05$) at 12 months of treatment. In summary, treatment with polyphenols produced little effects on cholesterol levels in the first year but accelerated the reduction of its levels associated with senescence.

Triglycerides

Triglyceride levels in control mice stayed around 40–60 mg/dL throughout the entire study. Mice fed HC diet showed an increase of these values of about 25–30%, which was homogeneous in mice treated or not with polyphenols (Fig. 4b). This increase was maintained during the first year of treatment and thereafter the difference became smaller and tended to disappear. In any case, there were no significant differences between the data obtained in mice treated with HC diet with or without polyphenols.

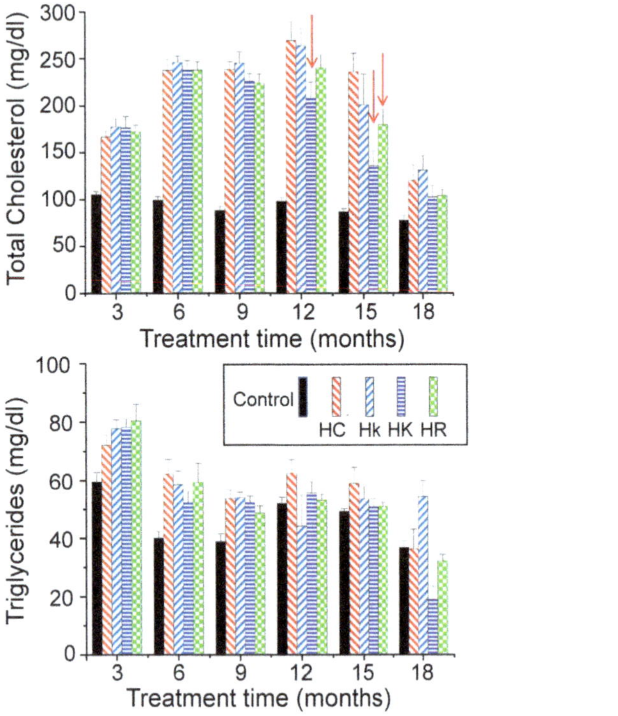

Figure 4. Mean blood total cholesterol (panel a) and triglycerides (panel b) values obtained every 3 months along the study, from the start of the hypercaloric diet. Arrows indicate the presence of differences statistically significant when the HC condition is compared to the HK and HR ones (see the text). Data are mean±s.e, n = 10 data for each value.

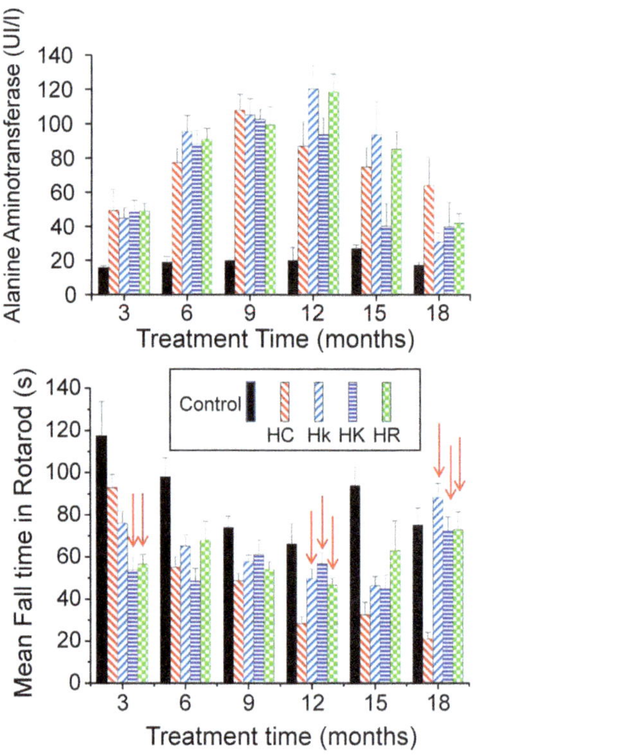

Figure 5. Mean blood alanine aminotransferase (panel a) and rotarod fall time (panel b) values obtained every 3 months along the study. Arrows indicate the presence of differences statistically significant when the HC condition is compared to the Hk, HK and HR ones (see the text). Data are mean±s.e, n = 10 data for each value.

Alanine aminotransferase

Alanine aminotransferase values in blood maintained at around 20–30 IU/L throughout the entire study in control mice. In mice treated with HC diet, there was a progressive increase in these values that reached a maximum of around 100 IU/L after 9 months of treatment (Fig. 5a). Again here, there were no significant differences between the data obtained in mice treated only with HC diet and in those that had also received polyphenols.

Motor coordination study with rotarod

In these studies, the time before fall of the mice from a rotating tube is a measure of the degree of coordination. In control mice, the time before fall decreased slightly with age, but remained between 80 and 120 seconds on average throughout the entire study. In mice treated with HC diet, there was a progressive decrease in that time, reaching values of only 30 seconds after a year of treatment (Fig. 5b). The effect of polyphenols was here quite surprising. In the first measurement, obtained after 3 months of treatment, mice treated with HC diet with kaempferol or resveratrol performed significantly worse (shorter times, $p<0.005$) than those treated only with diet HC. This effect disappeared at 6 and 9 months, because the values obtained for all mice with high-fat diet were here similar. Interestingly, after 12 months, data obtained by the HC diet treated mice continued to worsen, whereas those treated also with polyphenols remained stable or even improved. In fact, at 12 and 18 months, all the mice groups fed with diets containing polyphenols obtained significantly better marks ($p<0.001$) than those fed with HC diet.

Histological analysis

Histological studies of liver and heart samples were made at 6 and 12 months after the start of the hypercaloric diet. Fig. 6 shows typical Haematoxyline and Eosin stained sections from livers and hearts obtained 6 months after the start of the hypercaloric diet. Images obtained after 12 months provided similar results. The liver stained sections (Fig. 6a) show that all the mice under hypercaloric diet had clearly enlarged hepatocytes and a large degree of steatosis represented by the vacuolation of hepatocytes. However, after careful examination of a series of sections of each type we did not find any significant difference among the samples from mice fed only with plain hypercaloric diet and those from mice fed with hypercaloric diet plus any of the polyphenolic compounds. Regarding the heart stained sections (Fig. 6b), the hypercaloric diet induced little changes with respect to the controls, and they were not modified either by the presence of the polyphenols.

Gene expression

We have conducted an analysis of whole genome expression arrays in the 5 groups of mice after 1 year of treatment with the different diets. Treatment with HC diet produced a significant change in the pattern of gene expression of multiple genes with metabolic importance, as has been previously described. The list of genes showing a larger change, using a 10% false positives, is in the Table S3.

Concerning the effect of polyphenols, and this is a significant discrepancy with previous data [14], the group of genes that were

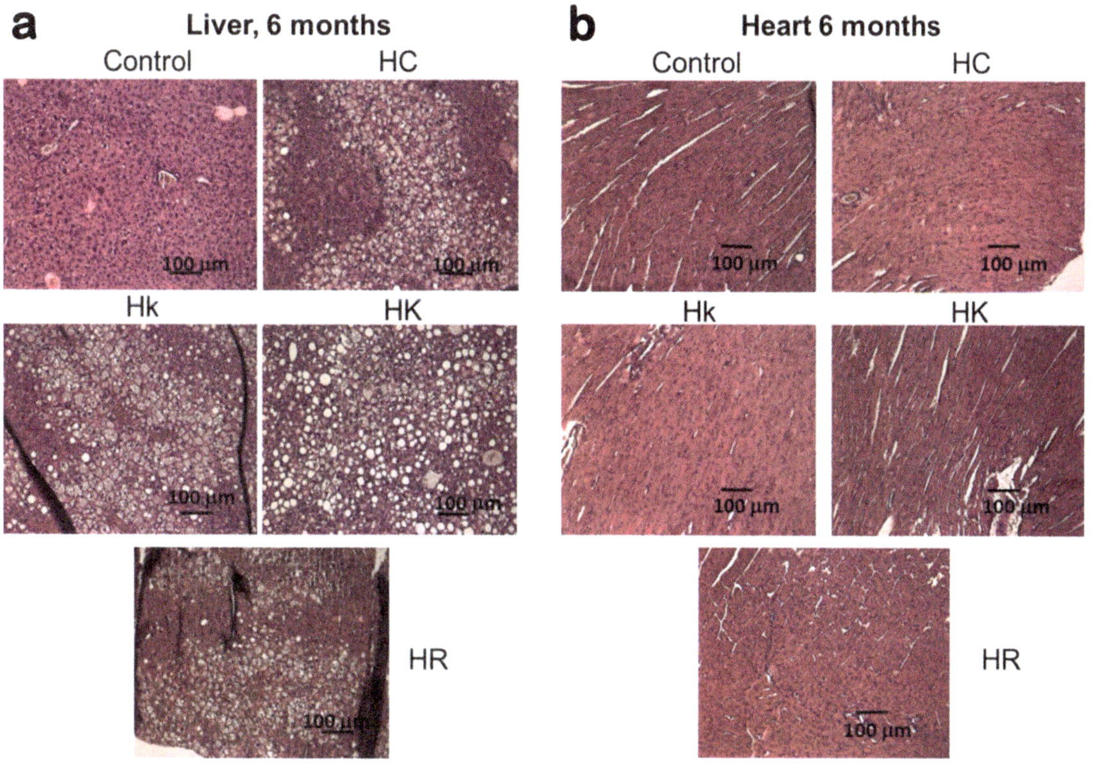

Figure 6. Haematoxylin and Eosin stained sections of liver (panel a) and heart (panel b), obtained from the five mice groups 6 months after the start of the hypercaloric diets and imaged in a Nikon Eclipse 80i upright microscope at 20×.

overexpressed or silenced was very similar in the group treated with hypercaloric diet alone and in the group fed with hypercaloric diet containing resveratrol. In fact, a direct comparison of the gene expression pattern obtained in both mice groups yielded no gene expression change between the two conditions (even using a maximum of 15% false positives).

Regarding the group fed with hypercaloric diet plus low dose of kaempferol, it was also not possible to find any gene changing expression when it was compared with the group fed only with hypercaloric diet. Similarly, in the case of the group fed with the high dose of kaempferol, just a slightly reduced expression of 6 genes by 20–30% was obtained, and only when the percentage of false positives was increased to 15% (see table S4). Some of them are mitochondrial proteins, so it may be interesting to study if they play any role in mitochondrial Ca^{2+} dynamics. However, the main conclusion of the gene expression studies is that the polyphenols added to the HC diet did not induce significant changes in the gene expression pattern generated by the HC diet.

Discussion

Our study has sought to shed light on the controversy over the role of polyphenols on health and survival in mice. We have used resveratrol, a potent activator of sirtuins [15], and kaempferol, which is a poor activator of sirtuins [15] but a potent antioxidant with strong effects on mitochondrial metabolism activation [25–27]. Our macro-study covers the entire lifetime of the mice (24 months) and includes a very high number of C57BL wild-type mice, 50 mice for each condition. This makes the results highly reliable.

Our data show that the main effect of mice treatment with hypercaloric diet containing polyphenols is an initial weight loss of 5–7%, when kaempferol or resveratrol are used at a dose of 25 mg/kg body weight per day. This decrease, which requires using the high dose of kaempferol, can be seen clearly from the beginning of the treatment and is maintained throughout the study. Food ingestion during the first year was similar or higher in the drug-treated groups than in the HC control, so that the weight loss cannot be attributed to a decreased food intake. The decrease in weight induced by resveratrol in hypercaloric diet-fed mice has been described previously [14]. However, the fact that the same effect is obtained with kaempferol is important, because this flavonoid has been shown to be a poor activator of sirtuins [15]. Its effects could rather be attributed to metabolic effects such as increase in oxygen consumption or thyroid hormones synthesis [25–27].

Regarding the weight loss associated with senescence, it occurred 3–4 months earlier in mice treated with polyphenols compared to controls with HC diet, even with the low dose of kaempferol. This decrease was not associated with increased toxicity or mortality because the survival curves of mice treated with HC diet with or without polyphenols were similar. It could be due in part to the 5–9% reduction in food intake observed in the senescence period in all the groups treated with either kaempferol or resveratrol.

As for the study of motor coordination in rotarod, the effects of polyphenols were variable in time: negative after 3 months of treatment, indifferent between 6 and 9 months and finally positive at longer times. Notably, however, the low doses of kaempferol increased rotarod times in the last months as much as the high doses, but hardly produced any alteration at short times. The improvement in rotarod performance after long times of treatment with resveratrol has been reported before [14]. Our data here show that the same findings were also obtained with kaempferol, suggesting again that mechanisms additional to sirtuin activation may be involved.

Regarding survival, our data do not confirm the previous report that resveratrol prolongs survival of mice fed with HC diet and makes it similar to that of control mice [14]. Instead, we find that survival in the groups of mice treated with HC diet and resveratrol or kaempferol was similar to that of the group fed HC diet only.

As for the biochemical parameters, it has been reported that treatment with HC diet produces a 30% increase in glucose levels in blood and a four times increase in blood insulin levels, and that both changes were reversed in the presence of resveratrol [14]. Our data, which track more completely the glucose levels at different times of treatment, show instead that glucose levels were doubled by the HC diet and that resveratrol and kaempferol treatments were only able to reduce in part that increase during senescence, after at least 1 year of treatment. As for the insulin levels, our data show a much higher increase, between 10 and 15 times the control values, in the groups treated with HC diet. Again in this case, the polyphenols were only able to partially reverse this effect after 1 year of treatment. The origin of these partial and very delayed effects is unclear, but it could be related to the reduction in food intake and faster decrease in weight we observe during senescence in the drug-treated groups. The lack of metabolic effects of resveratrol is consistent with recent data obtained in obese men [35].

Regarding gene expression, our data show that mice fed with hypercaloric diet show a large number of changes in gene expression, confirming data previously reported by other authors [36,37]. However, the presence of polyphenols in the hypercaloric diet hardly induced any change in gene expression with respect to the mice fed only with hypercaloric diet. These results are again contradictory with previous reports [14], which showed large changes in gene expression induced by resveratrol.

Conclusions

In summary, we have performed here a systematic macro-study of the effect of the polyphenols resveratrol and kaempferol included in a hypercaloric diet in groups of 50 mice for each condition, monitoring weight, survival and biochemical, neurological, histological and genetic parameters along the whole life of the mice. Our results indicate that these compounds reduced mice weight by 5–7% and prolonged treatments partially reversed some of the biochemical changes induced by the hypercaloric diet. However, the polyphenols did not significant modify survival or liver gene expression.

Supporting Information

Table S1 Food ingestion in the different groups measured in both g·mice^{-1}·day^{-1} or kcal·mice^{-1}·day^{-1}.

Table S2 Significance of mice weight differences between drug treated (Hk, HK and HR) and hypercaloric control HC (*, $p< 0.05$; **, $p<0.005$; ***, $p<0.001$).

Table S3 Differential gene expression obtained by comparing gene expression arrays for HC mice versus controls.

Table S4 Differential gene expression obtained by comparing gene expression arrays for HK versus HC mice.

Acknowledgments

We thank Pilar Alvarez and Laura González for excellent technical assistance, Dr. Encarna Fermiñán and Diego Alonso, Cancer Research Center (CSIC-University of Salamanca) for help with processing and analysis of the gene expression arrays, and Dr. Angel Barcia, the veterinary of the School of Medicine, for help with animal care.

Author Contributions

Conceived and designed the experiments: MM RIF AM JA. Performed the experiments: MM RIF AM SF. Analyzed the data: MM SF RIF AM JA. Wrote the paper: MM JA.

References

1. Middleton E Jr, Kandaswami C, Theoharides TC (2000) The effects of plant flavonoids on mammalian cells: implications for inflammation, heart disease, and cancer. Pharmacol Rev 52: 673–751.
2. Havsteen BH (2002) The biochemistry and medical significance of the flavonoids. Pharmacol Therap 96: 67–202.
3. Birt DF, Hendrich S, Wang W (2001) Dietary agents in cancer prevention: flavonoids and isoflavonoids. Pharmacol Ther 90: 157–177.
4. Nestel P (2003) Isoflavones: their effects on cardiovascular risk and functions. Curr Opin Lipidol 14: 3–8.
5. Scalbert A, Manach C, Morand C, Remesy C, Jimenez L (2005) Dietary polyphenols and the prevention of diseases. Crit Rev Food Sci Nutr 45: 287–306.
6. Grassi D, Necozione S, Lippi C, Croce G, Valeri L, et al. (2005) Cocoa reduces blood pressure and insulin resistance and improves endothelium-dependent vasodilation in hypertensives. Hypertension 46: 398–405.
7. Manach C, Mazur A, Scalbert A (2005) Polyphenols and prevention of cardiovascular diseases. Curr Opin Lipidol 16: 77–84.
8. Gates MA, Tworoger SS, Hecht JL, De Vivo I, Rosner B, et al. (2007) A prospective study of dietary flavonoid intake and incidence of epithelial ovarian cancer. Int J Cancer 121: 2225–2232.
9. Watanabe CM, Wolffram S, Ader P, Rimbach G, Packer L, et al. (2001) The in vivo neuromodulatory effects of the herbal medicine ginkgo biloba. Proc Natl Acad Sci U S A 98: 6577–6580.
10. Luo Y, Smith JV, Paramasivam V, Burdick A, Curry KJ, et al. (2002) Inhibition of amyloid-beta aggregation and caspase-3 activation by the Ginkgo biloba extract EGb761. Proc Natl Acad Sci U S A 99: 12197–12202.
11. Garcia-Mediavilla V, Crespo I, Collado PS, Esteller A, Sanchez-Campos S, et al. (2007) The anti-inflammatory flavones quercetin and kaempferol cause inhibition of inducible nitric oxide synthase, cyclooxygenase-2 and reactive C-protein, and down-regulation of the nuclear factor kappaB pathway in Chang Liver cells. Eur J Pharmacol 557: 221–229.
12. Kuppusamy UR, Das NP (1992) Effects of flavonoids on cyclic AMP phosphodiesterase and lipid mobilization in rat adipocytes. Biochem Pharmacol 44: 1307–1315.
13. Kuppusamy UR, Das NP (1994) Potentiation of beta-adrenoceptor agonist-mediated lipolysis by quercetin and fisetin in isolated rat adipocytes. Biochem Pharmacol 47: 521–529.
14. Baur JA, Pearson KJ, Price NL, Jamieson HA, Lerin C, et al. (2006) Resveratrol improves health and survival of mice on a high-calorie diet. Nature 444: 337–342.
15. Howitz KT, Bitterman KJ, Cohen HY, Lamming DW, Lavu S, et al. (2003) Small molecule activators of sirtuins extend Saccharomyces cerevisiae lifespan. Nature 425, 191–196.
16. Wood JG, Rogina B, Lavu S, Howitz K, Helfand SL, et al. (2004) Sirtuin activators mimic caloric restriction and delay ageing in metazoans. Nature 430: 686–689.
17. Viswanathan M, Kim SK, Berdichevsky A, Guarente L (2005) A role for SIR-2.1 regulation of ER stress response genes in determining C. elegans life span. Dev Cell 9: 605–615.
18. Jarolim S, Millen J, Heeren G, Laun P, Goldfarb DS, et al. (2004) A novel assay for replicative lifespan in Saccharomyces cerevisiae. FEMS Yeast Res 5: 169–177.
19. Valenzano DR, Terzibasi E, Genade T, Cattaneo A, Domenici L, et al. (2006) Resveratrol prolongs lifespan and retards the onset of age-related markers in a short-lived vertebrate. Curr Biol 16: 296–300.
20. Lee YE, Kim JW, Lee EM, Ahn YB, Song KH, et al. (2012) Chronic Resveratrol Treatment Protects Pancreatic Islets against Oxidative Stress in db/db Mice. PLoS One 7: e50412.
21. Burnett C, Valentini S, Cabreiro F, Goss M, Somogyvári M, et al. (2011) Absence of effects of Sir2 overexpression on lifespan in C. elegans and Drosophila. Nature 477: 482–485.
22. Canto C, Auwerx J (2011) Don't write sirtuins off. Nature 477: 411.

23. Lombard DB, Pletcher SD (2011) A valuable background check. Nature 477: 410.
24. Couzin-Frankel J (2011) Ageing genes: the sirtuin story unravels. Science 334: 1194–1198.
25. Montero M, Lobaton CD, Hernandez-SanMiguel E, SantoDomingo J, Vay L, et al. (2004) Direct activation of the mitochondrial calcium uniporter by natural plant flavonoids. Biochem J 384: 19–24.
26. da-Silva WS, Harney JW, Kim BW, Li J, Bianco SD, et al. (2007) The small polyphenolic molecule kaempferol increases cellular energy expenditure and thyroid hormone activation. Diabetes 56: 767–776.
27. Yu SF, Shun CT, Chen TM, Chen YH (2006) 3-O-beta-D-glucosyl-(1→6)-beta-D-glucosylkaempferol isolated from Sauropus androgenus reduces body weight gain in Wistar rats. Biol Pharm Bull 29: 2510–2513.
28. Lalonde R, Bensoula AN, Filali M (1995) Rotarod sensorimotor learning in cerebellar mutant mice. Neurosci Res 22: 423–426.
29. Shiotsukia H, Yoshimib K, Shimoa Y, Funayamaa M, Takamatsuc Y, et al. (2010) A rotarod test for evaluation of motor skill learning. J Neurosci Meth 189: 180–185.
30. Irizarry RA, Hobbs B, Collin F, Beazer-Barclay YD, Antonellis KJ, et al. (2003) Exploration, normalization, and summaries of high density oligonucleotide array probe level data. Biostatistics 4: 249–264.
31. Irizarry RA, Bolstad BM, Collin F, Cope LM, Hobbs B, et al. (2003) Summaries of Affymetrix GeneChip probe level data. Nucleic Acids Res 31: e15.
32. Bolstad BM, Irizarry RA, Astrand M, Speed TP (2003) A comparison of normalization methods for high density oligonucleotide array data based on variance and bias. Bioinformatics 19: 185–193.
33. Tusher VG, Tibshirani R, Chu G (2001) Significance analysis of microarrays applied to the ionizing radiation response. Proc Natl Acad Sci U S A 98: 5116–5121.
34. Benjamini Y, Drai D, Elmer G, Kafkafi N, Golani I (2001) Controlling the false discovery rate in behavior genetics research. Behav Brain Res 125: 279–284.
35. Poulsen MM, Vestergaard PF, Clasen BF, Radko Y, Christensen LP, et al. (2013) High-dose resveratrol supplementation in obese men: an investigator-initiated, randomized, placebo-controlled clinical trial of substrate metabolism, insulin sensitivity, and body composition. Diabetes 62: 1186–1195.
36. Shockley KR, Witmer D, Burgess-Herbert SL, Paigen B, Churchill GA (2009) Effects of atherogenic diet on hepatic gene expression across mouse strains. Physiol Genomics 39: 172–182.
37. Do GM, Oh HY, Kwon EY, Cho YY, Shin SK, et al. (2011) Long-term adaptation of global transcription and metabolism in the liver of high-fat diet-fed C57BL/6J mice. Mol Nutr Food Res 55: S173–S185.

A Dietary-Wide Association Study (DWAS) of Environmental Metal Exposure in US Children and Adults

Matthew A. Davis[1,2,3,4*], **Diane Gilbert-Diamond**[1,2,4], **Margaret R. Karagas**[1,2,4], **Zhigang Li**[1,2,4], **Jason H. Moore**[1,2,4,5], **Scott M. Williams**[2,5], **H. Robert Frost**[2,4,5]

1 Children's Environmental Health and Disease Prevention Research Center at Dartmouth, Hanover, New Hampshire, United States of America, **2** Institute for Quantitative Biomedical Sciences, Dartmouth College, Hanover, New Hampshire, United States of America, **3** University of Michigan School of Nursing, Ann Arbor, Michigan, United States of America, **4** Section of Biostatistics and Epidemiology, Department of Community and Family Medicine, Geisel School of Medicine at Dartmouth, Hanover, New Hampshire, United States of America, **5** Department of Genetics, Geisel School of Medicine at Dartmouth, Hanover, New Hampshire, United States of America

Abstract

Background: A growing body of evidence suggests that exposure to toxic metals occurs through diet but few studies have comprehensively examined dietary sources of exposure in US populations.

Purpose: Our goal was to perform a novel dietary-wide association study (DWAS) to identify specific dietary sources of lead, cadmium, mercury, and arsenic exposure in US children and adults.

Methods: We combined data from the National Health and Nutrition Examination Survey with data from the US Department of Agriculture's Food Intakes Converted to Retail Commodities Database to examine associations between 49 different foods and environmental metal exposure. Using blood and urinary biomarkers for lead, cadmium, mercury, and arsenic, we compared sources of dietary exposure among children to that of adults.

Results: Diet accounted for more of the variation in mercury and arsenic than lead and cadmium. For instance we estimate 4.5% of the variation of mercury among children and 10.5% among adults is explained by diet. We identified a previously unrecognized association between rice consumption and mercury in a US study population – adjusted for other dietary sources such as seafood, an increase of 10 g/day of rice consumption was associated with a 4.8% (95% CI: 3.6, 5.2) increase in blood mercury concentration. Associations between diet and metal exposure were similar among children and adults, and we recapitulated other known dietary sources of exposure.

Conclusion: Utilizing this combination of data sources, this approach has the potential to identify and monitor dietary sources of metal exposure in the US population.

Editor: Dana C Crawford, Case Western Reserve University, United States of America

Funding: This research project was supported by grants LM009012, LM010098, and GM103534 by the National Institutes of Health (NIH). Davis was supported by Award Number K01AT006162 from the NIH. Karagas and Gilbert-Diamond were supported by NIH NIEHS P01 ES022832 and EPA RD-83544201. Gilbert-Diamond was further supported by NIH NIGMS P20 GM104416. The NIH was not involved in the design and conduct of the study or collection, management, analysis, and interpretation of the data.

Competing Interests: The authors have declared that no competing interests exist.

* Email: mattadav@umich.edu

Introduction

Human environmental exposure to toxic metals such as lead, mercury, cadmium, and arsenic is associated with a wide array of immediate and long-term health effects. Upon exposure, lead, mercury, and cadmium accumulate in the nervous system, liver, kidneys, and lead accumulates within calcified tissues including bone and teeth [1–3]. While arsenic collects in keratin-rich tissues of the integumentary system [4], it is rapidly excreted by the urinary system [5].

The primary target organ for lead is the central and peripheral nervous systems and, as such, exposure is associated with neuropathies and neurobehavioral effects [6]. Infants and children, due to more rapid bone growth and differences in physiology [7], are most vulnerable to the neurotoxic effects of lead, and exposure is associated with a variety of effects on cognition and behavior even at low levels of exposure common in the US and elsewhere [1,8]. Likewise, methyl-mercury (the predominant form of mercury found in aquatic life [9]) exposure in animal studies is associated with developmental neurotoxic and immune-suppressive effects [2]. Cadmium in particular has a long-half life and is more widely distributed throughout the body but targets the kidney where cadmium accumulates in the epithelial cells of the proximal tubule that can result in reabsorption dysfunction [3,10]. Recent evidence indicates the potential for adverse health effects from arsenic exposure at the relatively low exposure levels common to populations worldwide, including an increased risk of cancer, cardiovascular and respiratory conditions, and diabetes [11–16].

The ingestion of contaminated food has become a well-known source of human exposure to toxic metals [2]. For instance, consumption of seafood has been associated with exposure to considerable amounts of methyl-mercury (especially in the consumption of predatory fish that are higher in the aquatic food chain [17]) and arsenic in adult populations [18,19]. Second only to smoking [20], dietary sources are considered the most significant route of non-occupational cadmium exposure; cereals, tubers, pulses, and rice are among the most recognized dietary sources of cadmium [21–23]. Contamination can occur if crops are grown in tainted soil or treated with metal-contaminated pesticides [2,24]. For example, arsenic contamination has been reported in rice, grains, fruits, and juices; presumably from both naturally occurring arsenic found in soil as well as use of arsenic-containing pesticides [25–28]. The exact mechanism of crop contamination differs based on both the specific environmental metal and crop. For instance, arsenic accumulates in rice [29] through the silicon transport system [30] because, to the rice plant, arsenous acid (the major form of arsenic in flooded rice paddies) is indistinguishable from silicic acid.

Despite considerable interest in identifying dietary sources of toxic metal exposure, environmental health studies typically examine only a few dietary sources at one time and broader approaches rely on less rigorous study designs such as market basket surveys. To our knowledge previous studies have not comprehensively examined dietary sources of environmental metal exposure in a large US study population. Examining associations between the various foods (particularly specific crops) and human exposure to metals could not only uncover sources of exposure, but could also potentially identify protective foods – foods whose nutritional composition might inhibit absorption of toxic metals.

Following in the footsteps of global investigations of associations such as genome-wide association studies (GWAS) [31,32] and the more recent environmental/exposure-wide association studies (EWAS) [33,34], we examined associations between 49 different foods and biomarkers of lead, mercury, cadmium, and arsenic exposure. To do so, we combined data from the National Health and Nutrition Examination Survey (NHANES) and the US Department of Agriculture's Food Intakes Converted to Retail Commodities Database (FICRCD) [35] that estimates the total food commodity intake for the individual foods reported by NHANES. As dietary patterns and metabolism differ according to age [36], we examined sources of dietary exposure to toxic metals among children (age <18 years) and adults (age ≥18 years) separately.

Methods and Materials

Study population

The NHANES is a nationally-representative, multi-stage random survey of the non-institutionalized US population that is conducted by the National Center for Health Statistics that gathers detailed information on diet and health from in-person interviews. NHANES study participants also undergo a rigorous clinical examination that includes the collection of blood and urine specimens. For this study, we used data from the NHANES demographics, in-person first day dietary questionnaire, laboratory, physical examination, and health questionnaire files. As our study used publically available and de-identified data, it was determined to be exempt from institutional board review by Dartmouth College's Committee for the Protection of Human Subjects.

We analyzed data from all study participants in the 2005–06 and 2007–08 NHANES surveys. During this period, a total of 20,497 individuals participated in the NHANES surveys (Figure 1) and the unweighted overall response rate was 77.4% and 75.4% for the 2005–06 and 2007–08 surveys respectively. NHANES study participants one year and older were eligible for blood lead, mercury, and cadmium laboratory analysis and approximately one-third of the participants were randomly selected for urinary biomarkers. For children (age <18 years), urinary laboratory analyses were restricted to ages between 6 to 17 years.

Biomarker measurements

After collection at an NHANES mobile examination site, whole blood specimens are stored frozen (−20°C) and transported to the National Center for Environmental Health (NCEH) at the Centers for Disease Control and Prevention for laboratory analysis. Diluted whole blood cadmium, lead, and mercury concentrations were determined using a quadruple inductively coupled plasma dynamic reaction cell mass spectrometry (ICP-DRC-MS) on a PerkinElmer ELAN DRC series (PerkinElmer Instruments Headquarters, Waltham, Massachusetts, USA). This laboratory analysis is an extension of ICP-MS that utilizes dynamic reaction technology to minimize argon-based interference. The interassay coefficient of variation (CV) across lots for blood lead, cadmium, mercury, and inorganic mercury ranged from 3.4 to 21.4% in the 2005–06 and 2007–08 NHANES surveys. The limit of detection for the various blood metals ranged from 0.20 to 0.40 µg/L.

For NHANES, urine was collected in containers from participants and shipped on dry ice (also frozen at −20°C) to the NCEH. At NCEH, urine samples were stored frozen and analyzed within three weeks of collection following standardized protocols. Urinary lead, cadmium, mercury, and total arsenic were also measured using inductively ICP-DRC-MS on a PerkinElmer ELAN DRC II or ELAN 6100 DRC Plus (PerkinElmer Headquarters, Waltham, Massachusetts, USA). Arsenic species and metabolites [arsenous acid, arsenic acid, monomethylarsonic acid (MMA), dimethylarsinic acid (DMA), arsenobetaine, and arsenocholine] were measured using a combination of high performance liquid chromatography and ICP-DRC-MS on a PerkinElmer Series 200 Pump and a PerkinElmer ELAN DRC II respectively (PerkinElmer Headquarters, Waltham, Massachusetts, USA).

The interassay CV among urinary lead, cadmium, total mercury, and total arsenic ranged from 2.3 to 19.9% and among the arsenic species and metabolites between 3.2 to 9.9%. The detection limit among lead, cadmium, total mercury, and total arsenic ranged from 0.04 to 0.74 µg/L. The detection limits for arsenous acid, arsenic acid, MMA, DMA, arsenobetaine, and arsenocholine were 1.20, 1.00, 0.64, 1.70, 0.40, and 0.59 µg/L respectively. Urinary concentration of arsenic is regarded as a valid measure of recent exposure, especially compared to methods that rely on models of exposure from dietary information [5].

24-hour dietary assessment

The in-person dietary questionnaire of NHANES collects detailed information on the study participant's diet for the 24-hour period proceeding the clinical and biomarker measurements and is a validated assessment of dietary consumption [37]. During the physical examination, NHANES participants are asked to recall everything they ate and drank in the previous day (24 hours) and trained NHANES personnel use these data to generate estimates of serving size. For children under the age of 12, the dietary component is conducted with the assistance of a proxy (i.e. a parent or other caregiver) and for children between the ages 12 and 17 the survey is administered without the assistance of a proxy.

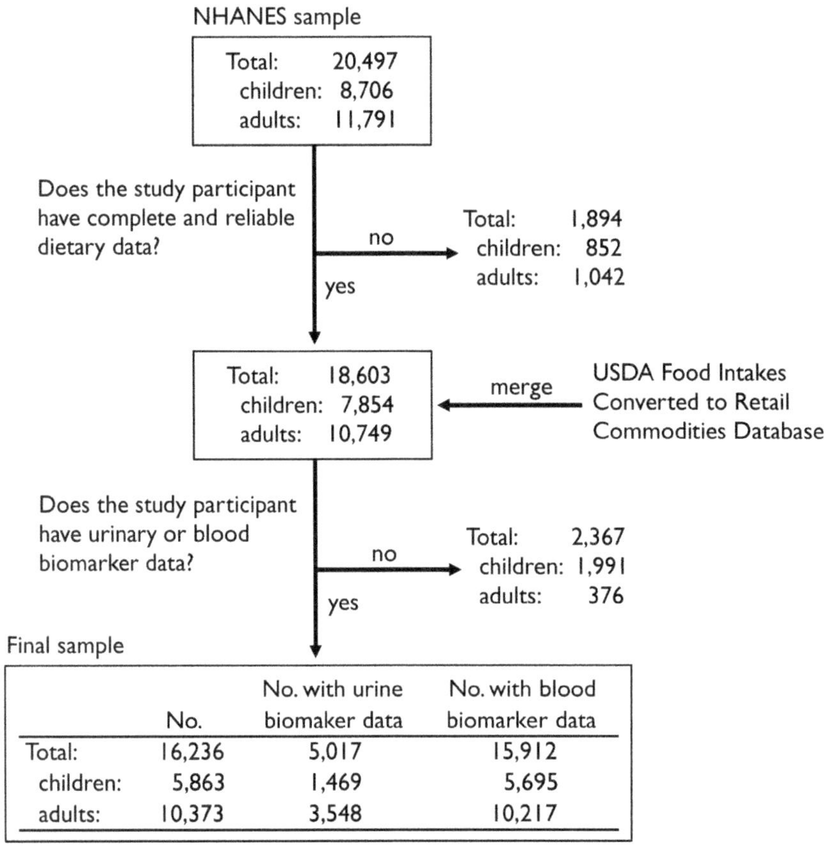

Figure 1. Flow diagram of inclusion for study participants and data sources. Abbreviations: NHANES, National Health and Nutrition Examination Survey; USDA, United States Department of Agriculture.

We used the USDA FICRCD for the corresponding NHANES years to convert the specific serving sizes reported to be consumed during the in-person 24-hour recall period into continuous measures of different food commodities [38]. The FICRCD provides conversion data to estimate the total content of food commodities such as tomatoes, beans, rice, beef etc. in each item with a USDA Food Code reported in NHANES data (e.g., the amount of beans or rice within a burrito). We estimated the total amount in grams of the various food servings consumed by each participant by multiplying the quantity of each food serving reported to be consumed during the 24-hour recall period by the FICRCD estimate of content (dry grams of food commodity per 100 grams of food serving) of the USDA Food Code, then summing across all foods consumed during the 24-hour recall period (Figure S1). As we were interested in identifying specific sources of dietary metal exposure we restricted our analyses to non-aggregate food commodities (i.e. excluded aggregated food groups such as "total diary" and "total meat" from our analyses). However, for the food commodity for eggs we combined the two reported measures "eggs with shell" and "eggs no shell". We specifically retained separate sources of fruit (e.g. "apples" versus "apple from juice") to examine potential differences in exposure that may occur from processing. Therefore, our final analyses consisted of 49 separate foods.

Other data

We also extracted data on sociodemographic characteristics (age, sex, race/ethnicity, marital status, educational attainment, and measures of socio-economic status), health status (self-reported health status and body mass index [BMI]), and information on other exposures (exposure to cigarette smoke, age of home, and drinking water source). We estimated the percentages of the population that were normal weight, overweight, and obese. To do so, for children we calculated the age- and sex- specific BMI Z-score using the 2006 growth curves from World Health Organization [39] for children five years and under. For children between the ages five and 18, we used the 2000 growth curves from the US Centers for Disease Control and Prevention [40] to calculate age- and sex- specific BMI Z-score. Based on the age- and sex- specific BMI Z-scores, children were classified as either normal weight ($<85^{th}$ percentile), overweight ($\geq 85^{th}$ to 95th percentile), or obese ($\geq 95^{th}$ percentile). Adults were also classified as normal weight, overweight, or obese based on a body mass index of <25.0 kg/m^2; ≥ 25.0 kg/m^2 to 30.0 kg/m^2; and $\geq$ 30.0 kg/m^2 respectively. We classified race/ethnicity as "Non-Hispanic White", "Non-Hispanic Black", "Hispanic or Mexican American" and "Other, multiple race/ethnicity." As a surrogate measure of potential occupational exposure to the four metals, we used self-reported employment status and reported hours working in the prior week to classify participants as not working (zero hours), part time (one to 40 hours), and full time (40 hours or more).

To account for lead exposure by contact with paint containing lead, we collapsed NHANES participant's self-reported age of home into those built prior to and after 1978 (the year lead paint was banned [41]). Because cigarette smoke is a source of cadmium and arsenic exposure [42,43], we used serum cotinine to account for active exposure to cigarette smoke. The NHANES measures serum cotinine using an isotope-dilution HPLC/atmospheric pressure chemical ionization mass spectrometry method.

In the US, arsenic exposure through drinking water is primarily found in private unregulated water systems and lead exposure can occur through drinking water contact with lead pipes [44]. Therefore we used the reported water consumed in the 24-hour dietary assessment period and self-reported drinking water source to create a measure of public (using a community water source) and private (defined as either a well, spring, or cistern water source) water consumption measured in grams per day.

In our analyses of urinary biomarkers, we used urinary creatinine to account for urinary dilution. In the 2005–06 NHANES survey, urinary creatinine was measured on a Beckman Synchron CX3 clinical analyzer (Beckman Instruments Inc., Brea, California, USA) using a Jaffe reaction and in the 2007–2008 survey it was measured on a Roche Modular P Chemistry Analyzer (Roche Diagnostics, Indianapolis, Indiana, USA) using an enzymatic method. Therefore, we adjusted 2005–06 urinary creatinine measurements to 2007–08 equivalents using a piecewise regression supplied by the NHANES [45].

Statistical analyses

Blood mercury level is an estimate of exposure to organic mercury (approximately 90% of blood mercury is methyl-mercury) and essentially all mercury in urine is inorganic [19]. We evaluated organic and inorganic forms of arsenic separately (i.e. blood versus urinary mercury), due to their differing toxicity [46]. For urinary arsenic, due to uncertain or negligible health impacts of arsenobetaine and arsenocholine exposure, we subtracted these components from the total urinary arsenic concentrations – thus our final definition of total urinary arsenic included arsenous acid, arsenic acid, MMA, and DMA [38,47]. For the 56 participants (1.1% of participants with urinary arsenic assessment) for whom the combination of arsenobetaine and arsenocholine exceeded the estimate of total arsenic reported by NHANES (presumably due to laboratory imprecision) we assigned a total arsenic value of zero.

We used an adjusted R-squared measure as our primary estimate of the overall contribution of diet to variation in the four biomarkers. We used several different approaches to examine the relationship between the reported consumption of specific foods and biomarker metal concentrations. First, we used Spearman correlation coefficients to explore relationships between the different foods and blood and urine biomarker concentrations. We then used linear models to adjust for confounding factors including all other foods in our analyses. For interpretation, our linear models estimate the effect of an increase of 10 grams per day of the various foods. We $\log_{10}$-transformed all biomarker variables to improve model fit and help normalize residuals and exponentiated all coefficients to represent the % change in biomarker concentration based on an increase of 10 grams per day for each food. Our linear models were based on complete case analysis. The analysis of NHANES data typically utilizes complex survey design methods in order to generate national estimates. As some of the analytic techniques used in our analyses are not yet fully developed in complex survey design methods (e.g., adjusted R-squared) and to maintain internal consistency, none of our analyses used complex survey methods.

To correct for multiple hypothesis testing across the various biomarkers for each food, we corrected for the false discovery rate [48]. For validation of potential associations between foods and environmental metal exposure, we also constructed a validation dataset (referred to herein as a validation study population) from 2003–04 NHANES and FICRCD data using the identical methods to that as our primary analytic dataset.

We used Stata version 13.0 (StatCorp, College Station, Texas, USA) for the management of NHANES data files and R (R Foundation for Statistical Computing, Vienna, Austria) for all statistical analyses.

Results

Characteristics of study participants

In the 2005–06 and 2007–08 NHANES surveys we identified 16,236 study participants (5,863 children and 10,373 adults) with complete dietary data and either a blood or urinary biomarker for lead, cadmium, mercury, or arsenic (Figure 1).

Among both children and adults the study population was approximately evenly distributed by sex. As expected, because NHANES oversamples minorities, racial/ethnic minorities were more heavily represented (e.g., 30.6% of children were of Hispanic or Mexican American background versus 29.1% who were Non-Hispanic White) in the study population (Table S1). Of the adults in our study, 46.0% reported not working in the past week, whereas 17.2% worked between one and 40 hours, and 36.7% reported 40 or more hours. The majority of study participants had serum cotinine levels in excess of 0.015 µg/L, and approximately 40% (35.8% of children and 43.3% of adults) were identified as residing in a house built before 1978. We classified 19.8% of children and 34.4% of adults as being obese.

Dietary sources of environmental metal exposure

Lead. Diet explained a greater amount of blood lead variation in children than in adults (2.9% of the variation in blood lead was explained by diet in children versus 1.6% in adults) (Table 1). While particularly in children a variety of foods were associated with blood lead concentration (e.g., for both whole milk and apple $r_s = 0.15$), consumption of rice among children was weakly associated with an increase in blood lead concentration in adjusted models; 10 g/day of dried rice was associated with a 1.6% (95% CI: 0.7, 2.5) increase in blood lead concentration. However, this association was not observed in our validation study population. Interestingly, consumption of oat flour was associated with a lower blood lead concentration in adults (a 10 g/day increase in oat flour was associated with a 1.8% decrease in blood lead concentration). Furthermore, an even stronger association (a 3.5% decrease per 10 g/day increase) between oat flour and lower blood lead concentration in adults was observed in our validation study population (Figure S2).

Cadmium. Among the four metals we examined, diet explained the least amount of detectable variation in cadmium exposure. Diet explained only 1.4% in children and 0.6% in adults of the variation in blood cadmium concentration (a short term biomarker) and less than 1.0% of variation in urinary cadmium concentration (a longer-term exposure biomarker) (Table 1).

Although weak positive associations between cheese, salad & cooking oils, and some vegetables were associated with blood cadmium concentration in children and negative associations were found between foods and blood cadmium levels in adults, few associations persisted in adjusted models and in our validation study population (Figure 2 versus Figure 3).

Mercury. We found stronger associations between diet and blood mercury concentration (a biomarker of primarily organic mercury) compared to lead and cadmium. Diet accounted for 4.5% of the variation in blood mercury concentration in children and 10.5% in adults.

In unadjusted and adjusted analyses, both seafood and rice consumption were associated with increases in blood mercury concentration. In adults, the Spearman correlation coefficient between fish & seafood and blood mercury concentration was 0.24 and the correlation between rice and blood mercury concentration was 0.14 (Figure 2). In models adjusted for other dietary sources, water, and sociodemographic characteristics, an increase of 10 g/day of rice and seafood consumption was associated with a 4.8% (95% CI: 3.6, 5.2) and 2.5% (95% CI: 2.2, 2.8) increase in blood mercury concentration respectively in adults (Figure 3). Both these associations were reproduced in our validation study population (Figure S2).

Arsenic. Diet had the strongest relationship to arsenic exposure among the four different metals we examined, and it accounted for 8.5% of the variation in total urinary arsenic (excluding arsenobetaine and arsenocholine) among children and 11.5% among adults (Table 1). When examining specific arsenic species, diet explained an even greater proportion of the variability in arsenic exposure (e.g., diet explained 13.7% of the variation in DMA in adults).

We found particularly strong associations between consumption of both rice and seafood and urinary arsenic concentration among both children and adults (Figure 2 and Figure 3). In adults, an increase of 10 g/day of dried rice was associated with an increase of 9.6% (95% CI: 8.2, 11.1) increase in total urinary arsenic and an 8.6% (95% CI: 7.6, 9.6) increase in DMA in adults. Similarly, an increase of 10 g/day of seafood in adults was associated with an increase of 3.4% (95% CI: 2.9, 3.9) in total urinary arsenic; similar associations were found in children as well. Although attenuated, we also found associations between rice consumption and MMA in both children and adults. All the associations between both rice and seafood and urinary arsenic concentration (both total urinary arsenic and DMA) were reproduced in our validation study population (Figure S2).

Discussion

To our knowledge, this is the first large-scale DWAS of environmental exposure to lead, cadmium, mercury, and arsenic. Using a combination of data from the NHANES and the USDA FICRCD, we were able to recapitulate known associations between dietary sources of metal exposure as well as uncover new potential sources of metal exposure. A particular strength of our approach to estimating intake of specific food types is the ability to adjust for other dietary sources to identify independent associations.

There is considerable interest in examining associations across many environmental factors including the contribution of diet and nutrient intake to human disease. Previous investigations have used NHANES data to perform nutrient-wide association studies (NWAS) and have examined associations between a wide array of nutrients and serum lipid levels [49] and blood pressure [50]. These studies are particularly well suited to disentangle biological underpinnings of disease (i.e. how different nutrients may affect health states); however, the strength of our approach lies in the ability to identify sources of metal exposure from specific foods. Up to this point, quantifying patterns of dietary consumption has been a challenge among researchers. While our analyses focused on identify sources of environmental metal exposure, combining NHANES and FICRCD data would also allow researchers the ability to explore associations between specific dietary profiles and health outcomes. Furthermore, because FICRCD data include information for a wide variety of foods, it may reduce bias in estimated associations by taking into account all dietary sources in

Table 1. Amount of variation of lead, cadmium, mercury, and arsenic exposure explained by diet among children versus adults.

	Children			Adults		
	Adjusted R-squared		% explained by Diet	Adjusted R-squared		% explained by Diet
Biomarker	Base model[a]	Base model + Diet[c]		Base model[a,b]	Base model + Diet[c]	
Blood						
Lead	0.17	0.20	2.9%	0.37	0.39	1.6%
Cadmium	0.36	0.38	1.4%	0.35	0.36	0.6%
Mercury	0.02	0.06	4.5%	0.04	0.14	10.5%
Urine[d]						
Lead	0.34	0.35	0.5%	0.43	0.44	1.3%
Cadmium	0.41	0.41	−0.2%	0.51	0.51	0.3%
Mercury	0.17	0.16	0.0%	0.24	0.27	2.5%
Total arsenic[e]	0.31	0.39	8.5%	0.32	0.43	11.5%
Arsenobetaine	0.01	0.16	14.8%	0.04	0.17	12.8%
DMA	0.29	0.40	11.5%	0.31	0.45	13.7%
MMA	0.20	0.23	2.6%	0.20	0.26	5.4%

Abbreviations: DMA, dimethylarsinic acid; MMA, monomethylarsonic acid.
[a]: base model covariates include age (continuous, years), sex, body mass index (continuous, for children Z-score and kg/m^2 for adults), serum cotinine (continuous, μg/L), and age of home (built before 1978 versus after 1978).
[b]: further adjusted for employment status (not working versus part- or full-time).
[c]: dietary data includes the 49 foods and water variables as independent variables (10 g/day).
[d]: further adjusted for urinary creatinine (continuous, mg/dL) to account for urinary dilution.
[e]: excludes arsenobetaine and arsenocholine.

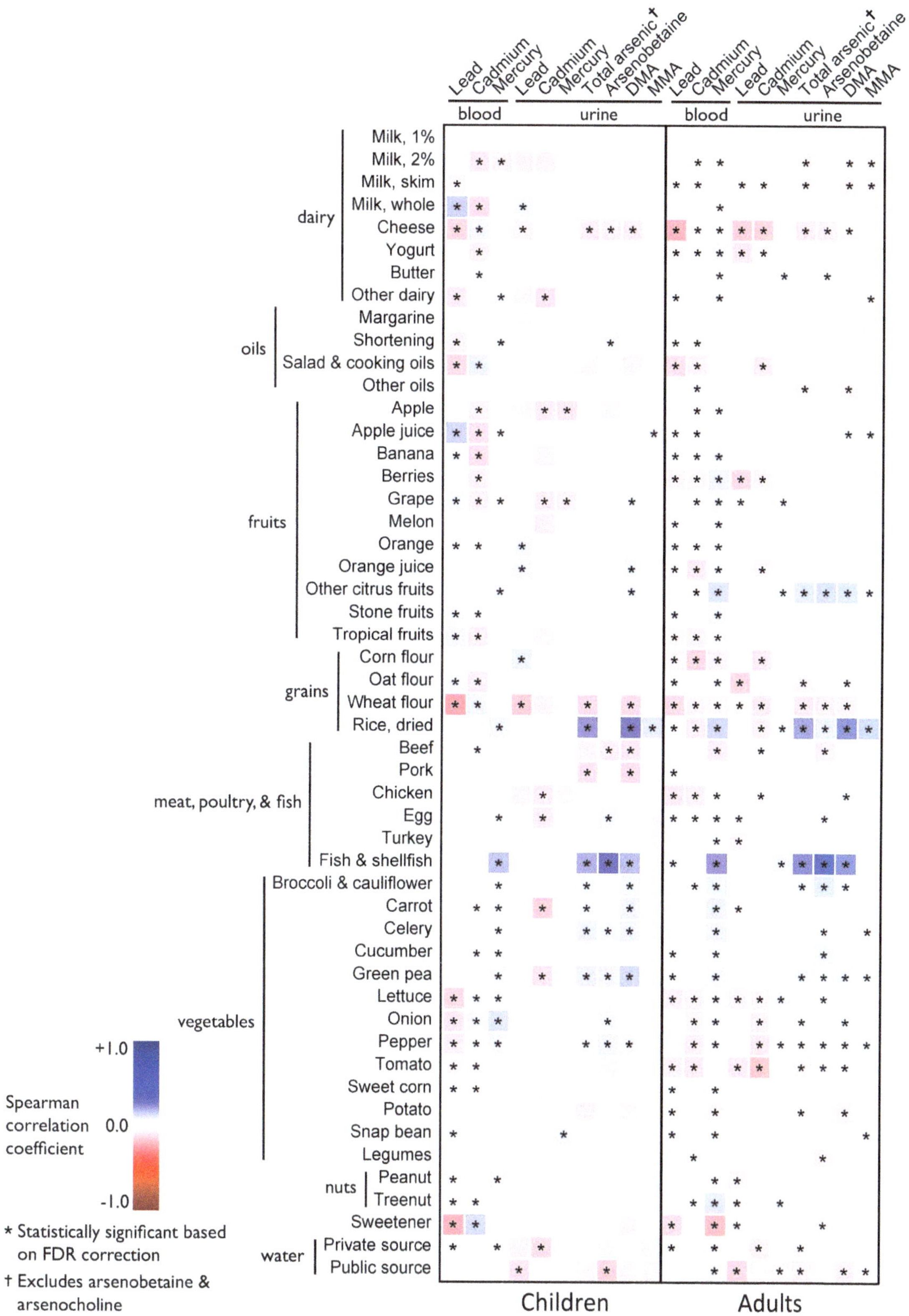

Figure 2. Spearman correlation coefficients between grams of food per day and lead cadmium, mercury, and arsenic biomarker concentrations among children versus adults. Abbreviations: DMA, dimethylarsinic acid; MMA, monomethylarsonic acid; FDR, false discovery rate.

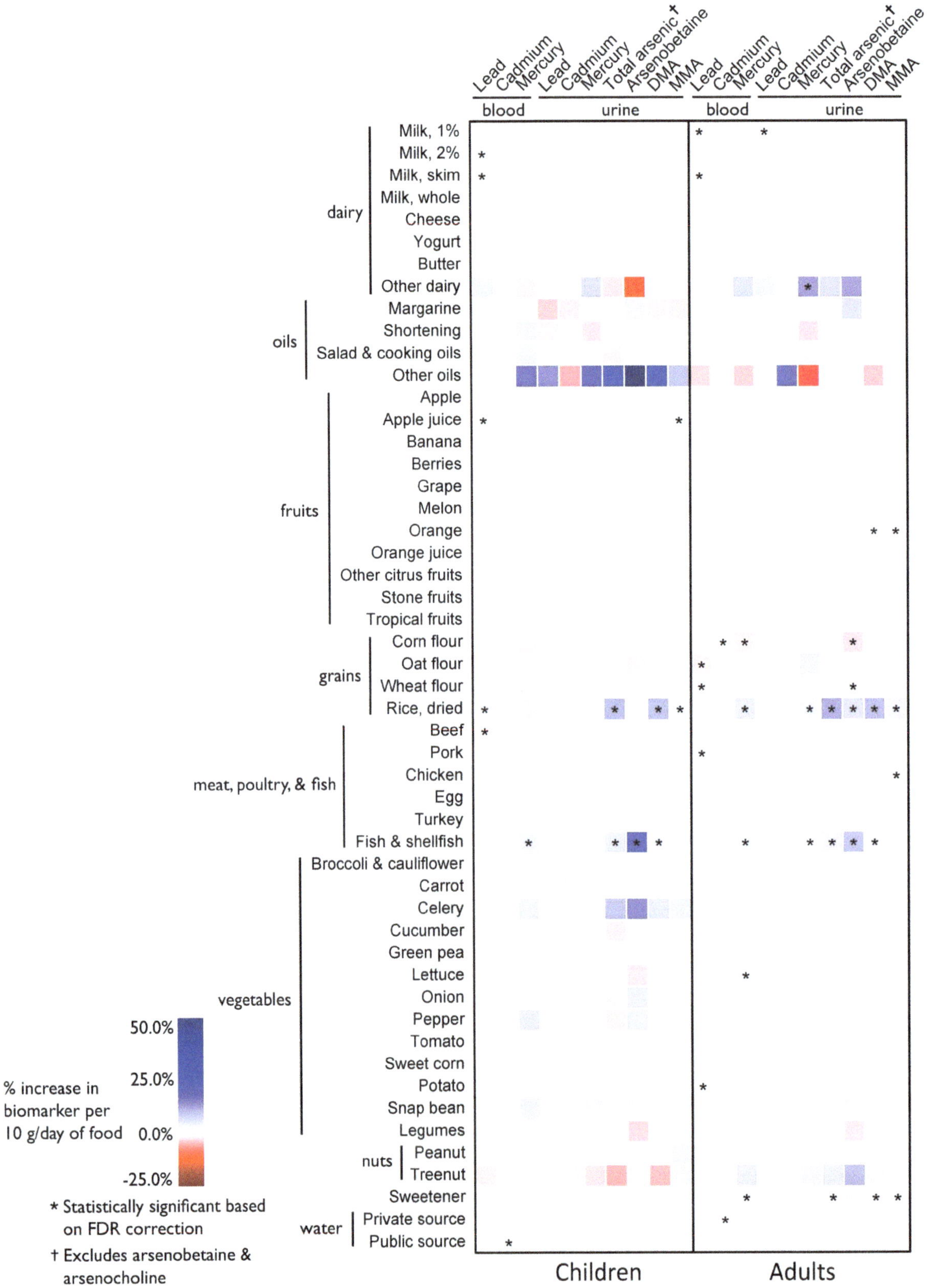

Figure 3. Percent change in lead, cadmium, mercury, and arsenic biomarker concentrations based on an increase of 10 grams of food per day among children versus adults. All models adjusted for age (continuous, years), sex, body mass index (continuous, Z-score for children and kg/m^2 for adults), serum cotinine (continuous, μg/L), and age of home (built before 1978 versus after 1978) and all other dietary sources in table (continuous, 10 g/day). Urinary biomarker models further adjusted for urinary creatinine (continuous, mg/dL) to account for urinary dilution and models restricted to adults also adjusted for employment status (not working versus full- or part-time). Abbreviations: DMA, dimethylarsinic acid; MMA, monomethylarsonic acid; FDR, false discovery rate.

statistical models. Lastly, our study begins to fill a gap in understanding the connection between environmental and internal measures of exposure.

As previously demonstrated in US populations, we found relationships between rice and seafood consumption with arsenic exposure [18,38,47,51] and determined that dietary patterns of metal exposure were similar between children and adults. Overall, we identified specific dietary sources of arsenic, mercury, and lead and detected a relative paucity of dietary exposure to cadmium in this study population. Because of the richness of the dietary data, we also uncovered potentially new dietary associations with metal exposures in this US population. In adjusted models, and validated in an independent study population, we found that rice consumption was associated with mercury exposure adults. This finding has particular relevance to future US safe food practices and may warrant further investigation. Previous studies have examined contaminated rice in China. In these studies, while most rice samples were below maximum allowable concentrations for toxic metals – estimates of lead for children and mercury for adults exceeded safe limits in some locales [52–55]. Interestingly, we also found evidence in our primary and validation study populations that certain foods may reduce exposure to toxic metals. For example, we found inverse associations between blood lead and oat flour suggesting that these foods (potentially due to their nutritional properties) may interfere with lead absorption.

Limitations

Our study has several limitations that must be acknowledged. First, our estimates of food consumption are based on self-report and therefore may be subject to misclassification. Despite the NHANES being known as reliable source of dietary data [37], due to measurement error our results are more likely biased towards the null. Second, as we did not apply the NHANES complex survey design methods to our analyses, our results are not necessarily generalizable to the entire US population. The NHANES sampling frame is the non-institutionalized population (i.e. excludes those in the military, nursing homes, etc.) and over samples minorities, thus our results should not be interpreted as representing the entire US population. However, while our estimates may not reflect the US, considering the more diverse sample, over-representation of minority groups may also be considered a strength. Third, because of wide variation in food growing practices and geology (e.g., there exists wide variation in arsenic concentration in rice due to both cultivation and species [56]), we are not able to draw conclusions regarding the specific amount of lead, cadmium, mercury, and arsenic exposure from the foods we examined.

Nonetheless, using a novel combination of data sources and methods from both informatics and epidemiology, we were able to observe known associations and identify potential new associations in a large US study population. This study provides an important demonstration of a DWAS of environmental metal exposures.

Supporting Information

Figure S1 National Health and Nutrition Examination Survey (2005–06 and 2007–08 surveys) first day dietary recall data converted to food commodities according to study participant sequence number.

Figure S2 Percent change in lead, cadmium, mercury, and arsenic biomarker concentrations based on an increase of 10 grams of food per day among children versus adults in validation study population. All models adjusted for age (continuous, years), sex, body mass index (continuous, Z-score for children and kg/m^2 for adults), serum cotinine (continuous, µg/L), and age of home (built before 1978 versus after 1978) and all other dietary sources in table (continuous, 10 g/day). Urinary biomarker models further adjusted for urinary creatinine (continuous, mg/dL) to account for urinary dilution and models restricted to adults also adjusted for employment status (not working versus full- or part-time). Abbreviations: DMA, dimethylarsinic acid; MMA, monomethylarsonic acid; FDR, false discovery rate.

Author Contributions

Conceived and designed the experiments: MAD MRK JHM SMW HRF. Analyzed the data: MAD JHM HRF. Wrote the paper: MAD DGD MRK ZL JHM SMW HRF.

References

1. Barbosa F Jr, Tanus-Santos JE, Gerlach RF, Parsons PJ (2005) A critical review of biomarkers used for monitoring human exposure to lead: advantages, limitations, and future needs. Environ Health Perspect 113: 1669–1674.
2. Borchers A, Teuber SS, Keen CL, Gershwin ME (2010) Food safety. Clin Rev Allergy Immunol 39: 95–141.
3. Prozialeck WC, Edwards JR (2010) Early biomarkers of cadmium exposure and nephrotoxicity. Biometals 23: 793–809.
4. Slotnick MJ, Nriagu JO (2006) Validity of human nails as a biomarker of arsenic and selenium exposure: A review. Environ Res 102: 125–139.
5. Orloff K, Mistry K, Metcalf S (2009) Biomonitoring for environmental exposures to arsenic. J Toxicol Environ Health B Crit Rev 12: 509–524.
6. Gidlow DA (2004) Lead toxicity. Occup Med (Lond) 54: 76–81.
7. Barry PS (1981) Concentrations of lead in the tissues of children. Br J Ind Med 38: 61–71.
8. Gulson BL, Mizon KJ, Korsch MJ, Howarth D, Phillips A, et al. (1996) Impact on blood lead in children and adults following relocation from their source of exposure and contribution of skeletal tissue to blood lead. Bull Environ Contam Toxicol 56: 543–550.
9. Lindberg A, Bjornberg KA, Vahter M, Berglund M (2004) Exposure to methylmercury in non-fish-eating people in Sweden. Environ Res 96: 28–33.
10. Jarup L, Akesson A (2009) Current status of cadmium as an environmental health problem. Toxicol Appl Pharmacol 238: 201–208.
11. Karagas MR, Stukel TA, Morris JS, Tosteson TD, Weiss JE, et al. (2001) Skin cancer risk in relation to toenail arsenic concentrations in a US population-based case-control study. Am J Epidemiol 153: 559–565.
12. Karagas MR, Tosteson TD, Morris JS, Demidenko E, Mott LA, et al. (2004) Incidence of transitional cell carcinoma of the bladder and arsenic exposure in New Hampshire. Cancer Causes Control 15: 465–472.
13. Amaral AF, Porta M, Silverman DT, Milne RL, Kogevinas M, et al. (2011) Pancreatic cancer risk and levels of trace elements. Gut 61: 1583–1588.
14. Leonardi G, Vahter M, Clemens F, Goessler W, Gurzau E, et al. (2012) Inorganic arsenic and basal cell carcinoma in areas of Hungary, Romania, and Slovakia: A case-control study. Environ Health Perspect 120: 721–726.
15. Sohel N, Persson LA, Rahman M, Streatfield PK, Yunus M, et al. (2009) Arsenic in drinking water and adult mortality: A population-based cohort study in rural Bangladesh. Epidemiology 20: 824–830.
16. International Agency for Research on Cancer (2004) Some Drinking Water Disinfectants and Contaminants, Including Arsenic. Lyon, France. Available online: http://monographs.iarc.fr/ENG/Monographs/vol84/volume84.pdf
17. Grandjean P, Weihe P, White RF, Debes F, Araki S, et al. (1997) Cognitive deficit in 7-year-old children with prenatal exposure to methylmercury. Neurotoxicol Teratol 19: 417–428.
18. Navas-Acien A, Francesconi KA, Silbergeld EK, Guallar E (2011) Seafood intake and urine concentrations of total arsenic, dimethylarsinate and arsenobetaine in the US population. Environ Res 111: 110–118.
19. Berglund M, Lind B, Bjornberg KA, Palm B, Einarsson O, et al. (2005) Inter-individual variations of human mercury exposure biomarkers: A cross-sectional assessment. Environ Health 4: 20.
20. Cho YA, Kim J, Woo HD, Kang M (2013) Dietary cadmium intake and the risk of cancer: A meta-analysis. PLoS One 8: e75087.

21. Llobet JM, Falco G, Casas C, Teixido A, Domingo JL (2003) Concentrations of arsenic, cadmium, mercury, and lead in common foods and estimated daily intake by children, adolescents, adults, and seniors of Catalonia, Spain. J Agric Food Chem 51: 838–842.
22. Watanabe T, Shimbo S, Nakatsuka H, Koizumi A, Higashikawa K, et al. (2004) Gender-related difference, geographical variation and time trend in dietary cadmium intake in Japan. Sci Total Environ 329: 17–27.
23. Satarug S, Garrett SH, Sens MA, Sens DA (2010) Cadmium, environmental exposure, and health outcomes. Environ Health Perspect 118: 182–190.
24. Islam E, Yang XE, He ZL, Mahmood Q (2007) Assessing potential dietary toxicity of heavy metals in selected vegetables and food crops. J Zhejiang Univ Sci B 8: 1–13.
25. Xue J, Zartarian V, Wang SW, Liu SV, Georgopoulos P (2010) Probabilistic Modeling of Dietary Arsenic Exposure and Dose and Evaluation with 2003–2004 NHANES Data. Environ Health Perspect 118: 345–350.
26. Yost IJ, Tao S-H, Egan SK, Barraj LM, Smith KM, et al. (2004) Estimation of dietary intake of inorganic arsenic in US children. Hum Ecol Risk Assess 10: 473–483.
27. Meacher DM, Menzel DB, Dillencourt MD, Bic LF, Schoof RA, et al. (2002) Estimation of multimedia inorganic arsenic intake in the US population. Hum Ecol Risk Assess 8: 1697–1721.
28. European Food Safety Authority (2009) Panel on Contaminants in the Food Chain (CONTAM): Scientific Opinion on Arsenic in Food. Available online: http://www.efsa.europa.eu/en/efsajournal/pub/1351.htm
29. Mitani N, Chiba Y, Yamaji N, Ma JF (2009) Identification and characterization of maize and barley Lsi2-like silicon efflux transporters reveals a distinct silicon uptake system from that in rice. Plant Cell 21: 2133–2142.
30. Ma JF, Yamaji N, Mitani N, Xu XY, Su YH, et al. (2008) Transporters of arsenite in rice and their role in arsenic accumulation in rice grain. Proc Natl Acad Sci U S A 105: 9931–9935.
31. Welcome Trust Case Control Consortium (2007) Genome-wide association study of 14,000 cases of seven common diseases and 3,000 shared controls. Nature 447: 661–678.
32. Haines JL, Hauser MA, Schmidt S, Scott WK, Olson LM, et al. (2005) Complement factor H variant increases the risk of age-related macular degeneration. Science 308: 419–421.
33. Lioy PJ, Rappaport SM (2011) Exposure science and the exposome: An opportunity for coherence in the environmental health sciences. Environ Health Perspect 119: A466–467.
34. Patel CJ, Bhattacharya J, Butte AJ (2010) An Environment-Wide Association Study (EWAS) on type 2 diabetes mellitus. PLoS One 5: e10746.
35. United States Department of Agriculture. Food Intakes Converted to Retail Commodities. Available: http://www.ars.usda.gov/Services/docs.htm?docid = 21993.
36. Drewnowski A, Rehm CD (2013) Energy intakes of US children and adults by food purchase location and by specific food source. Nutr J 12: 59.
37. Moshfegh AJ, Rhodes DG, Baer DJ, Murayi T, Clemens JC, et al. (2008) The US Department of Agriculture automated multiple-pass method reduces bias in the collection of energy intakes. Am J Clin Nutr 88: 324–332.
38. Davis MA, Mackenzie TA, Cottingham KL, Gilbert-Diamond D, Punshon T, et al. (2012) Rice consumption and urinary arsenic concentrations in U.S. children. Environ Health Perspect 120: 1418–1424.
39. The World Health Organization 2006 Child Growth Standards (2013) Available: http://www.who.int/childgrowth/en/
40. Centers for Disease Control and Prevention, 2000 Growth Charts (2010) Available: http://www.cdc.gov/growthcharts/cdc_charts.htm
41. Wakefield J (2002) The lead effect? Environ Health Perspect 110: A574–580.
42. Chen CL, Hsu LI, Chiou HY, Hsueh YM, Chen SY, et al. (2004) Ingested arsenic, cigarette smoking, and lung cancer risk: A follow-up study in arseniasis-endemic areas in Taiwan. JAMA 292: 2984–2990.
43. Adams SV, Newcomb PA (2014) Cadmium blood and urine concentrations as measures of exposure: NHANES 1999–2010. J Expo Sci Environ Epidemiol 24: 163–170.
44. Nathan VR (2006) Drinking water in Michigan: source, quality, and contaminants. J Water Health 4 Suppl 1: 67–73.
45. National Health and Nutrition Examination Survey. 2007–2008 Data Documentation, Codebook, and Frequencies: Urinary Albumin and Urinary Creatinine. Available: http://www.cdc.gov/nchs/nhanes/nhanes2007-2008/ALB_CR_E.htm
46. Meharg AA, Lombi E, Williams PN, Scheckel KG, Feldmann J, et al. (2008) Speciation and localization of arsenic in white and brown rice grains. Environ Sci Technol 42: 1051–1057.
47. Gilbert-Diamond D, Cottingham KL, Gruber JF, Punshon T, Sayarath V, et al. (2011) Rice consumption contributes to arsenic exposure in US women. Proc Natl Acad Sci U S A 108: 20656–20660.
48. Benjamini Y, Hochberg Y (1995) Controlling for false discovery rate: A practical and powerful approach to multiple testing. J R Stat Soc Series B 57: 289–300.
49. Patel CJ, Cullen MR, Ioannidis JP, Butte AJ (2012) Systematic evaluation of environmental factors: Persistent pollutants and nutrients correlated with serum lipid levels. Int J Epidemiol 41: 828–843.
50. Tzoulaki I, Patel CJ, Okamura T, Chan Q, Brown IJ, et al. (2012) A nutrient-wide association study on blood pressure. Circulation 126: 2456–2464.
51. Gamble MV, Liu X, Slavkovich V, Pilsner JR, Ilievski V, et al. (2007) Folic acid supplementation lowers blood arsenic. Am J Clin Nutr 86: 1202–1209.
52. Fang Y, Sun X, Yang W, Ma N, Xin Z, et al. (2014) Concentrations and health risks of lead, cadmium, arsenic, and mercury in rice and edible mushrooms in China. Food Chem 147: 147–151.
53. Huang Z, Pan XD, Wu PG, Han JL, Chen Q (2013) Health risk assessment of heavy metals in rice to the population in Zhejiang, China. PLoS One 8: e75007.
54. Rothenberg SE, Yu X, Zhang Y (2013) Prenatal methylmercury exposure through maternal rice ingestion: Insights from a feasibility pilot in Guizhou Province, China. Environ Pollut 180: 291–298.
55. Gilbert-Diamond D, Li Z, Perry AE, Spencer SK, Gandolfi AJ, et al. (2013) A population-based case-control study of urinary arsenic species and squamous cell carcinoma in New Hampshire, USA. Environ Health Perspect 121: 1154–1160.
56. Batista BL, Souza JM, De Souza SS, Barbosa F Jr. (2011) Speciation of arsenic in rice and estimation of daily intake of different arsenic species by Brazilians through rice consumption. J Hazard Mater 191: 342–348.

10

Differences in Muscle Transcriptome among Pigs Phenotypically Extreme for Fatty Acid Composition

Anna Puig-Oliveras[1,2]*, Yuliaxis Ramayo-Caldas[3], Jordi Corominas[1,2], Jordi Estellé[3,4,5], Dafne Pérez-Montarelo[6], Nicholas J. Hudson[7], Joaquim Casellas[2,8], Josep M. Folch[1,2], Maria Ballester[1,2]

1 Departament de Genètica Animal, Centre de Recerca en Agrigenòmica (CRAG), Bellaterra, Spain, **2** Departament de Ciència Animal i dels Aliments, Universitat Autònoma de Barcelona (UAB), Bellaterra, Spain, **3** Génétique Animale et Biologie Intégrative UMR1313 (GABI), Institut National de la Recherche Agronomique (INRA), Jouy-en-Josas, France, **4** Génétique Animale et Biologie Intégrative UMR1313 (GABI), AgroParisTech, Jouy-en-Josas, France, **5** Laboratoire de Radiobiologie et Etude du Génome (LREG), Commissariat à l'énergie atomique et aux énergies alternatives (CEA), Jouy-en-Josas, France, **6** Departamento de Genética Animal, Instituto Nacional de Investigación y Tecnología Agraria y Alimentaria (INIA), Madrid, Spain, **7** Computational and Systems Biology, Commonwealth Scientific and Industrial Research Organisation (CSIRO) Animal, Food and Health SciencesQLD, Brisbane, Australia, **8** Departament de Genètica i Millora Animal, Institut de Recerca i Tecnologies Agroalimentàries (IRTA), Lleida, Spain

Abstract

Background: Besides having an impact on human health, the porcine muscle fatty acid profile determines meat quality and taste. The RNA-Seq technologies allowed us to explore the pig muscle transcriptome with an unprecedented detail. The aim of this study was to identify differentially-expressed genes between two groups of 6 sows belonging to an Iberian × Landrace backcross with extreme phenotypes according to FA profile.

Results: We sequenced the muscle transcriptome acquiring 787.5 M of 75 bp paired-end reads. About 85.1% of reads were mapped to the reference genome. Of the total reads, 79.1% were located in exons, 6.0% in introns and 14.9% in intergenic regions, indicating expressed regions not annotated in the reference genome. We identified a 34.5% of the intergenic regions as interspersed repetitive regions. We predicted a total of 2,372 putative proteins. Pathway analysis with 131 differentially-expressed genes revealed that the most statistically-significant metabolic pathways were related with lipid metabolism. Moreover, 18 of the differentially-expressed genes were located in genomic regions associated with IMF composition in an independent GWAS study in the same genetic background. Thus, our results indicate that the lipid metabolism of FAs is differently modulated when the FA composition in muscle differs. For instance, a high content of PUFA may reduce FA and glucose uptake resulting in an inhibition of the lipogenesis. These results are consistent with previous studies of our group analysing the liver and the adipose tissue transcriptomes providing a view of each of the main organs involved in lipid metabolism.

Conclusions: The results obtained in the muscle transcriptome analysis increase the knowledge of the gene regulation of IMF deposition, FA profile and meat quality, in terms of taste and nutritional value. Besides, our results may be important in terms of human health.

Editor: Hervé Guillou, INRA, France

Funding: This work has been funded by MICINN project AGL2011-29821-C02 (Ministerio de Economía y Competitividad) and by the Innovation Consolider-Ingenio 2010 Program (CSD2007-00036). A. Puig-Oliveras was funded by a Personal Investigador en Formación (PIF) PhD grant from the Universitat Autònoma de Barcelona (458-01-1/2011). J. Corominas was funded by a Formación de Personal Investigador (FPI) PhD grant from Spanish Ministerio de Educación (BES-2009-018223), Y. Ramayo by a Formación del Profesorado Universitario (FPU) PhD grant (AP2008-01450). The funders had no role in study design, data collection and analysis, decision to publish, or preparation of the manuscript.

Competing Interests: The authors have declared that no competing interests exist.

* E-mail: anna.puig@cragenomica.es

Introduction

High-throughput sequencing technologies are rapidly evolving and its application to transcriptome analysis (RNA-Seq), with the adapted bioinformatic tools, allow the exploration of the transcriptome in an unprecedented manner in terms of accuracy and data insight [1]. In addition, RNA-Seq technology is useful, not only to detect variation in gene expression patterns, but also to identify new isoforms, splicing events, and different promoter and polyadenylation signal usage. Currently, only a few RNA-Seq studies have been conducted in livestock species such as pigs [2–6].

According to the Food and Agriculture Organization (FAO) [7], pork is the major source of meat intake by human, accounting for the 43% of the consumed meat worldwide. The taste and the quality of the cooked and the cured meat products depend on the oxidative stability of the muscle which is related to the fatty acid (FA) composition [8,9]. Furthermore, it is well known that genetic and environmental factors such as diet, are responsible for FA composition variation [10]. Besides its influence on meat taste, the FA composition in muscle has taken additional importance due to their nutritional value and human health-related benefits [11,12], particularly for its effects on human diseases such as cancers, coronary heart diseases and atherosclerosis [11]. It has been reported that omega-3 FAs, such as α-linolenic acid (C18:3 n-3), are associated with the reduction of low density lipoprotein (LDL) cholesterol and blood triacylglycerols, as well as with the modulation of immune functions and inflammatory processes [13,14]. Artificial selection to increase meat production in pigs has caused a reduction of intramuscular fat (IMF) and changes in meat FA composition in some breeds. Hereby, there is an increasing interest in the pork industry on producing meat products with a higher IMF content and with a healthier FA profile, while maintaining a reduced amount of backfat [15].

In a recent genome-wide association study (GWAS) [16], genomic regions associated with the IMF (*Longissimus dorsi*) FA composition were identified in a backcross population (BC1_LD; 25% Iberian and 75% Landrace). A combined linkage QTL scan and GWAS performed in the same backcross revealed significant pleiotropic regions with effects on both IMF and backfat tissues [17,18]. Moreover, the transcriptome of the other two major organs regulating lipid metabolism, liver and adipose tissue (backfat), have been studied using RNA-Seq in the BC1_LD animals [4,5]. In these studies, a shift towards the oxidation of FAs in liver [4] and an inhibition of *de novo* lipogenesis in adipose tissue [5] was observed in animals with higher content of polyunsaturated FA (PUFA). Since the adipose and liver tissues have previously been analysed using animals belonging to the same population, with the addition of the muscle transcriptome we aim to have a more complete view of the genetic regulation of lipid metabolism in pigs [4,5]. The goal of the current study was to identify differentially-expressed genes and pathways in the *Longissimus dorsi* muscle of Iberian × Landrace backcrossed pigs with extreme phenotypes for muscle FA profile to better understand the differences in this meat quality trait.

Results

Phenotypic differences among the analysed animals

In a previous work [4], a Principal Component Analysis (PCA) was performed to select animals of an Iberian × Landrace backcross (BC1_LD) with extreme phenotypes for IMF FA composition. Using the same classification and the first principal component, six females belonging to the extreme High (H) group and six from the Low (L) group were selected for muscle RNA-Seq analysis. Animal selection considered the parental genetic diversity according to the pedigree. Significant statistical differences (*P*-value <0.05) were identified between the H and L groups in 18 out of 26 evaluated traits (Table 1). The H group had, in comparison to the L group, a higher content of PUFA including linolenic (C18:2 n-6), α-linolenic, eicosadienoic (C20:2 n-6), eicosatrienoic (C20:3 n-6) and arachidonic (C20:4 n-6) FAs. Conversely, the L group had a higher content of monounsaturated FA (MUFA) like palmitoleic (C16:1 n-7) and oleic (C18:1 n-9) FAs and saturated FAs (SFA) such as myristic (C14:0) and palmitic (C16:0) FAs. The two groups of pigs did not differ significantly in either IMF content or backfat thickness.

Transcriptome analysis of swine muscle tissue

As described above, the *Longissimus dorsi* (LD) muscle transcriptome was sequenced in twelve sows (H = 6, L = 6) with extreme phenotypes for intramuscular FA composition. A total amount of 787.5 M of 75 bp paired-end reads were acquired from the RNA-Seq experiment. Sequence alignment was performed against the reference pig genome (Sscrofa10.2) by using Tophat [19]. About 85.1% (76.5%–86.6%) of reads were mapped to the reference genome, of which 14.5% (12.4%–16.1%) did not map to unique genomic locations. A total of 85.1% (84.0%–87.6%) of the mapped reads correspond to annotated genes, 79.1% (77.5%–84.1%) of them were located in exons and 6.0% (3.6%–6.8%) in introns. The remaining 14.9% (12.4%–16.0%) of reads mapped to intergenic regions, indicating that they were not annotated in the reference genome (Table S1).

The transcripts generated when assembling the short reads with Cufflinks [20] resulted in a mean of 43,255 transcripts expressed in muscle (Table S2). Transcripts were classified in different categories, being the most abundant the exonic transcripts (60.4%), the putative new isoforms (20.5%) and the intergenic transcripts (10.1%) (Table S2). A total of 9,887 new isoforms were identified corresponding to 9,805 known genes.

Transposable elements identification and novel coding gene discovery

The percentage of interspersed repeats identified with the Repeat Masker [21] in the intergenic transcripts was about 34.5%. Moreover, SINEs and LINEs were the most abundant repetitive elements identified (14.1% and 14.9%, respectively) (Table S3).

With the aim of improving the current porcine genome annotation, we took into account the intergenic transcripts identified with cufflinks (a mean of 4,440 transcripts) to determine whether these transcripts potentially codified for proteins. A total of 2,372 putative proteins were predicted by Augustus [22] corresponding to non-annotated transcripts of the Sscrofa10.2 genome assembly version. Among the 2,372 novel predicted proteins, only 1,406 (59.2%) had at least one orthologous gene identified with BLASTP option of Blast2GO, representing a total of 577 known genes (Table S4) [23]. These proteins corresponded to: 720 *Sus scrofa*, 17 *Homo sapiens* and 247 *Bos taurus in silico* predicted protein, and 476 *Sus scrofa*, 933 *Homo sapiens*, and 403 *Bos taurus* known proteins. The pig species was the only one showing a higher percentage of computationally predicted protein (60.2%) in comparison to known proteins (39.8%).

Moreover, 918 of the predicted novel proteins were successfully annotated with Blast2GO [23]. To summarize the functional annotation, a GO Slim analysis was performed. The most relevant molecular functions identified were "protein binding" (25%), "ion binding" (19%), "nucleic acid binding" (17%), "small molecular binding" (10%) and, interestingly, "lipid binding" (2%). These new transcripts were mainly involved in the following biological processes: "primary metabolic process" (9%), "cellular metabolic process" (9%), "macromolecule metabolic process" (8%) and "regulation of biological process" (7%). Using the Enzime code and KEGG, the main metabolic pathways represented were the "phosphatidylinositol signalling system" (12 sequences), "inositol phosphate metabolism" (11) and the "pyrimidine (9) and purine (8) metabolism".

Differential gene expression analysis

A high correlation (r = 0.98, *P*-value $<2.2\times10^{-16}$) between H and L groups in the mean gene expression was found, showing that most of the genes had a similar behaviour. A total of 11,945 transcripts were used to perform the differential expression analysis after filtering. Using EdgeR program [24], 314 genes were identified as significantly differentially expressed between H and L groups. Whereas, employing DESeq [25], 208 genes were detected. Figure 1 shows the *P*-value distribution and how among the transcripts accepted as differentially expressed the selected cut-off of *P*-value <0.01 is clearly departing from the expected *P*-value (equivalent to a FDR ≤0.12).

A total of 131 genes (Table S5) overlapping in both analyses were selected as differentially expressed between H and L groups

Table 1. Mean comparison between High and Low groups (six animals per group) of the traits included in the principal component analysis (PCA).

Characters	H Mean	L Mean	Significance	*P*-value
Carcass quality				
Carcass weight (CW) (kg)	66.22±10.52	70.50±7.91	NS	4.44×10^{-1}
Ham weight (HW) (kg)	18.79±2.32	18.97±2.41	NS	8.96×10^{-1}
Shoulder weight (SW) (kg)	6.6±0.95	6.32±0.97	NS	6.16×10^{-1}
Intramuscular fat (IMF) (%)	1.94±0.65	1.69±0.64	NS	5.25×10^{-1}
Fatty acids in intramuscular fat				
Saturated FA[a]				
Myristic acid (C14:0)	1.11±0.12	1.28±0.12	*	$3{,}08\times10^{-2}$
Palmitic acid (C16:0)	21.29±0.57	24.16±0.54	***	4.35×10^{-6}
Heptadecanoic acid (C17:0)	0.35±0.06	0.20±0.03	***	3.09×10^{-4}
Stearic acid (C18:0)	13.50±0.94	14.16±1.11	NS	2.91×10^{-1}
Arachidic acid (C20:0)	0.25±0.09	0.23±0.05	NS	5.83×10^{-1}
Monounsaturated FA[a]				
Palmitoleic acid (C16:1 n-7)	2.33±0.30	2.97±0.41	*	1.03×10^{-2}
Heptadecenoic acid (C17:1)	0.33±0.08	0.22±0.05	*	2.04×10^{-2}
Oleic acid (C18:1 n-9)	36.78±3.10	42.77±1.07	**	1.18×10^{-3}
Octadecenoic acid (C18:1 n-7)	3.85±0.20	4.14±0.27	NS	6.29×10^{-2}
Eicosenoic acid (C20:1 n-9)	0.82±0.13	0.82±0.07	NS	9.95×10^{-1}
Polyunsaturated FA[a]				
Linoleic acid (C18:2 n-6)	13.70±1.30	6.83±0.40	***	2.14×10^{-7}
α-Linolenic acid (C18:3 n-3)	1.14±0.42	0.47±0.07	**	3.23×10^{-3}
Eicosadienoic acid (C20:2 n-6)	0.61±0.16	0.38±0.05	**	8.39×10^{-3}
Eicosatrienoic acid (C20:3 n-6)	0.42±0.17	0.15±0.02	**	3.58×10^{-3}
Arachidonic acid (C20:4 n-6)	2.79±1.26	0.76±0.18	**	2.96×10^{-3}
Metabolic ratios				
Average Chain Length (ACL)	17.44±0.02	17.37±0.02	***	2.41×10^{-7}
Saturated FA (SFA)	36.49±1.08	40.02±1.28	***	4.20×10^{-4}
Monounsaturated FA (MUFA)	44.49±2.90	51.21±1.41	***	4.67×10^{-4}
Polyunsaturated FA (PUFA)	18.67±2.75	8.59±0.53	***	4.95×10^{-6}
Peroxidability index (PI)	30.92±6.66	13.53±1.02	***	8.60×10^{-5}
Double-bond index (DBI)	0.44±0.08	0.19±0.01	***	2.85×10^{-5}
Unsaturated index (UI)	0.89±0.06	0.70±0.01	***	1.82×10^{-5}

NS: *P*-value >0.05; * *P*-value <0.05; ** *P*-value <0.01; *** *P*-value <0.001
[a]The percentage of each FA, relative to the total FA

and, thereafter, used for pathway analysis (Figure 2). Fifty genes had a higher expression and 81 a lower expression in the H group (in comparison with L group). Remarkably, eighteen (*CLCA4, ANGPT1, PLEKHH1, SDR16C5, PIK3R1, INTU, MAL2, NCEH1, PLN, C4orf29, FABP3, TBX3, MCT1, ESF1, POLR3GL, DBT, C6orf165* and *CHAC1*) of the 131 genes were also present in the annotated QTL intervals of a GWAS study for the IMF FA profile performed in the same population [16]. Three of these genes (*PIK3R1, NCEH1* and *FABP3*) have been directly related with lipid metabolism [26], being clear candidate genes to study the genetic contribution of IMF FA composition. Intriguingly, only two (*C6orf165* and *CHAC1*) of the 18 genes were over-expressed in the H group. Moreover, two of the differentially-expressed genes in muscle (*AQP7* and *FOS*) were also identified as differentially expressed in liver [4], and seventeen of them (*AQP4, SCD, PLEKHB1, CTSF, CIDEC, ALDOC, CXCL2, KIAA0408, SLPI, ALB, C14H10orf116, ITPR2, TRIP10, BANF1, HIF1AN, CHAC1* and *FHL3*) were identified as differentially expressed in adipose tissue [5]. In addition, three of the differentially-expressed genes in our analysis (*ATF3, ENAH* and *SLPI*) were also identified in a muscle microarray study of extreme animals for FA composition from the same backcross [27]. Other genes such as *DNAJA4, ANKRD1, MYH10* and *TNFRSF12A* were also common, but they were only detected by the DESeq program [25] in the RNA-Seq data.

Functional analysis

With the aim of having a more complete functional view of our differentially-expressed genes in the H and L groups, we used Babelomics [28] and Ingenuity Pathways Analysis [29] programs, who have related capabilities but use different databases. The top canonical pathways overrepresented according to IPA were related with nitric oxide signalling in the cardiovascular system

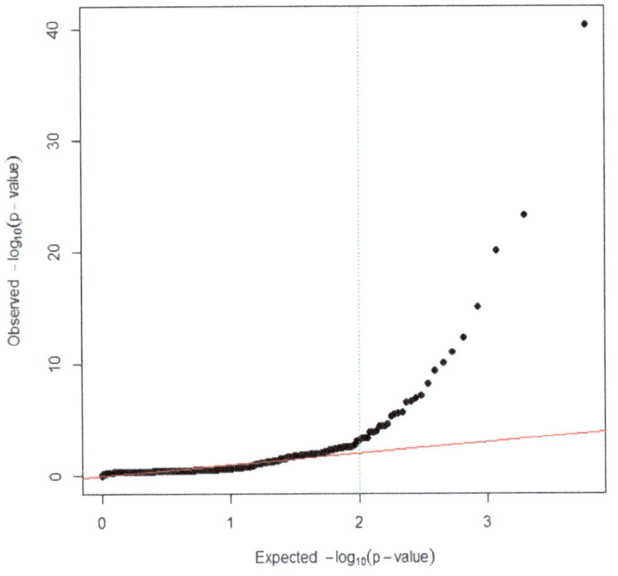

Figure 1. Q-Q plot representing the DESeq [25] ***P*-value distribution of the differentially expression analysis.** The expected distribution of the *P*-values is indicated with a red line, whereas black points represent the observed distribution. The selected cut-off is represented with a green discontinuous line (-log10 (*P*-value) >2).

(7 genes, *P*-value $=7.75\times10^{-7}$) and endothelial nitric oxide synthase signalling (*eNOS*, 8 genes, *P*-value $=2.34\times10^{-6}$). On the other hand, using Babelomics we observed an overrepresentation of lipids and lipoproteins metabolism (6 genes, *P*-value $=1.64\times10^{-3}$), and also the peroxisome proliferator-activated receptors (*PPAR*, 4 genes, *P*-value $=7.25\times10^{-4}$) and the insulin (5 genes, *P*-value $=1.00\times10^{-3}$) signalling and the hemostasis (7 genes, *P*-value $=1.64\times10^{-3}$) pathway (Table 2).

Among the top molecular and cellular functions significantly overrepresented when comparing H relative to L groups with Babelomics, we identified the response to organic substance (18 genes, *P*-value $=3.8\times10^{-7}$), the muscle organ development (5 genes, *P*-value $=3.8\times10^{-5}$), the energy derivation by oxidation of organic compounds (5 genes, *P*-value $=1.0\times10^{-4}$) and the response to hormone stimulus (9 genes, *P*-value $=2.6\times10^{-4}$). Whereas with IPA, the most relevant functions were involved in lipid metabolism (30 genes, *P*-value $=1.04\times10^{-6}$), molecular transport (36 genes, *P*-value $=1.04\times10^{-06}$), small molecule biochemistry (47 genes, *P*-value $=1.04\times10^{-6}$), cell death and survival (38 genes, *P*-value $=1.55\times10^{-6}$), carbohydrate metabolism (30 genes, *P*-value $=2.25\times10^{-6}$), energy production (10 genes, *P*-value $=5.8\times10^{-5}$) and skeletal and muscular system development and function (23 genes, *P*-value $=2.47\times10^{-4}$) (Table S6).

Among the related specific functions for lipid metabolism, the top molecular functions identified with IPA were the oxidation (*ACADVL, ACOX2, FABP3, PLIN1, PLIN5, PON2, SCD*; *P*-value $=3.59\times10^{-4}$), accumulation (*ACADVL, AQP7, FH, IDH1, PLIN1, PON2, RETSAT, SCD*; *P*-value $=7.90\times10^{-04}$), synthesis

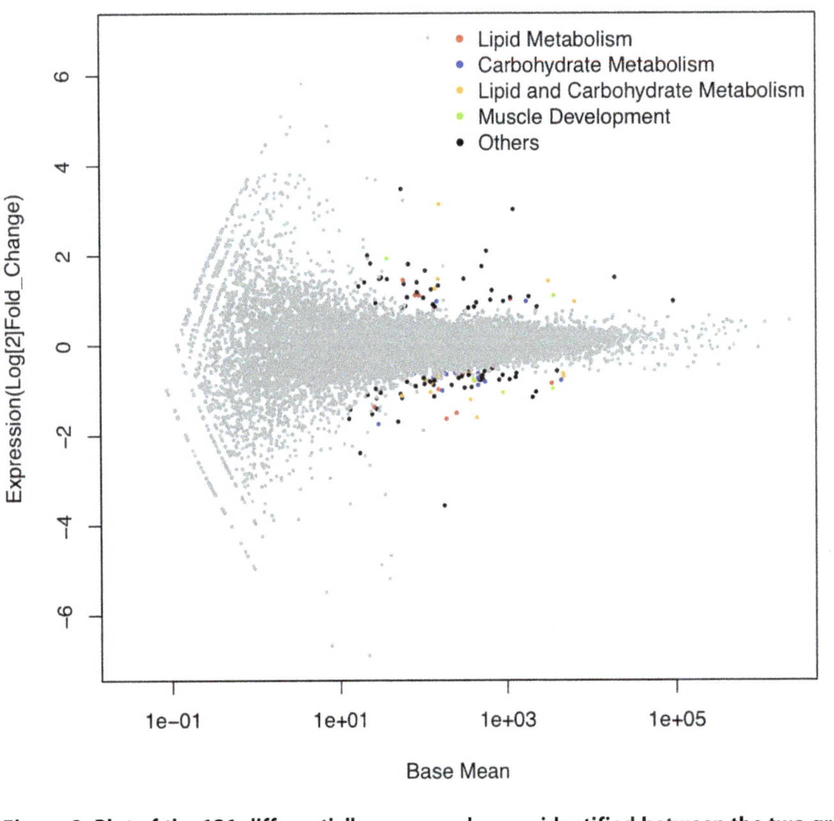

Figure 2. Plot of the 131 differentially-expressed genes identified between the two groups High and Low. X-axis values correspond to base mean expression values and y-axis values are the log2(fold change). The colour for the differentially-expressed genes is related to their function in lipid metabolism (red), carbohydrate metabolism (blue), both lipid and carbohydrate metabolism (orange), muscle development (green) or others (black).

Table 2. Summary of the most significantly-overrepresented pathways of the differentially-expressed genes in muscle between High and Low groups for fatty acid composition traits.

Babelomics			**IPA**		
Category	**Genes**	***P*-value**	**Category**	**Genes**	***P*-value**
Metabolism of Lipids and Lipoproteins	*SCD, ACADVL, ACOX2, IDH1, IDI1, ALB*	5.12×10^{-4}	Nitric Oxid Signalling in the Cardiovascular System	*BDKRB2, PIK3R3, PRKG1, PLN, ITPR2, PIK3R1, ATP2A2*	7.75×10^{-7}
Alanine, Aspartate and Glutamate Metabolism	*ABAT, GOT1, ASNS*	6.38×10^{-4}	eNOS Signalling	*BDK4B2, PIK3R3, AQP7, PRKG1, ITPR2, PIK3R1, CHRNA9, AQP4*	2.34×10^{-6}
PPAR Signalling Pathway	*ACOX2, AQP7, FABP3, SCD*	7.25×10^{-4}	Clathrin-mediated Endocytosis Signalling	*PIK3R3, ALB, CD2AP, TF, PIK3R1, TFRC, ITGB6, FGF1*	2.95×10^{-5}
Insulin Signalling Pathway	*GYS2, PIK3R1, TRIP10, PIK3R3, PPP1R3C*	1.00×10^{-3}	*ILK* Signalling	*PIK3R3, FOS, RND3, PIK3R1, ITGB6, MYL6B, MYH7B, ACTN3*	2.95×10^{-5}
Hemostasis	*ANGPT1, PIK3R1, ALDOA, ITPR2, PLEK, TF, ALB*	1.64×10^{-3}	*CXCR4* Signalling	*PIK3R3, FOS, RND3, ITPR2, PIK3R1, MYL6B*	4.79×10^{-4}

(*ACADVL, ACOX2, ALB, BDKRB2, CNTFR, FABP3, FGF1, FOS, IDI1, PIK3R1, PLIN1, PON2, SCD*; *P*-value $=2.28\times10^{-3}$), concentration (*DUSP1, EXTL1, FABP3, FOS, IDH1, NCEH1, PLIN1, PON2, PPP1R3C, SCD*; *P*-value $=2.48\times10^{-5}$) and homeostasis (*ACADVL, FABP3, GOT1, NCEH1, PIK3R1, PLIN1, SCD*; *P*-value $=1.96\times10^{-4}$) of lipids (Table S7). Other related pathways were identified such as concentration of bile acids (*ALB, ATF3, SCD*; *P*-value $=3.87\times10^{-4}$), obesity (*ABAT, AQP7 ARID5B, ATF3, DESP1, HBEGF, IDH1, PLIN1, RETSAT, SCD*; *P*-value $=5.76\times10^{-4}$), and insulin resistance (*ACOX2, ALB, AQP7, ATP2A2, FGF1, PIK3R1, PON2, PPP1R3C, SCD*; *P*-value $=5.41\times10^{-3}$) and sensitivity (*FABP3, HIF1AN, PIK3R1, SCD*; *P*-value $=7.39\times10^{-3}$). In addition, interesting functions such as heart disease, blood pressure, glucose tolerance, synthesis of carbohydrate and glucose metabolism disorder, biogenesis of cholesterol, differentiation of muscle cells and adiposity were also identified (Table S7).

Finally, a total of nine direct and nine indirect networks were obtained with IPA (Table S8). The top direct network was associated with cell death and survival, cellular development, connective tissue development and function (Figure 3). It showed a score of 55 and contained 29 molecules (Table S8). The top indirect network was related to metabolic disease, lipid metabolism and molecular transport (Figure S1). A total of 21 molecules were associated to this network having a score of 36 (Table S8).

Discussion

To date, muscle transcriptome analyses concerning meat quality in swine have mainly been conducted using microarrays [3,27,30–32]. Compared with microarrays, RNA-Seq enables to determine the transcript abundance with a larger dynamic range of expression levels, it is not limited by the available genomic sequencing information during microarray production and can provide information about new isoforms. However, the main RNA-Seq drawback when compared with microarrays is that the analysis relies on the current pig genome assembly (in this study 10.2), in which interesting genes involved in lipid metabolism are still incorrectly annotated or not present. Therefore, the improvement of the annotation is transcendental for further RNA-Seq studies.

Muscle transcriptome description

In the present study, using RNA-Seq analysis we were able to map a high percentage of reads to the current pig genome assembly (Sscrofa10.2). Our percentage of mapped reads (85.1%) was similar to the described in the pig adipose tissue transcriptome (80%–87%) [5] performed with the Sscrofa10.2 annotation version, however it was higher than the percentage found in the pig muscle transcriptome (64,8%) [6] performed with the Sscrofa9.2 version or the pig liver transcriptome (71.4%–77.7%) [4] using the Sscrofa9.61 annotation version. The high amount of transcripts mapping to intergenic regions and the novel coding gene discovery, showing a higher percentage of computationally predicted proteins (60.2%) versus known proteins (39.8%) in pig in comparison to other species such as bovine and human, reinforces the need to improve the current pig annotation. Similar results were shown in the porcine liver [4] and adipose tissue [5] transcriptomes, in which the 86.0% and 62.5% of the novel proteins identified respectively were computationally-predicted. As expected, the major overlap of predicted novel proteins was between muscle and adipose tissue [5] because unlike the liver and gonads [2,4], both analyses were performed using the most recent annotation of the genome. Hence, a total of 40% novel predicted proteins in the muscle tissue transcriptome have also been found in adipose tissue, either realised with the Sscrofa10.2. Of the 2,372 predicted novel proteins, 972 were validated *in silico* being present in at least one of the three tissues compared [2,4,5]. Interestingly, 36 of the novel predicted proteins were also identified in four different tissues (liver [4], gonads [2], adipose [5], and muscle tissue) (Figure 4). When analysing the main metabolic pathways for the novel transcripts identified, the "phosphatidylinositol signalling system" and "inositol phosphate metabolism" were among the most represented categories. The phosphatidylinositol signalling system plays a critical role in the regulation of diverse processes such as muscle contraction, cell secretion, cell growth and differentiation [33]. Moreover, phosphatidylinositol is an essential component of the lipid membrane, where the total amount of phospholipids remains fairly constant, or increases little, as the animal increases in fatness [9,34]. Not surprisingly, these pathways were also identified when analyzing the adipose tissue novel transcripts [5]. Interestingly, the phosphatidylinositol signalling was also found within the most significantly overrepresented pathways in animals differing in FA composition in an study using microarrays [35]. Finally, we detected a high percentage (34.5%) of new repetitive elements present in the porcine genome. This result was similar to those obtained in adipose tissue (36%) using the Sscrofa10.2 genome annotation, but higher than those obtained in gonads (7.3%) and liver (approximately 5.8–7.3%)

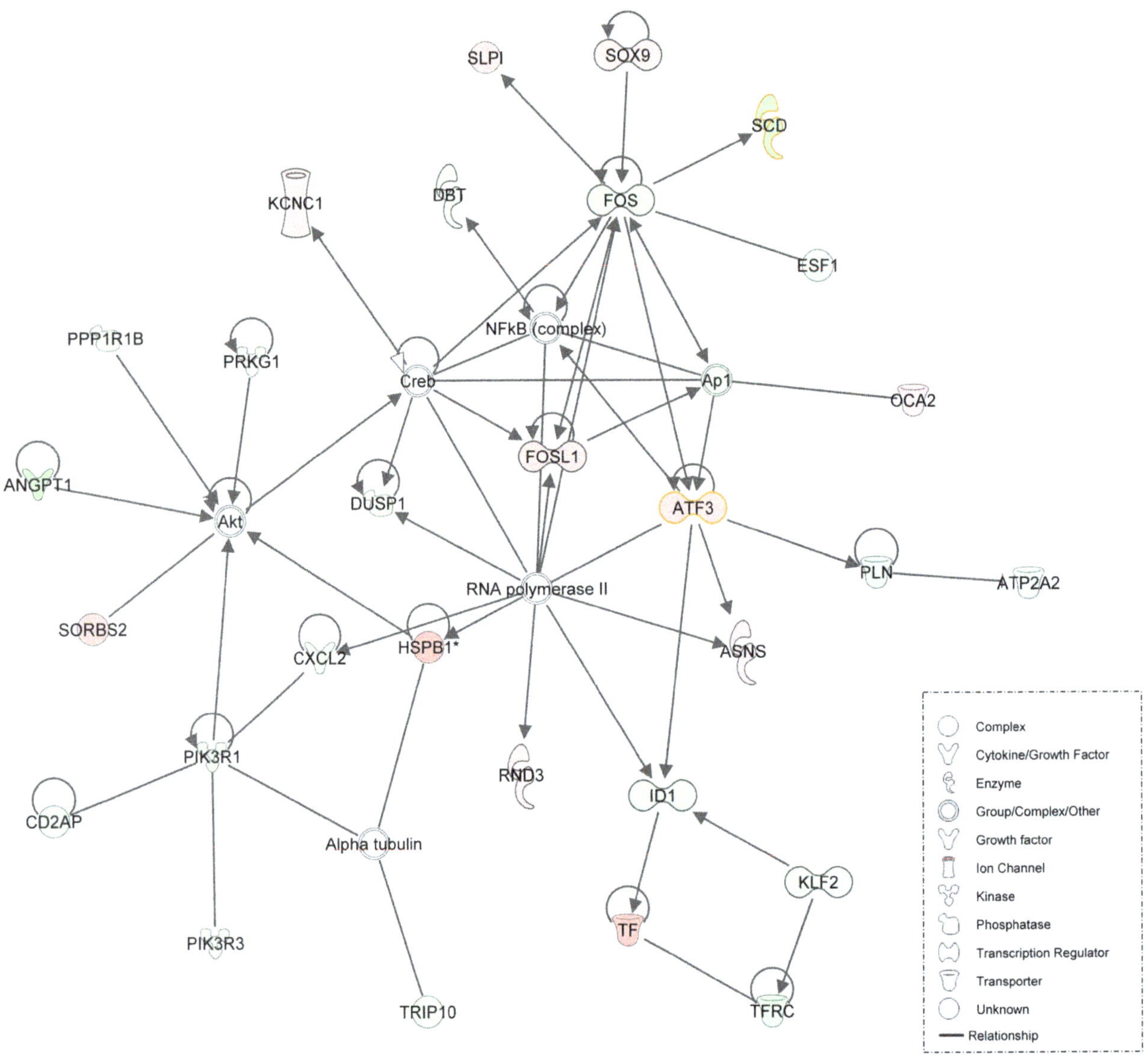

Figure 3. Network (direct, score 55) generated by IPA of 35 focus genes corresponding to the cell death and survival, cellular development, connective tissue and function pathways. Node colours indicate gene expression, being the red nodes higher-expressed genes and the green nodes lower-expressed genes in the H group relative to the L group. Colour intensity is related to the degree of expression. Node shapes indicate the biological function of the protein.

that used an older version of the pig genome assembly [2,4,5]. This higher content of repetitive elements can be explained by the improvement of the current assembly (Sscrofa10.2) of the pig genome being the repetitive regions the most difficult to assemble [36].

Differential Expression analysis

Apart from describing the transcriptome of the *Longissimus dorsi* muscle, this study aimed to identify genes that can be implicated in determining the phenotypic differences of animals with extreme IMF FA composition belonging to an Iberian x Landrace backcross (BC1_LD). Iberian pigs are a local Mediterranean breed, and in comparison with Landrace, they have an extreme trend to obesity, with a higher IMF content and a strongest development of backfat tissue [8]. In contrast to the Iberian pigs, commercial breeds such as Landrace have suffered a strong selection towards a lean meat content, muscularity and enhanced reproduction [37]. Moreover, these two breeds are extreme for FA composition, showing the Iberian pigs a higher content of SFA and MUFA (specially C16 and C18:1) and the Landrace pigs a higher content of PUFA [8,38]. In our study, animals belonging to L group had a higher content of SFA and MUFA similarly to the Iberian pigs, whereas animals from H group had higher content of PUFA, as observed in the Landrace animals. Thus, this animal material suits very well to studies aiming at identifying the molecular factors influencing the FA metabolism in pigs.

For the differential-expression analysis we intersected the two lists of genes, obtained by DEseq [25] and EdgeR [24], to obtain a

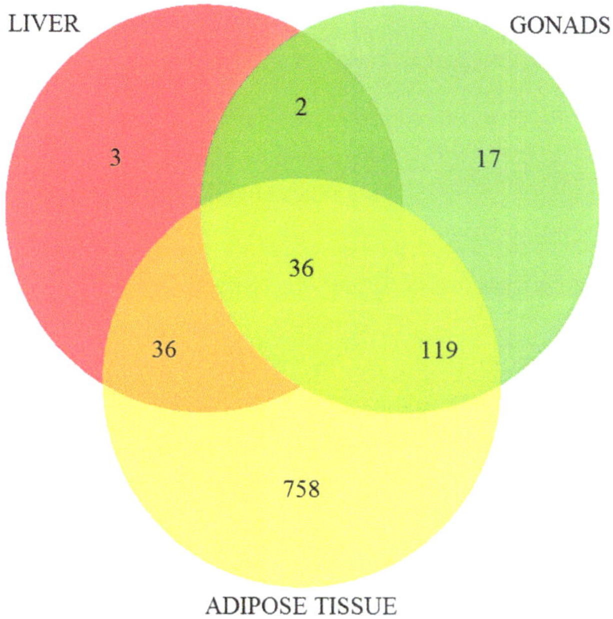

Figure 4. Venn diagram of the novel predicted proteins expressed in muscle, liver [4], gonads [2] and adipose tissue [5].

single list in order to avoid false positives [39]. For the same reason we used a strict *P*-value ≤0.01, based on the Q-Q plot and equivalent to a FDR ≤0.12, and a fold change ≥1.2 as used in the adipose transcriptome analysis [5,40]. We identified a lower number of differentially-expressed genes with DESeq (208 genes) when compared to EdgeR (314 genes) what is in accordance with the observations reported by Soneson & Delorenzi [40]. DESeq uses conservative default settings and performs well when outliers are introduced, having a better false discovery rate (FDR) control for large sample sizes than EdgeR [40]. Notice that some relevant genes identified using microarrays in the muscle transcriptome of animals extreme for FA metabolism [27,35] such as *ACACA*, *FABP4* or *PPARGC1A* remained incorrectly or non-annotated in the Sscrofa10.2 annotation version. On the other hand, interesting genes detected in our RNA-Seq study that may determine differences in FA composition in muscle such as *ChREBP*, *GYS2*, *PLIN1*, *PLIN5* and *AQP7* could not be detected in microarray studies since probes for these genes were not included.

Differentially modulated metabolic pathways between groups

Among the top canonical pathways overrepresented between both groups of animals, we found hemostasis, nitric oxide (NO), metabolism of lipids and lipoproteins and PPAR and insulin signalling pathways (Table 2). Remarkably, most of the genes represented in these pathways were down-expressed in the H group. When compared with a previous study using microarrays of animals of BC1_LD population [27], the insulin and the calcium signalling, the regulation of the cytoskeleton, the focal adhesion dynamics, the leukocyte accumulation and cardiomyopathies-related pathways (Table S7) were found in common. Interestingly, our analysis identified other relevant pathways related to lipid metabolism, PPAR and NO signalling. On the other hand, most of the main overrepresented pathways identified in our study were also present in Duroc animals displaying divergent MUFA and PUFA fatty acids percentages (Table 2) [35], thus supporting a relevant role of these metabolic pathways in determining intramuscular FA composition. However, a feedback loop in which FA composition modifies these metabolic pathways that in turn cause a change in FA composition cannot be ruled out as we described below (i.e. differences in C16:1 n-7 FA or PUFA). Besides, in our analysis two other interesting pathways were found: (i) the clathrin-mediated endocytosis signalling, which is used for molecules such as low density lipoproteins, transferrins or growth factors and (ii) the C-X-C chemokine receptor type 4 (CXCR4) signalling, involved in the endocytosis of the glucose transporter protein 4 (GLUT4), specially in myocytes [41].

In the following sections a detailed explanation of differentially-expressed genes belonging to each of the main overrepresented pathways will be discussed.

- **NO and insulin signalling pathways.** The skeletal muscle is a target organ for the insulin-induced glucose uptake and for the maintenance of glucose homeostasis in blood [42]. Insulin acts in the carbohydrate metabolism facilitating the glucose diffusion into adipose and muscle cells via glucose transporter proteins (GLUT) and stimulates FA synthesis and the storage of triglycerides by the esterification of glycerol phosphate. Notably, the C16:1 n-7 FA, observed to be decreased in the H group (Table 1), can act as a lipokine that jointly with the expression of the *peroxisome proliferator-activated receptor gamma* (*PPAR-γ*) can strongly stimulate the muscle insulin action [43,44]. Interestingly, *PPAR-γ* and *solute carrier family 2, member 4* (*SLC2A4*; also called *GLUT4*) were identified as over-expressed in the L group animals when using EdgeR program. Supporting these results, Cánovas *et al.* [35] identified a higher expression of *myocyte enhancer factor 2A* (*MEF2A*) gene which upregulates *GLUT4* in Duroc animals having a higher MUFA and SFA content. Furthermore, insulin stimulates eNOS, the enzyme responsible for synthesizing NO by calcium-independent phosphorylation via phosphoinositide 3-kinases (PI3 kinases) and the downstream effector serine/threonine kinase (Akt) [45]. NO is a signalling molecule synthesized from L-arginine that plays an important role in regulating energy metabolism in mammals [46]. It has been reported that a chronic exposure of NO may decrease whole-body energy metabolism, increasing the adiposity and obesity [46]. For instance, *PI3 kinases*, down-expressed in the H group, have been reported to be necessary for the insulin-stimulated glucose uptake and glycogen synthesis, meanwhile, *Akt* regulates cell growth and metabolism and it is involved in glucose transport and lipogenesis (Figure 4) [16,47]. In the same direction, the *glycogen synthase* (*GYS*) gene was down-expressed in animals belonging to the H group (Figure S1), what might be a downstream effect of the Akt pathway [48]. Thus, the *GYS* inhibition may decrease the synthesis of glycogen necessary for glucose storage.
- **PPAR and metabolism of lipids and lipoproteins pathways.** In concordance with the low glucose-uptake that seems to occur in the H group of animals, we observed a down-expression of lipogenic genes most probably due to the lack of activation of carbohydrate responsive-element binding protein (*ChREBP*) [49]. The *stearoyl-CoA desaturase* (*SCD*) gene (Table S5) is responsible for the biosynthesis of MUFA from SFA, and its deficiency has been associated with lean mice [50]. Furthermore, polymorphisms in *SCD* gene have been strongly associated with FA composition in pigs and cows [12,51–53]. It has been suggested that an inhibition of this enzyme produces an increase in fatty acid oxidation through the inhibition of *acetyl-CoA carboxylase* (*ACACA*), regulated via

ChREBP, and *de novo* lipogenesis [50,54]. Interestingly, the *SCD* gene was identified as down-expressed in the adipose tissue of animals with higher content of PUFA in the Iberian x Landrace crossbred [5] and over-expressed in animals with higher IMF accumulation [31,35]. Our results support the hypothesis of Corominas *et al.* [5], that suggested that higher PUFA content in the H group suppresses the *ChREBP* gene function in a LXR-dependent manner inhibiting glycolytic and lipogenic genes. Although not present in the overlapping list (Table S5), the *ChREBP* gene was identified as down-expressed in the H group for EdgeR program.

Another gene whose disruption is associated with lean mice and was also down-expressed in H group is the *perilipin* [55]. Perilipins modulate the hydrolysis of triglycerides by *hormone-sensitive lipase* (*LIPE*) [56]. Specifically, *perilipin 5* (*PLIN5*) may play a role of "master lipolytic regulator" in muscle, and its over-expression can increase lipid droplet size and triacylglycerol storage [57]. We also identified the lipid transporter *Fatty acid binding protein 3, muscle and heart* (*FABP3*) and the *Aquoporins* (*AQP4* and *AQP7*) as down-expressed in the H group (Table S4). *FABP3* is more expressed in the skeletal muscle than in other tissues and participates in FA uptake and cytosolic transport, having a high binding affinity for palmitic, oleic and stearic acids. Furthermore, *FABP3* acts as a transcription factor in the nucleus for the control of lipid-mediated transcriptional programs via nuclear hormone receptors or other transcription factors that respond to lipids [58]. This gene has also been found in a genomic region significantly associated with FA composition in a GWAS performed in the Iberian x Landrace cross, being a clear candidate to explain the differences in FA composition observed between the two groups of animals [16]. Besides, it has been suggested as a candidate gene for the control of IMF deposition as it was identified as over-expressed in animals with higher IMF content [59]. The *Aquaporins* are modulated by the PI3K/Akt signalling and they are involved in glycerol uptake, particularly *AQP4* is localized in muscle fibers and it is important for energy supply in the skeletal muscle [46,60,61]. The *AQP7* which is higher expressed in fat tissue was also identified in the liver transcriptome study as being also down-expressed in animals with a higher content of PUFA [4,61]. Another differentially-expressed gene between the two groups of animals was the *very long-chain specific acyl-CoA dehydrogenase* gene (*ACADVL*), a *PPAR* target gene which was down-expressed in the H group. This gene catalyzes the first step of the mitochondrial FA β-oxidation pathway, mainly in muscle, having preference for C16:0, C16:1, C18:0 and C18:1 [62,63]. Moreover, *ACADVL* deficiency in humans produced a defective oxidation of oleic FA and knock-out mice for *ACADVL* fed in high-fat diet had a decrease in whole body fat content [64]. Overall, these results agree with a previous study in which the transcriptome of two groups of Duroc pigs with different IMF composition was analysed using microarrays and concluded that the IMF accumulation in animals having more IMF, MUFA and SFA may result from a balance between uptake, synthesis and degradation of triglycerides [35].

- **Hemostasis.** Alterations in fat metabolism play a role in the development of cardiovascular disease. Not surprisingly, our data set revealed several differentially-expressed transcripts which could be classified as potential regulators of hemostasis (Table S2). For instance, the *angiopoietin-1* (*ANGPT1*) gene which has been reported to increase vessel formation causing an enhanced glucose uptake and also the glycogen and lipid synthesis [65] was over-expressed in the L group and present in a QTL interval of the GWAS for IMF FA profile in the same population (Table S5) [16]. Furthermore, and consistent with our results, the angiogenesis promoted by ANGPT1 has been reported to increase NO production accompanied by an activation of the Akt and the nuclear factor kappa-light-chain-enhancer of activated B cells (NF-κB) signalling pathways [66,67] (Figure 4). Accordingly, the *hypoxia-inducible factor-1, alpha subunit inhibitor* (*HIF1AN*), which is regulated through the NF-κB inflammatory pathway and serves as an oxygen sensor regulating heart's oxygen supply, was down-expressed in the L group (Table S5). Thus, the L group animals having more SFA and MUFA content may have boosted the angiogenesis and improved the inflammatory response through the activation of the *ANGPT1* gene. A decreased essential PUFA content may lead to a proinflammatory eicosanoids synthesis and vasoconstrictors activation as has been reported in other studies [68]. In this direction, an over-expression of genes encoding for the inositol 1,4,5-triphosphate receptor 2 (ITPR2) protein which activates the release of Ca(2+) in the vessels acting as vasoconstrictor and aldosterone A (ALDOA) which increases blood pressure when activated by angiotensin [69,70] was observed in L group.

Pig lipid metabolism affected by intramuscular FA composition

In general, our results show that differences in FA composition may influence the lipid metabolism determining the phenotypic variation observed between the two groups of animals. In previous studies of our group, we observed that in liver [4], a high content of PUFA (H group phenotype) shifted the metabolism towards the FA oxidation; meanwhile, in adipose tissue [5] inhibited lipogenesis. Accordingly, in other studies analyzing the muscle transcriptome using microarrays a favored FA oxidation and a reduced fatty acid uptake, lipogenesis and triacylglycerol synthesis was generally observed in the group with higher intramuscular PUFA content [27,35]. In our RNA-Seq study in muscle we observed an inhibition of glucose uptake and lipogenesis in the H group, which would produce a decrease in the triglyceride storage. Noteworthy, in adipose and muscle transcriptome analysis, the *albumin* (*ALB*) gene was identified as over-expressed in animals having a higher content of PUFA (H group) [5]. The ALB is a long chain FA transporter that enhances FA mobilization affecting cellular uptake and also plays an antioxidant function in plasma. In adipose tissue, we hypothesized that ALB was supplying the FFAs used for the oxidation in liver in pre-slaughtering fasting conditions [5]. In the same direction, our results suggested that in muscle there is also an increased input of FFAs from blood and adipose tissue in order to fulfil the high-energy requirements in the H group. We hypothesize that animals having a high content of SFA and MUFA such as the Iberian pig, which is a rustic and slow-growing breed, may have an enhanced adaptation to fasting thanks to their high availability of muscle energy stores. Thus, selection towards a fast growth in commercial pigs such as Landrace, may have affected the ability to adapt to food disposal fluctuations [71].

Implications

In conclusion, the genes identified here as differentially-expressed between extreme animals, the pathways and the gene networks, contribute to understand the differences in gene regulation between the two groups differing in the muscle FA composition. The functional analysis showed a different regulation of the lipid metabolism between groups, being more prone either to lipolisis or to lipogenesis depending on their FA composition. Moreover, the enrichment analysis showed that muscle plays a key role in energy metabolism, mainly in glucose and lipid metabolism, observing that animals having more PUFA, had a shift of the metabolism towards the lipolisis and also a lower glucose uptake. There are also evidences that the joint metabolism of the liver, adipose tissue and muscle may have an integrated role in determining the final FA composition of muscle. Therefore, the study of the muscle transcriptome may provide clues to decipher the genetic basis of meat quality traits. Moreover, this study may be of high relevance since FA composition in meat has important consequences in human health [72]. Besides, we observed that among the DE genes there was an overrepresentation of the obesity and the insulin resistance pathways. The results here exposed are particularly interesting because these diseases have a high prevalence and the pig has been described as a suitable biomodel for human lipid-related metabolic diseases [73].

Methods

Animal samples and phenotypes

The IBMAP population was originated by the cross of 3 Iberian boars (Guadyerbas) with 31 Landrace sows [74]. In this study we used 144 animals from the BC1_LD generation obtained by crossing five F1 boars with 26 Landrace sows. Animals were fed *ad libitum* with a cereal-based commercial diet (see [8] for diet details) and slaughtered at 179.8±2.6 days. Animal care and procedures were performed following national and institutional guidelines for the Good Experimental Practices and approved by the Ethical Committee of the Institution (IRTA- Institut de Recerca i Tecnologia Agroalimentàries). Samples of the *Longissimus dorsi* muscle were collected, snap frozen in liquid nitrogen and stored at −80°C until RNA extraction.

A Principal Component Analysis (PCA) was performed for characters related with the FA profile in muscle (see [4] for detailed description of this analysis). Twelve extreme animals were selected according to the first principal component (6 H and 6 L) [4]. Only females were taken into account in order to remove the sex effect on FA composition. The R language [75] was used to perform the statistical analysis of phenotypic mean comparison using a linear model.

RNA isolation

Total RNA was isolated from the *Longissimus dorsi* muscle of 12 samples with RiboPure Isolation of High Quality Total RNA (Ambion, Austin, TX, USA). Total RNA was quantified in a NanoDrop ND-1000 spectrophotometer (NanoDrop products, Wilmington, DE, USA) and Qubit (Invitrogen, Carlsbad, CA, USA). RNA purity and integrity was checked employing a Bioanalyzer-2100 (Agilent Technologies, Inc., Santa Clara, CA, USA). All samples had a RNA Integrity Number (RIN) above 8.5.

Paired-end raw sequences (75 bp) were generated using a Hi-Seq 2000 instrument (Illumina, Inc., San Diego, CA, USA) in CNAG institute (Centro Nacional de Análisis Genómico, Barcelona, España).

Mapping and annotation

We ran FastQC [76] for the quality control. Indexed reads were then mapped to the reference pig genome version 10.2 (Sscrofa10.2) and the annotation database Ensembl Genes 67 [77] using TopHat v2.0.1 [19] with an allowance of two mismatches for each read. The resulting bam files containing the aligned sequences, were subsequently merged with Samtools [78]. Reads were annotated using the intersectBed option of BEDtools [79]. Cufflinks v2.0.2 program [20] was used to assemble the transcripts with a minimum of 10 reads per alignment. Finally, Samtools [78] was employed to compute descriptive statistics.

Gene expression quantification and differential-expression analysis

The number of reads mapping to each gene was determined with the *comp-counts* option in Qualimap v5.0 program [80]. We discarded those genes with a group mean less than 20 counts. We calculated the Pearson correlation coefficient between the mean expression values of the H and L group using the *cor.test* function of R. For the differential expression analysis we used DESeq [25] and EdgeR [24] packages implemented in R. We considered as differentially expressed between H and L groups those genes identified by both programs (DESeq and EdgeR) with a fold change ≥1.2 and *P*-value ≤0.01, the same parameters used in Corominas *et al.* [5], these case for both programs. FDR was calculated using the R package qvalue [81].

Transposable elements and orthology analysis

We used RepeatMasker version open-3.3.0 [21] with the rm-20120418 database in order to identify repetitive and transposable elements in the pig muscle transcriptome. We used "quick search" and "pig" species options and the Search Engine NCBI/RMBLAST.

Intergenic expressed regions not annotated in the Sscrofa10.2 version assembly were identified using Cuffcompare [82] and extracted using our own Python and R scripts. Novel putative proteins were predicted with Augustus program [22]. Afterwards, using Blast2GO [23], we mapped and annotated the novel protein coding genes. Using BLASTP option (*E*-value hit filter 1.00E-6, annotation cutoff 55, gene ontology (GO) weight 5 and HSP-hit coverage cutoff 0) we checked their orthology with already annotated proteins in *Homo sapiens*, *Bos taurus* and *Sus scrofa* protein databases. The InterProScan specific tool implemented in Blast2GO was employed to refine the functional annotations. With the GO Slim options we selected the relevant GO terms belonging to the cellular component, biological process and molecular function categories. Parameters were set to 10 for the seq filter and 20 for node score filter. Finally the ontology level was set to 3.

Gene ontologies and pathways

The Ingenuity Pathways Analysis software [29] and FatiGO tools from Babelomics 4.3 [28] were used to identify the most relevant biological functions and pathways in which the differentially-expressed genes (between the H and L groups) were involved. IPA, which uses its own private databases, allowed us to identify biological relevant information, identifying overrepresented pathways using the BH multiple testing correction (FDR) at *P*-value <0.05, and generating biological networks. For FatiGO, we used KEGG [83] and Reactome [84] databases setting the cut-off FDR <0.1. The Mouse Genome Database (MGD) [26] was used in order to identify how mutant alleles driven in mice for the 18 identified genes common in GWAS and RNA-Seq analysis affected the phenotype.

Supporting Information

Figure S1 Network (indirect, score 36) generated by IPA of 35 focus genes corresponding to metabolic disease, lipid metabolism and molecular transport. Node colours indicate gene expression, being the red nodes higher-expressed genes and the green nodes lower-expressed genes in the H group relative to the L group. Colour intensity is related to the degree of expression. Node shapes indicate the biological function of the protein.

Table S1 Percentage of reads mapped for each sample and their localization (exonic, intronic or intergenic) regarding the pig reference genome sequence.

Table S2 Total number of assembled transcripts with cufflinks.

Table S3 Description of the repetitive elements identified in the intergenic transcripts of the swine muscle transcriptome.

Table S4 New predicted novel proteins with Augustus which have orthologous known genes identified with BLASTP option of Blast2GO.

Table S5 Differentially-expressed genes identified among extreme groups (High and Low) for fatty acid composition in muscle.

Table S6 Overrepresented categories identified with Babelomics and IPA for the differentially-expressed genes.

Table S7 Specific functions table identified with IPA for the differentially-expressed genes.

Table S8 Top networks identified with IPA from the differential expressed genes between High and Low animals.

Acknowledgments

We wish to thank Anna Castelló for RNA isolation and quantification.

Author Contributions

Conceived and designed the experiments: JMF MB. Performed the experiments: APO JMF MB. Analyzed the data: APO YRC MB JE. Contributed reagents/materials/analysis tools: JMF J. Corominas J. Casellas DPM JE YRC. Wrote the paper: APO JMF MB NH.

References

1. Trapnell C, Roberts A, Goff L, Pertea G, Kim D, et al. (2012) Differential gene and transcript expression analysis of RNA-seq experiments with TopHat and Cufflinks. Nat Protoc 7: 562–578. doi:10.1038/nprot.2012.016.
2. Esteve-Codina A, Kofler R, Palmieri N, Bussotti G, Notredame C, et al. (2011) Exploring the gonad transcriptome of two extreme male pigs with RNA-seq. BMC Genomics 12: 552.
3. Chen C, Ai H, Ren J, Li W, Li P, et al. (2011) A global view of porcine transcriptome in three tissues from a full-sib pair with extreme phenotypes in growth and fat deposition by paired-end RNA sequencing. BMC Genomics 12: 448.
4. Ramayo-Caldas Y, Mach N, Esteve-Codina A, Corominas J, Castelló A, et al. (2012) Liver transcriptome profile in pigs with extreme phenotypes of intramuscular fatty acid composition. BMC Genomics 13: 547. doi:10.1186/1471-2164-13-547.
5. Corominas J, Ramayo-Caldas Y, Puig-Oliveras A, Estellé J, Castelló A, et al. (2013) Analysis of porcine adipose tissue transcriptome reveals differences in de novo fatty acid synthesis in pigs with divergent muscle fatty acid composition. Press.
6. Jung WY, Kwon SG, Son M, Cho ES, Lee Y, et al. (2012) RNA-Seq Approach for Genetic Improvement of Meat Quality in Pig and Evolutionary Insight into the Substrate Specificity of Animal Carbonyl Reductases. PLoS ONE 7: e42198. doi:10.1371/journal.pone.0042198.
7. Food and Agriculture Organization (FAO). Available: http://www.fao.org. Accessed 2014 May 20.
8. Serra X, Gil F, Pérez-Enciso M, Oliver M, Vázquez J, et al. (1998) A comparison of carcass, meat quality and histochemical characteristics of Iberian (Guadyerbas line) and Landrace pigs. Livest Prod Sci 56: 215–223. doi:10.1016/S0301-6226(98)00151-1.
9. Wood JD, Enser M, Fisher AV, Nute GR, Sheard PR, et al. (2008) Fat deposition, fatty acid composition and meat quality: A review. Meat Sci 78: 343–358. doi:10.1016/j.meatsci.2007.07.019.
10. Reiter SS, Halsey CHC, Stronach BM, Bartosh JL, Owsley WF, et al. (2007) Lipid metabolism related gene-expression profiling in liver, skeletal muscle and adipose tissue in crossbred Duroc and Pietrain Pigs. Comp Biochem Physiol Part D Genomics Proteomics 2: 200–206. doi:10.1016/j.cbd.2007.04.008.
11. Zhang W, Xiao S, Samaraweera H, Lee EJ, Ahn DU (2010) Improving functional value of meat products. Spec Issue 56th Int Congr Meat Sci Technol 56th ICoMST 15–20 August 2010 Jeju Korea 86: 15–31. doi:10.1016/j.meatsci.2010.04.018.
12. Maharani D, Park H-B, Lee J-B, Yoo C-K, Lim H-T, et al. (2013) Association of the gene encoding stearoyl-CoA desaturase (SCD) with fatty acid composition in an intercross population between Landrace and Korean native pigs. Mol Biol Rep 40: 73–80. doi:10.1007/s11033-012-2014-0.
13. FAO (2008) Fats and fatty acids in human nutrition. Report of expert consultation.
14. Zhang S, Knight TJ, Stalder KJ, Goodwin RN, Lonergan SM, et al. (2009) Effects of breed, sex and halothane genotype on fatty acid composition of triacylglycerols and phospholipids in pork longissimus muscle. J Anim Breed Genet 126: 259–268. doi:10.1111/j.1439-0388.2008.00782.x.
15. Madeira MS, Pires VMR, Alfaia CM, Costa ASH, Luxton R, et al. (2013) Differential effects of reduced protein diets on fatty acid composition and gene expression in muscle and subcutaneous adipose tissue of Alentejana purebred and Large White × Landrace × Pietrain crossbred pigs. Br J Nutr FirstView: 1–14. doi:10.1017/S0007114512004916.
16. Ramayo-Caldas Y, Mercadé A, Castelló A, Yang B, Rodríguez C, et al. (2012) Genome-wide association study for intramuscular fatty acid composition in an Iberian × Landrace cross. J Anim Sci 90: 2883–2893. doi:10.2527/jas.2011-4900.
17. Muñoz M, Rodríguez MC, Alves E, Folch JM, Ibañez-Escriche N, et al. (2013) Genome-wide analysis of porcine backfat and intramuscular fat fatty acid composition using high-density genotyping and expression data.
18. Revilla M, Ramayo-Caldas Y, Castelló A, Corominas J, Puig-Oliveras A, et al. (2014) New insight into the SSC8 genetic determination of fatty acid composition in pigs. Genet Sel Evol In Press.
19. Trapnell C, Pachter L, Salzberg SL (2009) TopHat: discovering splice junctions with RNA-seq. Bioinformatics 25: 1105–1111.
20. Trapnell C, Williams BA, Pertea G, Mortazavi A, Kwan G, et al. (2010) Transcript assembly and quantification by RNA-Seq reveals unannotated transcripts and isoform switching during cell differentiation. Nat Biotechnol 28: 511–515.
21. RepeatMasker version open-3.3.0. Available: http://www.repeatmasker.org. Accessed 2014 May 20.
22. Stanke M, Diekhans M, Baertsch R, Haussler D (2008) Using native and syntenically mapped cDNA alignments to improve de novo gene finding. Bioinformatics 24: 637–644.
23. Conesa A, Götz S, García-Gómez JM, Terol J, Talón M, et al. (2005) Blast2GO: a universal tool for annotation, visualization and analysis in functional genomics research. Bioinformatics 21: 3674–3676. doi:10.1093/bioinformatics/bti610.
24. Robinson M, Oshlack A (2010) A scaling normalization method for differential expression analysis of RNA-seq data. Genome Biol 11: R25.
25. Anders S, Huber W (2010) Differential expression analysis for sequence count data. Genome Biol 11: R106.
26. Mouse Genome Informatics. Available: http://www.informatics.jax.org. Accessed 2014 May 20.
27. Pena RN, Noguera JL, Casellas J, Díaz I, Fernández AI, et al. (2013) Transcriptional analysis of intramuscular fatty acid composition in the longissimus thoracis muscle of Iberian × Landrace back-crossed pigs. Anim Genet: n/a–n/a. doi:10.1111/age.12066.
28. Medina I, Carbonell J, Pulido L, Madeira SC, Goetz S, et al. (2010) Babelomics: an integrative platform for the analysis of transcriptomics, proteomics and genomic data with advanced functional profiling. Nucleic Acids Res 38: W210–W213. doi:10.1093/nar/gkq388.
29. Ingenuity Pathways Analysis software. Available: www.ingenuity.com. Accessed 2014 May 20.

30. Yu K, Shu G, Yuan F, Zhu X, Gao P, et al. (2013) Fatty Acid and Transcriptome Profiling of Longissimus Dorsi Muscles between Pig Breeds Differing in Meat Quality. 9 1: 108–118. doi:doi:10.7150/ijbs.5306.
31. Hamill R, Aslan O, Mullen A, O'Doherty J, McBryan J, et al. (2013) Transcriptome analysis of porcine M. semimembranosus divergent in intramuscular fat as a consequence of dietary protein restriction. BMC Genomics 14: 453.
32. Zhao X, Mo D, Li A, Gong W, Xiao S, et al. (2011) Comparative Analyses by Sequencing of Transcriptomes during Skeletal Muscle Development between Pig Breeds Differing in Muscle Growth Rate and Fatness. PLoS ONE 6: e19774. doi:10.1371/journal.pone.0019774.
33. Putney JW, Bird GSJ (1993) The Inositol Phosphate-Calcium Signaling System in Nonexcitable Cells. Endocr Rev 14: 610–631. doi:10.1210/edrv-14-5-610.
34. Lagace TA, Ridgway ND (2013) The role of phospholipids in the biological activity and structure of the endoplasmic reticulum. Funct Struct Divers Endoplasmic Reticulum 1833: 2499–2510. doi:10.1016/j.bbamcr.2013.05.018.
35. Canovas A, Quintanilla R, Amills M, Pena R (2010) Muscle transcriptomic profiles in pigs with divergent phenotypes for fatness traits. BMC Genomics 11: 372.
36. Quesneville H, Bergman CM, Andrieu O, Autard D, Nouaud D, et al. (2005) Combined Evidence Annotation of Transposable Elements in Genome Sequences. PLoS Comput Biol 1: e22. doi:10.1371/journal.pcbi.0010022.
37. Wilkinson S, Lu ZH, Megens H-J, Archibald AL, Haley C, et al. (2013) Signatures of Diversifying Selection in European Pig Breeds. PLoS Genet 9: e1003453. doi:10.1371/journal.pgen.1003453.
38. Estévez M, Morcuende D, Cava López R (2003) Physico-chemical characteristics of M. Longissimus dorsi from three lines of free-range reared Iberian pigs slaughtered at 90 kg live-weight and commercial pigs: a comparative study. Meat Sci 64: 499–506. doi:10.1016/S0309-1740(02)00228-0.
39. Yendrek C, Ainsworth E, Thimmapuram J (2012) The bench scientist's guide to statistical analysis of RNA-Seq data. BMC Res Notes 5: 506.
40. Soneson C, Delorenzi M (2013) A comparison of methods for differential expression analysis of RNA-seq data. BMC Bioinformatics 14: 91.
41. Antonescu CN, Díaz M, Femia G, Planas JV, Klip A (2008) Clathrin-Dependent and Independent Endocytosis of Glucose Transporter 4 (GLUT4) in Myoblasts: Regulation by Mitochondrial Uncoupling. Traffic 9: 1173–1190. doi:10.1111/j.1600-0854.2008.00755.x.
42. Kubota T, Kubota N, Kadowaki T (2013) The role of endothelial insulin signaling in the regulation of glucose metabolism. Rev Endocr Metab Disord 14: 207–216. doi:10.1007/s11154-013-9242-z.
43. Cao H, Gerhold K, Mayers JR, Wiest MM, Watkins SM, et al. (2008) Identification of a Lipokine, a Lipid Hormone Linking Adipose Tissue to Systemic Metabolism. Cell 134: 933–944. doi:10.1016/j.cell.2008.07.048.
44. Leonardini A, Laviola L, Perrini S, Natalicchio A, Giorgino F (2009) Cross-Talk between PPAR and Insulin Signaling and Modulation of Insulin Sensitivity. PPAR Res 2009. Available: http://dx.doi.org/10.1155/2009/818945.
45. Wilcox G (2005) Insulin and Insulin Resistance. Clin Biochem Rev 2: 19–39.
46. Dai Z, Wu Z, Yang Y, Wang J, Satterfield MC, et al. (2013) Nitric oxide and energy metabolism in mammals. BioFactors 39: 383–391. doi:10.1002/biof.1099.
47. Summers SA, Garza LA, Zhou H, Birnbaum MJ (1998) Regulation of Insulin-Stimulated Glucose Transporter GLUT4 Translocation and Akt Kinase Activity by Ceramide. Mol Cell Biol 18: 5457–5464.
48. Luo J, Sobkiw CL, Hirshman MF, Logsdon MN, Li TQ, et al. (2006) Loss of class IA PI3K signaling in muscle leads to impaired muscle growth, insulin response, and hyperlipidemia. Cell Metab 3: 355–366. doi:10.1016/j.cmet.2006.04.003.
49. Herman MA, Peroni OD, Villoria J, Schon MR, Abumrad NA, et al. (2012) A novel ChREBP isoform in adipose tissue regulates systemic glucose metabolism. Nature 484: 333–338. doi:10.1038/nature10986.
50. Cohen P, Miyazaki M, Socci ND, Hagge-Greenberg A, Liedtke W, et al. (2002) Role for Stearoyl-CoA Desaturase-1 in Leptin-Mediated Weight Loss. Science 297: 240–243. doi:10.1126/science.1071527.
51. Jiang Z, Michal J, Tobey D, Daniels T, Rule D, et al. (2008) Significant associations of stearoyl-CoA desaturase (SCD1) gene with fat deposition and composition in skeletal muscle. Int J Biol Sci 4: 345–351.
52. Renaville B, Prandi A, Fan B, Sepulcri A, Rothschild MF, et al. (2013) Candidate gene marker associations with fatty acid profiles in heavy pigs. Meat Sci 93: 495–500. doi:10.1016/j.meatsci.2012.11.019.
53. Estany J, Ros-Freixedes R, Tor M, Pena RN (2014) A Functional Variant in the Stearoyl-CoA Desaturase Gene Promoter Enhances Fatty Acid Desaturation in Pork. PLoS ONE 9: e86177. doi:10.1371/journal.pone.0086177.
54. Benhamed F, Denechaud P-D, Lemoine M, Robichon C, Moldes M, et al. (2012) The lipogenic transcription factor ChREBP dissociates hepatic steatosis from insulin resistance in mice and humans. J Clin Invest 122: 2176–2194. doi:10.1172/JCI41636.
55. Martinez-Botas J, Anderson JB, Tessier D, Lapillonne A, Chang BH-J, et al. (2000) Absence of perilipin results in leanness and reverses obesity in Leprdb/db mice. Nat Genet 26: 474–479. doi:10.1038/82630.
56. Dalen KT, Dahl T, Holter E, Arntsen B, Londos C, et al. (2007) LSDP5 is a PAT protein specifically expressed in fatty acid oxidizing tissues. Biochim Biophys Acta BBA - Mol Cell Biol Lipids 1771: 210–227. doi:10.1016/j.bbalip.2006.11.011.
57. Bosma M, Sparks LM, Hooiveld GJ, Jorgensen JA, Houten SM, et al. (2013) Overexpression of PLIN5 in skeletal muscle promotes oxidative gene expression and intramyocellular lipid content without compromising insulin sensitivity. Biochim Biophys Acta BBA - Mol Cell Biol Lipids 1831: 844–852. doi:10.1016/j.bbalip.2013.01.007.
58. Furuhashi M, Hotamisligil GS (2008) Fatty acid-binding proteins: role in metabolic diseases and potential as drug targets. Nat Rev Drug Discov 7: 489–503. doi:10.1038/nrd2589.
59. Damon M, Wyszynska-Koko J, Vincent A, Hérault F, Lebret B (2012) Comparison of Muscle Transcriptome between Pigs with Divergent Meat Quality Phenotypes Identifies Genes Related to Muscle Metabolism and Structure. PLoS ONE 7: e33763. doi:10.1371/journal.pone.0033763.
60. Basco D, Blaauw B, Pisani F, Sparaneo A, Nicchia GP, et al. (2013) AQP4-Dependent Water Transport Plays a Functional Role in Exercise-Induced Skeletal Muscle Adaptations. PLoS ONE 8: e58712. doi:10.1371/journal.-pone.0058712.
61. Rodríguez A, Catalán V, Gómez-Ambrosi J, García-Navarro S, Rotellar F, et al. (2011) Insulin- and Leptin-Mediated Control of Aquaglyceroporins in Human Adipocytes and Hepatocytes Is Mediated via the PI3K/Akt/mTOR Signaling Cascade. J Clin Endocrinol Metab 96: E586–E597. doi:10.1210/jc.2010-1408.
62. He M, Rutledge S, Kelly D, Palmer C, Murdoch G, et al. (2007) A new genetic disorder in mitochondrial fatty acid beta-oxidation: ACAD9 deficiency. Am J Hum Genet 81: 87–103.
63. Rakhshandehroo M, Knoch B, Müller M, Kersten S (2010) Peroxisome Proliferator-Activated Receptor Alpha Target Genes. PPAR Res 2010. Available: http://dx.doi.org/10.1155/2010/612089.
64. Chegary M, Brinke H te, Ruiter JPN, Wijburg FA, Stoll MSK, et al. (2009) Mitochondrial long chain fatty acid β-oxidation in man and mouse. Biochim Biophys Acta BBA - Mol Cell Biol Lipids 1791: 806–815. doi:10.1016/j.bbalip.2009.05.006.
65. Sung HK, Kim Y-W, Choi SJ, Kim J-Y, Jeune KH, et al. (2009) COMP-angiopoietin-1 enhances skeletal muscle blood flow and insulin sensitivity in mice. Am J Physiol - Endocrinol Metab 297: E402–E409. doi:10.1152/ajpendo.00122.2009.
66. Chen J-X, Stinnett A (2008) Ang-1 Gene Therapy Inhibits Hypoxia-Inducible Factor-1α (HIF-1α)-Prolyl-4-Hydroxylase-2, Stabilizes HIF-1α Expression, and Normalizes Immature Vasculature in db/db Mice. Diabetes 57: 3335–3343. doi:10.2337/db08-0503.
67. Oubaha M, Gratton J-P (2009) Phosphorylation of endothelial nitric oxide synthase by atypical PKCζ contributes to angiopoietin-1–dependent inhibition of VEGF-induced endothelial permeability in vitro. Blood 114: 3343–3351. doi:10.1182/blood-2008-12-196584.
68. Novgorodtseva T, Kantur T, Karaman Y, Antonyuk M, Zhukova N (2011) Modification of fatty acids composition in erythrocytes lipids in arterial hypertension associated with dyslipidemia. Lipids Health Dis 10: 18.
69. Xi Q, Adebiyi A, Zhao G, Chapman KE, Waters CM, et al. (2008) IP3 Constricts Cerebral Arteries via IP3 Receptor–Mediated TRPC3 Channel Activation and Independently of Sarcoplasmic Reticulum Ca2+ Release. Circ Res 102: 1118–1126. doi:10.1161/CIRCRESAHA.108.173948.
70. Bayorh MA, Ganafa AA, Emmett N, Socci RR, Eatman D, et al. (2005) Alterations in Aldosterone and Angiotensin II Levels in Salt-Induced Hypertension. Clin Exp Hypertens 27: 355–367. doi:10.1081/CEH-57423.
71. Merlot E, Vincent A, Thomas F, Meunier-Salaün M-C, Damon M, et al. (2012) Health and immune traits of Basque and Large White pigs housed in a conventional or enriched environment. animal 6: 1290–1299.
72. Webb EC, O'Neill HA (2008) The animal fat paradox and meat quality. 54th Int Congr Meat Sci Technol 54th ICoMST 10-15August 2008 Cape Town South Afr 80: 28–36. doi:10.1016/j.meatsci.2008.05.029.
73. Lunney JK (2007) Advances in Swine Biomedical Model Genomics. Int J Biol Sci 3: 179–184. doi:doi:10.7150/ijbs.3.179.
74. Pérez-Enciso M, Clop A, Noguera JL, Ovilo C, Coll A, et al. (2000) A QTL on pig chromosome 4 affects fatty acid metabolism: evidence from an Iberian by Landrace intercross. J Anim Sci 78: 2525–2531.
75. Ihaka R, Gentleman R (1996) R: A Language for Data Analysis and Graphics. J Comput Graph Stat 5: 299–314. doi:10.2307/1390807.
76. FastQC. Available: http://www.bioinformatics.bbsrc.ac.uk/projects/fastqc/.Accessed 2014 May 20.
77. Ensembl Genes 67. Available: http://www.ensembl.org/info/data/ftp/index.html.Accessed 2014 May 20.
78. Li H, Handsaker B, Wysoker A, Fennell T, Ruan J, et al. (2009) The Sequence Alignment/Map format and SAMtools. Bioinformatics 25: 2078–2079. doi:10.1093/bioinformatics/btp352.
79. Quinlan AR, Hall IM (2010) BEDTools: a flexible suite of utilities for comparing genomic features. Bioinformatics 26: 841–842. doi:10.1093/bioinformatics/btq033.
80. García-Alcalde F, Okonechnikov K, Carbonell J, Cruz LM, Götz S, et al. (2012) Qualimap: evaluating next-generation sequencing alignment data. Bioinformatics 28: 2678–2679. doi:10.1093/bioinformatics/bts503.
81. Storey JD, Tibshirani R (2003) Statistical significance for genomewide studies. Proc Natl Acad Sci 100: 9440–9445. doi:10.1073/pnas.1530509100.
82. Mortazavi A, Williams BA, McCue K, Schaeffer L, Wold B (2008) Mapping and quantifying mammalian transcriptomes by RNA-seq. Nat Methods 5: 621–628.
83. Kyoto Encyclopedia of Genes and Genomes. Available: http://www.genome.jp/kegg/pathway.html. Accessed 2014 May 20.
84. Reactome. Available: http://www.reactome.org. Accessed 2014 May 20.

MLST Subtypes and Population Genetic Structure of *Cryptosporidium andersoni* from Dairy Cattle and Beef Cattle in Northeastern China's Heilongjiang Province

Wei Zhao[1], Rongjun Wang[2], Weizhe Zhang[1], Aiqin Liu[1]*, Jianping Cao[3], Yujuan Shen[3], Fengkun Yang[1], Longxian Zhang[2]*

1 Department of Parasitology, Harbin Medical University, Harbin, Heilongjiang, China, **2** College of Animal Science and Veterinary Medicine, Henan Agricultural University Zhengzhou, Henan, China, **3** National Institute of Parasitic Diseases, Chinese Center for Disease Control and Prevention, Key Laboratory of Parasite and Vector Biology, Ministry of Health, WHO Collaborating Centre for Malaria, Schistosomiasis and Filariasis, Shanghai, China

Abstract

Cattle are the main reservoir host of *C. andersoni*, which shows a predominance in yearlings and adults of cattle. To understand the subtypes of *C. andersoni* and the population genetic structure in Heilongjiang Province, fecal specimens were collected from 420 dairy cattle and 405 beef cattle at the age of 12–14 months in eight cattle farms in five areas within this province and were screened for the presence of *Cryptosporidium* oocysts by microscopy after Sheather's sugar flotation technique. The average prevalence of *Cryptosporidium* spp. was 19.15% (158/825) and all the *Cryptosporidium* isolates were identified as *C. andersoni* by the SSU rRNA gene nested PCR-RFLP using *SspI*, *VspI* and *MboII* restriction enzymes. A total of 50 *C. andersoni* isolates were randomly selected and sequenced to confirm the RFLP results before they were subtyped by multilocus sequence typing (MLST) at the four microsatellite/minisatellite loci (MS1, MS2, MS3 and MS16). Four, one, two and one haplotypes were obtained at the four loci, respectively. The MLST subtype A4,A4,A4,A1 showed an absolute predominance and a wide distribution among the six MLST subtypes obtained in the investigated areas. Linkage disequilibrium analysis showed the presence of a clonal population genetic structure of *C. andersoni* in cattle, suggesting the absence of recombination among lineages. The finding of a clonal population genetic structure indicated that the prevalence of *C. andersoni* in cattle in Heilongjiang Province is not attributed to the introduction of cattle. Thus, prevention and control strategies should be focused on making stricter measures to avoid the occurrence of cross-transmission and re-infection between cattle individuals. These molecular data will also be helpful to explore the source attribution of infection/contamination of *C. andersoni* and to elucidate its transmission dynamics in Heilongjiang Province, even in China.

Editor: Yung-Fu Chang, Cornell University, United States of America

Funding: The study was supported partially by the National Natural Science Foundation of China (No. 31110103901) (Longxian Zhang) and the National S & T Major Program for Infectious Disease of China Nos. 2012ZX10004-201 and 2009ZX10004-201 (Jianping Cao). The funders had no role in study design, data collection and analysis, decision to publish, or preparation of the manuscript.

Competing Interests: The authors have declared that no competing interests exist.

* Email: liuaiqin1128@126.com (AL); zhanglx8999@gmail.com (LZ)

Introduction

Cryptosporidium spp. are the important intestinal pathogens in both humans and animals with a global distribution. The parasites can cause diarrhea in both immune-compromised and immune-competent individuals, and show a high mortality in patients with HIV-infection [1–4]. Numerous studies of molecular characterizations of *Cryptosporidium* isolates confirm the presence of extensive genetic variations within the genus *Cryptosporidium*. To date, 26 species and more than 70 genotypes of *Cryptosporidium* have been identified with new genotypes being found, and 13 species and three genotypes of *Cryptosporidium* have been isolated from humans [5–8].

Various subtyping tools have been developed and proven to be useful in molecular epidemiological and population genetic studies for *Cryptosporidium* spp, with GP60 gene sequencing being the most commonly used tool for *Cryptosporidium* subtyping. However, gp60 subtyping is restricted to *C. parvum* and *C. hominis* as well as other *Cryptosporidium* species/genotypes, which are genetically closely related to both of them [5,9–12]. A high-resolution multilocus sequence typing (MLST) technique has also been applied to characterize the genetics and population structure of *C. parvum* and *C. hominis* based on length polymorphism and single nucleotide polymorphism (SNP) [5,13–15]. For *C. muris* and *C. andersoni* as rare *Cryptosporidium* species in humans, the genetic data were available only at a genotype level. Take *C. andersoni* for example, to date, the identification of human-derived *C. andersoni* isolates was only based on the analysis of SSU rRNA gene or COWP gene, including a recent study conducted in Shanghai, China, where all the 34 *Cryptosporidium*-positive patients were confirmed to be infected with *C. andersoni* [16–20]. Recently, an MLST tool used for subtyping *C. muris* and *C. andersoni* has been established by Feng et al. [21]. It will be helpful in solving the problems on tracking the source of infection/contamination and elucidating transmission dynamics of human cryptosporidiosis caused by *C. muris* and *C. andersoni* by providing more genetic data.

Epidemiological data from different hosts have documented the host range or the host specificity of *C. andersoni*. Cattle are considered to be the main animal reservoir hosts of *C. andersoni*, although it is also occasionally detected in other animals such as bactrian camels, sheep, and hamsters [11,22,23]. Studies of age-associated distribution of *C. andersoni* in cattle reveal that *C. andersoni* is the predominant *Cryptosporidium* species responsible for cattle cryptosporidiosis in yearlings and adults [24–28]. Recent studies subtyped successfully *C. andersoni* isolates from cattle by MLST, including some isolates from a few areas in China [21,29,30]. In northeast's China, Heilongjiang Province, cattle are one of the most important economic animals and have been reported to be infected with *C. andersoni*, even in preweaned calves [12,31]. In addition, *C. andersoni* oocysts have been detected in raw wastewater from urban wastewater treatment plants [32]. The aims of the present study were to subtype C. *andersoni* isolates from yearlings of dairy cattle and beef cattle in Heilongjiang Province by MLST, and to elucidate population genetic structure of *C. andersoni* by diversity statistical test, and measurements of linkage disequilibrium. Meanwhile, we explored the relationship between MLST subtypes and breeds of cattle. The MLST data will be helpful to avoid or reduce the occurrence of cattle cryptosporidiosis in the investigated areas by making efficient control strategies based on characterization of population genetic structure. They will also be valuable to assess the risk that cattle infected with *C. andersoni* pose to humans by comparing population genetics of *C. andersoni* from humans and cattle in the future.

Materials and Methods

Ethics statement

This study was strictly performed in accordance with the recommendations of the Regulations for the Administration of Affairs Concerning Experimental Animals of Harbin Medical University/the Ministry of Health, China. All the fecal samples were obtained by the collection of feces excreted from cattle under the permission of farm owners to have their animals involved, with no specific permits being required by the authority. The protocol of the present study was reviewed and approved by the Animal Ethical Committee of Harbin Medical University (HMUIRB20130009).

Collection of *C. andersoni* isolates

Between May 2012 and July 2013, a total of 825 fecal specimens (420 from dairy cattle and 405 from beef cattle) were randomly collected from yearlings in eight cattle farms in five areas within Heilongjiang Province, including Harbin, Qiqihar, Mudanjiang, Jiamusi and Daqing. Their ages ranged from 12 to 14 months. All the fecal samples were taken immediately from fresh feces deposited on the ground after cattle defecation, and Sheather's sugar flotation technique was used to concentrate *Cryptosporidium* oocysts. The concentrates were detected by bright-field microscopy under ×400 and ×1,000. All the fecal samples microscopy-positive for *Cryptosporidium* oocysts were stored in 2.5% potassium dichromate at 4°C prior to being used in molecular biologic characterizations.

DNA Extraction and molecular identification of *C. andersoni*

Potassium dichromate was washed off *Cryptosporidium* oocyst-positive fecal samples with distilled water by centrifugation at 1500 g for 10 minutes at room temperature four times. Genomic DNA was extracted from 200 mg of each fecal sample using a QIAamp DNA Mini Stool Kit (Qiagen, Hilden, Germany) according to the manufacturer recommended procedures. Eluted DNA was stored at −20°C until further use in PCR analysis. All DNA preparations were confirmed molecularly for the presence of *Cryptosporidium* spp. by a nested PCR amplification of an approximate 830 bp fragment of the SSU rRNA gene as previously described, followed by RFLP analysis with *Ssp*I, *Vsp*I and *Mbo*II restriction enzymes to determine *Cryptosporidium* species/genotypes [33–35]. Not all positive specimens were sequenced to further confirm the RFLP results, and we only sequenced *C. andersoni* isolates used for the MLST study.

Molecular characterizations of *C. andersoni* at MS1, MS2, MS3 and MS16 loci

Approximate 30% of *C. andersoni* positive-samples of each farm were subtyped by amplifying the four minisatellite/microsatellite markers by nested PCRs, respectively. Target genes were MS1 coding for hypothetical protein, MS2 coding for 90 kDa heat shock protein, MS3 coding for hypothetical protein, and MS16 coding for leucine rich repeat family protein. The expected fragment lengths were approximate 550 bp, 450 bp, 530 bp and 590 bp, respectively, and primers and amplification conditions in nested PCR analysis were used as Feng et al described previously[21].

Nucleotide sequence analysis

All purified secondary PCR products were directly sequenced with secondary PCR primers on an ABI PRISMTM 3730 DNA Analyzer (Applied Biosystems, USA), using a BigDye Terminator v3.1 Cycle Sequencing kit (Applied Biosystems, USA). Accuracy of the sequencing data was confirmed by sequencing in both directions and additional PCR products if necessary. All the gene sequences obtained in the present study were aligned with each other and reference sequences obtained from GenBank by the Basic Local Alignment Search Tool (BLAST) and Clustal X 1.83. *C. andersoni* subtypes were named according to the numbers in microsatellite/minisatellite repeats or/and nucleotide diversity in non-repeat regions at each locus (Table 1), and a novel subtype was designated if no identical sequences were obtained.

Data analysis

DnaSP version 5.10.01 (http://www.ub.edu/dnasp/) was used to analyze the genetic diversity of *C. andersoni* isolates. Sequences from four loci were combined in a single contig and analyzed for linkage disequilibrium (LD) across the entire composite sequence by DnaSP 5.10.01 [36]. D' was calculated for all pairs of sites. Both the two-tailed Fisher's exact test and the χ^2 test were used to determine significance of the associations between polymorphic sites. The average LD was estimated by using the Z*n*S statistic, which averages LD over all pairwise comparisons for S polymorphisms in N sequences.

Results

Prevalence of *C. andersoni* in yearlings

A total of 420 and 405 fecal samples of 12–14-month-old dairy cattle and beef cattle, respectively, were screened for the presence of *Cryptosporidium* oocysts by microscopy. The average prevalence of *Cryptosporidium* spp. was 19.15% (158/825). *Cryptosporidium* oocysts were detected in 20.71% (87/420) dairy cattle and 17.53% (71/405) beef cattle, with no statistical difference in the prevalence between them ($\chi^2 = 1.35$, $P = 0.25$). Meanwhile, cattle

Table 1. Genetic characterizations of haplotypes of *C. andersoni* at MS1, MS2, MS3 and MS16 loci.

Haplotype	MS1			MS2				MS3					MS16	
	Accession No.[a]	Repeats[b]		Accession No.[a]	Repeat[b]	Polymorphic site		Accession No.[a]	Repeats[b]		Polymorphic site		Accession No.[a]	Repeat[b]
		a (n)	b (n)		c (n)	278	489		d (n)	e (n)	220	473		f (n)
A1	HM565067	3	14	HM565078	11	T	G	HM565095	2	2	A	C	HM565086	14
A2	JF732838	3	13	HM565079	10	T	G	HM565097	2	3	G	C	JF732872	12
A3	JF732836	3	12	HM565080	10	C	A	HM565094	2	3	G	T		
A4	JF732843	3	15	JF732853	10	C	G	HM565096	2	2	G	C		
A5	JF732845	3	16	JF732851	11	C	G							
A6	JF732846	3	17											

[a]Accession numbers of all the reference sequences from GenBank.
[b]The small letters a to f in the horizontal subheading represent the repeats at the four loci: a = (TAAAGGGCGAGA); b = (GAACGAGATAGG); c = (CCATACCTC); d = (TGTTGGTGTTGCTGT); e = (TGCTGCAGCTGC); f = (CTTCTTCAT).

were found to be infected with *Cryptosporidium* in all eight farms from the five investigated areas (Table 2). All the *Cryptosporidium* isolates were molecularly confirmed as *C. andersoni* by SSU rRNA nested PCR-RFLP using *SspI*, *VspI* and *MboII* restriction enzymes. Additionally, 50 *C. andersoni* isolates randomly selected for the MLST analysis were sequenced to further confirm the RFLP results.

Multilocus subtypes and polymorphism of *C. andersoni*

Approximate 30% of *C. andersoni* isolates were collected from each cattle farm and a total of 50 *C. andersoni* isolates (27 from dairy cattle and 23 from beef cattle) were used for analysis of MLST subtypes. At the four microsatellite/minisatellite loci (MS1, MS2, MS3 and MS16), 47, 48, 46 and 45 DNA preparations were sequenced successfully, respectively, and four, one, two and one haplotypes were identified, respectively. Representative nucleotide sequences were deposited in the GenBank under accession numbers KJ001678 to KJ001689.

A total of 45 out of 50 *C. andersoni* isolates were successfully subtyped at all the four loci, with six MLST subtypes being found. The MLST subtype A4,A4,A4,A1 showed a predominance, accounting for a high prevalence (73.33%, 33/45) in cattle with 79.16% (19/24) for dairy cattle versus 66.67% (14/21) for beef cattle. This subtype appeared in seven out of eight cattle farms, showing an extensive distribution in the investigated areas. However, the other three MLST subtypes, A2,A4,A4,A1 (n = 2), A2,A4,A2,A1 (n = 1) and A4,A4,A2,A1 (n = 2) were only found in dairy cattle while the remaining two MLST subtypes, A5,A4,A4,A1 (n = 5) and A1,A4,A4,A1 (n = 2) were only found in beef cattle (Table 2).

Sequence data of all four loci were concatenated making a multilocus gene of 1864 bp length. Genetic diversity of sequences was analyzed using DnaSP 5.10.01. The 45 sequences produced 18 polymorphic sites and two haplotypes with one haplotype diversity of 0.202±0.073, nucleotide diversity of 0.00200, and average number of nucleotide differences of 3.636.

Linkage disequilibrium analysis

A total of 45 *C. andersoni* isolates subtyped successfully at all the four loci were included in LD analysis. To examine LD within and between loci, we analyzed pairwise associations of polymorphism across the concatenated sequences. LD was estimated using the *ZnS* statistic, which calculates the average correlation among alleles in all pairs of polymorphic sites. *ZnS* value of 1.0000 indicated that the *C. andersoni* isolates had a clonal population structure, suggesting the absence of recombination among lineages, which was supported by the D' statistic (Figure S1).

Discussion

Cattle are considered as the main reservoir hosts of *C. andersoni* although the parasite has also been isolated from sheep, bactrian camels and hamsters [11,22,23]. Using the MLST tool for subtyping *C. muris* and *C. andersoni* developed by Feng et al. (2011) [21], a total of 14 MLST subtypes have been identified in *C. muris* isolates from animals and humans [21,29], while 18 MLST subtypes have been found in *C. andersoni* isolates from animals with 14 subtypes in cattle [21,29,30] (details seen in Table 3). In the present study, we investigated the occurrence of *Cryptosporidium* spp. in 12–14-month-old yearlings of dairy cattle and beef cattle by microscopy. The average prevalence of *Cryptopsoridium* spp. was 19.15% (157/825) with 20.71% (87/420) for dairy cattle versus 17.35% (71/405) for beef cattle, and all the *Cryptosporidium* isolates were identified as *C. andersoni*. Among the 50 *C. andersoni* isolates selected for MLST

Table 2. Prevalence and MLST subtypes of *C. andersoni* from dairy cattle and beef cattle.

Collection site	Dairy cattle			Beef cattle		
	Positive no./ Examined no.(%)	Subtyped no./ Amplified no.[a]	MLST subtypes (n)[b]	Positive no./ Examined no. (%)	Subtyped no./ Amplified no.[a]	MLST subtypes (n)[b]
Daqing	22/112 (19.64)	6/7	A4,A4,A4,A1 (5), A2,A4,A4,A1 (1)	11/89 (12.36)	3/3	A5,A4,A4,A1 (2), A1,A4,A4,A1 (1)
Harbin	13/83 (15.66)	4/4	A4,A4,A4,A1 (4)	NE		
Jiamusi	NE			7/108 (6.48)	2/2	A4,A4,A4,A1 (2)
Mudanjiang	40/153 (26.14)	10/12	A4,A4,A4,A1 (6), A2,A4,A4,A1 (1), A2,A4,A2,A1 (1), A4,A4,A2,A1 (2)	13/142 (9.15)	3/4	A4,A4,A4,A1 (2), A1,A4,A4,A1 (1)
Qiqihaer	12/72 (16.67)	4/4	A4,A4,A4,A1 (4)	40/66 (60.60)	13/14	A4,A4,A4,A1 (10), A5,A4,A4,A1 (3)
Total	87/420 (20.71)	24/27	A4,A4,A4,A1 (19), A2,A4,A4,A1 (2), A2,A4,A2,A1 (1), A4,A4,A2,A1 (2)	71/405 (17.53)	21/23	A4,A4,A4,A1 (14), A5,A4,A4,A1 (5), A1,A4,A4,A1 (2)

Note: NE = not examined.
[a]Subtyped no. indicating the number of *C. andersoni* isolates subtyped successfully by PCR at all the four loci (MS1, MS2, MS3 and MS16); Amplified no. indicating the number of *C. andersoni* isolates analyzed by PCR at all the four loci (MS1, MS2, MS3 and MS16).
[b]The haplotypes were arranged in accordance with the order of gene loci amplified, MS1, MS2, MS3 and MS16.

analysis, only 45 *C. andersoni* isolates were successfully subtyped at all the four microsatellite/minisatellite loci (MS1, MS2, MS3 and MS16) and six MLST subtypes have been obtained (Table 2). The MLST subtype A4,A4,A4,A1 was the most prevalent and the most widespread compared to other five subtypes in the investigated areas, based on the fact that this subtype could be found in 73.33% (33/45) of *C. andersoni* isolates and in 87.5% (7/8) of cattle farms. According to the present and previous data, *C. andersoni* MLST subtype (A4,A4,A4,A1) was also the most common in cattle in China among 10 subtypes identified (Table 4). Meanwhile, *C. andersoni* MLST subtypes in China were noticed to be different from those found in cattle in other countries, accounting for subtypes A2,A3,A2,A1, A2,A3,A1,A1 and A2,A3,A4,A1 in the USA, A2,A3,A4,A1 in Canada, and A2,A3,A4,A1 and A1,A3,A4,A1 in the Czech Republic [21]. The differences in genetic characterizations of *C. andersoni* might be related to the geographic separation just like *C. parvum* and *C. hominis* [5]. The results above suggested that occurrence of *C. andersoni* in cattle in China is not attributable to the introduction of cattle.

All but MLST subtype A4,A4,A4,A1 were subtypes apparently associated to either dairy or beef cattle (Table2). However, three subtypes (A2,A4,A4,A1, A2,A4,A2,A1 and A4,A4,A2,A1) in dairy cattle and one subtype (A1,A4,A4,A1) in beef cattle obtained in the present study were also described in beef cattle and dairy cattle in Shaanxi, China, respectively [30], suggesting that cross transmission of *C. andersoni* might occur between two breeds of cattle. However, to date, the MLST subtype A5,A4,A4,A1 has only been found in beef cattle in Heilongjiang and Henan of China [29]. Whether MLST subtypes are related to cattle breeds needs to be confirmed by a larger sample size of *C. andersoni* from cattle. The fact that the MLST subtype A2,A4,A2,A1 of *C. andersoni* in cattle was also reported in sheep further evidences that *C. andersoni* might circulate between cattle and sheep [29].

The intra-genetic variations of cattle-derived *C. andersoni* were observed in the present study based on multilocus DNA sequence analysis of a 1864 bp length fragment for 45 *C. andersoni* isolates by DnaSP. We could see 18 polymorphic sites and two haplotypes, with one haplotype diversity of 0.202 ± 0.073, nucleotide diversity of 0.00200, and average number of nucleotide differences of 3.636. In fact, genetic polymorphism has been described within *C. andersoni* at a subtype level. The present data, together with previous studies of MLST subtypes of *C. andersoni*, revealed the nucleotide differences of each haplotype at any locus in the number of microsatellite/minisatellite repeats or/and in the base variation in the non-repeat regions. In general, nucleotide sequences are the most conservative at the MS16 locus compared to the other three loci analyzed based on the fact that only two haplotypes have been currently found at this locus: A1 in cattle, sheep and camels, and A2 only in hamsters (Table 3). Thus, we can subtype *C. andersoni* isolates from a specific host at the other loci except MS16 locus to study intra-genetic variations of this parasite. Currently, six, five and four haplotypes of *C. andersoni* from different hosts have been identified worldwide at MS1, MS2 and MS3 loci, respectively (Table 3). At the MS1 locus, the genetic difference of six subtypes of *C. andersoni* (A1 to A6) is totally reflected in the copy number of microsatellite/minisatellite repeats. In contrast, at the MS2 and MS3 loci, the haplotypes of *C. andersoni* are named based on the copy number of microsatellite/minisatellite repeats, and in the case of the same number of repeats, the haplotypes of *C. andersoni* are distinguished from each other according to base variations in the non-repeat regions. The genetic characterizations of each haplotype at each locus has been summarized in Table 1.

In the present study, significant LD (Z_nS value of 1.0000) showed that *C. andersoni* had a clonal population genetic structure. The result suggested the absence of recombination among lineages of *C. andersoni* in cattle in Heilongjiang Province, which was consistent with *C. andersoni* isolates from other areas in China [29,30]. A clonal population genetic structure indicates the multilocus subtypes are relatively stable in time and place, and thus can be used effectively in the longitudinal tracking of the transmission and in the investigation of cryptosporidiosis outbreaks caused by *C. andersoni* in the areas investigated. Wang et al. (2012) conducted LD analysis of *C. andersoni* population in cattle in China [29]. When the isolates showing the same MLST subtype were scored as one individual, the result of I^S_A value ($I^S_A = 0.0290$,

Table 3. MLST subtypes of *C. andersoni* from different hosts worldwide.

Host	Subtyped no.	MS1	MS2	MS3	MS16	Reference
sheep	1	A2	A4	A2	A1	[29]
	1	A2	A5	A2	A1	[29]
hamster	2	A3	A4	A2	A2	[29]
bactrian camel	1	A6	A4	A2	A1	[29]
	1	A6	A5	A2	A1	[29]
cattle	3	A1	A2	A4	A1	[21]
	1	A1	A3	A4	A1	[21]
	34	A1	A4	A4	A1	[29,30]; this study
	2	A2	A1	A2	A1	[21]
	1	A2	A1	A3	A1	[21]
	1	A2	A3	A1	A1	[21]
	1	A2	A3	A2	A1	[21]
	3	A2	A3	A4	A1	[21]
	6	A2	A4	A2	A1	[29,30]; this study
	6	A2	A4	A4	A1	[29,30]; this study
	1	A3	A4	A4	A1	[29]
	3	A4	A4	A2	A1	[30]; this study
	82	A4	A4	A4	A1	[29,30]; this study
	6	A5	A4	A4	A1	[29]; this study

$V_D<L$) suggested that cattle-derived *C. andersoni* isolates had an epidemic population structure, which might result from the clonal expansion of two MLST subtypes (A4,A4,A4,A1 and A1,A4,A4,A1) [29].

In conclusion, six MLST subtypes of *C. andersoni* were found in cattle in Heilongjiang Province, with the subtype A4,A4,A4,A1 being predominant in both dairy and beef cattle. The finding of the same MLST subtypes in dairy cattle, beef cattle and sheep in the present and previous studies suggest the likelihood of cross transmission of *C. andersoni* between these hosts [29,30]. The MLST subtype A5,A4,A4,A1 has only been found in beef cattle. Nevertheless, we cannot draw a definitive conclusion about the relationship between *C. andersoni* MLST subtypes and breed of cattle due to the small sample size. The characterization of a clonal population genetic structure of *C. andersoni* indicates that the prevalence of *C. andersoni* in cattle is not attributed to the introduction of cattle. Thus, a key component to avoid or reduce cattle cryptosporidiosis is to prevent the occurrence of cross-transmission and re-infection between cattle individuals by making effective control strategies. The MLST data will be helpful to explore the source attribution of infection/contamination of

Table 4. MLST subtypes of *C.andersoni* in cattle in different provinces of China.

Location	Subtyped no.	MLST subtype (no.)	Reference
Guangxi	4	A1,A4,A4,A1 (2); A2,A4,A2,A1 (1); A4,A4,A4,A1 (1)	[29]
Heilongjiang	50	A4,A4,A4,A1 (37); A5,A4,A4,A1 (5); A2,A4,A4,A1 (2); A2,A4,A2,A1 (2) A4,A4,A2,A1 (2); A1,A4,A4,A1 (2)	[29]; this study
Henan	22	A4,A4,A4,A1 (9); A1,A4,A4,A1 (3); A1,A2,A4,A1 (3); A2,A4,A2,A1 (2); A2,A1,A2,A1 (2); A2,A1,A3,A1 (1); A3,A4,A4,A1 (1); A5,A4,A4,A1 (1)	[29,21]
Jilin	1	A4,A4,A4,A1 (1)	[29]
Shaanxi	57	A4,A4,A4,A1 (26); A1,A4,A4,A1 (26); A2,A4,A4,A1 (3); A2,A4,A2,A1 (1); A4,A4,A2,A1 (1)	[30]
Shanxi	5	A4,A4,A4,A1 (5)	[29]
Sichuan	5	A4,A4,A4,A1 (3); A2,A4,A4,A1 (1); A1,A4,A4,A1 (1)	[29]
Total	144	A4,A4,A4,A1 (82); A1,A4,A4,A1 (34); A2,A4,A4,A1 (6); A2,A4,A2,A1 (6); A5,A4,A4,A1 (6); A4,A4,A2,A1 (3); A3,A4,A4,A1 (1); A1,A2,A4,A1 (3); A2,A1,A2,A1 (2); A2,A1,A3,A1 (1)	

human cryptosporidiosis caused by *C. andersoni* and its transmission dynamics in Heilongjiang Province, even in China.

Supporting Information

Figure S1 Linkage disequilibrium among different populations by DnaSP analysis of concatenated sequences from four genetic loci. Sequences from four loci were combined in a single contig and analyzed for linkage disequilibrium (LD) across the entire composite sequence by DnaSP 5.10.01 software.

Author Contributions

Conceived and designed the experiments: AL LZ. Performed the experiments: Wei Zhao Weizhe Zhang FY. Analyzed the data: RW Wei Zhao. Contributed reagents/materials/analysis tools: JC YS. Contributed to the writing of the manuscript: AL LZ Wei Zhao RW.

References

1. Goldstein ST, Juranek DD, Ravenholt O, Hightower AW, Martin DG, et al. (1996) Cryptosporidiosis: an outbreak associated with drinking water despite state-of-the-art water treatment. Ann Intern Med 124: 459–468.
2. Mor SM, DeMaria A Jr, Griffiths JK, Naumova EN (2009) Cryptosporidiosis in the elderly population of the United States. Clin Infect Dis 48: 698–705.
3. Nahrevanian H, Assmar M (2008) Cryptosporidiosis in immunocompromised patients in the Islamic Republic of Iran. J Microbiol Immunol Infect 41: 74–77.
4. Sodqi M, Marih L, Lahsen AO, Bensghir R, Chakib A, et al. (2012) Causes of death among 91 HIV-infected adults in the era of potent antiretroviral therapy. Presse Med 41: 386–390.
5. Xiao L (2010) Molecular epidemiology of cryptosporidiosis: an update. Exp Parasitol 124: 80–89.
6. Fayer R (2010) Taxonomy and species delimitation in *Cryptosporidium*. Exp Parasitol 124: 90–97.
7. Helmy YA, Krücken J, Nöckler K, von Samson-Himmelstjerna G, Zessin KH (2013) Molecular epidemiology of *Cryptosporidium* in livestock animals and humans in the Ismailia province of Egypt. Vet Parasitol 193: 15–24.
8. Elwin K, Hadfield SJ, Robinson G, Crouch ND, Chalmers RM (2012) *Cryptosporidium viatorum* n. sp. (Apicomplexa: Cryptosporidiidae) among travellers returning to Great Britain from the Indian subcontinent, 2007–2011. Int J Parasitol 42: 675–682.
9. Plutzer J, Karanis P (2009) Genetic polymorphism in *Cryptosporidium* species: an update. Vet Parasitol 165: 187–199.
10. Hijjawi N, Ng J, Yang R, Atoum MF, Ryan U (2010) Identification of rare and novel *Cryptosporidium* GP60 subtypes in human isolates from Jordan. Exp Parasitol 125: 161–164.
11. Lv C, Zhang L, Wang R, Jian F, Zhang S, et al. (2009) *Cryptosporidium* spp. in wild, laboratory, and pet rodents in China: prevalence and molecular characterization. Appl Environ Microbiol 75: 7692–7699.
12. Zhang W, Wang R, Yang F, Zhang L, Cao J, et al. (2013) Distribution and genetic characterizations of *Cryptosporidium* spp. in pre-weaned dairy calves in Northeastern China's Heilongjiang Province. PLoS One 8: 54857.
13. Gatei W, Das P, Dutta P, Sen A, Cama V, et al. (2007) Multilocus sequence typing and genetic structure of *Cryptosporidium hominis* from children in Kolkata, India. Infect Genet Evol 7: 197–205.
14. Robinson G, Chalmers RM (2012) Assessment of polymorphic genetic markers for multi-locus typing of *Cryptosporidium parvum* and *Cryptosporidium hominis*. Exp Parasitol 132: 200–215.
15. Quílez J, Vergara-Castiblanco C, Monteagudo L, Del Cacho E, Sánchez-Acedo C (2011) Multilocus fragment typing and genetic structure of *Cryptosporidium parvum* Isolates from diarrheic preweaned calves in Spain. Appl Environ Microbiol 77: 7779–7786.
16. Leoni F, Amar C, Nichols G, Pedraza-Díaz S, McLauchlin J (2006) Genetic analysis of *Cryptosporidium* from 2414 humans with diarrhoea in England between 1985 and 2000. J Med Microbiol 55: 703–707.
17. Morse TD, Nichols RA, Grimason AM, Campbell BM, Tembo KC, et al. (2007) Incidence of cryptosporidiosis species in paediatric patients in Malawi. Epidemiol Infec 135: 1307–1315.
18. Waldron LS, Dimeski B, Beggs PJ, Ferrari BC, Power ML (2011) Molecular epidemiology, spatiotemporal analysis, and ecology of sporadic human cryptosporidiosis in Australia. Appl Environ Microbiol 77: 7757–7765.
19. Agholi M, Hatam GR, Motazedian MH (2013) HIV/AIDS-associated opportunistic protozoal diarrhea. AIDS Res Hum Retroviruses 29: 35–41.
20. Liu H, Shen Y, Yin J, Yuan Z, Jiang Y, et al. (2014) Prevalence and genetic characterization of *Cryptosporidium*, *Enterocytozoon*, *Giardia* and *Cyclospora* in diarrheal outpatients in China. BMC Infect Dis 14: 25.
21. Feng Y, Yang W, Ryan U, Zhang L, Kvác M, et al. (2011) Development of a multilocus sequence tool for typing *Cryptosporidium muris* and *Cryptosporidium andersoni*. J Clin Microbiol 49: 34–41.
22. Wang R, Zhang L, Ning C, Feng Y, Jian F, et al. (2008) Multilocus phylogenetic analysis of *Cryptosporidium andersoni* (Apicomplexa) isolated from a bactrian camel (Camelus bactrianus) in China. Parasitol Res 102: 915–920.
23. Yang R, Jacobson C, Gardner G, Carmichael I, Campbell AJ, et al. (2014) Longitudinal prevalence, oocyst shedding and molecular characterisation of *Cryptosporidium* species in sheep across four states in Australia. Vet Parasitol 200: 50–58.
24. Feng Y, Ortega Y, He G, Das P, Xu M, et al. (2007) Wide geographic distribution of *Cryptosporidium bovis* and the deer-like genotype in bovines. Vet Parasitol 144: 1–9.
25. Fayer R, Santín M, Trout JM, Greiner E (2006) Prevalence of species and genotypes of *Cryptosporidium* found in 1–2-year-old dairy cattle in the eastern United States. Vet Parasitol 135: 105–112.
26. Santín M, Trout JM, Xiao L, Zhou L, Greiner E, et al. (2004) Prevalence and age-related variation of *Cryptosporidium* species and genotypes in dairy calves. Vet Parasitol 122: 103–117.
27. Langkjaer RB, Vigre H, Enemark HL, Maddox-Hyttel C (2007) Molecular and phylogenetic characterization of *Cryptosporidium* and *Giardia* from pigs and cattle in Denmark. Parasitology 134: 339–350.
28. Wang R, Ma G, Zhao J, Lu Q, Wang H, et al. (2011) *Cryptosporidium andersoni* is the predominant species in post-weaned and adult dairy cattle in China. Parasitol Int 60: 1–4.
29. Wang R, Jian F, Zhang L, Ning C, Liu A, et al. (2012) Multilocus sequence subtyping and genetic structure of *Cryptosporidium muris* and *Cryptosporidium andersoni*. PLoS One 7: 43782.
30. Zhao GH, Ren WX, Gao M, Bian QQ, Hu B, et al. (2013) Genotyping *Cryptosporidium andersoni* in cattle in Shaanxi Province, Northwestern China. PLoS One 8: 60112.
31. Liu A, Wang R, Li Y, Zhang L, Shu J, et al. (2009) Prevalence and distribution of *Cryptosporidium* spp. in dairy cattle in Heilongjiang Province, China. Parasitol Res 105: 797–802.
32. Liu A, Ji H, Wang E, Liu J, Xiao L, et al. (2011) Molecular identification and distribution of *Cryptosporidium* and *Giardia duodenalis* in raw urban wastewater in Harbin, China. Parasitol Res 109: 913–918.
33. Xiao L, Singh A, Limor J, Graczyk TK, Gradus S, et al. (2001) Molecular characterization of *Cryptosporidium* oocysts in samples of raw surface water and wastewater. Appl Environ Microbiol 67: 1097–1101.
34. Xiao L, Bern C, Limor J, Sulaiman I, Roberts J, et al. (2001) Identification of 5 types of *Cryptosporidium* parasites in children in Lima, Peru. J Infect Dis 183: 492–497.
35. Xiao L, Feng Y (2008) Zoonotic cryptosporidiosis. FEMS Immunol Med Microbiol 52: 309–323.
36. Rozas J, Sanchez-DelBarrio JC, Messeguer X, Rozas R (2003) DnaSP, DNA polymorphism analyses by the coalescent and other methods. Bioinformatics 19: 2496–2497.

12

A Prospective Cohort Study to Examine the Association between Dietary Patterns and Depressive Symptoms in Older Chinese People in Hong Kong

Ruth Chan[1]*, Dicken Chan[2], Jean Woo[1]

1 Department of Medicine and Therapeutics, The Chinese University of Hong Kong, Shatin, Hong Kong, **2** The Jockey Club School of Public Health and Primary Care, The Chinese University of Hong Kong, Shatin, Hong Kong

Abstract

Introduction: Dietary patterns are culturally specific and there is limited data on the association of dietary patterns with late-life depression in Chinese. This study examined the associations between dietary patterns and baseline and subsequent depressive symptoms in community-dwelling Chinese older people in Hong Kong.

Methods: Participants aged ≥65 year participating in a cohort study examining the risk factors for osteoporosis completed a validated food frequency questionnaire at baseline between 2001 and 2003. Factor analysis was used to identify three dietary patterns: "vegetables-fruits" pattern, "snacks-drinks-milk products" pattern, and "meat-fish" pattern. Depressive symptoms were measured at baseline and 4-year using the validated Geriatric Depression Scale. Multiple logistic regression was used for cross-sectional analysis (n = 2,902) to assess the associations between dietary patterns and the presence of depressive symptoms, and for longitudinal analysis (n = 2,211) on their associations with 4-year depressive symptoms, with adjustment for socio-demographic and lifestyle factors.

Results: The highest quartile of "vegetables-fruits" pattern score was associated with reduced likelihood of depressive symptoms [Adjusted OR = 0.55 (95% CI: 0.36–0.83), $p_{trend} = 0.017$] compared to the lowest quartile at baseline. Similar inverse trend was observed for the highest quartile of "snacks-drinks-milk products" pattern score [Adjusted OR = 0.41 (95% CI: 0.26–0.65), $p_{trend} < 0.001$] compared to the lowest quartile. There was no association of "meat-fish" pattern with the presence of depressive symptoms at baseline. None of the dietary patterns were associated with subsequent depressive symptoms at 4-year.

Conclusion: Higher "vegetables-fruits" and "snacks-drinks-milk products" pattern scores were associated with reduced likelihood of baseline depressive symptoms in Chinese older people in Hong Kong. The longitudinal analyses failed to show any causal relationship between dietary patterns and depressive symptoms in this population.

Editor: Robert Stewart, Institute of Psychiatry, United Kingdom

Funding: This study was supported by grants from the Research Grants Council of Hong Kong, CUHK 4101/02M; the Hong Kong Jockey Club Charities Trust; the SH Ho Centre for Gerontology and Geriatric and the Centre for Nutritional Studies, The Chinese University of Hong Kong. The funders had no role in study design, data collection and analysis, decision to publish, or preparation of the manuscript.

Competing Interests: The authors have declared that no competing interests exist.

* Email: ruthchansm@cuhk.edu.hk

Introduction

Depression is a common mental health disorder. It affects over 350 million people worldwide and it is expected that depression will become the world's leading cause of disease burden by the year 2030 [1]. Depression is less prevalent among older adults than among younger counterparts [2]. However, late-life depression is considered as an important public health problem due to its devastating consequences, including increased risk of morbidity and reduced physical, cognitive, and social functioning [3,4]. As a result, to identify modifiable risk factors for depression is inevitably important [5].

Recent evidence suggests that diet modifies key biological factors associated with the development of depression, and diet rich in fruits, vegetables, whole grains and fish is in general associated with lower risk of depression [6,7]. Studies have shown that the antioxidant compounds in fruit and vegetables could reduce neuronal damage induced by oxidative-stress whereas long-chain omega-3 polyunsaturated fatty acids could possibly affect mood by an alteration of the brain serotonergic function and its immune-neuroendocrine effects [6,7]. However, the examination of diet as a risk factor for depression has traditionally focused on the effect of single foods and nutrients, and the findings thus far are inconsistent [8]. Since diet is a combination of food and nutrients, there has been an increasing interest in using dietary pattern analysis in epidemiological studies [9]. There are two main approaches to define dietary patterns [9,10]. One approach is the *a priori* approach in which dietary indices are constructed based on prevailing dietary recommendations. Another approach is the *a posteriori* approach in which dietary patterns are derived from statistical modeling, such as factor analysis, using data from dietary records or food frequency questionnaires (FFQ).

Data on the association between dietary patterns and depression are limited. Some cross-sectional studies have been carried out in Caucasians and Japanese to evaluate the association between dietary patterns and depression or depressive symptoms in adulthood [11–16]. To our knowledge, nine prospective studies have examined the role of dietary patterns and depression or depressive symptoms in adulthood [17–25] and two prospective studies have evaluated this association in adolescents [26,27]. Few studies have investigated the association between depression and diet in Chinese older people, and these studies mainly focused on the effect of single foods and nutrients [28,29]. Only one cross-sectional study has examined the association of dietary patterns with depressive symptoms in Chinese but it was done in adolescents [27].

Since dietary patterns are culturally specific and there is limited data on the association of dietary patterns with late-life depression in Chinese, we evaluated the association between dietary patterns and baseline and subsequent depressive symptoms in older Chinese people, using data from a sample of community-dwelling men and women aged 65 and over participating in a prospective study in Hong Kong. We hypothesized that dietary patterns are associated with baseline and subsequent depressive symptoms in this population.

Methods

Study population

Subjects were participants of a cohort study examining the risk factors for osteoporosis in Hong Kong [30]. 2,000 men and 2,000 women aged 65 years and over living in the community were recruited in a health survey between August 2001 and December 2003 by recruitment notices and talks in community centers and housing estates. Participants were volunteers and were able to walk or take public transport to the study site. They were recruited using a stratified sample so that approximately 33% would be in each of these age groups: 65–69, 70–74, 75+. Compared with the official population statistics, participants had higher educational level than the overall older population in Hong Kong (12–18% vs. 3–9% with tertiary education in the age groups 80+, 75–79,70–74, and 65–69 years) [31]. The 4-year follow-up was held between August 2005 and November 2007. Follow-up was done by a mailed reminder for a follow-up body check appointment. Phone reminders were given again close to the appointment dates, and defaulters were given a second appointment to enhance attendance rates. Mean (SD) follow-up year was 3.9 (0.1) years.

We excluded participants who did not have dietary data (n = 5), those with extreme daily energy intake at the first- and last-half percentiles of the sex-specific range (n = 37), those who had missing data for the variables included for the analyses (n = 6), and those who were probable dementia defined using the cognitive part of the Community Screening Instrument for Dementia (CSI-D) with the cutoff point of ≤28.4 [32] (n = 1,050). The baseline analysis was performed on 2,902 participants. For the longitudinal analysis, we further excluded 218 participants who had depressive symptoms at baseline and 473 participants who did not attend the 4-year follow-up. 2,211 participants were therefore included for the 4-year incidence analysis (Figure 1). This study was conducted in accordance with the Declaration of Helsinki. This study was approved by the Clinical Research Ethics Committee of the Chinese University of Hong Kong. Written informed consent was obtained from all participants.

Demographic and overall health characteristics

A standardized interview was performed to collect information on age, gender, education level, marital status, smoking habit, alcohol use and medical history. Information on the duration and

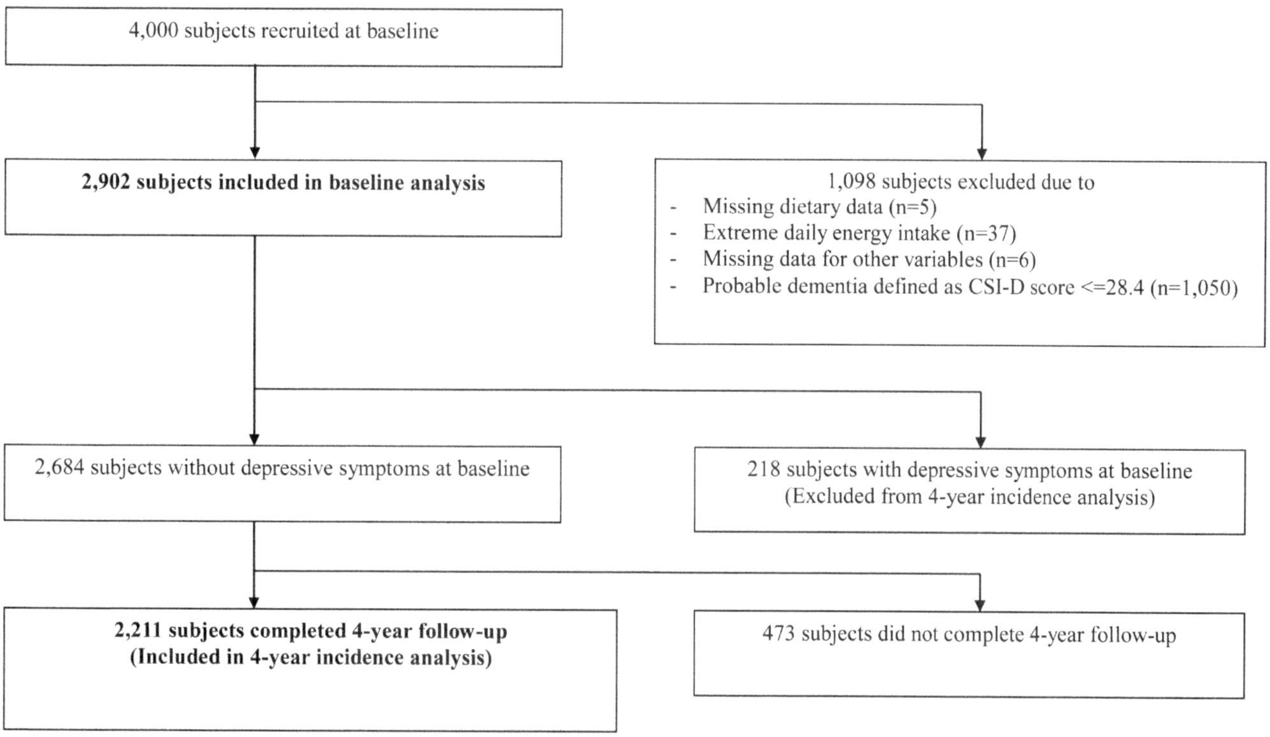

Figure 1.Number of subjects included and excluded for baseline and 4-year follow-up analyses.

level of past and current use of cigarettes, cigars and pipes was obtained. Smoking history was classified in terms of former smoking (at least 100 cigarettes smoked in a lifetime), current smoking and never smoking. Drinking status was defined as never, former (ever drank at least 5 drinks daily in a lifetime) or current drinker. Baseline disease status was obtained by self-report of their doctors' diagnoses, supplemented by the identification of drugs brought to the interviewers.

Anthropometric data

Body weight was measured to the nearest 0.1 kg with participants wearing a light gown, using the Physician Balance Beam Scale (Healthometer, Illinois, USA). Height was measured to the nearest 0.1 cm using the Holtain Harpenden stadiometer (Holtain Ltd, Crosswell, UK). Body mass index (BMI) was calculated as body weight in kg / (height in m)^2.

Physical activity assessment

Physical activity was assessed by the Physical Activity Scale for the Elderly (PASE) [33], which was adapted for use in elderly Hong Kong Chinese [34]. This is a 12-item scale measuring the average number of hours per day spent in leisure, household, and occupational physical activities over the previous 7-day period. Activity weights for each item were determined based on the amount of energy spent, and each item score was calculated by multiplying the activity weight with daily activity frequency. A composite PASE score of all the items was yielded. A higher PASE score reflects higher physical activity level.

Number of instrumental activities of daily living (IADLs) were assessed using specific questions and participants were asked to self-report of any impairment in walking two to three blocks outdoors on level ground, climbing 10 steps without resting, preparing own meals, doing heavy housework like scrubbing floors or washing windows, and shopping for groceries or clothes. A summed score from 0 to 5 was calculated from these activities as the degree of impairment in IADLs, with higher score indicating greater impairment.

Assessment of cognitive function

Since depression may be associated with cognitive impairment, in the analysis of factors associated with depression, the presence of cognitive impairment was adjusted for as a confounding factor. Cognitive function was assessed by trained research staff using the cognitive part of the Community Screening Instrument for Dementia (CSI-D) [32], validated in different cultural and educational settings [32]. The cognitive part of the CSI-D consists of 32 items in six cognitive domains: orientation to time, orientation to place, praxis, abstract thinking, language and memory. A summary score ranged from 0 to 33 was generated, with higher score meaning better cognitive function. The cutoff point for probable dementia is $\leq$28.4.

Assessment of depressive symptoms

Depressive symptoms was assessed by face-to-face interviews using a validated Chinese version of the Geriatric Depression Scale (GDS) [35,36]. The GDS short form was found to be a highly reliable (reliability coefficient of 0.90) and valid screening device (sensitivity of 96.3% and specificity of 87.5%) for assessing geriatric depression in Hong Kong Chinese [36]. The GDS short form consists of 15 questions relevant to depression, such as motivation, self-image, losses, agitation and mood. A yes/no format was designed for each question. A summary score ranged from 0 to 15 was generated, and a cut-off of 8 or more was used to define the presence of depressive symptoms.

Dietary assessment

Baseline dietary intake was assessed using a validated FFQ developed in a population survey [37]. Daily nutrient intake was calculated using food tables derived from McCance and Widdowson [38] and the Chinese Medical Sciences Institute [39]. The FFQ consisted of 280 food items. Each participant reported the frequency and the usual amount of consumption of each food item over the past year. For each food 9 different categories were given from never or seldom to more than once a day. Portion size was explained to participants using a catalogue of pictures of individual food portions. For seasonally consumed vegetables and fruits, participants were asked about the months of food consumption over the past year. The amount of cooking oil was estimated according to the usual cooking methods of preparing standardized portion of different foods and the usual portion of different foods consumed by the participants.

Dietary patterns derived by factor analysis

Details of dietary pattern scores derived by the factor analysis have been described elsewhere [40]. In brief, individual food items from the FFQ were aggregated into 32 food groups based on similarity of type of food and nutrient composition. The food groups were energy adjusted by dividing the energy intake from each food group by total energy intake and multiplying by 100, and were expressed as percentage contribution to total energy [41]. Factor analysis was conducted with varimax rotation using the 32 food groups [9]. Factors were retained based on an eigenvalues greater than 1.0, a scree plot, and the interpretability [42]. The factor scores for each pattern were calculated for each participant by summing intakes of food items weighted by their factor loadings. A higher score indicated greater conformity with the pattern being calculated.

Statistical analysis

Statistical analyses were performed using the statistical package SPSS version 21.0 (SPSS Inc., Illinois, US). Data were checked for normality using histograms and logarithmic transformation was applied whenever appropriate. Dietary pattern scores derived by factor analysis were stratified into quartiles based on the distribution of each sex. Pearson's correlation was used to examine the correlation between each dietary pattern score and intakes of various nutrients. Independent *t* test and chi square test were used to examine baseline differences in mean age, BMI, PASE, CSI-D score, energy intake, and also differences in the distribution of sex, education level, smoking status, alcohol use, number of IADLs, self-reported disease status, quartiles of each dietary pattern score between participants with depressive symptoms and participants without depressive symptoms at baseline. These tests were also used to examine differences in baseline characteristics between participants who included and excluded in the baseline analysis, and between participants who completed and participants who did not complete the 4-year follow-up.

Multivariate logistic regression was used to estimate the odds ratio (OR) and 95% confidence intervals (CIs) for both the baseline and the subsequent depressive symptoms according to quartiles of each dietary pattern score. Model 1 was adjusted for baseline age (years), sex, and daily energy intake (kcal). Model 2 was further adjusted for baseline BMI, PASE, number of IADLs (no difficulty/some difficulties), smoking habit (never/past/current), alcohol use (never/past/current), education level (no education/primary or below/secondary or matriculation/University or above), and marital status (married or living with a partner/ widowed, separated or divorced/single). Model 3 was further adjusted for baseline self-reported history of diabetes (yes/no), hypertension (yes/no), and CVD or stroke (yes/no), and CSI-D score. Test for trend was examined by entering quartiles of each dietary pattern score in all models. An α level of 5% was used as the level of significance. Interaction between sex and quartiles of each dietary pattern score was tested by addition of cross-product terms to the multivariate models. Interactions were not significant, thus all analyses are presented in the total population.

To check the possibility of reverse causation, a sensitivity analysis excluding participants with extreme GDS at the top two percentiles (GDS≥11) was performed for the cross-sectional data. Considering that GDS is a screening scale and may be limited as a case-defining instrument compared to other diagnostic instruments [43], multivariate logistic regression models were repeated using a group whose depressive symptom levels had clearly increased over 4-year (i.e. with an increase in GDS score at 4 and over from baseline to four years) as an outcome variable. This cut-off value was chosen because 142 participants (6.4%) could be classified as the worsening cases and this number of cases may be more sufficient and powerful for statistical analysis than using an increase in GDS score at 5 and over as a cut-off value (i.e. n = 85). All models were adjusted for the same variables mentioned above.

Results

Dietary patterns of the participants

Factor analysis identified three dietary patterns (Table 1). The first factor (vegetables-fruits pattern) was dominated by frequent intake of vegetables, fruits, soy and soy products, and legumes. The second factor (snacks-drinks-milk products pattern) was composed of a mixture of healthy and unhealthy food groups. It was characterized by frequent intake of condiments, drinks, fast food, French fries, potato chips, sweets and desserts, nuts, milk products, and whole grains. The third factor (meat-fish pattern) included frequent intake of dim sum, red and processed meats, poultry, fish and seafood, and wine.

'Vegetables-fruits' dietary pattern scores were inversely associated with total fat, saturated fat, monounsaturated fat and polyunsaturated fat intakes, and positively associated with intakes of protein, fiber, isoflavones, most vitamins and minerals. 'Snacks-drinks-milk products' dietary pattern scores were inversely associated with intakes of polyunsaturated fat and vitamin K, and positively associated with intakes of carbohydrates, protein, total fat, saturated fat, monounsaturated fat, cholesterol, fiber, most minerals and vitamins. Whilst 'snacks-drinks-milk products' dietary pattern scores were also positively associated with intakes of fiber and most minerals and vitamins, the associations were less strong than those with 'vegetables-fruits' dietary pattern scores. 'Meat-fish' dietary pattern scores were weakly positively associated with intakes of polyunsaturated fat and most micronutrients, moderately positively associated with intakes of protein, total fat and monounsaturated fat, and strongly positively associated with saturated fat and cholesterol intakes. The positive associations of protein, total fat, different kinds of fat and cholesterol with 'meat-fish' dietary pattern scores were stronger than those with 'snacks-drinks-milk products' dietary pattern scores (Table 2).

Participants' characteristics by baseline depressive status

Participants who were excluded in the cross-sectional analysis were older and less physically active, had lower education level, and were more likely to be female, widowed, separated, divorced or single, and to have self-reported history of diabetes than those who were included in the cross-sectional analysis ($p<0.05$). Those who discontinued the 4-year follow-up were older, less physically active, and were more likely to be divorced or single as compared to those who completed the 4-year follow-up ($p<0.05$) (details not shown).

Among 2,902 participants included in the cross-sectional analysis, there were 218 (7.5%) participants who were classified as having depressive symptoms at baseline. For the longitudinal analysis, 81 (3.7%) cases were newly identified as having depressive symptoms out of 2,211 participants at the 4-year follow-up. The characteristics of participants with depressive symptoms and participants without depressive symptoms at baseline are shown in Table 3. Those who had depressive symptoms had lower CSI-D score, lower education level, more impairments in IADLs, and were more likely to be widowed, separated, divorced or single, and current smokers, and were more likely to have self-reported history of heart diseases or stroke. Those who had depressive symptoms also showed lower 'vegetables-fruits' dietary pattern scores and lower 'snacks-drinks-milk products' dietary pattern scores.

Dietary patterns and the presence of depressive symptoms at baseline and 4-year

In the cross-sectional analysis, participants in the highest quartile of "vegetables-fruits" pattern score had reduced likelihood of depressive symptoms [Adjusted OR = 0.55 (95% CI: 0.36–0.83), $p_{trend} = 0.017$] compared to participants in the lowest quartile. Participants in the highest quartile of "snacks-drinks-milk products" pattern score also showed reduced likelihood of depressive symptoms [Adjusted OR = 0.41 (95% CI: 0.26–0.65), $p_{trend} < 0.001$] compared to those in the lowest quartile. There was no association of "meat-fish" pattern with depressive status at baseline (Table 4). Longitudinal analysis showed that none of the dietary patterns were associated with the presence of depressive symptoms at 4-year (Table 5).

Sensitivity analysis excluding participants with extreme GDS (i.e. GDS≥11 (n = 56)) showed similar results for the cross-sectional data (details not shown). Multivariate logistic regression models that were repeated using a group with an increase in GDS score >= 4 over four years as an outcome also showed no association between each dietary pattern and the presence of depressive symptoms at 4-year (details not shown).

Discussion

This study found an inverse association between "vegetables-fruits' and 'snacks-drinks-milk products' dietary pattern scores and baseline depressive symptoms. However, no significant associations between 'meat-fish' dietary pattern scores and baseline depressive symptoms were observed. Moreover, we did not observe significant associations between baseline dietary pattern scores and subsequent depressive symptoms at 4-year.

Previous cross-sectional studies have evaluated the association between dietary patterns and depression or depressive symptoms. However, the results are inconclusive [13–16,22]. Similar to our findings, two recent studies from Japan showed that a healthy Japanese dietary pattern characterized by high intakes of plant foods including vegetables, fruit, mushrooms and soy products was associated with fewer depressive symptoms [14,16]. Our results were also consistent with the findings from an Australian study which showed that a diet characterized by high intakes of fruits, vegetables, and plant based foods was associated with fewer depressive symptoms[13]. Compared to the "snacks-drinks-milk products" pattern and the "meat-fish" pattern, the "vegetables-fruits" pattern showed the highest correlations with fiber and other

Table 1. Food group factor loading[a] for three dietary patterns.

Food groups	Dietary patterns		
	Factor 1: Vegetables-fruits	**Factor 2: Snacks-drinks-milk products**	**Factor 3: Meat-fish**
Other vegetables	**0.60**	-0.08	0.03
Cruciferous vegetables	**0.48**	−0.08	−0.06
Tomatoes	**0.47**	0.05	−0.04
Soy	**0.43**	0.03	0.10
Dark green & leafy vegetables	**0.42**	−0.27	−0.04
Starchy vegetables	**0.42**	0.07	−0.03
Fruits	**0.39**	0.06	0.03
Legumes	**0.35**	−0.06	0.02
Mushroom & fungi	**0.25**	0.07	−0.06
Fats and oils	**−0.39**	−0.20	0.11
Condiments	−0.06	**0.48**	−0.06
Coffee	−0.15	**0.41**	−0.15
Nuts	0.12	**0.39**	−0.03
Fast food	−0.02	**0.35**	0.14
French fries and potato chips	−0.02	**0.34**	0.14
Milk and milk products	0.11	**0.33**	−0.10
Whole grains	0.16	**0.32**	−0.16
Sweets and desserts	0.01	**0.27**	0.19
Beverages	−0.02	**0.22**	0.10
Eggs	0.08	**0.22**	0.05
Dim sum	−0.17	−0.17	**0.51**
Red and processed meats	−0.07	−0.03	**0.47**
Poultry	0.06	0.03	**0.47**
Fish and seafood	0.20	−0.26	**0.33**
Cakes, cookies, pies and biscuits	0.07	0.12	**0.24**
Wine	−0.15	0.07	**0.22**
Refined grains	−0.24	−0.42	**−0.74**
Organ meats	−0.08	0.13	0.12
Others	0.01	0.07	0.05
Preserved vegetables	0	0.10	0.01
Soups	0	0	−0.01
Tea	−0.03	0.17	0.05
% variance explained	**6.5**	**5.2**	**5.2**

[a]Factor loadings with absolute value ≥0.2 are shown in bold (Field 2005). For food group loads more than one dietary pattern, only the highest absolute value of loading is bolded.

nutrients, such as vitamin C that are considered as beneficial for brain health [6]. It is possible that the "vegetables-fruits" pattern is associated with reduced oxidative stress, higher anti-inflammatory property, and higher antioxidant capacity, the potential biological mechanisms that are linked with better mood and brain health [44]. The potential protective effect of the 'vegetables-fruits' pattern could also come from folate that is rich in some cruciferous vegetables, leafy vegetables, and other green vegetables. There has been evidence to suggest that folate deficiency impairs the synthesis of homocysteine to methionine and S-adenosyl-methionine. The latter is a methyl donor and is involved in the synthesis and metabolism of neurotransmitters [45]. There is also substantial evidence from observational studies and randomized controlled trials to suggest that folate deficiency is associated with increased risk of depression [7,46].

Our study showed that 'snacks-drinks-milk products' dietary pattern was linked to a fewer depressive symptoms. Such an inverse association was less easy to interpret. In comparison to the 'vegetable-fruit' dietary pattern, the positive association of this pattern with intakes of fiber and most minerals and vitamins was less strong. However, this pattern was composed of healthy and unhealthy food groups. This pattern was dominated by the intake of condiments, drinks, sweets and desserts, fast food, French fries, potato chips, nuts, milk and milk products, and whole grains. Past studies have examined the role of these food groups in depression [47–49]. Greater intake of high-calorie sweet foods and fast foods appeared to be associated with more depressive symptoms [47,48].

Table 2. Pearson's correlations between each dietary pattern score and nutrient intakes at baseline (n = 2,902).

Nutrients	Vegetables-fruits		Snacks-drinks-milk products		Meat-fish	
	r	p	r	p	r	P
Energy (kcal)	−0.05	0.006	0.21	<0.001	0.22	<0.001
Carbohydrates (g)	−0.01	0.456	0.17	<0.001	−0.11	<0.001
Protein (g)	0.13	<0.001	0.21	<0.001	0.39	<0.001
Fat (g)	−0.12	<0.001	0.18	<0.001	0.48	<0.001
SFA (% energy)	−0.17	<0.001	0.14	<0.001	0.57	<0.001
MUFA (% energy)	−0.06	0.001	0.06	0.001	0.36	<0.001
PUFA (% energy)	−0.13	<0.001	−0.11	<0.001	0.15	<0.001
Cholesterol (mg) †	0.03	0.168	0.15	<0.001	0.55	<0.001
Fiber (g) †	0.60	<0.001	0.17	<0.001	0.04	0.019
Vitamin A (IU) †	0.57	<0.001	0.05	0.006	0.11	<0.001
Vitamin C (mg) †	0.52	<0.001	0.03	0.103	0.12	<0.001
Calcium (mg)	0.36	<0.001	0.31	<0.001	0.02	0.258
Phosphorus (mg)	0.19	<0.001	0.33	<0.001	0.07	<0.001
Iron (mg) †	0.28	<0.001	0.26	<0.001	0.18	<0.001
Potassium (mg) †	0.24	<0.001	0.08	<0.001	0.33	<0.001
Magnesium (mg) †	0.38	<0.001	0.07	<0.001	−0.01	0.645
Sodium (mg) †	0.12	<0.001	0.23	<0.001	0.31	<0.001
Zinc (mg)	0.20	<0.001	0.15	<0.001	0.28	<0.001
Isoflavones (mg) †	0.35	<0.001	0.09	<0.001	0.13	<0.001
Vitamin K (μg) †	0.52	<0.001	−0.13	<0.001	0.07	<0.001
Vitamin D (IU) †	0.10	<0.001	0.30	<0.001	0.06	0.001

SFA, Saturated fatty acids; MUFA, Monounsaturated fatty acids; PUFA, Polyunsaturated fatty acids.
†log transformed nutrient intake.

In contrast, there is evidence to suggest that increased intake of milk and dairy products, in particular the low-fat milk and dairy products is associated with better brain function and mood [49].

Our longitudinal analysis did not show significant associations between baseline dietary pattern scores and subsequent depressive symptoms at 4-year. Sensitivity analysis by repeating the multivariate logistic regression models with an outcome of a group with an increase in GDS score >= 4 over four years also confirmed these negative findings. Furthermore, in order to investigate the relationship between diet and depression persistence at 4-year, we tried to repeat the multivariate logistic regression models for participants with depressive symptoms at baseline. No association between dietary patterns and the presence of depressive symptoms was observed at 4-year among this group of baseline depressive participants and these findings further confirmed our negative longitudinal findings. Several prospective studies have examined the role of dietary patterns and incident depression or depressive symptoms in adulthood [17–25], and the findings generally support the role of dietary patterns in the development of depression. Most studies reported significant associations between dietary patterns and incident depression or depressive symptoms [17–19,21–25], but one recent study showed no clear associations between dietary patterns and depression incidence [20]. Using data of 3,486 men and women of the Whitehall II prospective cohort, Akbaraly and colleagues showed a higher odds of depressive symptoms with a "processed food pattern" which was heavily loaded by high intake of sweetened desserts, chocolates, fried food, processed meat, pies, refined grains, high-fat dairy products and condiments [18]. In the GAZEL cohort, Le Port et al. [19] reported that healthy pattern (characterized by vegetables consumption) were associated with fewer depressive symptoms in men and women, and traditional pattern (characterized by fish and fruit consumption) were associated with lower risk of incident depression in women. Furthermore, the highest quartile of low-fat, western, high snack and high fat-sweet diets in men and low-fat and high snack diets in women were associated with higher likelihood of depressive symptoms compared to the lowest quartile. However, recent findings among women in the Nurses' Health Study did not suggest clear associations between dietary Prudent and Western pattern scores and incident depression risk [20]. Differences in the study design, such as tools for assessing depression (i.e. self-reported scale vs. clinical diagnosis), inclusion and exclusion criteria for the subjects, and covariates that were included in the statistical models may account for the variations in the study findings [50]. Recent findings from a multicenter, randomized, primary prevention filed trial suggest that a Mediterranean diet supplemented with nuts could possibly reduce the risk of depression in patients with type 2 diabetes [51]. Therefore, the role of diet in depression warrants further investigation.

Strengths of our study are inclusion of both cross-sectional and longitudinal study design, and adjustment for several potential confounders. However, our study had several limitations. First, the use of the self-reported measure of depression (GDS) and cognitive impairment (CSI-D) may be one of the limitations. However, the sensitivity of these measures is high and has been validated in Chinese populations [32,36]. Second, the low number of participants with depressive symptoms at the 4-year follow-up

Table 3. Subject characteristics by baseline depressive status (n = 2,902).

	Subjects without depressive symptoms (GDS<8) (n = 2,684)		Subjects with depressive symptoms (GDS>=8) (n = 218)		*P value*[1]
	Mean/n	**(SD/%)**	**Mean/n**	**SD/%**	
Age (years)	71.8	(4.8)	72.2	(5.0)	0.310
BMI (kg/m^2)	23.6	(3.2)	23.4	(3.3)	0.203
PASE score	94.1	(44.7)	91.5	(40.2)	0.399
CSI-D score	31.2	(0.9)	31.0	(0.8)	**0.001**
Daily energy intake (kcal)	1913.8	(571.4)	1876.3	(556.7)	0.351
Dietary pattern scores					
Vegetables-fruits	0.015	(1.002)	−0.187	(0.958)	**0.004**
Q1	651	(24.3)	76	(34.9)	**0.002**
Q2	677	(25.2)	49	(22.5)	
Q3	669	(24.9)	55	(25.2)	
Q4	687	(25.6)	38	(17.4)	
Snacks-drinks-milk products	0.022	(1.004)	−0.272	(0.915)	**<0.001**
Q1	646	(24.1)	81	(37.2)	**<0.001**
Q2	662	(24.7)	62	(28.4)	
Q3	684	(25.5)	43	(19.7)	
Q4	692	(25.8)	32	(14.7)	
Meat-fish	0.004	(0.996)	−0.045	(1.051)	0.487
Q1	669	(24.9)	56	(25.7)	0.441
Q2	665	(24.8)	61	(28.0)	
Q3	670	(25.0)	56	(25.7)	
Q4	680	(25.3)	45	(20.6)	
Female (%)	1075	(40.1)	87	(39.9)	0.967
Education level (%)					
Primary or below	1697	(63.2)	157	(72.0)	**0.014**
Secondary / Matriculation	636	(23.7)	45	(20.6)	
University or above	351	(13.1)	16	(7.3)	
Marital status (%)					
Married or living with a partner	2085	(77.7)	155	(71.1)	**0.004**
Widowed, separated or divorced	546	(20.3)	52	(23.9)	
Single	53	(2.0)	11	(5.0)	
Smoking status (%)					
Never smoke	1583	(59.0)	110	(50.5)	**0.003**
Ex-smoker	910	(33.9)	80	(36.7)	
Current smoker	191	(7.1)	28	(12.8)	
Alcohol use (%)					
Never	2203	(82.1)	181	(83.0)	0.191
Ex-drinker	55	(2.0)	8	(3.7)	
Current drinker	426	(15.9)	29	(13.3)	
Self-reported medical history (%)					
Diabetes mellitus	350	(13.0)	38	(17.4)	0.067
Hypertension	1118	(41.7)	100	(45.9)	0.225
Heart diseases or stroke	552	(20.6)	71	(32.6)	**<0.001**
IADLs					
No impairment	2141	(79.8)	138	(63.3)	**<0.001**
Some impairments	543	(20.2)	80	(36.7)	

[1]Differences between groups were assessed by independent *t* test or chi square test.

Table 4. Odds ratios (95% CI) for the cross-sectional association between dietary patterns and depressive symptoms (GDS> = 8) at baseline (n = 2,902).

Dietary pattern	Case / Control	Crude		P_{trend}[1]	Model 1[2]		P_{trend}	Model 2[3]		P_{trend}	Model 3[4]		P_{trend}
		OR	(95% CI)		OR	(95% CI)		OR	(95% CI)		OR	(95% CI)	
Vegetables-fruits													
Q1	76/651	1		**0.001**	1		**0.001**	1		**0.019**	1		**0.017**
Q2	49/677	0.62	0.43–0.90		0.62	0.43–0.91		0.67	0.46–0.98		0.68	0.46–0.99	
Q3	55/669	0.70	0.49–1.01		0.71	0.49–1.02		0.81	0.56–1.18		0.83	0.57–1.20	
Q4	38/687	0.47	0.32–0.71		0.48	0.32–0.72		0.56	0.37–0.84		0.55	0.36–0.83	
Snacks- drinks-milk products													
Q1	81/646	1		**<0.001**	1		**<0.001**	1		**<0.001**	1		**<0.001**
Q2	62/662	0.75	0.53–1.06		0.75	0.53–1.06		0.76	0.53–1.09		0.77	0.54–1.10	
Q3	43/684	0.50	0.34–0.74		0.51	0.34–0.74		0.51	0.34–0.76		0.52	0.35–0.78	
Q4	32/692	0.37	0.24–0.56		0.37	0.24–0.57		0.40	0.25–0.62		0.41	0.26–0.65	
Meat-fish													
Q1	56/669	1		0.221	1		0.273	1		0.269	1		0.199
Q2	61/665	1.10	0.75–1.60		1.10	0.76–1.61		1.18	0.80–1.73		1.18	0.80–1.73	
Q3	56/670	1.00	0.68–1.47		1.01	0.69–1.49		1.08	0.73–1.61		1.06	0.71–1.58	
Q4	45/680	0.79	0.53–1.19		0.81	0.54–1.22		0.80	0.53–1.22		0.77	0.51–1.18	

[1]Test for trend was examined by entering dietary pattern score quartiles as a fixed factor and testing the contrast by using the polynomial option in all models.
[2]Model 1: adjusted for age, sex and daily energy intake.
[3]Model 2: further adjusted for BMI, PASE, number of IADLs, smoking status, alcohol use, education and marital status.
[4]Model 3: further adjusted for self-reported history of diabetes mellitus, hypertension, heart disease and stroke, and CSI-D score.

Table 5. Odds ratios (95% CI) for the longitudinal association between baseline dietary patterns and 4-year incidence of depressive symptoms (GDS>=8) (n=2,211).

Dietary pattern	Case / Control	Crude		P_{trend}[1]	Model 1[2]		P_{trend}	Model 2[3]		P_{trend}	Model 3[4]		P_{trend}
		OR	(95% CI)		OR	(95% CI)		OR	(95% CI)		OR	(95% CI)	
Vegetables-fruits													
Q1	25/494	1		0.415	1		0.432	1		0.903	1		0.931
Q2	17/547	0.61	0.33–1.15		0.62	0.33–1.17		0.71	0.38–1.35		0.73	0.38–1.38	
Q3	18/534	0.67	0.36–1.24		0.66	0.36–1.24		0.77	0.41–1.45		0.80	0.42–1.50	
Q4	21/555	0.75	0.41–1.35		0.76	0.42–1.37		0.94	0.51–1.73		0.94	0.51–1.74	
Snacks- drinks-milk products													
Q1	24/494	1		0.430	1		0.569	1		0.845	1		0.824
Q2	13/514	0.52	0.26–1.03		0.54	0.27–1.07		0.61	0.31–1.21		0.62	0.31–1.24	
Q3	27/550	1.01	0.58–1.77		1.07	0.61–1.89		1.28	0.71–2.29		1.28	0.71–2.31	
Q4	17/572	0.61	0.33–1.15		0.65	0.34–1.24		0.84	0.43–1.65		0.85	0.43–1.68	
Meat-fish													
Q1	23/530	1		0.880	1		0.822	1		0.935	1		0.957
Q2	17/530	0.74	0.39–1.40		0.74	0.39–1.41		0.78	0.41–1.49		0.79	0.41–1.50	
Q3	16/533	0.69	0.36–1.32		0.71	0.37–1.36		0.74	0.38–1.44		0.75	0.39–1.45	
Q4	25/537	1.07	0.60–1.91		1.09	0.61–1.97		1.05	0.57–1.92		1.04	0.56–1.90	

[1]Test for trend was examined by entering dietary pattern score quartiles as a fixed factor and testing the contrast by using the polynomial option in all models.
[2]Model 1: adjusted for age, sex and daily energy intake at baseline.
[3]Model 2: further adjusted for BMI, PASE, number of IADLs, smoking status, alcohol use, education and marital status at baseline.
[4]Model 3: further adjusted for self-reported history of diabetes mellitus, hypertension, heart disease and stroke, and CSI-D score at baseline.

may have limited the power of the longitudinal analysis. Although we found significant associations between "vegetables-fruits" and "snacks-drinks-milk products" patterns and depressive symptoms in the cross-sectional analysis, the directionality of the associations was uncertain. The possibility of reverse causation may not be ruled out. People with major depression may change their eating behavior and food choices, either adopting an unhealthy diet (i.e. high-caloric foods) or reducing food intake [47,52], thus interpreting the relationship between diet and depression may be difficult in view of the bidirectional changes in diet as a consequence of mental health symptoms. We tried to conduct a sensitivity analysis excluding participants with extreme GDS (i.e. GDS≥11 (n = 56)) and the significant association between dietary patterns and depressive symptoms remained at baseline. These results possibly suggest that reverse causation seems an unlikely explanation for the significant findings in our cross-sectional analysis. Furthermore, we did not have dietary data at the 4-year follow-up whereas dietary patterns may have changed between baseline and follow-up. Moreover, although we controlled for various common factors and major chronic conditions in the analysis, residual potential confounding from some other factors related to the development of depression, such as family history of depression and recent life stress events might still be present. In addition, our sample as a whole was of a higher educational standard compared with the general Hong Kong population, and there were some differences in the baseline characteristics between those who included and those who excluded in the analysis, and between those who completed and those who discontinued the 4-year follow-up. Therefore, the results may not be generalized to the general population.

In conclusion, our cross-sectional analysis suggested significant associations between 'vegetables-fruits' dietary pattern and 'snacks-drinks-milk products' dietary pattern and the presence of depressive symptoms in the community-dwelling Chinese older people in Hong Kong. However, the longitudinal analyses did not support that dietary patterns are predictive of the occurrence of depressive symptoms.

Acknowledgments

We would like to give thanks for Ms Kay Yuen for coordination of this study.

Author Contributions

Conceived and designed the experiments: RC JW. Analyzed the data: RC DC JW. Contributed to the writing of the manuscript: RC DC JW

References

1. World Health Organization (2008) Global Burden of Disease: 2004 Update. Geneva: World Health Organization.
2. Hasin DS, Goodwin RD, Stinson FS, Grant BF (2005) Epidemiology of major depressive disorder: results from the National Epidemiologic Survey on Alcoholism and Related Conditions. Arch Gen Psychiatry 62: 1097–1106.
3. Blazer DG (2003) Depression in late life: review and commentary. J Gerontol A Biol Sci Med Sci 58: 249–265.
4. Fiske A, Wetherell JL, Gatz M (2009) Depression in older adults. Annu Rev Clin Psychol 5: 363–389.
5. Collins PY, Patel V, Joestl SS, March D, Insel TR, et al. (2011) Grand challenges in global mental health. Nature 475: 27–30.
6. Rogers PJ (2001) A healthy body, a healthy mind: long-term impact of diet on mood and cognitive function. Proc Nutr Soc 60: 135–143.
7. Stanger O, Fowler B, Piertzik K, Huemer M, Haschke-Becher E, et al. (2009) Homocysteine, folate and vitamin B12 in neuropsychiatric diseases: review and treatment recommendations. Expert Rev Neurother 9: 1393–1412.
8. Murakami K, Sasaki S (2010) Dietary intake and depressive symptoms: a systematic review of observational studies. Mol Nutr Food Res 54: 471–488.
9. Hu FB (2002) Dietary pattern analysis: a new direction in nutritional epidemiology. Curr Opin Lipidol 13: 3–9.
10. van Dam RM (2005) New approaches to the study of dietary patterns. Br J Nutr 93: 573–574.
11. Jacka FN, Pasco JA, Mykletun A, Williams LJ, Hodge AM, et al. (2010) Association of Western and traditional diets with depression and anxiety in women. Am J Psychiatry 167: 305–311.
12. Samieri C, Jutand MA, Feart C, Capuron L, Letenneur L, et al. (2008) Dietary patterns derived by hybrid clustering method in older people: association with cognition, mood, and self-rated health. J Am Diet Assoc 108: 1461–1471.
13. Crichton GE, Bryan J, Hodgson JM, Murphy KJ (2013) Mediterranean diet adherence and self-reported psychological functioning in an Australian sample. Appetite 70: 53–59.
14. Nanri A, Kimura Y, Matsushita Y, Ohta M, Sato M, et al. (2010) Dietary patterns and depressive symptoms among Japanese men and women. Eur J Clin Nutr 64: 832–839.
15. Sugawara N, Yasui-Furukori N, Tsuchimine S, Kaneda A, Tsuruga K, et al. (2012) No association between dietary patterns and depressive symptoms among a community-dwelling population in Japan. Ann Gen Psychiatry 11: 24 doi: 10.1186/1744-859X-11-24.
16. Suzuki T, Miyaki K, Tsutsum A, Hashimoto H, Kawakami N, et al. (2013) Japanese dietary pattern consistently relates to low depressive symptoms and it is modified by job strain and worksite supports. J Affect Disord 150: 490–498.
17. Sa' nchez-Villegas A, Delgado-Rodrı'guez M, Alonso A, Schlatter J, Lahortiga F, et al. (2009) Association of the Mediterranean Dietary Pattern With the Incidence of Depression The Seguimiento Universidad de Navarra/University of Navarra Follow-up (SUN) Cohort. Arch Gen Psychiatry 66: 1090–1098.
18. Akbaraly TN, Brunner EJ, Ferrie JE, Marmot MG, Kivimaki M, et al. (2009) Dietary pattern and depressive symptoms in middle age. Br J Psychiatry 195: 408–413.
19. Le Port A, Gueguen A, Kesse-Guyot E, Melchior M, Lemogne C, et al. (2012) Association between dietary patterns and depressive symptoms over time: a 10-year follow-up study of the GAZEL cohort. PLOS ONE 7: e51593.
20. Chocano-Bedoya PO, O'Reilly EJ, Lucas M, Mirzaei F, Okereke OI, et al. (2013) Prospective study on long-term dietary patterns and incident depression in middle-aged and older women. Am J Clin Nutr 98: 813–820.
21. Lucas M, Chocano-Bedoya P, Shulze MB, Mirzaei F, O'Reilly EJ, et al. (2013) Inflammatory dietary pattern and risk of depression among women. Brain Behav Immun 36: 46–53.
22. Rienks R, Dobson AJ, Mishra GD (2013) Mediterranean dietary pattern and prevalence and incidence of depressive symptoms in mid-aged women: results from a large community-based prospective study. Eur J Clin Nutr 67: 75–82.
23. Hodge A, Almeida OP, English DR, Giles GG, Flicker L (2013) Patterns of dietary intake and psychological distress in older Australians: benefits not just from a Mediterranean diet. Int Psychogeriatr 25: 456–466.
24. Jacka FN, Cherbuin N, Anstey KJ, Butterworth P (2014) Dietary Patterns and Depressive Symptoms over Time: Examining the Relationships with Socioeconomic Position, Health Behaviours and Cardiovascular Risk. PLOS ONE 9: e87657.
25. Ruusunen A, Lehto SM, Mursu J, Tolmunen T, Tuomainen TP, et al. (2014) Dietary patterns are associated with the prevalence of elevated depressive symptoms and the risk of getting a hospital discharge diagnosis of depression in middle-aged or older Finnish men. J Affect Disord 159: 1–6.
26. Jacka FN, Kremer PJ, Berk M, de Silva-Sanigorski AM, Moodie M, et al. (2011) A prospective study of diet quality and mental health in adolescents. PLOS ONE 6: e24805.
27. Weng TT, Hao JH, Qian QW, Cao H, Fu JL, et al. (2011) Is there any relationship between dietary patterns and depression and anxiety in Chinese adolescents? Public Health Nutr 15: 673–682.
28. Tsai AC, Chang TL, Chi SH (2012) Frequent consumption of vegetables predicts lower risk of depression in older Taiwanese - results of a prospective population-based study. Public Health Nutr 15: 1087–1092.
29. Woo J, Lynn H, Lau WY, Leung J, Lau E, et al. (2006) Nutrient intake and psychological health in an elderly Chinese population. Int J Geriatr Psychiatry 21: 1036–1043.
30. Wong SY, Kwok T, Woo J, Lynn H, Griffith JF, et al. (2005) Bone mineral density and the risk of peripheral arterial disease in men and women: results from Mr. and Ms Os, Hong Kong. Osteoporos Int 16: 1933–1938.
31. Census and Statistics Department (2006) Hong Kong 2006 Population Bycensus Thematic Report: Older Persons. Hong Kong: Census and Statistics Department.
32. Prince M, Acosta D, Chiu H, Scazufca M, Varghese M, et al. (2003) Dementia diagnosis in developing countries: a cross-cultural validation study. Lancet 361: 909–917.
33. Washburn RA, Smith KW, Jette AM, Janney CA (1993) The Physical Activity Scale for the Elderly (PASE): development and evaluation. J Clin Epidemiol 46: 153–162.
34. Liu B, Woo J, Tang N, Ng K, Ip R, et al. (2001) Assessment of total expenditure in a Chinese population by a physical activity questionnaire: examination of validity. Int J Food Sci Nutr 52: 269–282.

35. Yesavage JA, Brink TL, Rose TL, Lum O, Huang V, et al. (1983) Development and validation of a geriatric depression screening scale. A preliminary report. J Psychiatr Res 17: 37–49.
36. Lee HB, Chiu HFK, Kwok WY, Leung CM, Kwong PK, et al. (1993) Chinese elderly and the GDS short form: a preliminary study. Clin Gerontol 14: 37–39.
37. Woo J, Leung SSF, Ho SC, Lam TH, Janus ED (1997) A food frequency questionnaire for use in the Chinese population in Hong Kong: Description and examination of validity. Nutr Res 17: 1633–1641.
38. Paul AA, Southgate DAT (1978) McCance & Widdowson's: The Composition of Foods. London: HMSO.
39. Yang Y, Wang G, Pan X (2002) China Food Composition 2002; Institute of Nutrition & Food Safety CC, editor. Peking: University Medical Press.
40. Chan R, Chan D, Woo J (2012) Associations between dietary patterns and demographics, lifestyle, anthropometry and blood pressure in Chinese community-dwelling older men and women. J Nutr Sci 1: e20 doi:10.1017/jns.2012.19
41. Reedy J, Wirfalt E, Flood A, Mitrou PN, Krebs-Smith SM, et al. (2010) Comparing 3 dietary pattern methods–cluster analysis, factor analysis, and index analysis–With colorectal cancer risk: The NIH-AARP Diet and Health Study. Am J Epidemiol 171: 479–487.
42. Field A (2005) Discovering Statistics Using SPSS; Wright DB, editor. London: Sage Publications.
43. Roman MW, Callen BL (2008) Screening instruments for older adult depressive disorders: updating the evidence-based toolbox. Issues Ment Health Nurs 29: 929–941.
44. Bodnar LM, Wisner KL (2005) Nutrition and depression: implications for improving mental health among childbearing-aged women. Biol Psychiatry 58: 679–685.
45. Bottiglieri T (2005) Homocysteine and folate metabolism in depression. Prog Neuro-Psychopharmacol Biol Psychiatry 29: 1103–1112.
46. Fava M, Mischoulon D (2009) Folate in depression: efficacy, safety, differences in formulations, and clinical issues. J Clin Psychiatry 70 Suppl 5: 12–17.
47. Jeffery RW, Linde JA, Simon GE, Ludman EJ, Rohde P, et al. (2009) Reported food choices in older women in relation to body mass index and depressive symptoms. Appetite 52: 238–240.
48. Crawford GB, Khedkar A, Flaws JA, Sorkin JD, Gallicchio L (2011) Depressive symptoms and self-reported fast-food intake in midlife women. Prev Med 52: 254–257.
49. Camfield DA, Owen L, Scholey AB, Pipingas A, Stough C (2011) Dairy constituents and neurocognitive health in ageing. Br J Nutr 106: 159–174.
50. Quirk SE, Williams;L.J.;, O'Neil A, Pasco JA, Jacka FN, et al. (2013) The association between diet quality, dietary patterns and depression in adults: a systematic review. BMC Psychiatry 175.
51. Sánchez-Villegas A, Martínez-González MA, Estruch R, Salas-Salvadó J, Corella D, et al. (2013) Mediterranean dietary pattern and depression: the PREDIMED randomized trial. BMC Medicine 11.
52. Lai JS, Hiles S, Bisquera A, Hure AJ, McEvoy M, et al. (2014) A systematic review and meta-analysis of dietary patterns and depression in community-dwelling adults. Am J Clin Nutr 99: 181–197.

13

Hunter-Gatherer Inter-Band Interaction Rates: Implications for Cumulative Culture

Kim R. Hill[1]*, Brian M. Wood[2], Jacopo Baggio[1], A. Magdalena Hurtado[1], Robert T. Boyd[1]

1 School of Human Evolution and Social Change, Arizona State University, Tempe, Arizona, United States of America, **2** Department of Anthropology, Yale University, New Haven, Connecticut, United States of America

Abstract

Our species exhibits spectacular success due to cumulative culture. While cognitive evolution of social learning mechanisms may be partially responsible for adaptive human culture, features of early human social structure may also play a role by increasing the number potential models from which to learn innovations. We present interview data on interactions between same-sex adult dyads of Ache and Hadza hunter-gatherers living in multiple distinct residential bands (20 Ache bands; 42 Hadza bands; 1201 dyads) throughout a tribal home range. Results show high probabilities (5%–29% per year) of cultural and cooperative interactions between randomly chosen adults. Multiple regression suggests that ritual relationships increase interaction rates more than kinship, and that affinal kin interact more often than dyads with no relationship. These may be important features of human sociality. Finally, yearly interaction rates along with survival data allow us to estimate expected lifetime partners for a variety of social activities, and compare those to chimpanzees. Hadza and Ache men are estimated to observe over 300 men making tools in a lifetime, whereas male chimpanzees interact with only about 20 other males in a lifetime. High intergroup interaction rates in ancestral humans may have promoted the evolution of cumulative culture.

Editor: R. Alexander Bentley, Bristol University, United Kingdom

Funding: This research was funded by a Late Lessons Grant from Arizona State University and National Science Foundation Grant BCS1062879. The funders had no role in study design, data collection and analysis, decision to publish, or preparation of the manuscript.

Competing Interests: The authors have declared that no competing interests exist.

* Email: Kim.Hill@asu.edu

Introduction

It has been hypothesized that cumulative culture and extensive non-kin cooperation allowed Homo sapiens to replace other hominin species in the Pleistocene and facilitated the biological dominance of our species in the Holocene [1]. In order to understand the emergence of these features we must examine aspects of social behavior in our ancestors that may have favored their evolution. Observations of modern hunter-gatherers offer the opportunity to examine features of that lifestyle that may be associated with important evolved human traits. Within-band interactions such as non-kin food sharing [2], cooperative food acquisition, and provisioning of multiple goods and services [3] are well documented for recent hunter-gatherers [4,5] and part of a cooperative breeding life history that may be critical for explaining human success. But, between-band interactions may also be important for understanding the unique nature of our species. Inter-band social networks are hypothesized to explain evolved brain expansion [6,7], extensive non-kin cooperation [8,9,10] and the emergence of cumulative culture [11,12,13].

Early ethnographers suggested that hunter-gatherer societies were primarily kin based [14,15], and hence between-group interactions might be primarily associated with genetic kinship. More recently however, large interaction networks in our species are hypothesized to derive from pair bonding in ancestral hunter-gatherer societies, with recognition of affines producing a unique metaband (ie. tribal) social structure, not found in any other primate [16,17]. Finally, cultural institutions such as ritualized partnerships and complex marriage rules have been hypothesized as features designed to promote between-band interaction in foragers [18,19,20]. In this paper we examine the effects of all three of these on interband interactions. While recent studies have examined reported preferential association networks [21], scientists still have no quantitative measure from any hunter-gatherer society of actual interaction rates between individuals residing in different bands. Here we present the first study designed to provide quantitative estimates of inter-band interaction rates and examine the impact of genetic and affinal kinship and ritual relationships on these rates.

Methods

Ethics statement

This study was reviewed and approved by the institutional Review Board of Arizona State University and Stanford University. Because informants were illiterate and spoke only native languages, general consent was obtained in community meetings and subsequent individual verbal consent was obtained from all participants as per IRB approval.

Study populations

Ache hunter-gatherers roamed the forests of eastern Paraguay exploiting palm starch and hunting mammals with bow and arrow until pacification in the 1970s [22]. The Ache "tribe" is defined by a single mutually intelligible language and shared cultural features absent from the surrounding Guarani horticultural tribes (see Text S1, for details). The Ache had no pan-tribal political or religious leaders and the entire tribe never gathered together in one place for any political or religious functions. Within the Ache tribe, there were four regional "sub-tribes" in the 20th century (Figure S1 in File S1), defined by dialect and minor cultural differences. Ache sub-tribes were further subdivided into multiple residential bands that camped together and formed the basis of daily living. Because of visiting and migration, band composition was stable over periods of months but not years.

The Northern Ache were the largest Ache sub-tribe, consisting of about 560 people living in 18–20 residential bands during the last decade before peaceful outside contact [17]. Northern Ache bands were usually dispersed throughout their core home range of ~5,270 km^2 (Figure 1) and informants report that the different residential bands were generally located at distances of 10–30 km from each other. Occasionally these bands roamed as far as 150 km apart when they made temporary use of distant areas in their ~14,630 km^2 maximal home range.

The Hadza of Tanzania continue to forage on foot with bows, small axes, digging sticks, and carrying slings, without the aid vehicles, guns or other modern equipment. They share a common isolate click language and a set of unique customs (see File S1 for details). The Hadza were first encountered by Europeans in the late 19th century, and have been the subject of extensive anthropological research [23]. Archaeological evidence from Mumba cave attests to hunter-gatherers living in the Lake Eyasi area for at least 60,000 years [24], and genetic studies of the Hadza reveal their high genetic distance from other east African populations, their ancient shared ancestry with other African hunter-gatherers, and evidence of recent intermarriage with neighboring Bantu and Cushitic speaking neighbors [25]. The tribe now resides in an area of about 3,000 km^2 and the Eastern Hadza sub-tribe dwells southeast of Lake Eyasi, in three distinct regional clusters, (MH, YS, TM). During the 2012 interview period, the Eastern Hadza consisted of approximately 950 individuals living in 49 named bands. GPS coordinates show these bands ranged in distance from 200 meters to ~80 km apart, with mean distance about 35 km (Figure 2, S2 in File S1).

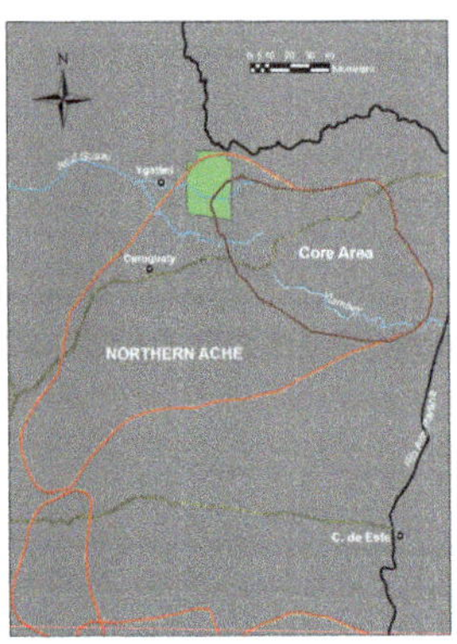

Figure 1. Northern Ache maximal boundaries and core use area during the second half of the 20th century. Bands were distributed throughout the core area, occassionally visiting more remote tribal home range in the Southwest. Band location moved almost daily with no restricted localities. The construction of the road passing through Curuguaty and the core Ache territualory was the impetus for permanent peaceful outside contact in the 1970s. The green square shows the modern day Mbarcayu reserve.

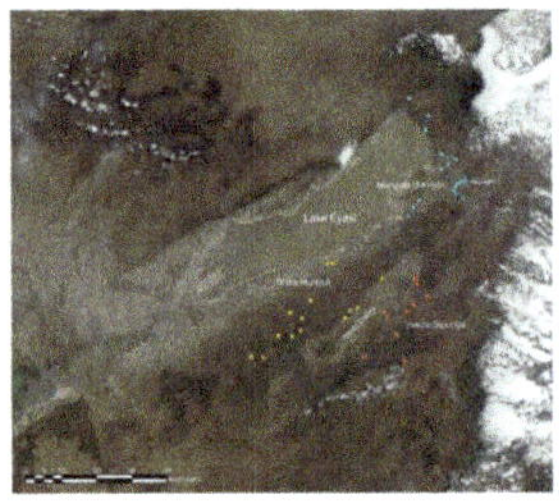

Figure 2. Eastern Hadza camps where interview subjects and target individuals resided in 2012, with the three regions defined by point color. In the Center is Lake Eyasi, Tanzania. Satellite image from NASA Earth Observatory.

Interviews

Inter-band interaction was assayed by asking Ache and Hadza subjects "yes/no" questions about social contacts with randomly chosen same-sex "target" adults (1201 same sex dyads) during specified time periods [see File S1 for more details]. Interaction rates reported in this paper represent the probability of random same sex adult dyads having interacted in the specified way at least once during a specified time period.

Between 2009–2010 KH and a native assistant conducted interviews with Northern Ache adults who had been ≥15 years old in 1970 (the year prior to first peaceful contact). Each taped interview consisted of one subject and one same-sex "target" who was chosen randomly from a list of all adults that were alive between 1965–1970 (169 men, 146 women). At the beginning of each interview we identified the "target" individual to the subject by specifying the target's unique nickname, or identifying a unique set of the target's close kin. We interviewed subjects asking 40 questions about the target's prior interaction with the subject. Seven questions on the interview are not reported in this paper because they refer only to agonistic interaction which address a different set of issues than we consider here. The final list of questions is shown in Table S1 in File S1. Each interview question could be answered as "yes" or "no". Informants were asked about interactions only during the time period during which the interviewee was adult, and prior to first peaceful outside contact. Previous reliability studies have shown that informant recall over this time period, for group co-membership is quite accurate [17,26], and that life history event data (births, deaths, marriages, ages, cause of death) obtained by interviews covering this time period are very reliable when reports by multiple informants are compared [22]. The interview questions asked of each subject included items like "Did target ever share meat with you?", "Did you ever have a conversation with target?", "Did target ever hunt or gather with you"? The final sample from the Ache consists of 351 interviews with 32 different subjects and 88 different target individuals (see Table 1).

In 2012 BW and assistants administered a modified shorter version of the interaction survey to Eastern Hadza subjects. That interview contained 15 questions, 13 of which were identical to questions KH had asked the Ache (Table S1 in File S1), and these questions constituted the database for all subsequent analyses. 850 interviews were conducted with 39 men and 36 women over age 25, residing in 22 separate residential bands. Subjects were asked to report only interactions that had taken place after the widely remembered 2005 presidential election (Jakaya Kikwete) in Tanzania.

Each Hadza interview subject was shown photos of 12 same-sex target individuals. Targets included 213 different women and 187

Table 1. Characteristics of the Ache and Hadza study samples.

	Ache	Hadza
Population during study period	560	950
Residential bands during study period	~20	49
Band location	mobile	tethered
Metaband rituals	yes	no
Tribal core home range	5,270 km^2	3,000 km^2
Same sex dyads interviewed	351	850
Different interview subjects	32	75
Different targets	88	400
Percent male dyads in sample	72%	52%
Target identified by	nickname, kin	photo
Interaction period	before 1970	2005–2012
Interaction questions	40	15

different men residing in 42 different residential bands. The target sample was stratified to include equal numbers of individuals from all three Eastern Hadza regions (Figure S2 in File S1 shows the connection between the camps of each subject and target). To begin the interview, researchers showed facial photographs of the target individual to the interview subject. 72% of men and 60% of women were able to name the target individual after seeing a photograph, while most others knew something about the target individual but not their name. Interview questions analyzed here were identical to those asked of the Ache (eg. "Did you ever hear target X sing a song?", "Does target X have a affinal kin relationship to you?").

The final interview database and key are provided (Database S1, DatabaseKey S1) with the Supporting Information.

Models and statistical analysis

Inter-band interactions take place when members of different residential groups meet and engage in social activity. Interactions often result from targeted visits, but may also occur by chance through unintended encounters between visitors and third parties. For example, individual *A* from band 1 may visit *B* from band 2 and fortuitously encounter both individual *C* residing in band 2 (not an intended target) and individual *D* from band 3 who is simultaneously visiting band 2. In this way all *As*, *Cs*, and *Ds* in the population may eventually encounter and interact with each other. For this reason, we have assumed this process can be simplified to a random encounter model. Because the elapsed time over which an interaction could take place was variable and higher for the Ache on average (mean = 11.2 years; range = 1–24 years) than for the Hadza (a constant 7 years) we need to estimate rates of interaction per unit time for direct comparison. To estimate yearly rates of interaction for both groups, we assumed that the interaction rate of each pair of individuals was constant through time, and then examined whether the baseline yearly rates are higher when subject and target were genetic or affinal kin or were partners in a ritual relationship. This was formalized by setting

$$p_i = \frac{1}{1+e^{-(a+bu_i+cv_i+dw_i)}} \qquad \text{(eqn. 1)}$$

where p_i is the probability of an interaction each year for pair i, and u_i, v_i and w_i are dummy variables representing close genetic kinship, affinal kinship, and ritual relationship. We converted genetic coefficient of relatedness into a binary variable, close kin vs. distant or non-kin, so that the magnitude of effect of this variable could be compared directly to affine, and ritual relationship, which are also binary variables. In the statistical model u_i equals one when the relatedness between pair i is greater than or equal to 0.125 (first cousin) and zero otherwise, v_i is one when an affinal kinship term was reported for pair i, and zero if not, w_i is one when a ritual relationship was reported for pair i, and zero otherwise. Positive values of the parameters b, c and d mean that genetic or affinal kinship or ritual relationship increase the rate of interaction. The parameter a gives the baseline yearly rate of interaction between individuals who are neither kin, affines, nor in a ritual relationship. With these assumptions, the probability that a pair of individuals has a least one interaction during t years, P_i, is given by:

$$P_i = 1-(1-p_i)^t \qquad \text{(eqn. 2)}$$

and this can be used to calculate the likelihood of the observed data from a sample of dyads.

The values of the coefficients a, b, c and d were estimated by finding the values that maximize this likelihood (see File S1 for computational details). Bootstrapped standard errors for these coefficients were calculated by resampling with replacement from the full dataset (1000 repetitions). The estimated yearly rates of interaction for each pair of individuals and each activity were then computed by substituting the estimated coefficients and the reported kinship and ritual relationship values for that dyad into equation 1. Mean yearly rates of interaction for each population were computed by averaging the rates for all dyads in that population. Confidence intervals for the yearly rate estimates were calculated using the joint distribution of coefficient values derived from the bootstrap analysis. The mean yearly rate of interaction was computed for each combination of coefficients with support, and the probabilities of each interaction rate were summed yielding probability distributions for the estimated mean rates of interaction for Ache and Hadza. As a guide to the significance of differences between the Ache and Hadza mean rates of interaction, we used these distributions to calculate whether the probability that the means were actually the same was less than the conventional threshold value 0.05.

Results

Correlates of interaction

Reported interactions were divided for convenience into five categories: 1) simple association, 2) intimate association, 3) caretaker, 4) cooperator, and 5) cultural model. Statistical analyses (below) suggest that ritual relationship in the most important predictor of increased interaction in all categories. The proportions of subjects that reported specific types of interaction with target individuals are quite high for both study populations, with probabilities of having camped together, conversed, shared meat, shared vegetable, or watched target make a tool at least once, all around 90% for Ache dyads who were adults during an average elapsed time of ~11 years prior to peaceful contact (Table S1 in File S1, Figure S3 in File S1). Hadza dyadic interaction probabilities reported for the same activities (over the 7 year period covered by interviews) were all lower than the Ache, but still in the range of 30–40%.

Ache and Hadza interaction data were fit to eqn. 1 in order to estimate yearly interaction rates and determine if genetic or affinal kinship or ritual relationships are associated with higher interaction rates between random adult dyads in each group. These independent variables are not collinear (Table S3 in File S1). In both groups 5–10% of random dyadic pairs were "closekin" ($r \geq 0.125$), and another 15–20% were "affines" (Table 2, Table S2 in File S1). Ritual relationships were also reported in both groups. Just under 20% of Ache adults call each other by ritual terms such as "jary", "chave", "upiare", "tapare", "mondoare", "kaviru", "kmanove", "mubuare" etc. All these terms are associated with birth and puberty rituals and are associated with a specific ritual role (eg. the one who cut the umbilical cord, the one who washed the newborn, the one who held the newborn, etc.). These named dyadic relationships imply rights and obligations of mutual support according to Ache social norms. Hadza dyadic named ritual partners do not exist, but people do sometimes participate together in sacred epeme dance and meat consumption rituals. Co-participants in these rituals made up about 16% of the dyads in the Hadza sample. While Ache and Hadza ritual relationships are different in character, both types of ritual relationships define and reinforce patterns of behavior between individuals, and hence may influence patterns of inter-band interaction.

Maximum Likelihood estimates of the coefficients b, c, and d, measure the effect of each of the independent variables with the other two variables controlled. These are presented in Table 3 for the 13 interaction types recorded for both groups (detailed analyses of alternative models are provided in Tables S4–S13 in File S1). The most important predictor of dyadic interaction in the Ache interviews was simply the elapsed time that subject and target were adults in the precontact period (the model in Tables S4–S8 in File S1 that contains only the constant term). Genetic kinship was not associated with significantly higher interaction rates for the Ache, but affinal kin did show significantly higher interaction rates for two questions. Ache dyads with ritual relationships interact significantly more often for 5 of the 13 questions analyzed. Among the Hadza elapsed time was constant and genetic kinship was significantly associated with higher interaction rates for 12 of 13 questions. Affinal kin experienced higher interaction rates for 11 of 13 questions, while Hadza dyads with common participation in the epeme ritual showed higher interaction rates for all 13 questions.

When we compare the overall effects of kinship and ritual, it is clear that ritual relationship is far more associated with interaction than is kinship for both study populations. The effect size (beta coefficient) is greater for ritual than kin for 11 of the 13 questions for the Ache, and 13 of 13 questions for the Hadza. Because most Ache ritual relationships were intiated at birth or puberty but interaction took place in adulthood, we can assume that the ritual relationship promoted interaction (not vice versa). Among the Hadza, individuals must spend at least some time in the same camp in order to jointly participate in the epeme ritual, hence common coresidence might produce an association between ritual co-participation and interaction frequency in other realms. However, co-residing in the same camp is not always a significant predictor of interaction for the Hadza, and even when coresidence is controlled by multiple regression, ritual relationship is still an important predictor of interaction (Tables S9–S13 in File S1). In most cases for either Ache or Hadza the effect of ritual on interaction rates is more than twice as great as that of either type of kinship (eg. Figure 3).

Yearly Interaction Rates

Yearly interaction rates for each of the sample dyads were calculated by solving for p_i in equation 2 with the effects of the three independent variables determined by the maximum likelihood estimates for eqn. 1 as reported in Table 3. These yearly interaction rate estimates were then averaged for all dyads to obtain a population mean yearly interaction rate for each type of interaction covered by the interviews.

Table 2. Values for independent variables in dyadic interaction interviews.

Indep	Question from which is derived	Percentage of sample		
Var.		All	Ache	Hazda
Closekin	Ego and target closely related (genetic coefficient $r \geq 0.125$)	5.86	9.4	4.47
Affine	Ego employs affinal term for target (ie. spouse's sibs or parents)	16.31	19.94	14.88
Ritual	Ego and target have ritual relationship	17.07	20.23	15.76
Elapsed	Mean years at risk of adult interaction with target	8.17	11.16	7
	(during pre-contact forest period for Ache)			
Sex	Female to Female dyadic relationship	42.41	27.92	48.1
	Male to Male dyadic relationship	57.59	72.08	51.9
Ethnicity	Ache	28.19	(100)	(0)
	Hazda	71.81	(0)	(100)

Table 3. Maximum Liklihood Estimates of the beta coefficients for genetic kin (closekin), affinal kin, and ritual relations from equation 1.

Group	Dep Var	Question	Ache			Hazda		
			closekin	affine	ritual	closekin	affine	ritual
Associate	q6	Have you spoken with target?	0.525	0.031	0.413	1.490*	1.308*	2.862*
			(0.942)	(0.268)	(0.433)	(0.323)	(0.169)	(0.695)
	q8	Did target sleep in your camp?	0.048	−0.003	0.358	1.133*	0.834*	2.193*
			(0.971)	(0.351)	(0.469)	(0.348)	(0.218)	(0.176)
	q10	Have you joked with target?	−0.313	0.409*	−0.114	0.637	1.444*	1.671*
			(0.288)	(0.205)	(0.204)	(0.376)	(0.213)	(0.219)
Intimate Associate	q22	Has target given you a non food gift?	−0.131	−0.340	0.478*	1.098*	0.534*	2.098*
			(0.342)	(0.268)	(0.232)	(0.364)	(0.212)	(0.165)
	q34	Did target ever groom you?	−0.298	−0.287	0.772*	1.053*	0.079	2.245*
			(0.820)	(0.340)	(0.273)	(0.367)	(0.287)	(0.220)
Caretaker	q39	Did target give you food when you were sick or injured?	0.406	0.264*	0.705	1.015*	0.368	1.988*
			(0.388)	(0.297)	(0.270)	(0.348)	(0.227)	(0.190)
Cooperator	q18	Has target shared non meat foods with you?	−0.074	−0.026	0.888	0.973*	0.566*	2.087*
			(0.385)	(0.302)	(0.457)	(0.374)	(0.208)	(0.163)
	q19	Has target shared meat with you?	−0.071	−0.210	0.962*	1.262*	0.709*	2.133*
			(0.377)	(0.259)	(0.474)	(0.339)	(0.216)	(0.167)
	q23	Did target ever lend you something?	−0.178	−0.528*	0.490*	1.122*	0.650*	1.994*
			(0.285)	(0.231)	(0.202)	(0.297)	(0.201)	(0.158)
	q24	Did you ever hunt/collect roots with target?	−0.216	−0.103	0.188	0.843*	0.696*	2.189*
			(0.281)	(0.202)	(0.190)	(0.384)	(0.196)	(0.168)
Cultural Model	q9	Have you heard target sing?	−0.414	−0.277	0.272	0.965*	0.850*	1.988*
			(0.294)	(0.219)	(0.213)	(0.361)	(0.192)	(0.164)
	q17	Has target shared news with you?	0.174	−0.186	0.416*	1.565*	0.935*	2.299*
			(0.297)	(0.236)	(0.207)	(0.318)	(0.218)	(0.207)
	q31.1	Did you ever watch target make a tool?	0.045	−0.146	1.229	1.075*	1.176*	2.358*
			(0.967)	(0.349)	(0.713)	(0.413)	(0.197)	(0.209)

Note = Bootstrapped standard errors in parenthesis (over 1000 repetitions).
*= estimate significantly different from zero at the 5% level.

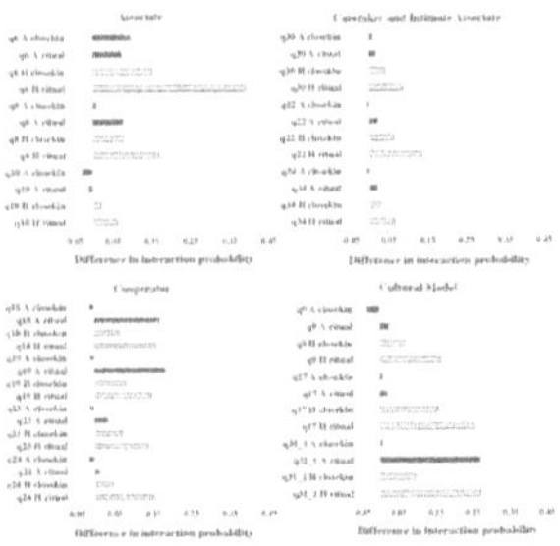

Figure 3. Comparison of the effect of "closekin" and "ritual relationship" on the predicted probability of engaging in specified interaction types. Each bar represents a the average difference in the probability of interaction calculated as: (P(y)|closekin = 1) – (P(y)|closekin = 0) for "closekin", and (P(y)|ritual = 1) – (P(y)|ritual = 0) for "ritual relationship". Probabilities are calculated by averaging values over all dyads while keeping closekin or ritual fixed at 1 or 0, and $t = 1$. Dark bars represent Ache, light bars represent Hadza.

Ache yearly probability of interaction for common activity types (conversing, sleeping in same camp, sharing food, watching tool manufacture) ranged from about 0.20 to 0.30 per anum, and were generally significantly higher (2–5 fold) than Hadza rates (Table 4, Figure S4 in File S1). Medium frequency interactions (joking, listening to the target sing) showed probabilities of 0.10 to 0.12 per year among Ache, about 2 to 4 times higher than the Hadza. Finally, rare interaction types (hunting/collecting together, giving non-food gifts, grooming, lending a tool, sharing important news, and caring for sick/injured individuals) showed generally low annual probabilities for both the Ache and the Hadza (0.02–0.08 per dyad per year), with each group showing some higher rates for specific interactions (Table 4). In sum, 9 of 13 Ache yearly rates were significantly higher than for the Hadza and 2 of 13 of the Hadza rates (transmitting news, feeding when incapacitated) were significantly higher than for the Ache.

Lifetime Interaction Partners

Our model assumes that interactions take place at a constant rate, hence the cumulative probability of at least one interaction over time is a negatively accelerated monotonically increasing function. For many of the interaction types that we examined the probability of at least one interaction between random same sex adult dyads becomes quite substantial after ten years or more (Figures S5, S6 in File S1). Combining estimated yearly interaction rates with the population size and life tables (Table S15 in File S1) allows us to estimate the expected number of lifetime adult interaction partners for Ache and Hadza adults.

Assuming a stable age-structured population the mean number of lifetime adult interactants (N) can be expressed as:

$$N = (n_1 - 1)P_1 + 2n_1 \sum_{\tau=2}^{T} P_\tau \qquad \text{(eqn. 3)}$$

Where n_1 is the number of adults in the first yearly adult age cohort of the interacting population, T is the maximum age to which an adult survives, and P_τ, the yearly probability of an interaction with a target individual that is $\underline{\tau}$ years older than the subject, is a function of both adult survival rates and yearly interaction rates (see File S1 for derivation). Since the number of individuals who enter the first age cohort is proportional to the total size of a stable population, the number of expected lifetime interactants is approximately a linear function of size of the potential interaction population. With moderate interaction rates and low mortality, the number of lifetime interactants approaches $2n$ since there are n older interactants when ego reaches adulthood and ego will meet about n younger new interactants before dying (Figure 4).

Because recent theoretical work suggests that interaction network size can determine whether cultural traits accumulate complexity [11,12] we are particularly interested to compare the social universe of hunter-gatherers to chimpanzees. Our calculations suggest that the lifetime number of interactants for male Ache and Hadza hunter-gatherers is more than an order of magnitude higher than that expected for male chimpanzees (female dispersal from the natal community makes this calculation difficult for chimpanzee females). Precontact Northern Ache men, for example, are expected to have hunted with 206 men, conversed with 290 men, and watch tool making by 302 different men in a lifetime (Table S16 in File S1). Eastern Hadza men are expected to converse with 427 other Hadza men, hunt with 303 men, and watch tool making by 395 different men in a lifetime. In contrast, chimpanzees living in typical communities of 11 adult males are expected to interact with a mean of only 21 other adult males in a lifetime (Table S16 in File S1).

The relationship between yearly probability of interaction and expected proportion of the population that will interact in a lifetime asymptotes quickly, and even low rates of interpersonal interaction among hunter-gatherers lead to lifetime interactions with most other adults (Figure 4). This is because the human adult lifespan is so much longer than that of chimpanzees. The average expected time that both members of an Ache or Hadza dyad who enter adulthood together will both still be alive is about 27 years while the average expected time that two male chimpanzees from the same community, entering adulthood together, are still both alive is only 6 years.

Discussion

Among the Ache and Hadza, frequent visiting and long lifespans mean that adults typically interact with more than three hundred same-sex adults during their lifetimes. This implies a social universe of about a thousand individuals, when opposite-sex adults and children are included. Recent work on the San Bushmen also suggests a similarly high number of significant interactants [27]. Additionally, close companions often interact with a somewhat different set of individuals, so that the total number of indirect interactants that each individual hears about repeatedly in detailed stories, and could expect to possibly meet some time during their lifetime is clearly more than 1,000. This is a much higher number of individually known social interactants than reported for any other primate, and possibly more than any other species on earth. It is also much greater than the predicted 150 significant social interactants (known as "Dunbar's number") that was extrapolated from primate brain by social group size regressions [6,7]. It should not surprise us that humans have more relationships than their brain size alone predicts, as humans alone use language and symbolic devices to store information about potential relationships. The main reason why human's interact with so many more individuals than other apes is because: 1) human lifespans are much longer, and 2) interaction between neighboring and distant residential social units is extensive.

An important question is when and how the meta-band social structure arose in hominin evolution. We agree with other authors that pair-bonding, paternal investment, and habitual marital

Table 4. Proportion of dyads reporting interaction of specified type, and the yearly interaction rate estimated from equation 2, with effects of kinship and ritual relationship controlled.

Dep Var.	Question to Interviewee	Proportion of sample interacting#		Yearly interaction probability##	
		Ache	Hadza	Ache	Hadza
	Associate				
q6	Have you spoken with target?	0.87	0.40	0.215*	0.119
q8	Did target sleep in your camp?	0.93	0.28	0.293*	0.058
q10	Have you joked with target?	0.71	0.17	0.117*	0.028
	Intimate Associate				
q22	Has target given you a non food gift?	0.37	0.24	0.040	0.047
q34	Did target ever groom you?	0.22	0.13	0.022	0.020
	Caretaker				
q39	Did target give you food when you were sick or injured?	0.21	0.19	0.021*	0.031
	Cooperator				
q18	Has target shared non meat foods with you?	0.88	0.28	0.219*	0.055
q19	Has target shared meat with you?	0.87	0.26	0.217*	0.051
q23	Did target ever lend you something?	0.54	0.26	0.075*	0.050
q24	Did you ever hunt/collect roots with target?	0.78	0.26	0.068*	0.051
	Cultural Model				
q9	Have you heard target sing?	0.69	0.31	0.102*	0.063
q17	Has target shared news with you?	0.44	0.36	0.051*	0.089
q31.1	Did you ever watch target make a tool?	0.90	0.38	0.277*	0.093

*Note: # = raw proportion of sample interacting for each interaction type. ## = mean yearly probability of interaction based on eqn 1 & 2 with variables ritual, closekin and affine, plus a constant term and averaged over all dyads. * = Hazda and Ache mean rates are significantly different at the 5% level (see File S1 for details on calculations).*

exchange between kin groups [16,28] are probably the key to this shift. Our results suggest that affinal kinship is about as important as genetic kinship for interactions between hunter-gatherer adults. Likewise, the fact that ritual relationship is a strong predictor of inter-band interaction in the Ache and Hadza is congruent with the idea that cultural institutions often expand interaction networks in hunter-gatherer societies [18,29]. For example, the fact that the Ache organize multi-band club fight rituals each year whereas the Hadza have no multi-band rituals is an important reason why Ache inter-band yearly interaction rates are higher.

We are not yet certain to what extent the Ache and Hadza are representative of other hunter-gatherers. First, both study populations are small and encapsulated, with hostile relations with neighbors. In other regions of the world, relations with surrounding ethnic groups may be more peaceful allowing even larger interaction networks. Additionally, the Hadza and Ache practiced no long distance trade and the spheres of interaction with outsiders may be narrower than among other world foragers where trade networks were important. On the other hand, the Ache and Hadza exhibit no land ownership or territoriality. In other foraging societies land ownership was important and structured inter-group interaction in ways that might restrict interaction networks.

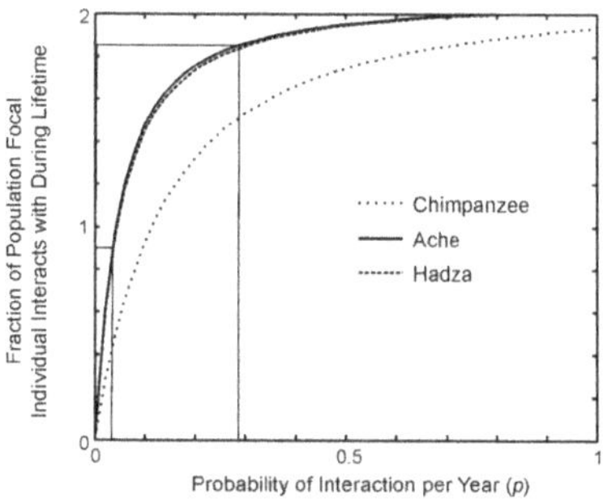

Figure 4. Fraction of the adult male standing population that interact at least once over a lifetime plotted by different yearly rates of interaction (p) covering the range of yearly interaction rates listed in Table 4, based on the adult survival table for Ache, Hadza, and Chimpanzees. The shaded area shows the range of yearly interaction rates of the hunter-gatherer populations.

We should also note that the Ache and Hadza differ between themselves. Ache maintained higher yearly interaction rates, yet the Hadza live in a larger ethnolinguistic unit with more total interactions possible over long time periods. The higher Ache yearly interaction rates appear to be due to both ritual activities (mentioned above) and different spatial social structure. Hadza bands are geographically localized but Ache bands ranged freely throughout the entire tribal territory. Hadza, but not Ache foragers also show a more consistent sex difference with Hadza women generally showing lower interaction rates than Hadza men (Table S14 in File S1, Tables S9–S13 in File S1).

The difference in lifetime interaction partners between humans and other apes has important implications. First, hominin brain expansion may be primarily explained by the memory requirements of storing critical details about an increasingly large number of social partners [6]. Second, mathematical models of cultural evolution suggest that a tenfold increase in the number of potential cultural models, can allow populations with skills and technologies that are difficult to copy to achieve a ratcheting up of cultural adaptation while populations with fewer individuals to imitate

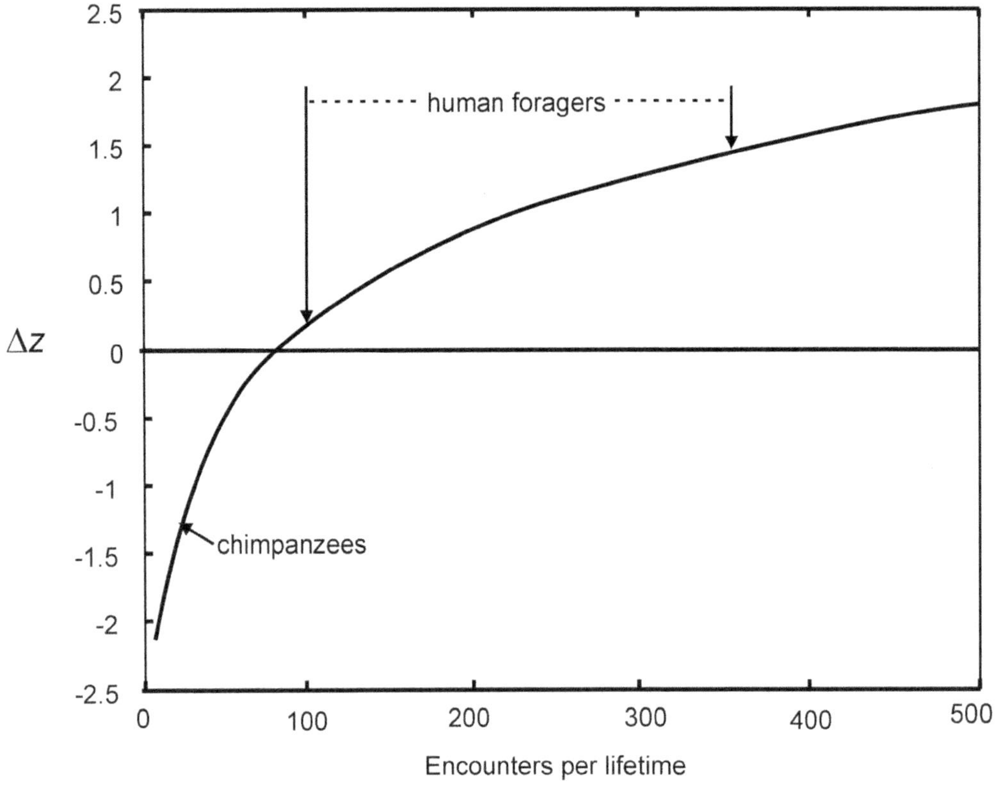

Figure 5. Mean change across one generation of social learning, in the cultural adaptiveness of a trait of moderate complexity following Henrich (*11*: Fig. 3). The α/β ratio of the model is 5, indicating a moderate mean decrease in cultural adaptedness through initial copy error followed by moderate dispersion of cultural adaptedness (z values) of copiers due to random error and guided innovation. With success-biased imitation, human foragers, with their large number of observed models (range from Table S16 File S1 is indicated), accumulate improvements each generation ($\Delta z>0$), whereas chimpanzees, with a smaller number of lifetime interactants are not able to maintain or improve the initial cultural traits ($\Delta z<0$).

would never succeed in doing so [11]. For example, our simulation shows that for a cultural trait of medium difficulty (moderate imitation error and moderate innovation), hunter-gatherers that prefer to copy the most competent individual they observe, could easily maintain and improve the practice or technology whereas chimpanzees, would not be able to maintain the trait nor improve on it through time (Text in File S1, Figure 5). Simply put, chimpanzees are unlikely to observe a cultural trait much better than that displayed by the previous generation. Humans, by observing more individuals in a lifetime, are more likely to ecounter one person who has innovated a significantly better cultural trait than was present in the previous generation. By imitation of the best trait, progressive improvement is possible. Thus, the reason why humans, but not chimpanzees have cumulative culture may be partially due to social structure as well as cognitive differences.

Third, many of the inter-band interactions we recorded were cooperative in nature. This should lead researchers to focus on mechanisms that can explain cooperation in groups of hundreds of unrelated individuals. Finally, the large interaction networks that characterize ancestral hunter-gatherers have important implications for infectious disease transmission. How this affected the evolution of the human immune system and health practices in our ancestors remains to be investigated.

Acknowledgments

We thank the Northern Ache of Paraguay and the Eastern Hadza of Tanzania. We also thank Rob Walker for estimating genetic coefficients between Ache dyads.

Author Contributions

Conceived and designed the experiments: KH BW. Performed the experiments: KH BW AMH. Analyzed the data: KH JB RB. Wrote the paper: KH BW JB AMH RB.

References

1. Hill K, Barton M, Hurtado AM (2009) The emergence of human uniqueness: underlying characteristics of behavioral modernity. Evol Anthropol 18: 187–200.
2. Gurven MD (2004) To give and to give not: the behavioral ecology of human food transfers. Behav Brain Sci 27: 543–559.
3. Hill K (2002) Altruistic cooperation during foraging by the Ache, and the evolved human predispostion to cooperate. Hum Nat 13: 105–128.
4. Hrdy SB (2009) Mothers and others. Cambridge, MA: Belknap Press. 422 p.
5. Hill KR, Hurtado AM (2009) Cooperative breeding in South American hunter-gatherers. Proc Roy Soc B 276: 3863–3870.
6. Dunbar R (2003) The social brain: mind, language, and society in evolutionary perspective. Annu Rev. Anthropol 32: 163–81.
7. Dunbar R (2010) How many friends does one person need? Dunbar's number and other evolutionary quirks. Cambridge, MA: Harvard University Press. 312 p.
8. Boyd R, Richerson PJ (1988) The evolution of reciprocity in sizable groups. J Theor Biol 132: 337–356.
9. Eshel I, Cavalli-Sforza LL (1982) Assortment of encounters and evolution of cooperativeness. Proc Natl Acad Sci USA 79: 1331–1335.
10. Ohtsuki H, Hauert C, Lieberman E, Nowak MA (2006) A simple rule for the evolution of cooperation on graphs and social networks. Nature 441: 502–505.
11. Henrich J (2004) Demography and cultural evolution: how adaptive cultural processes can produce maladaptive losses: the Tasmanian case. Am Antiq 69: 197–214.
12. Powell A, Shennan S, Thomas MG (2009) Late Pleistocene demography and the appearance of modern human behavior. Science 324: 1298–1301.
13. Boyd R, Richerson PJ (1996) Why culture is common but cultural evolution is rare. Proc British Acad 88: 77–93.
14. Radcliffe-Brown AR (1952) Structure and function in primitive society: essays and addresses by AR Radcliffe-Brown. London: Taylor & Francis. 234 p.
15. Service ER (1962) Primitive social organization: an evolutionary perspective. New York: Random House. 221 p.
16. Chapais B (2008) Primeval kinship: how pair-bonding gave birth to human society Cambridge, MA: Harvard University Press. 368 p.
17. Hill KR, Walker RS, Božičević M, Eder J, Headland T, et al. (2011) Co-residence patterns in hunter-gatherer societies show unique human social structure. Science 331: 1286–1289.
18. Wiessner PW (1977) Hxaro: A regional system of reciprocity for reducing risk among the Kung San. Ph.D. dissertation, Ann Arbor: University of Michigan.
19. Wiessner P (1998) On network analyses: the potential for understanding (and misunderstanding) !Kung hxaro. Curr Anthropol 39: 514–517.
20. Yengoyan A (1968) Demographic and ecological influences on Australian aborigine marriage sections. In Lee RB, DeVore I, editors. Man the hunter. Chicago: Aldine Press. pp. 185–199.
21. Apicella CL, Marlowe FW, Fowler JH, Christakis NA (2012) Social networks and coooperation in hunter-gatherers. Nature 481: 497–501.
22. Hill K, Hurtado AM (1996) Ache life history: the ecology and demography of a foraging people. New York: Transaction Publishers. 561 p.
23. Marlowe FW (2010) The Hadza: Hunter-gatherers of Tanzania. Berkeley: University of California Press. 336 p.
24. Gliganic L, Jacobs Z, Roberts R, Domínguez-Rodrigo M, Mabulla A (2012) New ages for Middle and Later Stone Age deposits at Mumba rockshelter, Tanzania: optically stimulated luminescence dating of quartz and feldspar grains. J. Hum Evol 62: 533–547.
25. Tishkoff S, Reed FA, Friedlander FR, Ehret C, Ranciarro A, et al. (2009) The genetic structure and history of Africans and African Americans. Science 324: 1035–1044.
26. McMillan GP (2001) Ache residential grouping and social foraging. PhD Dissertion, Albuquerque: University of New Mexico.
27. Wiessner P (2014) The Embers of Society: Firelight Talk among the Ju/'hoansi Bushmen. Proc Natl Acad Sci USA, In press.
28. Wiessner P (2009) Parent offspring conflict in marriage. In Shennan S, editor. Pattern and process in cultural evolution. Berkeley: University of California Press. pp. 251–263.
29. Guemple DL (1972) Alliance in Eskimo Society. Seattle: University of Washington Press.

14

Dorsal Striatal Dopamine, Food Preference and Health Perception in Humans

Deanna L. Wallace[1]*, Esther Aarts[1,2], Linh C. Dang[1,3], Stephanie M. Greer[1], William J. Jagust[1], Mark D'Esposito[1]

1 Helen Wills Neuroscience Institute, University of California, Berkeley, California, United States of America, **2** Center for Cognitive Neuroimaging, Donders Institute for Brain, Cognition and Behaviour, Radboud University, Nijmegen, The Netherlands, **3** Department of Psychology, Vanderbilt University, Nashville, Tennessee, United States of America

Abstract

To date, few studies have explored the neurochemical mechanisms supporting individual differences in food preference in humans. Here we investigate how dorsal striatal dopamine, as measured by the positron emission tomography (PET) tracer [^{18}F]fluorometatyrosine (FMT), correlates with food-related decision-making, as well as body mass index (BMI) in 16 healthy-weight to moderately obese individuals. We find that lower PET FMT dopamine synthesis binding potential correlates with higher BMI, greater preference for perceived "healthy" foods, but also greater healthiness ratings for food items. These findings further substantiate the role of dorsal striatal dopamine in food-related behaviors and shed light on the complexity of individual differences in food preference.

Editor: J Bruce Morton, University of Western Ontario, Canada

Funding: This work was generously funded by NIH grants DA20600, AG044292 and F32DA276840, and the Tanita Healthy Weight Community Fellowship. The funders had no role in study design, data collection and analysis, decision to publish, or preparation of the manuscript.

Competing Interests: The authors have declared that no competing interests exist.

* E-mail: deanna_wallace@berkeley.edu.

Introduction

Modern society is surrounded by an overabundance and a wide-variety of food choices, which in part contributes to the growing overweight population in the United States [1]. Yet, the underlying neurochemical mechanisms supporting individual differences in food preferences are not well-understood. Some individuals naturally base their food preferences more on the health value of food items versus the taste value of food items, and the ventromedial prefrontal cortex (vmPFC) has been shown to play a role in goal values related to influences of "health" and "taste" [2]. Furthermore, there is a wide variation in individuals' judgment of caloric content and perceived "healthiness" of food items [3], and studies show perceived "healthy" foods are over-consumed as compared to perceived "unhealthy" foods, despite equal nutritional value [3,4].

Dorsal striatal dopamine has been shown to play a role in motivation for food in both human and animal models [5,6,7], yet the relationship between dopamine and food desirability or preferences in humans has not been thoroughly explored. Additionally, studies that utilize PET ligands that bind dopamine receptors have shown correlations with BMI, however, in both positive [8] and negative [9] directions, and not all studies find significant associations (for review see [10]). Also, due to the nature of these PET ligands that are dependent on the state of endogenous dopamine release, it is difficult to interpret relationships between striatal dopamine and BMI. Lower dopamine receptor binding could represent fewer existing striatal dopamine receptors (i.e. a negative relationship between PET binding and BMI, as found in [9]), or greater dopamine receptor binding could represent lower endogenous dopamine release, allowing more available receptors in which the PET ligand could bind (i.e. a positive relationship between binding and BMI, as found in [8]). To complement previous studies that have utilized PET ligands that bind dopamine receptors, here we used a stable measurement of presynaptic dopamine synthesis capacity with the PET ligand [^{18}F]fluorometatyrosine (FMT) that has been extensively studied in human and animal models [11,12,13,14].

The aims of our study were to investigate the relationship between dorsal striatal PET FMT dopamine synthesis measures and BMI and to study how these PET FMT dopamine synthesis measures may correlate with individual differences in food preference. We hypothesized that lower PET FMT dopamine synthesis binding would correspond with higher BMI, as suggested by previous work [15]. We also predicted that individuals with lower endogenous striatal dopamine would have greater overall preference for food items (i.e. both "healthy" and "unhealthy" foods) as compared to individuals with higher striatal dopamine and that an individual's health perception of food items may also influence preference.

Methods and Materials

Subjects

Thirty-three healthy, right-handed subjects who previously received PET FMT dopamine synthesis scans were invited to participate in the behavioral study presented here and were given no prior knowledge to the study, only informed that it involved studying complex decision-making. Of these 33, 16 subjects agreed to participate (8 M, age 20–30). BMI ((weight in kilograms)/

(height in meters)^2)) was calculated for all subjects (range: 20.2–33.4, with 1 obese, 4 overweight and 11 healthy-weight subjects). Subjects had no history of drug abuse, eating disorders, major depression and anxiety disorders. Subjects were also asked to if they were in very poor, poor, average, good or excellent health. All reported to be in overall average to excellent health and not currently dieting or trying to lose weight. Socioeconomic status (SES) was also collected from individuals using the Barratt simplified measure of social status (BSMSS) [16].

Ethics Statement

All subjects gave written informed consent and were paid for participation according to institutional guidelines of the local ethics committee (University of California Berkeley (UCB) and Lawrence Berkeley National Laboratory (LBNL) Committee for the Protection of Human Participants (CPHP) and Lawrence Berkeley National Laboratory Institutional Review Boards (IRB)). UCB's and LBNL's CPHPs and IRBs specifically approved the studies presented here

PET data acquisition and analysis

PET imaging and FMT binding were performed at Lawrence Berkeley National Laboratory, as described previously [17]. FMT is a substrate of aromatic L-amino acid decarboxylase (AADC), a dopamine-synthesizing enzyme whose activity corresponds to the capacity of dopaminergic neurons to synthesize dopamine [13] and has been shown to be indicative of pre-synaptic dopamine synthesis capacity [18]. FMT is metabolized by AADC to [^{18}F]fluorometatyramine, which is oxidized to [^{18}F]fluorohydroxyphenylacetic acid (FPAC), remains in the dopaminergic terminals and is visible on PET FMT scans. Thus, signal intensity on PET FMT scans has been shown to be comparable with [^{18}F]fluorodopa [18], in which tracer uptake is highly correlated ($r = 0.97$, $p<0.003$) with striatal dopamine protein levels in post-mortem patients, as measured by high performance liquid chromatographic (HPLC) methods [19]. Moreover, in comparison to [^{18}F]fluorodopa, FMT is also not a substrate for O-methylation and therefore provides higher signal-to-noise images than [^{18}F]fluorodopa [18]. Additionally, FMT measures have been shown to directly correspond with dopamine measures in animal Parkinson's disease models [14].

Scans were conducted either from 9AM-12PM or 1PM-4PM. The average delay between acquisition of the PET FMT dopamine synthesis data and the behavioral data was 2.37 ± 0.26 years, comparable to the delay reported in a previous study from our lab utilizing PET FMT [11]. Although this delay is not ideal, a study by Vingerhoets et al. [20] has shown that striatal Ki related to presynaptic dopamine is a relatively stable measurement, having a 95% chance of remaining within 18% of its original value within individual healthy subjects over a 7-year time-span. Therefore, FMT measures, comparable to [^{18}F]fluorodopa [13], are thought to reflect relatively stable processes (i.e. synthesis capacity) and therefore not particularly sensitive to small state-related changes. Additionally, BMI was not significantly different between the acquisition of the PET and behavioral data (average change in BMI: 0.13 ± 1.45, $T(15) = 0.2616$, $p = 0.79$, two-tailed paired t-test). Also, all subjects were screened for any lifestyle changes in the time since last testing (i.e. change in diet and exercise/daily activity, smoking or drinking, mental health or medication status). Finally, change in BMI from time of the PET FMT scan to behavioral testing as well as the time elapsed between PET scan and behavioral testing were used as variables in the multiple regression data analysis.

PET scans were performed using the Siemens ECAT-HR PET camera (Knoxville, TN). Approximately 2.5 mCi of high specific activity FMT was injected as a bolus into an antecubital vein and a dynamic acquisition sequence in 3D mode was obtained for a total of 89 min scan time. Two high-resolution anatomical images (MPRAGE) were acquired in each participant on a Siemens 1.5 T Magnetom Avanto MRI scanner (Siemens, Erlangen, Germany), using a 12-channel head coil ($TE/TR = 3.58/2120$ ms; voxel size $= 1.0 \times 1.0 \times 1.0$ mm, 160 axial slices; $FOV = 256$ mm; scanning time ~9 minutes). The two MPRAGEs were averaged to obtain one high-resolution structural image, which was used to generate individual caudate and cerebellum regions of interest (ROI).

Left and right caudate and cerebellum ROIs (used as reference region, as in previous studies [11]) were manually drawn on each participant's anatomical MRI scan using FSLView (http://www.fmrib.ox.ac.uk/fsl/), as described previously [21]. Both inter- and intra-rater reliability were above 95% (from ratings made by two lab members). To avoid contamination of FMT signal from dopaminergic nuclei, only the posterior three-fourths of the gray matter were included in the cerebellar reference region. After co-registration to PET FMT space, only the voxels with an above 50% chance to lie in the ROIs were included to ensure high grey matter probability.

PET FMT images were reconstructed with an ordered subset expectation maximization algorithm with weighted attenuation, scatter corrected, motion-corrected and smoothed with a 4 mm full width half maximum kernel, using Statistical Parametric Mapping version 8 (SPM8) (www.fil.ion.ucl.ac.uk/spm/). The anatomical MRI scan was coregistered to the mean image of all realigned frames in the PET FMT scan using FSL-FLIRT (http://www.fmrib.ox.ac.uk/fsl/, version 4.1.2). Using an in-house graphical analysis program implementing Patlak plotting [22,23], K_i images, representing the amount of tracer accumulated in the brain relative to the reference region (cerebellum [11,12], a standard practice in PET analysis to minimize potential confounds of noise from PET data), were created. K_i values were obtained separately from the left and right caudate ROIs and associations were computed between K_i values, BMI, and the behavioral measures. Additionally, since age and sex have been shown to have an effect on FMT binding [15,24], correlations between FMT and BMI were corrected for age and sex (as well as any changes in BMI from time of PET scan to behavioral testing) by control variables in a Pearson's partial correlation.

Behavioral paradigm

Subjects were asked to eat a typical, but not too heavy meal an hour prior to the testing session. In order to encourage compliance with this request, testing sessions were scheduled after typical meal times (i.e. 9AM, 2PM and 7:30PM), and time of last meal was recorded. Food items consumed prior to testing and the elapsed time from last meal eaten to testing session were recorded, (as determined by the resource www.caloriecount.com and meal and serving sizes self-reported by individual). To ensure hunger was not influencing the task, we also measured hunger and fullness with a visual analog scale [25].

Pictures of eighty food items were used in which subjects were asked to rate the items in 3 separate blocks based on 1) desirability, 2) healthiness and 3) tastiness in the program E-Prime Professional (Psychology Software Tool, Inc., Sharpsburg, PA, USA) (see **Figure 1**). In order to create a task with balanced numbers of healthy, unhealthy and neutral food items, we first created an objective health value for each of the eighty food items by assigning a standardized, objective score of -3 (very unhealthy) to +

3 (very healthy) to each food based on a letter grade (ranging from F-minus (very unhealthy) to A-plus (very healthy)) and nutritional information from the on-line resource www.caloriecount.com. These letter grades incorporate several factors (i.e. calories, grams of fat, fiber etc.) and are listed as an on-line reference for "choices for healthy eating," as stated on the website. We then balanced the task with approximately equal numbers of healthy (i.e. foods with objective scores of 2 or 3, such as fruit and vegetables), neutral (i.e. foods with objective scores of 1 and −1, such as saltine crackers) and unhealthy items (i.e. foods with negative objective scores of −2 or −3 such as highly processed candy bars).

Subjects were first asked to rate the degree to which they "desired" or "wanted" each item (scale of 1 (strongly do not want) to 4 (strongly want)), referred to throughout the text as "preferred", a term consistent with the literature [2]. The food item would appear and the subject would have up to 4 seconds to respond, and they rated all eighty food items before continuing to the subsequent "health" and "taste" blocks (see below). Because humans have the capacity to modulate food choices based not only on taste for certain foods, but also on perceptions of healthiness [26], we only asked the subject to rate how much they would want the food or find the food desirable and the preference block was always presented first. In an attempt to capture how much the subject actually preferred the food items presented, subjects were informed they would receive a food item from the task at the end of testing based on their "desirability" ratings. The subjects also did not know in the upcoming second and third blocks (described below), they would be asked to judge how healthy and tasty they found each food item.

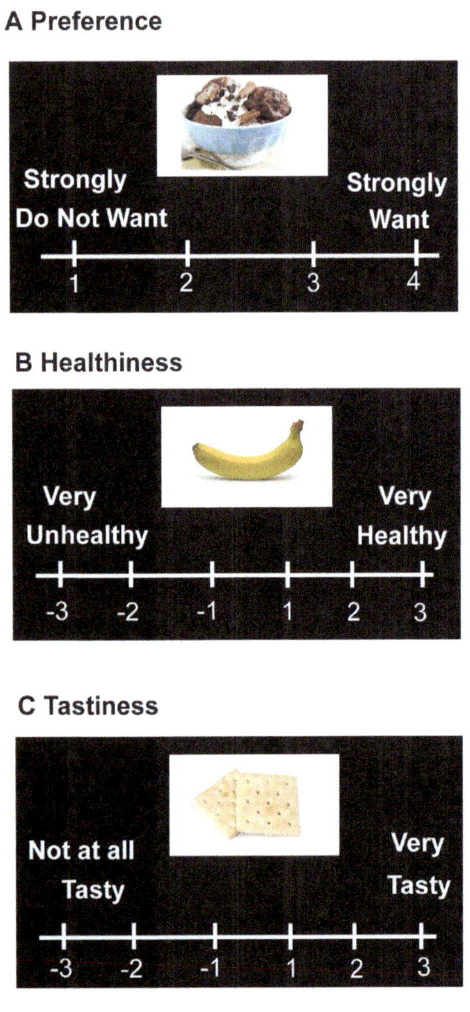

Figure 1. Behavioral Task. Subjects rated food items based on **A)** Preference (i.e. "wanting/desirability"), rated on a scale of 1–4 **B)** Perceived healthiness, rated on a scale of −3 to +3 and **C)** Tastiness, rated on scales −3 to +3. Food items rated 3 or 4 in the preference/desirability block were scored as "preferred", while those rated 2 or 3 in the healthiness/tastiness blocks were rated as perceived "healthy"/"tasty" and −2 or −3 as perceived "unhealthy"/"untasty".

In the second block, subjects rated how much they perceived the eighty food items as healthy or unhealthy (−3 for very unhealthy to 3 for very healthy) and in a third block, how tasty they found the eighty food items (−3 for not at all tasty to 3 for very tasty). The order of these blocks was consistent for all subjects, as we did not want to influence health ratings in a potential order effect. The subjects were informed that the ratings of health and taste would not affect the item they would receive based on their answers in the "desirability" block. We chose a 6-point scale for health and taste values to allow a wider range of measuring taste/health perception, including a "neutral" rating corresponding to −1 and +1, whereas the 4-point scale of the desirability/preference block would reflect only preferred or non-preferred food items. The total task lasted approximately 25 minutes. Subjects were asked at the end of the task if there were any food items that were unfamiliar that may have led to non-responses. All subjects reported familiarity with food items and all items were given ratings for all three blocks by all subjects.

Dopamine in the dorsal striatum has been shown to have a strong association in motivation for food [5,6,7]. Taste perception is also highly correlated with desirability of food, in that most humans prefer foods that they also find tasty [27]. Because there are many combinations of the preference, taste and health blocks that could be examined, to eliminate multiple comparisons and the potential for spurious correlations, based on this literature, we examined the number of food items that were self-rated as 1) preferred, tasty, and perceived "healthy" and 2) preferred, tasty, and perceived "unhealthy". (Preferred items rated as 3 or 4 in the "desirability" block; tasty items rated as 2 or 3 in the "tastiness" block; perceived "healthy" items rated as 2 or 3 and perceived "unhealthy" items rated as −2 or −3 in the "healthiness" block). Post-hoc analysis also investigated the ratio of perceived "healthy"-to-"unhealthy" food items, the number of preferred perceived "healthy" food items that were not actually objectively rated as healthy (i.e preferred items that the individual rated as healthy minus items the subject rated as preferred that were actually healthy as determined by the assigned objective health score. (For example, if a subject rated "crackers" as a preferred perceived healthy food with a healthy score of 3 (very healthy), and the assigned objective health score was a 1 (neutral-healthy), this would be counted as a preferred perceived healthy food that was not actually healthy). Average calories for preferred items from each individual subject were also calculated.

Statistical Analysis

Step-wise multiple linear regression was used to test the relationships between the two separate dependent variables: 1) preferred, tasty and perceived healthy and 2) preferred, tasty and perceived unhealthy food items, and the independent variables: right caudate PET FMT values, left caudate PET FMT values, BMI, age, sex, socio-economic status, any changes in BMI between PET and behavioral testing and time elapsed between PET and behavioral testing in SPSS version 19 (IBM, Chicago, Ill., USA), with inclusion of the independent variable to the model set at $p<0.05$ and excluded with $p>0.1$. The perceived "healthy"-to-"unhealthy" ratio was highly correlated with the dependent variable of preferred perceived "healthy" items ($r=0.685$, $p<0.003$), and therefore, we were unable to enter this variable into the model. However, Pearson's partial correlations, corrected for age, sex and any BMI changes, were used to test direct relationships between right caudate PET FMT and 1) BMI, 2) perceived "healthy"-to-"unhealthy" ratio and 3) average calories of preferred items, conducted with SPSS version 19 (IBM, Chicago, Ill., USA). We also further tested the relationship between PET FMT dopamine synthesis values, the number of preferred perceived "healthy" food items that were not rated as healthy by the calculated score, and preferred items that were rated as healthy by the calculated score in a step-wise multiple regression model. (The number of preferred perceived "healthy" food items not rated as healthy by the calculated score, and preferred items rated as healthy by the calculated score were not significantly correlated ($r=0.354$, $p=0.23$). We also tested if there was a relationship between change in BMI and the dependent variables: left and right caudate PET FMT values, SES, age, sex, time between PET imaging and behavioral testing, number of preferred perceived "healthy" foods and preferred perceived "unhealthy" foods using step-wise linear regression. Data are shown as Pearson r-values.

Results

Relationship between PET FMT dopamine synthesis values and BMI

We first tested whether a significant relationship exists between caudate PET FMT dopamine synthesis values and BMI measurements across 16 individuals (average-to-moderately overweight/obese individuals). We found a significant negative correlation between caudate PET FMT dopamine synthesis values and BMI, with higher BMI individuals having lower dopamine synthesis (**Figure 2A**: PET FMT raw images of higher (left) and lower (right) BMI individuals; **Figure 2B**: right caudate, $r=-0.66$, $p=0.014$, left caudate: $r=-0.22$, $p=0.46$ (not significant (n.s.)), controlled for age, sex and any changes in BMI from PET FMT dopamine synthesis scan to behavioral testing).

Relationship between PET FMT dopamine synthesis values and food preference

Subjects rated eighty food items in 3 separate blocks based on the their perception of 1) desirability, 2) healthiness and 3) tastiness of each food item (see **Figure 1**). Approximately 50% of the items were healthy and unhealthy, as set forth by health information (See **Methods and Materials**). Dopamine in the dorsal striatum has been shown to have a strong association in motivation for food [5,6,7], while hedonic properties of food are mediated through other neuronal mechanisms [7,27]. However, taste perception is highly correlated with desirability of food, in that most humans prefer foods that they also find tasty [27]. Here we also find that taste perception and preference are highly correlated, in that items preferred are also rated as tasty ($r=0.707$, $p<0.002$).

Therefore, to examine how health perception may influence food-related decision-making, we utilized step-wise multiple linear regression to model the relationships between the dependent variable of the number of food items rated as preferred, tasty and perceived healthy and the independent variables of FMT in the left and right caudate, BMI, age, sex, SES, change in BMI from time of PET scan to behavioral testing and time elapsed from time of PET to behavioral testing. Right caudate PET FMT dopamine synthesis values significantly contribute to the regression model for the number of preferred, tasty items that were perceived as healthy (Beta: -0.696; $t(15)=-3.625$, $p<0.003$, **Figure 3**), while all other independent variables were excluded from the model as non-significant ($t(15)<1.216$, $p>0.246$). We also tested the hypothesis that the number of preferred, perceived "unhealthy" items would also show a relationship with these independent variables, but no independent variable was entered into the model as significant ($F<2.7$, $p>0.1$). Thus, individuals with lower caudate PET FMT dopamine synthesis values have greater preferences for perceived "healthy" but not perceived "unhealthy" food items.

Relationship between PET FMT dopamine synthesis values and health perception of food items

We hypothesized that the relationship between caudate PET FMT dopamine synthesis values and preference for perceived "healthy" items may be due to individual differences in the health perception of food items. Although we designed the task with an approximate 1:1 ratio of healthy to unhealthy food items, individuals varied widely in their perception of the healthiness of the items, with ratios of healthy to unhealthy items ranging from 1.83:1 to 0.15:1. Therefore, as a post-hoc analysis, we investigated the relationship between right caudate PET FMT dopamine synthesis and the ratio of perceived "healthy" to "unhealthy" items, and found a significant negative correlation ($r=-0.534$, $p=0.04$), with lower caudate PET FMT dopamine synthesis values corresponding to greater numbers of items perceived as "healthy" compared to "unhealthy".

We therefore utilized step-wise multiple linear regression to investigate the relationships between caudate PET FMT dopamine synthesis and preference for perceived healthy but not actual healthy foods (as determined by the objective calculated score, see **Methods**), and preference for healthy foods as determined by the objective calculated score. We found a significant relationship between caudate PET FMT dopamine synthesis values and preference for perceived healthy but not actual healthy foods (Beta: -0.631, $t(15)=-3.043$, $p<0.01$), but no significant relationship between caudate PET FMT dopamine synthesis values and preference for actual calculated healthy foods ($t(15)=-1.54$, $p>0.148$), indicating preference for over-perceived "healthy" foods correlated more strongly in lower FMT individuals. Furthermore, there was no significant relationship between caudate PET FMT dopamine synthesis values and the average calories of preferred items ($r=0.288$, $p>0.34$), indicating that lower PET FMT dopamine synthesis individuals did not differ in the caloric content of preferred foods.

We also did not find any relationship between change in BMI and PET FMT dopamine synthesis values, SES, age, sex, time between PET imaging and behavioral testing, number of preferred perceived "healthy" foods or preferred perceived "unhealthy" foods ($p>0.1$).

Time of testing session, time elapsed since last meal, and number of calories eaten at the last meal were not significantly correlated with any behavioral measures ($p>0.13$). Hunger and fullness measures also did not correlate with any of the behavioral measures ($p>0.26$).

Discussion

The aim of this study was to investigate the relationship between endogenous caudate dopamine synthesis, BMI and food-related behavior. We found that lower caudate dopamine synthesis as measured by PET FMT dopamine synthesis correlated with 1) greater BMI and 2) greater preference for perceived "healthy" foods. We also found a relationship between lower caudate PET

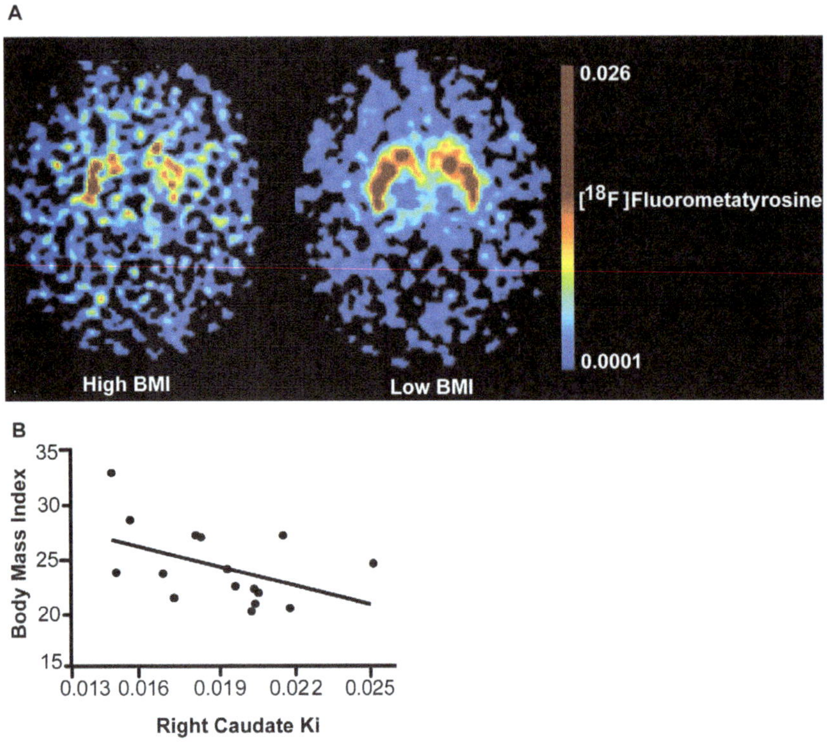

Figure 2. Dorsal striatal dopamine and BMI. A) PET imaging with FMT showed lower dorsal striatal dopamine synthesis capacity in a representative higher BMI individual (left) than a representative lower BMI individual (right, raw images for illustration purposes only). **B**) BMI and dorsal striatal dopamine were negatively correlated as measured by the PET ligand FMT, a measure of presynaptic dopamine synthesis capacity, relative to the cerebellum ($r = -0.66$, $p = 0.014$, $n = 16$, controlled for age, sex and any changes in BMI from PET scan to behavioral testing).

FMT dopamine synthesis values and greater over-rating of the healthiness of food items, as well as a significant correlation with greater preferred perceived "healthy" foods that were not actually healthy. We found no significant relationship between PET FMT dopamine synthesis and the average caloric content of preferred food items.

Research suggests that preference for and overconsumption of unhealthy foods are two of the many contributors to weight gain and higher BMI (Centers for Disease Control and Prevention; http://www.cdc.gov/obesity/index.html). Interestingly, we found lower dorsal striatal dopamine synthesis correlated with greater numbers of preferred, perceived "healthy" food items. Although this correlation cannot imply causation, this finding suggests

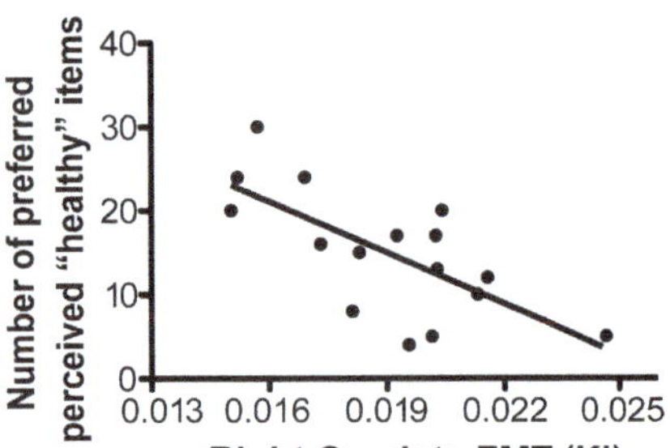

Figure 3. Dorsal striatal dopamine and food-related behaviors. A significant relationship was found between lower caudate PET FMT dopamine synthesis values and greater preference for perceived "healthy" food items (Beta: -0.696; $t(15) = -3.625$, $p < 0.003$).

endogenous differences in dorsal striatal dopamine synthesis may in part play a role in individual differences for food preference. Here we propose that lower caudate PET FMT dopamine synthesis values represent lower tonic dopamine, which in response to palatable stimuli, allows for greater phasic bursting [28] and perhaps altered responsivity to foods. Additionally, these differences in dorsal striatal dopamine may affect processing of gustatory stimuli in somatosensory cortex, as a previous study has shown altered activation in both dorsal striatal and somotosensory regions with food intake in individuals susceptible to obesity [29]. Lower dorsal striatal dopamine may also result in connectivity differences between the dorsal striatum and dorsolateral prefrontal cortex (DLPFC), as suggested by our recent findings [30]. Therefore, we hypothesize dopamine-related dorsal striatal mechanisms may influence health perception differences through either connectivity with somatosensory processing (i.e. altered taste sensation properties) or perhaps connectivity with DLPFC, which has been shown to play a role in over-evaluation of previously preferred choice items [31]. Functional magnetic resonance imaging (fMRI) could elucidate these potential mechanisms of individual differences in food preferences and over-rating of health values.

Initially, we predicted that individuals with lower dorsal striatal dopamine would have greater overall food preference (i.e. prefer more number of items self-rated as "healthy" and "unhealthy"), as compared to individuals with higher dorsal striatal dopamine. However, another finding of our study was that over-rating the healthiness of foods (i.e. an increased sense of healthiness), but not the caloric content of the preferred food items or preference for objectively-defined healthy food items, was significantly related to endogenous dorsal striatal dopamine measures. Therefore, one explanation for our findings of a significant relationship with only perceived "healthy" foods may be that foods perceived as "healthy" are more justified as preferred. This may especially be the case since our study purposely was conducted after the subjects' mealtimes when overall desire for food should be minimal. Therefore, subjects had greater preference for over-rated "healthy" foods even though they were satiated and not hungry at the time. Future studies investigating the relationship between endogenous striatal dopamine and food preferences in hungry versus sated states would further substantiate this hypothesis.

It can also be argued that health perception requires exposure and experience with food items to gain a sense of health value, and it may be the case that dietary lifestyle differences have influenced or modified underlying dorsal striatal dopamine synthesis. Furthermore, differences with familiarity of food items could have attributed to differences in food preference or over-rating of foods as healthy. However, subjects did report at the end of the task that they were familiar with all food items (see **Methods**). Although we did not investigate differences in diet, we purposely screened subjects that were not dieting at the time of the study. Additionally, all of the subjects were young (age range 19–30) without any history of eating disorders and rated themselves as in average to excellent health. We also assessed socioeconomic status, and found no influence. However, there are other environmental influences on food preferences that in addition to striatal dopamine could be explored further in future studies.

We hypothesize that the subtle individual differences in health perception may contribute to increased BMI over time, as it has been reported that minor increases in caloric intake on a daily basis (whether perceived as "healthy" or "unhealthy") contribute to overall weight gain [32]. Although we found no relationship between BMI and health perception here, perhaps with a greater range of BMI, over-rating of the healthiness of food items may be more pronounced in higher BMI subjects. Our lack of significant findings between BMI and food-related behaviors may also suggest that endogenous striatal dopamine is more closely related to food-related behavior than BMI itself as a phenotype, since BMI is influenced by various complicated factors and may not be the best predictor of behavior or neuroimaging findings (see [10] for review). We also did not find any predictors for the change in BMI for time elapsed between PET acquisition and behavioral testing, although the change in BMI for subjects was small and not significantly different between time points. However, future studies utilizing PET FMT dopamine synthesis measures, along with food preferences and health perception measures, in a population with greater BMI fluctuation would be of great interest.

To complement previous studies that utilized PET ligands that bind dopamine receptors, we utilized a measure of dopamine synthesis capacity and show that lower dopamine synthesis in the dorsal striatum (i.e. caudate) corresponds with higher BMI. Though it should be noted, due to the cross-sectional nature of our study, we cannot definitively conclude a cause or effect relationship to lower dorsal striatal FMT dopamine synthesis values corresponding with higher BMI. However, our study used healthy-weight to moderately overweight/obese (i.e. non-morbidly obese) individuals, and therefore our results may suggest that lower dorsal striatal presynaptic dopamine measures could correspond with a propensity towards obesity. On the other hand, it may also be the case that downregulation of presynaptic dopamine in the caudate has occurred in response to moderately higher BMI, as it has been shown that dopaminergic signaling is decreased in response to overconsumption of food in animal models [5,33], and overconsumption of food is typically associated with weight gain leading to higher BMI. Although we used individuals with a limited range of BMI in our study, perhaps viewed as a limitation of the study, we actually find the results even more compelling in that a relationship between PET FMT dopamine synthesis and BMI is present without including morbidly obese individuals. Moreover, although our sample size ($n = 16$) was greater than or comparable to other sample sizes in PET FMT studies ([11,12,15]), replication of our findings with a larger sample size and a broader range of BMI would further substantiate our results and may find greater preferences for unhealthy food items correlating with lower PET FMT dopamine synthesis values, which were not detected in our study.

In summary, although other neurotransmitter systems are involved in feeding and weight regulation [7], our study finds a role for dorsal striatal dopamine in food preferences as well as health perception of food in humans. Future prospective studies utilizing dopamine-related PET measures are of great interest to investigate how endogenous dopamine, as well individual differences in food-related behavior, might correlate with body weight fluctuation in humans.

Author Contributions

Conceived and designed the experiments: DLW EA SMG LCD. Performed the experiments: DLW EA LCD. Analyzed the data: DLW LCD. Wrote the paper: DLW. Edited and revised the manuscript: EA SMG LCD WJJ MD.

References

1. Swinburn BA, Sacks G, Hall KD, McPherson K, Finegood DT, et al. (2011) The global obesity pandemic: shaped by global drivers and local environments. Lancet 378: 804–814.
2. Hare TA, Camerer CF, Rangel A (2009) Self-control in decision-making involves modulation of the vmPFC valuation system. Science 324: 646–648.
3. Provencher V, Polivy J, Herman CP (2009) Perceived healthiness of food. If it's healthy, you can eat more! Appetite 52: 340–344.
4. Gravel K, Doucet E, Herman CP, Pomerleau S, Bourlaud AS, et al. (2012) "Healthy," "diet," or "hedonic". How nutrition claims affect food-related perceptions and intake? Appetite 59: 877–884.
5. Johnson PM, Kenny PJ (2010) Dopamine D2 receptors in addiction-like reward dysfunction and compulsive eating in obese rats. Nat Neurosci 13: 635–641.
6. Szczypka MS, Kwok K, Brot MD, Marck BT, Matsumoto AM, et al. (2001) Dopamine production in the caudate putamen restores feeding in dopamine-deficient mice. Neuron 30: 819–828.
7. Volkow ND, Wang GJ, Baler RD (2011) Reward, dopamine and the control of food intake: implications for obesity. Trends Cogn Sci 15: 37–46.
8. Dunn JP, Kessler RM, Feurer ID, Volkow ND, Patterson BW, et al. (2012) Relationship of dopamine type 2 receptor binding potential with fasting neuroendocrine hormones and insulin sensitivity in human obesity. Diabetes Care 35: 1105–1111.
9. Wang GJ, Volkow ND, Logan J, Pappas NR, Wong CT, et al. (2001) Brain dopamine and obesity. Lancet 357: 354–357.
10. Ziauddeen H, Farooqi IS, Fletcher PC (2012) Obesity and the brain: how convincing is the addiction model? Nat Rev Neurosci 13: 279–286.
11. Cools R, Frank MJ, Gibbs SE, Miyakawa A, Jagust W, et al. (2009) Striatal dopamine predicts outcome-specific reversal learning and its sensitivity to dopaminergic drug administration. J Neurosci 29: 1538–1543.
12. Cools R, Gibbs SE, Miyakawa A, Jagust W, D'Esposito M (2008) Working memory capacity predicts dopamine synthesis capacity in the human striatum. J Neurosci 28: 1208–1212.
13. DeJesus O, Endres C, Shelton S, Nickles R, Holden J (1997) Evaluation of fluorinated m-tyrosine analogs as PET imaging agents of dopamine nerve terminals: comparison with 6-fluoroDOPA. J Nucl Med 38: 630–636.
14. Eberling JL, Bankiewicz KS, O'Neil JP, Jagust WJ (2007) PET 6-[F]fluoro-L-m-tyrosine Studies of Dopaminergic Function in Human and Nonhuman Primates. Front Hum Neurosci 1: 9.
15. Wilcox CE, Braskie MN, Kluth JT, Jagust WJ (2010) Overeating Behavior and Striatal Dopamine with 6-[F]-Fluoro-L-m-Tyrosine PET. J Obes 2010.

16. Barratt W (2006) The Barratt Simplified Measure of Social Status (BSMSS) measureing SES.
17. VanBrocklin HF, Blagoev M, Hoepping A, O'Neil JP, Klose M, et al. (2004) A new precursor for the preparation of 6-[18F]Fluoro-L-m-tyrosine ([18F]FMT): efficient synthesis and comparison of radiolabeling. Appl Radiat Isot 61: 1289–1294.
18. Jordan S, Eberling J, Bankiewicz K, Rosenberg D, Coxson P, et al. (1997) 6-[^{18}F]fluoro-L-m-tyrosine: metabolism, positron emission tomography kinetics, and 1-methyl-4-phenyl-1,2,3,6-tetrahydropyridine lesions in primates. Brain Res 750: 264–276.
19. Snow BJ (1996) Fluorodopa PET scanning in Parkinson's disease. Adv Neurol 69: 449-457.
20. Vingerhoets FJ, Snow BJ, Tetrud JW, Langston JW, Schulzer M, et al. (1994) Positron emission tomographic evidence for progression of human MPTP-induced dopaminergic lesions. Ann Neurol 36: 765–770.
21. Mawlawi O, Martinez D, Slifstein M, Broft A, Chatterjee R, et al. (2001) Imaging human mesolimbic dopamine transmission with positron emission tomography: I. Accuracy and precision of D(2) receptor parameter measurements in ventral striatum. J Cereb Blood Flow Metab 21: 1034–1057.
22. Logan J (2000) Graphical analysis of PET data applied to reversible and irreversible tracers. Nucl Med Biol 27: 661–670.
23. Patlak C, Blasberg R (1985) Graphical evaluation of blood-to-brain transfer constants from multiple-time uptake data. Generalizations. J Cereb Blood Flow Metab 5: 584–590.
24. Laakso A, Vilkman H, Bergman J, Haaparanta M, Solin O, et al. (2002) Sex differences in striatal presynaptic dopamine synthesis capacity in healthy subjects. Biol Psychiatry 52: 759–763.
25. Parker BA, Sturm K, MacIntosh CG, Feinle C, Horowitz M, et al. (2004) Relation between food intake and visual analogue scale ratings of appetite and other sensations in healthy older and young subjects. Eur J Clin Nutr 58: 212–218.
26. Hare TA, Malmaud J, Rangel A (2011) Focusing attention on the health aspects of foods changes value signals in vmPFC and improves dietary choice. J Neurosci 31: 11077–11087.
27. Berridge KC (2009) 'Liking' and 'wanting' food rewards: brain substrates and roles in eating disorders. Physiol Behav 97: 537–550.
28. Goto Y, Otani S, Grace AA (2007) The Yin and Yang of dopamine release: a new perspective. Neuropharmacology 53: 583–587.
29. Stice E, Yokum S, Burger KS, Epstein LH, Small DM (2011) Youth at risk for obesity show greater activation of striatal and somatosensory regions to food. J Neurosci 31: 4360–4366.
30. Wallace DL, Vytlacil JJ, Nomura EM, Gibbs SE, D'Esposito M (2011) The dopamine agonist bromocriptine differentially affects fronto-striatal functional connectivity during working memory. Front Hum Neurosci 5: 32.
31. Mengarelli F, Spoglianti S, Avenanti A, di Pellegrino G (2013) Cathodal tDCS Over the Left Prefrontal Cortex Diminishes Choice-Induced Preference Change. Cereb Cortex.
32. Katan MB, Ludwig DS (2010) Extra calories cause weight gain—but how much? JAMA 303: 65–66.
33. Thanos PK, Michaelides M, Piyis YK, Wang GJ, Volkow ND (2008) Food restriction markedly increases dopamine D2 receptor (D2R) in a rat model of obesity as assessed with in-vivo muPET imaging ([11C] raclopride) and in-vitro ([3H] spiperone) autoradiography. Synapse 62: 50–61.

15

Urinary Sodium Excretion and Dietary Sources of Sodium Intake in Chinese Postmenopausal Women with Prehypertension

Zhao-min Liu[1]*, Suzanne C. Ho[2], Nelson Tang[1], Ruth Chan[1], Yu-ming Chen[3], Jean Woo[1]*

1 Department of Medicine &Therapeutics, the Chinese University of Hong Kong, Hong Kong Special Administrative Region, PR, China, **2** Division of Epidemiology, The Jockey Club School of Public Health and Primary Care, the Chinese University of Hong Kong, Hong Kong Special Administrative Region, PR, China, **3** Department of Medical Statistics and Epidemiology, School of Public Health, Sun Yat-sen University, Guangzhou, PR, China

Abstract

Background: Reducing salt intake in communities is one of the most effective and affordable public health strategies to prevent hypertension, stroke and renal disease. The present study aimed to determine the sodium intake in Hong Kong Chinese postmenopausal women and identify the major food sources contributing to sodium intake and urine excretion.

Methods: This was a cross-sectional study among 655 Chinese postmenopausal women with prehypertension who were screened for a randomized controlled trial. Data collection included 24 h urine collection for the measurement of sodium, potassium and creatinine, 3-day dietary records, anthropometric measures and questionnaire survey on demographic data and dietary habits.

Results: The average salt intake estimated from urinary excretion was 7.8±3.2 g/d with 82.1% women above WHO recommendation of 5 g/day. Food groups as soup (21.6%), rice and noodles (13.5%), baked cereals (12.3%), salted/preserved foods (10.8%), Chinese dim sum (10.2%) and sea foods (10.1%) were the major contributors of non-discretionary salt. Discretionary salt use in cooking made a modest contribution to overall intake. Vegetable and fruit intake, age, sodium intake from salted foods, sea foods and soup were the independent determinants of urinary sodium excretion.

Conclusions: Our data revealed a significant room for reduction of the sodium intake. Efforts to reduce sodium from diets in Hong Kong Chinese postmenopausal women should focus on both processed foods and discretionary salt during cooking. Sodium reduction in soup and increase in fruit intake would be potentially effective strategy for reducing sodium.

Editor: Pal Bela Szecsi, Gentofte University Hospital, Denmark

Funding: The study was funded by the Chinese University of Hong Kong Research Committee Direct Grant No. 2041783. The funders had no role in study design, data collection and analysis, decision to publish, or preparation of the manuscript.

Competing Interests: The authors have declared that no competing interests exist.

* Email: liuzhaomin@cuhk.edu.hk (ZML); jeanwoowong@cuhk.edu.hk (JW)

Introduction

Reducing salt intake in communities is one of the most effective and affordable public health strategies to prevent hypertension, decrease the risk of stroke, heart and renal diseases,the three major causes of mortality globally as well aslocally [1]. Elevated blood pressure (BP) may also aggravate the positive association between urinary sodium excretion and risk of coronary heart disease [2]. Despite campaigns that encourage reduced sodium intake, excessive consumption remains a major public health problem in most populations [3].

In addition to the sodium naturally present in foods and drinking water, other important sources of sodium in our diet come from the salt used during cooking or at the table (discretionary salt), salt added in processed foods, as well as non-salt sodium containing ingredients such as monosodium glutamate (MSG) (flavor enhancer), sodium nitrate (preservative) and sodium carbonate (tenderizers) etc. Dietary survey methods tend to underestimate sodium intakes since only a portion of sodium can be captured by dietary assessment. The timed 24-hour urinary sodium excretion is considered the gold standard method to estimate intake since 85–90% of ingested sodium is excreted through the kidneys and provide an estimate of total sodium intake from all sources.

Dietary sodium intake and the major sources vary among different regions and populations, largely determined by cultural preference [3]. Awareness of contemporaneous sodium intake and identification of food sources of sodium in diets will inform more specific tailoring of salt reduction policies in local population. However, studies estimating salt consumption using timed urine samples, characterizing the food groups to assess contributions to the source of sodium as well as the associations with urinary sodium excretion are limited in Asian population. No study had been conducted among postmenopausal women with pre-hypertension or early hypertension, a population at high risk of cardiovascular diseases (CVD), declining renal function as well as osteoporosis (the major adverse medical conditions [4] [5] [6] linked with excessive sodium intake). Furthermore, potassium has been recognized as a protective factor for hypertension [7] and a proposed modifier of the association between sodium intake and CVD [8]. However, studies on the potassium intake and the contribution to urinary potassium excretion are still limited.

Thus, understanding the sodium and potassium intake among high risk populations would have enormous public health implications. The major purpose of present study was to determine the sodium intake in Hong Kong Chinese postmenopausal women with prehypertension and identify the major food groups contributing to sodium and potassium intake and urine excretion. The study will provide the basis for public health initiatives to achieve population-wide reductions in salt intake.

Methods

The study protocol has been approved by the Ethical Research Committee of the Chinese University of Hong Kong (CRE Ref. No. 2012.201) and conducted according to the Declaration of Helsinki. Written informed consent has been obtained from all participants.

Subjects and recruitment

This was a cross-sectional study among 726 Chinese postmenopausal women who attended a screening visit for a randomized controlled trial testing the effect of soy products supplementation on BP. Subjects were recruited from the local community by advertisement in newspapers or health talks from April to Dec, 2011. Women after prescreening interview were invited to health center for an introduction talk and training for 24 h urine collection and 3 days dietary records.

Inclusion and exclusion criteria

Subjects were Hong Kong Chinese women aged 48–70 y; at least 1 year after the cessation of menstruation; with mean systolic BP 120~180 mmHg or diastolic BP above 80~100 mmHg or both. Subjects were excluded if they were on anti-hypertensive medication, hormone therapy or hypoglycemic agents in recent 3 months; medical history or presence of certain chronic diseases such as stroke, cardiac infarction, severe liver and renal diseases; breast or uterine or ovarian cancer or other malignancies in recent 5 years. More details regarding subjects recruitment were published elsewhere [9].

Twenty-four hours urine collection

Participants were provided with a standable and graduated urine collection bag and instructed on the method of 24 h urine collection. They were required to void their bladder before starting the collection and save all urines voided from that moment onwards for the following 24 h. Participants were asked about the completeness of urine collection and to record the starting and the final collection times. The total volume of urine was measured and mixed thoroughly before aliquots. Aliquoted urine samples were immediately frozen to −85°C until analysis.

Dietary survey, food groups and sodium intake calculation

We used 3-day food records questionnaire to estimate dietary nutrients intake. Food items were those most frequently consumed based on previous local surveys [10,11]. The food items and reference portion size (Chinese bowl) in our dietary records were similar to our previously validated one-week food frequency questionnaire [6]. Subjects received a 30-min training on estimation of food amounts, portion and utensil sizes. Three-day food diary was completed by subjects before the visit for urine submission and checked by trained research staff. Cooked dishes and non-commercial processed foods with multiple ingredients were disaggregated into individual food items. Dietary nutrients including energy, protein, total fat, cholesterol and fiber were calculated based on the China Food Composition Table [12].

From the 3-day dietary data, the sodium consumption of the following 15 food groups was calculated: rice and noodles; Chinese dim sum; baked cereals; preserved/salted foods; dairy products; animal meat; sea foods; vegetables; soy foods; fruits; nuts; chips and cookies; beverages; soups and others. Total sodium intake was calculated by summing the estimates from all contributory food items or groups. Sodium content in each food item was adopted from Chinese Composition Table [12] and a local food sodium database [13]. We also asked participants to estimate their domestic salt consumption per month, dietary habit on preserved vegetables, fried foods, roasted meat and pickled meat, as well as their salt taste preference (in comparison with general restaurants).

Demographic, anthropometric data and BP measurement

Individual information was collected by trained interviewers by face-to-face interview based on pretested and structured questionnaires on socio-demographic data, medical history, medication and dietary habits. Anthropometric measures such as body weight, height, waist and hip circumferences were performed according to standard protocols. BP was measured according to standard methods using a validated oscillometric technique (Omron M4-I Intellisense, Omron Corporation, Japan). Subjects were seated quietly for at least 5 minutes with the non-dominant arm supported at heart level. A cuff bladder encircling at least 80% of the arm was used to ensure accuracy. Two readings were obtained with 1 minute interval. A third BP was measured if more than 5 mmHg difference in systolic BP between two readings was noted, and the mean of the two closest was taken as the valid BP.

Urinary biochemical testing

Twenty four hours urine samples were obtained for measurement of sodium, potassium and creatinine. The analyses were performed on Hitachi 7101 automated analyzer (Japan) at a certified clinical lab. Urine sodium and potassium were measured by ion selective electrode methods, and creatinine was measured by enzymatic colorimetric assay. The intra and inter assay coefficients of variation (CV) were 0.42% and 1.69% for urinary sodium, 0.60% and 2.01% for urinary potassium, 1.25% and 2.17% for urinary creatinine. Urinary sodium excretion was analyzed as a proxy of salt intake (g/d) calculated by the equation: 24 h urine volume (L)×urinary sodium (mmol/L)×58.4 [3].

Statistical analysis

Analyses were performed using SPSS, version 17.0 (SPSS Inc., Chicago, IL, USA). $P<0.05$ was considered statistically significant. All variables were tested for normality using the Kolmogorov–Smirnov test and variables with skewed distribution were reported as median and quartiles. The relative contribution of food groups to the salt and potassium intake in diet were expressed as percentages. Pearson correlation and partial correlation (controlling for age, BMI and energy) analyses were performed to assess the correlations of sodium intake from various food groups with urinary sodium excretion and creatinine corrected sodium excretion (urinary sodium to creatinine ratio). Multiple linear regression analyses were used to evaluate the independent determinants of creatinine corrected urinary sodium excretion as well as urinary sodium to potassium ratio by inclusion of variables

Table 1. Characteristics of participants.

Characteristics	n	Mean±SD or number (%)
Age (y)	596	57.7±4.7
Age at menopause (y)	596	50.3±4.3
Years after menopause (y)	596	8.5±5.6
Body weight (kg)	596	56.2±9.0
BMI (kg/m^2)	596	23.2±3.3
WHR	596	0.837±0.049
SBP (mmHg)	596	136.9±19.4
DBP (mmHg)	596	82.9±10.6
Hypertension (%)		268 (45.2%)
Education	596	%
Primary school and below		128 (21.6%)
Middle school		358 (60.4%)
University and above		107 (18.0%)
Occupation	596	%
Housewife		291 (50.3%)
Part-time		135 (23.3%)
Full-time		153 (26.4%)
Dietary intake	655	
Total energy (kcal/d)		2033±186
Protein (g/d)		119±102
Fat (g/d)		41.0±22.2
Cholesterol (mg/d)		259.9±132.5
Dietary vegetable intake (rice bowl)		1.5±0.8
Dietary fruit intake (small bowl)		1.6±0.8
24 h urine collection and biochemical testing	655	
24 h urine volume (ml)		2082.4±633.6
Urine Na excretion (mmol/d)		133.9±55.5
Urine K excretion (mmol/d)		57.7±19.9
Urinary sodium to potassium molar ratio		2.44±0.96
Urine Cr excretion (mmol/d)		8.5±2.7

Data are presented as mean ± standard deviation for continuous variables or number (%) for categorical variables. BMI, body mass index; WHR, waist to hip ratio; SBP, systolic blood pressure; DBP, diastolic blood pressure; Hypertension: SBP≥140 mm Hg, DBP≥90 mm Hg, or both; Na, sodium; K, potassium; Cr, creatinine. Dietary analyses were from food frequency questionnaires. 1 rice bowl of vegetable is equal to 200 g; 1 small bowl of fruit is equal to 100 g.

displaying significant correlations with urinary sodium by a stepwise approach. Sensitivity analyses were performed by excluding women with potentially incomplete 24 h urine collection.

The level of agreement between total dietary salt intake (salt estimated from dietary records and additional salt in home cooking) and urinary salt excretion was assessed using the Bland and Altman method [14] to identify the mean difference between the two measures.

Results

Of the 726 women who attended the screening visit, 655 (90.2%) donated 24 h urine sample and provided 3-day dietary records, 596 (82.1%) completed anthropometric measures and questionnaire survey. Basic characteristics were indicated in **Table 1**. The mean age of the participants was 57.7±4.7 years. Of the 655 women who provided 24 h urine samples, 86 (13.1%) reported incompleteness with misses of 1–2 voids, 10 (1.5%) with total urine volume <1000 ml and 491 (74.8%) with urinary creatinine excretion in the normal range (7–18 μmol/24 h) [15]. We conducted several sensitivity analyses by excluding subjects with missed voids (n = 86) or subjects with 30% or higher coefficients of variation (n = 78) in weight corrected creatinine (Cr/Wt [16], 24 h creatinine excretion in milligrams divided by body weight in kilograms). However, there was no marked difference in the urinary salt excretion (7.6±2.9 and 7.8±3.1 g/d, respectively) in comparison with the uncorrected data (7.8±3.2 g/d).

Dietary habit and preference were indicated in **Table 2**. Most of the women (69.5%) favored light taste diet which is less salty than foods generally provided in restaurants. The average urinary salt excretion, dietary records estimated salt intake and self-reported additional salt intake were 7.8±3.2, 5.3±2.3 and 2.2±1.9 g/d respectively (**Table 3**). According to the estimates of urinary salt excretion, 17.9% women met the WHO target of < 5 g salt/d [17] and 31.6% met the China Nutrition Society target

Table 2. Dietary habit and taste preference among participants.

Dietary habit and preference	Mean±SD or number (%)
Numbers of dining out per month (not including breakfast)	11.2±10.1
Salt taste preference compared with general restaurants	
More salty	4 (7%)
Similar	25 (4.3%)
A little less salty	147 (25.5%)
Less salty	341 (59.2%)
Much less salty	55 (9.5%)
Almost no salt	4 (0.7%)
Preserved vegetables intake	
≥3 times/week	21 (3.7%)
1~2 times/week	42 (7.3%)
1~3 times/month	144 (25.1%)
2~11 times/yr	150 (26.2%)
<1 time/yr	216 (37.7%)
Fried foods intake	
≥3 times/week	50 (8.7%)
1~2 times/week	169 (29.4%)
1~3 times/month	187 (32.6%)
2~11 times/yr	102 (17.8%)
<1 time/yr	66 (11.5%)
Roasted meat intake	
≥3 times/week	38 (6.6%)
1~2 times/week	119 (20.8%)
1~3 times/month	222 (38.7%)
2~11 times/yr	124 (21.6%)
<1 time/yr	70 (12.2%)
Pickled meat/fish/sausages intake	
≥3 times/week	36 (6.3%)
1~2 times/week	95 (16.6%)
1~3 times/month	173 (30.2%)
2~11 times/yr	154 (26.9%)
<1 time/yr	115 (20.1%)
Regular alcohol drinking	56 (8.5%)
Regular tea drinking	454 (80.2%)
Regular coffee drinking	208 (36.8%)

Data are presented as mean ± standard deviation for continuous variables or number (%) for categorical variables. Regular drinking means drinking alcohol, tea or coffee more than 1 time per week.

of <6 g salt/d. The urinary potassium excretion and average dietary potassium intake were 2.3±0.8 and 4.2±4.1 g/d respectively.

Figure 1 indicated the percentiles of the food groups' contributions to dietary records estimated sodium consumption (non-discretionary salt). Of the 15 food groups, soup, rice and noodles, baked cereals, salted/preserved foods, Chinese dim sum and sea foods were the major contributors to non-discretionary salt. **Figure S1** indicated the percentiles of the food groups' contributions to dietary potassium intake. Rice and noodles, fruits and vegetables are the major contributors to the dietary potassium consumption.

Person correlation analyses (**Table 4**) indicated that creatinine corrected urinary sodium excretion was positively associated with total salt intake, sodium from Chinese dim sum, soup, preserved/salted foods and sea foods. Similar findings were observed when further controlling for age, body weight and total energy. While sodium from rice and noodles was negatively correlated with urinary sodium excretion, further adjustment for creatinine and other variables, the associations became statistically non-significant. Creatinine corrected urinary potassium excretion was also positively associated with dietary potassium intake ($r = 0.09$, $p = 0.04$) and the association remained significant after adjustment of age, BMI and total energy ($r = 0.10$, $p = 0.03$) (data not shown).

Table 3. Sodium and potassium intake estimated by dietary records and 24 h urinary excretion.

Salt and potassium intake estimation by dietary record and 24 h urinary estimation		
	Sodium (Salt, sodium chloride)	**Potassium**
24 h urinary excretion		
Mean±SD (g/d)	3.1±1.3 (7.8±3.2)	2.3±0. 8
Median (g/d)	3.0 (7.5)	2.1
25th~75th percentile (g/d)	2.2~3.7 (5.6~9.5)	1.7~2.6
<5 g salt/d	17.9%	-
<5.8 g salt/d	27.8%	-
<6 g salt/d	31.6%	-
>9 g salt/d	31.1%	-
Dietary records estimated intake		
Mean±SD (g/d)	2.1±0.9 (5.3±2.3)	4.2±4.1
Median (g/d)	2.0 (5.1)	4.0
25th~75th percentile (g/d)	1.5~2.5 (3.7~6.4)	2.4~6.1
Self-reported additional intake		
Mean±SD (g/d/person)	0.9±0.7 (2.2±1.9)	-
Median (g/d/person)	0.7 (1.7)	-
25th~75th percentile (g/d)	0.4±1.2 (0.9~3.0)	-

<5 g salt/d: WHO recommendation; <5.8 g salt/d (2300 mg sodium/d): American CDC and FDA recommendation; <6 g salt/d: Chinese Nutrition Society recommendation; The conversion factor of salt from g/d to mmol/d is to multiply 17.1.

Multiple linear stepwise regression analysis (**Table 5**) indicated that age, dietary vegetable intake, sodium from salted foods, soup and sea foods were positively, while total fruit intake were negatively associated with creatinine adjusted urinary salt excretion. Similar regression analysis on urinary sodium and potassium ratio (**Table S1**) indicated that BMI, sodium intake from salted foods and animal meat were positively, while dietary fruits intake, sodium intake from vegetables were negatively associated with urinary sodium and potassium ratio.

The 95% limit of agreement, defined as the mean difference between total dietary salt intake (non-discretional plus additional) and urinary salt excretion was −3.5 g (95% CI: −10.9 to 3.9 g).

Discussion

Salt intake estimated from 24 h urinary excretion indicated that most (>80%) Hong Kong Chinese postmenopausal women had salt consumption above WHO recommendation of 5 g/d [17]. Food groups such as soup, salted foods, Chinese dim sum and sea foods were the major contributors to urinary sodium excretion. Discretionary salt intake made a modest contribution to overall intake. The study presents a comprehensive overview on salt intake in Hong Kong Chinese postmenopausal women and provides the basis for public health initiatives on the primary targets for salt reduction at a population level.

In our report, urinary salt excretion was 7.8 g/d; however if approximately 15% non-renal loss [18] were to be included, the overall salt intake would be 9.0 g/d. Studies have estimated that decreasing salt intake from 10 g to 5 g per day would reduce overall stroke rate by 23% and CVD by 17% [19]. A recent meta-analysis reported a small salt reduction of 2.0–2.3 g/day was associated with a 20% decrease in cardiovascular events [20]. The favorable effect was even observed in normotensive population [21] [22]. If sodium intake of the population can be decreased, such important health gains can be achieved with relatively small economic commitment [23]. An economic modeling study estimated that 8.5 million cardiovascular deaths could be prevented over 10 years for a 15% (1.7 g/day) reduction in salt intake achievable with a low cost of US$0.40~1.00/person/year. With the high prevalence of hypertension in Chinese population and the heavy burden of CVD on health resources, reducing sodium intake would be an effective and affordable public health strategy.

Two international studies, INTERSALT (10079 men and women aged 20–59 y from 1985 to 1987) and INTERMAP (4680 men and women aged 40–59 years from 1996 to 1999) were by far the largest studies around the world with collection of standardized data on 24-hour urinary sodium excretion. INTERSALT [24] reported that the highest urinary sodium excretion were found in China, ranging up to 299 mmol/d (17.5 g salt/d) in men and 253 mmol/d (14.8 g salt/d) in women in the Beijing, northern China. The sodium excretion in southern China (Guangxi) was much lower with 150 mmol/d (8.8 g salt/d) in men and 128 mmol/d (7.5 g salt/d) in women. INTERMAP [25] investigated 3 counties in rural China and reported an average of sodium intake of 3.6 g/d (9.1 g salt/d) in the North and 2.5 g/d (6.35 g salt/d) in the South. Both studies reported that sodium intake in China was greatly above the international recommended intake and considerably varied by geographic regions. Our results in salt intake are in line with the data in South China. However, the two studies were conducted 20~30 years ago and did not include samples from urban areas of China.

A number of studies have been published since then giving data on sodium intake from different regions in China. However, most of the reports were based on dietary survey methods and studies without timed urine collections. The China Health and Nutrition Survey cohort [26] which included 16,869 adults aged 20–60 y from 1991 to 2009 reported that sodium intake is decreasing but remains double the Institute of Medicine recommendations (1.5 g sodium or 3.8 g salt/d). The study reported a lower proportion of

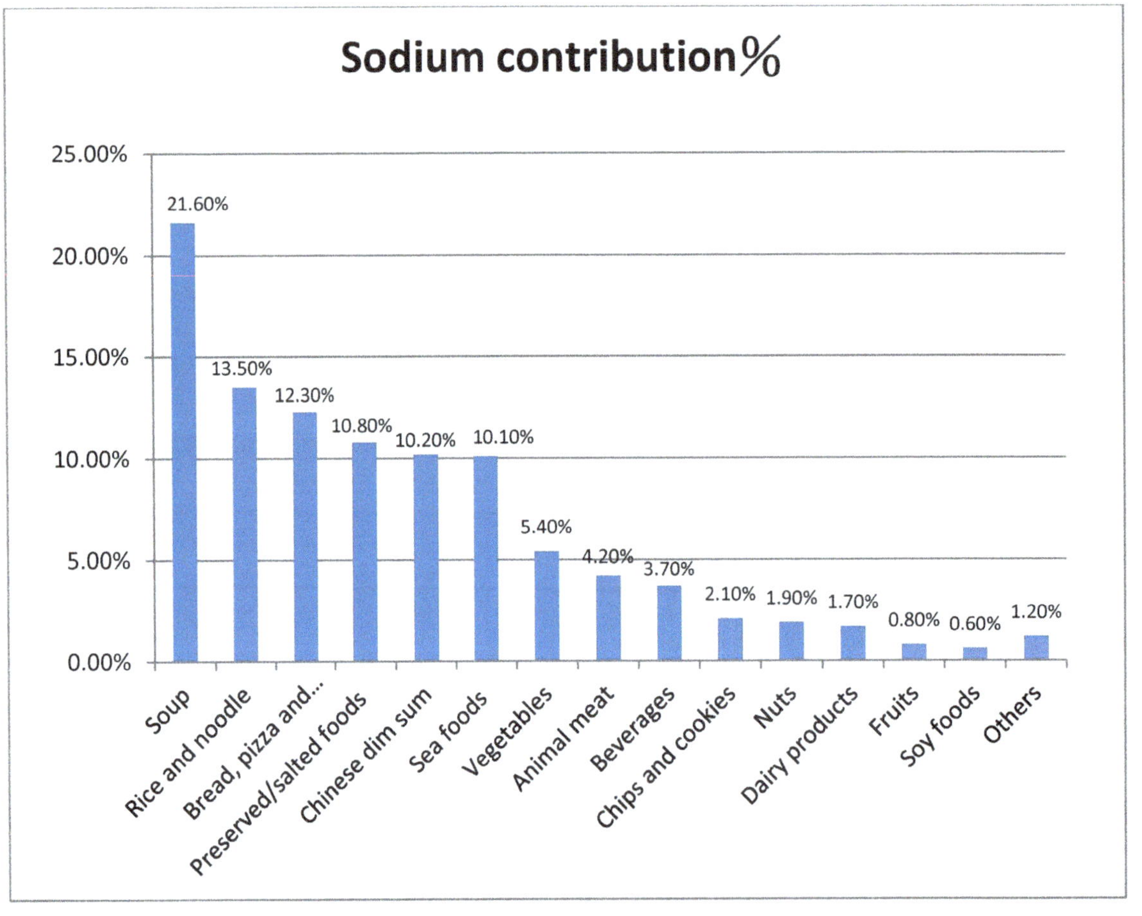

Food groups and non-discretionary dietary sodium intake were derived from 3-day food records. Sodium contribution expressed as percentage of total dietary sodium intake. For food groups, soup included canton soup and cream soup; baked cereals include bread, cake, pizza and hamburger etc.; Preserved/salted foods included preserved/salted /pickled vegetable, meat, fish etc..

Figure 1. Percentage contributions of food groups to non-discretionary dietary sodium intake. Food groups and non-discretionary dietary sodium intake were derived from 3-day food records. Sodium contribution expressed as percentage of total dietary sodium intake. For food groups, soup included canton soup and cream soup; baked cereals include bread, cake, pizza and hamburger etc.; Preserved/salted foods included preserved/salted/pickled vegetable, meat, fish etc.

sodium from added salt (69.7% in 2009) than in other studies. The sodium intake was 4.7 g/d (11.9 g salt) in 2009 and 4.4 g/d (11.2 g salt) in South China. However, the sodium intake in this study was estimated by 3 consecutive 24-h dietary recalls and condiments.

In 1995/96, the Hong Kong Adult Dietary Survey [27] interviewed a random sample of 1010 Chinese adults aged 25~74 and estimated the sodium intake by spot urinary excretion. Results showed that 78% of participants had a daily sodium intake of more than 2.3 g/d (5.8 g salt), and sodium intake increased with age with about 5.2 g/day (13.2 g salt/d) in men and 4.5 g/day (11.4 g salt/d) in women aged 55 and above. However, the study using spot urine to estimate sodium intake which could be less accurate than timed urine sample.

Our results in Hong Kong postmenopausal women indicated that the sodium intake in our study (7.8 g salt/d), while lower than several previous reports [26–28] in China, was still generally higher (>80%) than WHO recommendation [17]. The discrepancies between our results and other studies could be due to different methods for salt estimation and the different population characteristics investigated (such as region, age or health status etc.). For example, the participants in INTERMAP Chinese samples were from rural areas, younger than ours (49 vs 56) and less hypertensive patients (17%) than our subjects (45%).

In Asian countries (mainland China and Japan) [29,30], discretionary salt use accounted for most (>70%) sodium intake and only a small proportion of sodium is intrinsic in foods. In contrast, in European and Northern American diets [31,32], an estimated 75% of sodium intake comes from non-discretionary source such as processed or restaurant-prepared foods. Our study of source of salt intake among Hong Kong postmenopausal women showed that the pattern is intermediate between typical Asian and western diets. Our dietary survey showed that non-discretionary salt intake was 5.3 g/d accounting for 59% (5.3/9)

Table 4. Pearson correlations and partial correlations (controlling for age, weight and dietary energy) between salt intake and 24 h urinary sodium excretion.

	24 h Urinary Na excretion	Cr corrected Na excretion	Partial correlation with Cr corrected Na excretion
Salt taste preference#	−0.224**	−0.161**	−0.163**
Total salt intake†	0.112*	0.097*	0.088*
Self-estimated additional salt intake	0.064	0.050	0.061
Non-discretionary salt intake (dietary records)	0.090*	0.112*	0.116*
Dietary sodium from food groups			
Baked cereals	−0.049	−0.035*	0.054
Chinese dim sum	0.079*	0.087*	0.087*
Soup	0.026	0.083*	0.101*
Preserved/salted foods	0.113**	0.117**	0.116**
Sea foods	0.123**	0.128*	0.125*
Animal meat	0.073	0.028	0.035
Dairy products	−0.033	0.020	0.024
Chips and cookies	0.058	−0.036	−0.047
Soy foods	−0.011	−0.021	−0.050
Nuts	−0.055	−0.044	−0.042
Vegetables	−0.044	0.059	0.036
Fruits	−0.014*	0.026	0.052
Rice and noodles	−0.100*	0.010	0.014
Beverages	0.062	0.053	0.053

#The salt taste preference was in comparison with general restaurants, 1 to 5 categories corresponded to saltiest to least salty taste;
†Total salt intake was estimated from both non-discretionary salt (3 days dietary records) and discretionary salt (additional salt intake); Na, sodium; Cr, creatinine; Cr corrected Na excretion, urinary sodium to creatinine ratio;
*, $p<0.05$;
**, $P<0.01$.

total salt intake, thus the discretionary salt was estimated to be 41% (4.7 g/d). Since participants reported a 2.2 g/d additional salt in home cooking, the other discretionary sodium was likely from other condiments (soy sauce, MSG etc.) or non-salt sodium ingredients that we have not investigated. The relatively lower discretionary salt use in Hong Kong women compared with typical Asian diet could be due to the westernization of Hong Kong cultures, increasing consumption of western foods, processed foods and eating away from home. Thus, unlike strategies in many Asian and western countries, the efforts to reduce sodium from diets in Hong Kong population should focus on both non-discretionary salt such as processed foods and discretionary salt used during home cooking.

In our study, food groups such as soup, salted foods, Chinese dim sum, sea foods and baked cereals made major contributions to the non-discretionary sodium intake. The findings are similar to Japan [29], in which the major source of non-discretionary sodium was from commercially processed fish/seafood (15%), salted soups (15%) and preserved vegetables (13%). However, data from UK and USA [29,33] showed that cereal and meat products accounted

Table 5. Stepwise regression analysis with creatinine adjusted 24 h urine Na excretion as dependent variable and selected variables.

Variables	β	SE	P value
Dietary fruit intake	−1.200	0.323	0.001
Dietary vegetable intake	0.931	0.322	0.004
Sodium intake from sea foods	1.972	0.797	0.014
Sodium intake from salted foods	1.868	0.747	0.013
Sodium intake from soup	1.077	0.439	0.014
Age	0.121	0.055	0.029

BMI, body mass index; β, standardized coefficient; SE, standard error;
Only dependent variables with $P<0.05$ were shown. Variables excluded include: body mass index (BMI), dietary energy (by FFQ), dietary sodium intake from bread, Chinese dim sum, animal meat, rice and noodles, and self-reported additional salt intake.

for the greatest proportion (38%) of household sodium intake. The discrepancies in food groups' contributions could be due to the cultural difference in dietary pattern. In western countries, bread and meat are staple foods and made substantial contribution to dietary sodium [33], while in South China, Chinese dim sum, double-stewed soup, sea foods and salted fish and egg are popular in Cantonese cuisines and are the essential contributors to salt intake. However, in the regression model, only salted foods, soup and sea foods are independent contributory factors to urinary sodium excretion. One possible reason could be that Chinese dim sum and baked cereals are significantly related with total energy intake, so that these variables become non-significant to the overall model when adjusting for energy and BMI.

In the regression model, we observed that fruit intake was negatively while vegetable intake was positively associated with urinary sodium excretion. The possible reason could be related to the colinearity of some dietary components. The Chinese style of cooking vegetables involves liberal use of salt, which would increase urinary salt excretion. At the same time fruits contains higher amount of potassium which may ameliorate the negative impact of salt intake [34]. Our study provided evidence that decrease additional salt in vegetable dishes and increase fruit intake could be effective in sodium reduction.

The observed correlation coefficient ($r = 0.11$, $p<0.01$) between sodium intake estimated from 3-day dietary records and urinary sodium excretion in our study was lower than INTERMAP study ($r = 0.42$), but is still similar to studies in Finland women [35] ($r = 0.13$) and African adults ($r = 0.15$) [36]. The relative weak correlation of dietary sodium intake and urinary excretion may be explained by measurement error of dietary assessment, the single instead of multiple 24 h urine collection, variable excretion rates, and sodium losses through other metabolic pathways such as sweat and feces etc. [37]. Error in sodium intake estimated from dietary survey may occur due to inaccurate reporting, day-to-day variation or omission of added salt or other condiments during cooking or at the table.

In contrast with the underestimation of sodium intake using urinary sodium collection, dietary estimates of potassium intake often exceeded those of urinary collection which was also suggested in our data. This is because 15~20% of potassium is lost in the feces and another portion is excreted from sweat [37]. Compared with previous urinary data in Chinese population [38,39], our subjects had a relatively lower urinary sodium/potassium ratio (2.4 vs 3.4 [39]) and higher potassium excretion (2.3 vs 1.9 g/24 h [38]). The relatively high potassium excretion and intake in our study might be explained by the fact that our participants were at high risk of hypertension and might be following medical advice in restricting sodium intake and increasing fruits and vegetable intake.

To our knowledge, this is the first study in Hong Kong to report findings on the major dietary sources contributing to dietary and urinary sodium and potassium. The study evaluated the characteristics of sodium and potassium intake in a population with high risk for hypertension and other chronic diseases such as CVD, declining renal function and osteoporosis. The population may benefit significantly from the reduction in sodium intake. The other strengths include the relatively large number of participants with 24 h urinary based estimates of sodium and potassium intake, high completeness of urine collection, the availability of detailed covariates to adjust for a range of potential confounders. In addition, none of the participants were on antihypertensive treatment, which may confound the relationship between intake and urinary mineral excretion and therefore reverse causation seemed unlikely.

The present study has several limitations. First, dietary survey in estimation of sodium and potassium intake is prone to a number of errors. Accurate measurement of sodium and potassium intake by dietary survey is difficult due to extensive sodium and potassium distribution in foods, and widespread use of salt or sodium compounds in food processing [31,40]. As with 3-day food records, the included food items may not necessarily be inclusive of all the sources of sodium and potassium. The other specific sources of error in sodium include: difficulties in estimating the amount of sodium added during cooking; variation in the proportion of salt retained in food; salt loss in cooking water or left behind on the plate [31]; variation in the sodium content of manufactured foods [13]. In addition, we did not specifically investigate the consumption of other condiments except for salt, such as soy sauce, MSG etc. in cooking or at the table.

Second, urinary sodium was assessed by a single 24 h urine collection and a possible regression dilution bias may be introduced due to the daily individual variability. However, a single urine measurement is considered a more accurate measure of sodium intake at a population level [41], though possibly less accurate for individuals.

Third, our study was conducted among Chinese postmenopausal women with prehypertension. Thus, the findings may not be extrapolated to the broader populations. The participants were aware of their elevated BP and willing to register for a randomized controlled trial. This population is likely to be more health consciousness in following medical advice to reduce their dietary sodium intake [31]. However, the urinary sodium data still revealed that more than 80% women had excess salt intake above WHO recommendation. The data is likely to be higher in sodium intake among general population. In addition, our participants were mainly housewives and responsible for cooking for family. Thus, health promotion regarding salt intake and health effort targeting women of this group may be effective in community in salt reduction.

Conclusions

Our data in Hong Kong Chinese postmenopausal women with prehypertension revealed that most women had salt consumption above the international recommendation, suggesting a significant room for reduction of the sodium intake. Efforts to reduce sodium from diets in this population should focus on both discretional salt uses during home cooking and processed foods such as Chinese dim sum, salted foods, and baked cereals etc. Sodium reduction in soup and increase in fruit intake would be potentially effective strategy for reducing sodium. Further studies are necessary in other life stage of populations to provide definitive data on salt intake, and to act as a baseline against which to monitor the impact of future salt reduction initiatives.

Supporting Information

Figure S1 Percentage contributions of food groups to dietary potassium intake. Food groups and dietary potassium intake were derived from 3-day food records. Potassium contribution expressed as percentage of total dietary potassium intake. For food groups, soup included canton soup and cream soup; baked cereals include bread, cake, pizza and hamburger etc.; Preserved/salted foods included preserved/salted/pickled vegetable, meat, fish etc.

Table S1 Stepwise regression analysis with urinary Na/K ratio as dependent variable and selected variables.

BMI, body mass index; β, standardized coefficient; SE, standard error; Only dependent variables with $P<0.05$ were shown. Variables excluded include: age, dietary energy, sodium intake from soup, baked cereals, sea foods, Chinese dim sum, fruits, rice and noodles.

Acknowledgments

We are indebted to our study participants and our research assistant Miss Anna Tsang. Without their effort this investigation would not have been possible.

Author Contributions

Conceived and designed the experiments: JW ZML SCH RC. Performed the experiments: ZML. Analyzed the data: ZML. Contributed reagents/materials/analysis tools: NT YMC. Wrote the paper: ZML.

References

1. Meneton P, Jeunemaitre X, de Wardener HE, MacGregor GA (2005) Links between dietary salt intake, renal salt handling, blood pressure, and cardiovascular diseases. Physiol Rev 85: 679–715.
2. Joosten MM, Gansevoort RT, Mukamal KJ, Lambers Heerspink HJ, Geleijnse JM, et al. (2014) Sodium excretion and risk of developing coronary heart disease. Circulation 129: 1121–1128.
3. Brown IJ, Tzoulaki I, Candeias V, Elliott P (2009) Salt intakes around the world: implications for public health. Int J Epidemiol 38: 791–813.
4. Forman JP, Scheven L, de Jong PE, Bakker SJ, Curhan GC, et al. (2012) Association between sodium intake and change in uric acid, urine albumin excretion, and the risk of developing hypertension. Circulation 125: 3108–3116.
5. Massey LK, Whiting SJ (1995) Dietary salt, urinary calcium, and kidney stone risk. Nutr Rev 53: 131–139.
6. Ho SC, Chen YM, Woo JL, Leung SS, Lam TH, et al. (2001) Sodium is the leading dietary factor associated with urinary calcium excretion in Hong Kong Chinese adults. Osteoporos Int 12: 723–731.
7. Koliaki C, Katsilambros N (2013) Dietary sodium, potassium, and alcohol: key players in the pathophysiology, prevention, and treatment of human hypertension. Nutr Rev 71: 402–411.
8. Morris RC Jr, Schmidlin O, Frassetto LA, Sebastian A (2006) Relationship and interaction between sodium and potassium. J Am Coll Nutr 25: 262S–270S.
9. Liu Z-m, Ho SC, Chen Y-m, Woo J (2013) A Six-Month Randomized Controlled Trial of Whole Soy and Isoflavones Daidzein on Body Composition in Equol-Producing Postmenopausal Women with Prehypertension. Journal of Obesity 2013: 9.
10. Woo J, Leung SSF, Ho SC, Lam TH, Janus ED (1997) A food frequency questionnaire for use in the Chinese population in Hong Kong: Description and examination of validity. Nutrition Research 17: 1633–1641.
11. Ho SC, Donnan S, Sham A (1988) Dietary intake among elderly Chinese in Hong Kong. Journal of Human Nutrition and Dietetics 1: 205–215.
12. Yue-xin Y (2002) China Food Composition 2002. Institute of Nutrition and Food Safety. Beijing, PR China Peking University Medical Press.
13. Centre for Food Safety (2012) Study on Sodium Content in Local Foods. Hong Kong: Centre for Food Safety, Food and Environmental Hygiene Department, The Government of the Hong Kong Special Administrative Region.
14. Bland JM, Altman DG (1986) Statistical methods for assessing agreement between two methods of clinical measurement. Lancet 1: 307–310.
15. Siersbaek-Nielsen K, Hansen JM, Kampmann J, Kristensen M (1971) Rapid evaluation of creatinine clearance. Lancet 1: 1133–1134.
16. Cook NR, Appel LJ, Whelton PK (2014) Lower levels of sodium intake and reduced cardiovascular risk. Circulation 129: 981–989.
17. World Heatlh Organization (October, 2010) Strategies to monitor and evaluate population sodium consumption and sources of sodium in the diet. Geneva (CHE): WHO.
18. Ovesen L, Boeing H (2002) The use of biomarkers in multicentric studies with particular consideration of iodine, sodium, iron, folate and vitamin D. Eur J Clin Nutr 56 Suppl 2: S12–17.
19. Cook NR, Cutler JA, Obarzanek E, Buring JE, Rexrode KM, et al. (2007) Long term effects of dietary sodium reduction on cardiovascular disease outcomes: observational follow-up of the trials of hypertension prevention (TOHP). BMJ 334: 885–888.
20. He FJ, MacGregor GA (2011) Salt reduction lowers cardiovascular risk: meta-analysis of outcome trials. Lancet 378: 380–382.
21. He FJ, MacGregor GA (2002) Effect of modest salt reduction on blood pressure: a meta-analysis of randomized trials. Implications for public health. J Hum Hypertens 16: 761–770.
22. He FJ, MacGregor GA (2003) How far should salt intake be reduced? Hypertension 42: 1093–1099.
23. Asaria P, Chisholm D, Mathers C, Ezzati M, Beaglehole R (2007) Chronic disease prevention: health effects and financial costs of strategies to reduce salt intake and control tobacco use. Lancet 370: 2044–2053.
24. Stamler J (1997) The INTERSALT Study: background, methods, findings, and implications. Am J Clin Nutr 65: 626S–642S.
25. Zhao L, Stamler J, Yan LL, Zhou B, Wu Y, et al. (2004) Blood pressure differences between northern and southern Chinese: role of dietary factors: the International Study on Macronutrients and Blood Pressure. Hypertension 43: 1332–1337.
26. Du S, Neiman A, Batis C, Wang H, Zhang B, et al. (2013) Understanding the patterns and trends of sodium intake, potassium intake, and sodium to potassium ratio and their effect on hypertension in China. Am J Clin Nutr.
27. Woo J (1998) Nutrition and health issues in the general Hong Kong population. Hong Kong Med J 4: 383–388.
28. (2011) China NCD Report 2011. Beijing, China: Bureau of Disease Control and Prevention MOH and China CDC.
29. Anderson CA, Appel LJ, Okuda N, Brown IJ, Chan Q, et al. (2010) Dietary sources of sodium in China, Japan, the United Kingdom, and the United States, women and men aged 40 to 59 years: the INTERMAP study. J Am Diet Assoc 110: 736–745.
30. Zhai FY, XG Y (2006) Part 2: diet and nutrition intake (in Chinese). Report of National Nutrition and Health Survey of China Residents in 2002. Beijing: People's Health Press.
31. James WP, Ralph A, Sanchez-Castillo CP (1987) The dominance of salt in manufactured food in the sodium intake of affluent societies. Lancet 1: 426–429.
32. Mattes RD, Donnelly D (1991) Relative contributions of dietary sodium sources. J Am Coll Nutr 10: 383–393.
33. Webster JL, Dunford EK, Neal BC (2010) A systematic survey of the sodium contents of processed foods. Am J Clin Nutr 91: 413–420.
34. Weaver CM (2013) Potassium and health. Adv Nutr 4: 368S–377S.
35. Reinivuo H, Valsta LM, Laatikainen T, Tuomilehto J, Pietinen P (2006) Sodium in the Finnish diet: II Trends in dietary sodium intake and comparison between intake and 24-h excretion of sodium. Eur J Clin Nutr 60: 1160–1167.
36. Charlton KE, Steyn K, Levitt NS, Jonathan D, Zulu JV, et al. (2008) Development and validation of a short questionnaire to assess sodium intake. Public Health Nutr 11: 83–94.
37. Espeland MA, Kumanyika S, Wilson AC, Reboussin DM, Easter L, et al. (2001) Statistical issues in analyzing 24-hour dietary recall and 24-hour urine collection data for sodium and potassium intakes. Am J Epidemiol 153: 996–1006.
38. O'Donnell MJ, Yusuf S, Mente A, Gao P, Mann JF, et al. (2011) Urinary sodium and potassium excretion and risk of cardiovascular events. JAMA 306: 2229–2238.
39. Kwok TC, Chan TY, Woo J (2003) Relationship of urinary sodium/potassium excretion and calcium intake to blood pressure and prevalence of hypertension among older Chinese vegetarians. Eur J Clin Nutr 57: 299–304.
40. Sanchez-Castillo CP, Warrender S, Whitehead TP, James WP (1987) An assessment of the sources of dietary salt in a British population. Clin Sci (Lond) 72: 95–102.
41. Luft FC, Fineberg NS, Sloan RS (1982) Estimating dietary sodium intake in individuals receiving a randomly fluctuating intake. Hypertension 4: 805–808.

16

How State Taxes and Policies Targeting Soda Consumption Modify the Association between School Vending Machines and Student Dietary Behaviors

Daniel R. Taber[1]*, Jamie F. Chriqui[1], Renee Vuillaume[2], Frank J. Chaloupka[1,3]

1 Institute for Health Research and Policy, University of Illinois at Chicago, Chicago, Illinois, United States of America, **2** John F. Kennedy School of Government, Harvard University, Cambridge, Massachusetts, United States of America, **3** Department of Economics, University of Illinois at Chicago, Chicago, Illinois, United States of America

Abstract

Background: Sodas are widely sold in vending machines and other school venues in the United States, particularly in high school. Research suggests that policy changes have reduced soda access, but the impact of reduced access on consumption is unclear. This study was designed to identify student, environmental, or policy characteristics that modify the associations between school vending machines and student dietary behaviors.

Methods: Data on school vending machine access and student diet were obtained as part of the National Youth Physical Activity and Nutrition Study (NYPANS) and linked to state-level data on soda taxes, restaurant taxes, and state laws governing the sale of soda in schools. Regression models were used to: 1) estimate associations between vending machine access and soda consumption, fast food consumption, and lunch source, and 2) determine if associations were modified by state soda taxes, restaurant taxes, laws banning in-school soda sales, or student characteristics (race/ethnicity, sex, home food access, weight loss behaviors.)

Results: Contrary to the hypothesis, students tended to consume 0.53 fewer servings of soda/week (95% CI: -1.17, 0.11) and consume fast food on 0.24 fewer days/week (95% CI: -0.44, -0.05) if they had in-school access to vending machines. They were also less likely to consume soda daily (23.9% vs. 27.9%, average difference = -4.02, 95% CI: -7.28, -0.76). However, these inverse associations were observed primarily among states with lower soda and restaurant tax rates (relative to general food tax rates) and states that did not ban in-school soda sales. Associations did not vary by any student characteristics except for weight loss behaviors.

Conclusion: Isolated changes to the school food environment may have unintended consequences unless policymakers incorporate other initiatives designed to discourage overall soda consumption.

Editor: Andrea S. Wiley, Indiana University, United States of America

Funding: Support for this research was provided by the Robert Wood Johnson Foundation to the Bridging the Gap program located within the Health Policy Center at the University of Illinois at Chicago (PI: Frank Chaloupka), and by grant number 4R00HD073271-02 from the National Institute of Child Health and Human Development (PI: Daniel Taber). The views expressed herein are solely those of the authors and do not reflect the official views or positions of the Robert Wood Johnson Foundation, the National Institute of Child Health and Human Development, or the National Institutes of Health. The funders had no role in study design, data collection and analysis, decision to publish, or preparation of the manuscript.

Competing Interests: The authors have declared that no competing interests exist.

* Email: Daniel.Taber@uth.tmc.edu

Introduction

Sugar-sweetened beverage (SSB) consumption has become one of the primary targets of childhood obesity prevention efforts in the United States (U.S.) [1]. The negative health effects of SSB consumption are well-documented [2,3], including recent randomized trials that found SSB consumption was associated with higher weight gain [4,5]. Sodas are the most popular SSB among adolescents in the U.S. [6,7] and were the biggest source of calories of any food/beverage group among 14–18 year-olds in 2005–06 [8]. Recent evidence suggests that adolescents have gradually been replacing soda with other SSBs, but soda remains the most heavily consumed sweetened beverage [6].

Numerous policy initiatives have been proposed to reduce consumption of soda and other SSBs, including taxes, marketing regulations, limits on portion sizes, and limits on sugar content [9–12]. One of the most widespread initiatives is banning the sale of SSBs within schools [13,14]. Evidence at all grade levels suggests that policies that ban SSBs have succeeded in reducing students' access to SSBs [15–18], though policies at the high school level tend to focus exclusively on soda. Nationally, the proportion of high school students who could purchase soda in school declined steadily from 53.6% in 2006–07 to 25.3% in 2010–11, but most high school students could purchase some type of SSB in school in 2010–11 (87.8%) [19].

Policies have achieved their direct goal of reducing SSB access, but there is relatively little evidence that such changes influence students' consumption of soda or overall SSBs. Several studies reported that consumption was unaffected [16,20–22] even if policies reduced in-school access [16]. These studies utilized several independent data sources that sampled students nationwide. In contrast, however, studies in specific states or districts reported that sweetened beverage restrictions succeeded in reducing sweetened beverage intake [23,24].

These inconsistent findings could be explained by numerous demographic, behavioral, environmental, or policy characteristics. Previous studies have already suggested that the effects of policies on student behavior may be modified by race/ethnicity [21,22], or whether the policy targets SSBs other than soda [16] and whether it targets all school venues [24,25]. Additionally, experts have pointed out that students can easily obtain SSBs from other sources (e.g., home, convenience stores) [10,20,26] and thus improvements to the school food environment may be less successful among students who have more access outside of school. The impact of school nutrition policies could also depend on whether school-based changes are complemented by policies in other sectors (e.g., soda taxes). Finally, health consciousness could play a role, as a recent study of calorie labels found that this initiative was more effective among consumers who were less health conscious [27].

To enhance school policy effectiveness, policymakers must consider how effects are modified by factors at the individual, local, or state level. The objective of this study was to determine if the association between school vending machine access and soda consumption varies by demographic, environmental, or policy measures in a nationally representative sample of high school students. We further analyzed dietary behaviors outside of school (e.g., fast food consumption) to assess whether students who do not have access to vending machines in school obtain more unhealthy foods/beverages elsewhere.

Methods

This cross-sectional study linked student data from the National Youth Physical Activity and Nutrition Study (NYPANS), conducted by the Centers for Disease Control and Prevention (CDC) in Spring 2010, with state-level data on soda taxes, restaurant taxes, and laws governing the sale of soda in schools, collected as part of the Bridging the Gap (BTG) research program. The study was approved by the Institutional Review Boards of the University of Illinois at Chicago and the University of Texas Health Science Center at Houston.

Student sample

The objective of NYPANS was to measure diet, physical activity, and sedentary behaviors, and environmental determinants of such behaviors, in a nationally representative of 9th–12th grade students [28]. Students were sampled using a 3-stage cluster sample design; school and student participation was voluntary, and local permission procedures were followed. The school response rate was 82%, the student response rate was 88%, and the overall response rate was 73%. In total, 10887 public school students participated in NYPANS.

For the purpose of our study, students were excluded because they were missing data on vending machine access within school (n = 691), soda consumption (n = 42), fast food consumption (n = 10), lunch source (n = 496), or other variables of interest (n = 209), or if they were unsure if vending machines that sold sweetened beverages were available in school (n = 1194). Students who were excluded did not differ from the study sample with respect to weight status, soda consumption, or gender, but they were more likely to be racial/ethnic minorities ($p<0.001$), tended to be in lower grade levels ($p<0.001$), were less likely to have access to vending machines ($p<0.001$), were more likely to obtain lunch away from home/school ($p = 0.02$) and reported more fast food intake ($p<0.001$). The final study sample included 8245 students in 27 states.

Student-level measures

All data were obtained using a written questionnaire completed in class. The independent variable of interest was whether the school had "a vending machine that students can use to purchase soda or pop, sports drinks, or fruit drinks that are not 100% juice, such as Coke, Gatorade, or Sunny Delight?" Hereafter, we use the term "vending machines" to refer specifically to this type of vending machine.

Our dependent variables of interest were soda consumption, fast food consumption, and whether students obtained their lunch away from home or school on schooldays. We focused only on soda, not other SSBs, because soda has been the primary target of policy changes on the high school level. Soda consumption was modeled as both a continuous measure of the number of servings consumed in the past 7 days (ranging from none to "4 or more per day") and a binary measure of whether students consumed at least one soda per day in the past 7 days (hereafter referred to as "daily consumption"). The questionnaire explicitly told students to report consumption of diet soda separately; analyses in this study only utilized data on regular soda consumption. Fast food was modeled as a continuous measure of the number of days in which students consumed fast food in the past 7 days. Students were instructed to include consumption of soda and fast food from all sources regardless of time or location.

Analyses for this study also utilized data on race/ethnicity, sex, grade, availability of food at home, and weight loss behaviors. Students' race/ethnicity was categorized as non-Hispanic White (ref), non-Hispanic Black, Hispanic, and non-Hispanic Other. Home food access was categorized based on whether students usually or always had access to fruits/vegetables or unhealthy snacks ("chips, cookies, or cake") at home; we cross-classified students as having access to fruits/vegetables only (ref), unhealthy snacks only, both, or neither. Weight loss behaviors were measured using a series of 10 questions that asked students if they had tried to lose weight in the past 30 days through various behaviors. For our purpose, we classified 5 of the 10 behaviors as healthy (exercising, consuming less food or fewer high-fat foods, consuming fewer calories, consuming more fruits/vegetables, drinking more water) and the remaining 5 as unhealthy (skipping meals, fasting, smoking, vomiting or taking laxatives, taking diet pills/powders/liquids without a doctor's advice). Note that these classifications reflect the general health of the behaviors, not the behaviors' effectiveness as weight loss methods. Students were then grouped into 3 mutually exclusive categories of weight loss behavior – those trying to lose weight only through healthy behaviors, those trying to lose weight through at least one unhealthy behavior, and those not trying to lose weight.

We considered analyzing whether the association between vending machine access and dietary behaviors varied by weight status (normal weight, overweight, obese) based on height and weight data obtained by CDC staff. However, this analysis was dropped because the quantity of missing height/weight data was relatively large and exploratory analyses suggested that the associations of interest did not vary by weight status.

State data

The study included analyses of whether the associations of interest varied by state tax rates for soda sold in grocery stores, state tax rates for foods sold in restaurants, or state laws governing the availability of soda in all school venues. Tax rates were compiled from state statutory and administrative law using primary legal research methods [29,30] and were confirmed by the state [31,32]. They were modeled as a continuous measure of the difference between soda/restaurant tax rates versus the general food tax rates (i.e., "disfavored" amount) [33]. Laws regarding the availability of soda in high school vending machines, school stores, and cafeterias (a la carte) in the 2009–10 school year were obtained from the Westlaw and Lexis-Nexis legal research databases and verified against secondary sources [34–36]. Laws for the 3 venues were combined to create one binary indicator of whether the state prohibited soda in all 3 venues. Of the 27 states that were sampled as part of NYPANS, eight banned soda in high schools in the 2009–10 school year; of these 8, four states implemented the ban starting in 2009–10 and four states implemented the ban prior to 2009–10. We explored categorizing states based on the length of their ban, but judged that the sample sizes were insufficient for such an analysis.

Both the state tax rate data and the state laws governing soda availability in schools were compiled by the Bridging the Gap research program at the University of Illinois at Chicago.

Statistical analysis

Due to their respective distributions, the 4 dependent variables were analyzed using different types of regression models – a negative binomial model for total servings of soda in the past 7 days, a Poisson model for fast food consumption in the past 7 days, and a logistic model for daily soda consumption and lunch source. All analyses accounted for the complex sampling design in NYPANS and utilized the 'margin' command in Stata, Version 12, to calculate the average marginal effects (AME) of interest.

First, we estimated the association between vending machine access and each dependent variable. Students with no access to school vending machines were the referent, and thus the parameters of interest were hypothesized to be positive (e.g., higher soda consumption in students with access to school vending machines). These models controlled for race/ethnicity, sex, grade, home food access, state median household income (obtained from the 2010 Census), and Census region (Northeast, Midwest, South, West).

Subsequently, we added interaction terms between vending machine access and race/ethnicity, sex, grade, home food access, weight loss behaviors, disfavored soda tax (when modeling soda), disfavored restaurant tax (when modeling fast food and lunch source), and state law banning soda in all school venues. Interaction terms for each variable were modeled separately. When modeling interactions with variables that were not in the original model (e.g., soda tax), the main effect of these variables was also added. Weight loss behavior was initially modeled as a 3-category variable, as described earlier, but we combined 2 of the categories – students who were trying to lose weight through unhealthy behaviors and students who were not trying to lose weight – after analyses revealed that the associations of interest were virtually identical in these 2 groups. When modeling interactions with state taxes and state soda bans, Census region was modeled as a 3-category variable (South/Midwest, Northeast, West) due to the limited distributions of region within categories of state taxes/laws. Home food access was removed from models that included state soda taxes because it may mediate any effect of taxes on soda consumption.

One state, Colorado, was excluded from all analyses of lunch source because it had an extraordinarily high proportion of students who obtained lunch away from school or home (42.0%, versus 6.1% in the remaining sample) and had unusually high leverage as a result.

Results

Table 1 displays characteristics of the study sample overall and by vending machine access. Nearly all categorical measures had similar distributions regardless of vending machine access. The exception was that students with vending machines were more likely to be from the Midwest (30.0%) and less likely to be from the Northeast (11.1%) relative to students without vending machines (15.8% and 24.9%, respectively.) Students without vending machines were less likely to be obese but more likely to be overweight, and they reported slightly more servings of fast food and soda, relative to students with vending machines.

The adjusted associations between vending machine access and soda consumption, fast food consumption, and lunch source are displayed in Table 2. The negative associations indicate that, contrary to the hypothesis, overall soda and fast food consumption were lower among students who had access to vending machines in school. Most notably, students were less likely to report consuming at least 1 soda per day if they had access to school vending machines (23.9%) compared to those who did not have access (27.9%). Students also reported eating fast food on fewer days per week, on average, if they had access to school vending machines (1.82 versus 2.06, AME = -0.24, 95% CI: -0.44, -0.05). They were slightly less likely to obtain a lunch away from home or school, but the difference was more modest.

The associations represented in Table 2 were consistently modified by state tax rates and, to a lesser degree, state laws regarding soda sales in school (Table 3). Results suggested that the unexpected negative associations in Table 2 were generally limited to students in states with no disfavored taxes – i.e., states that taxed soda and restaurant food at the same rate as other foods. For example, in states with no disfavored soda tax, vending machine access was associated with 1.14 fewer servings of soda per week (95% CI: -1.92, -0.36), but this difference became progressively smaller as tax rates increased. The implications of this are displayed in Figure 1. In short, model estimates predict that the inverse association between vending machine access and soda consumption is eliminated if the state tax rate for soda exceeded the general food tax rate by 7.25% (the maximum amount in the study sample.) Similar patterns were observed across all four outcomes.

Similar patterns were also observed when modeling the interaction between vending machine access and state laws banning soda in all venues. In the lower portion of Table 3, the "main effect" of vending machine access represents the association between access and the outcomes of interest in states that did not ban soda; for example, the probability of students drinking soda every day was 6.23 percentage points lower if they had access to vending machines (95% CI: -9.52, -2.93), relative to students without access, in states with no ban. However, the interaction between vending machine access and in-school soda ban was of approximately the same magnitude (AME = 5.79, 95% CI: 0.00, 11.6), essentially meaning that the inverse association between vending machine access and daily consumption was eliminated in states that banned soda. The same pattern was observed for fast food consumption and lunch source – i.e., the inverse "main effect" of vending machine access was balanced by the interaction

Table 1. Descriptive statistics of study sample, National Youth Physical Activity and Nutrition Study.

Variable	Overall	Vending machine [a] Yes	Vending machine [a] No
N	8245	6467	1909
Sex (%)			
Female	49.1	49.1	49.0
Race/ethnicity (%)			
Non-Hispanic White	58.7	60.2	52.8
Non-Hispanic Black	14.6	14.3	15.6
Hispanic	18.3	17.0	23.2
Non-Hispanic Other	8.5	8.5	8.3
Census region			
South	37.2	37.6	35.7
Northeast	13.9	11.1	24.9
Midwest	27.1	30.0	15.8
West	21.9	21.4	23.6
Weight status			
Overweight (%)	18.0	17.6	19.3
Obese (%)	18.9	19.9	15.3
BMI percentile (mean)	64.2	64.5	63.2
Dietary behaviors			
Servings of soda/week (mean)	5.3	5.3	5.6
Days of fast food/week (mean)	1.9	1.8	2.0
Weight loss behavior (%)			
Not trying to lose weight	29.2	29.0	30.0
Healthy weight loss behaviors	43.2	43.3	42.7
Unhealthy weight loss behaviors	27.6	27.7	27.3
Home food access (%)			
Fruits/vegetables	31.9	31.0	35.5
Unhealthy snacks	13.1	13.0	13.5
Both	37.3	38.5	32.6
Neither	17.7	17.6	18.4
Where students obtain lunch (%)			
None	7.0	6.7	8.4
Home	20.0	20.4	18.5
School	67.0	67.3	65.8
Elsewhere	6.0	5.6	7.2

[a]School vending machine that sells "soda or pop, sports drinks, or fruit drinks that are not 100% juice, such as Coke, Gatorade, or Sunny Delight"

Table 2. Adjusted measures of student soda/fast food consumption and lunch source, by school vending machine access [a].

	Vending machine access in school Yes	Vending machine access in school No	AME [b]	95% CI	p
Soda servings per week (mean)	5.27	5.80	-0.53	-1.17, 0.11	0.11
Daily soda consumption (%)	23.9	27.9	-4.02	-7.28, -0.76	0.02
Days of fast food per week (mean)	1.82	2.06	-0.24	-0.44, -0.05	0.01
Lunch obtained away from home/school (%)	5.15	7.19	-2.03	-4.59, 0.52	0.12

[a]Adjusted for race/ethnicity, age, sex, state median income, Census region, and home food access.
[b]AME = Average marginal effect; represents average difference associated with the presence of vending machines that sell sugar-sweetened beverages in school.

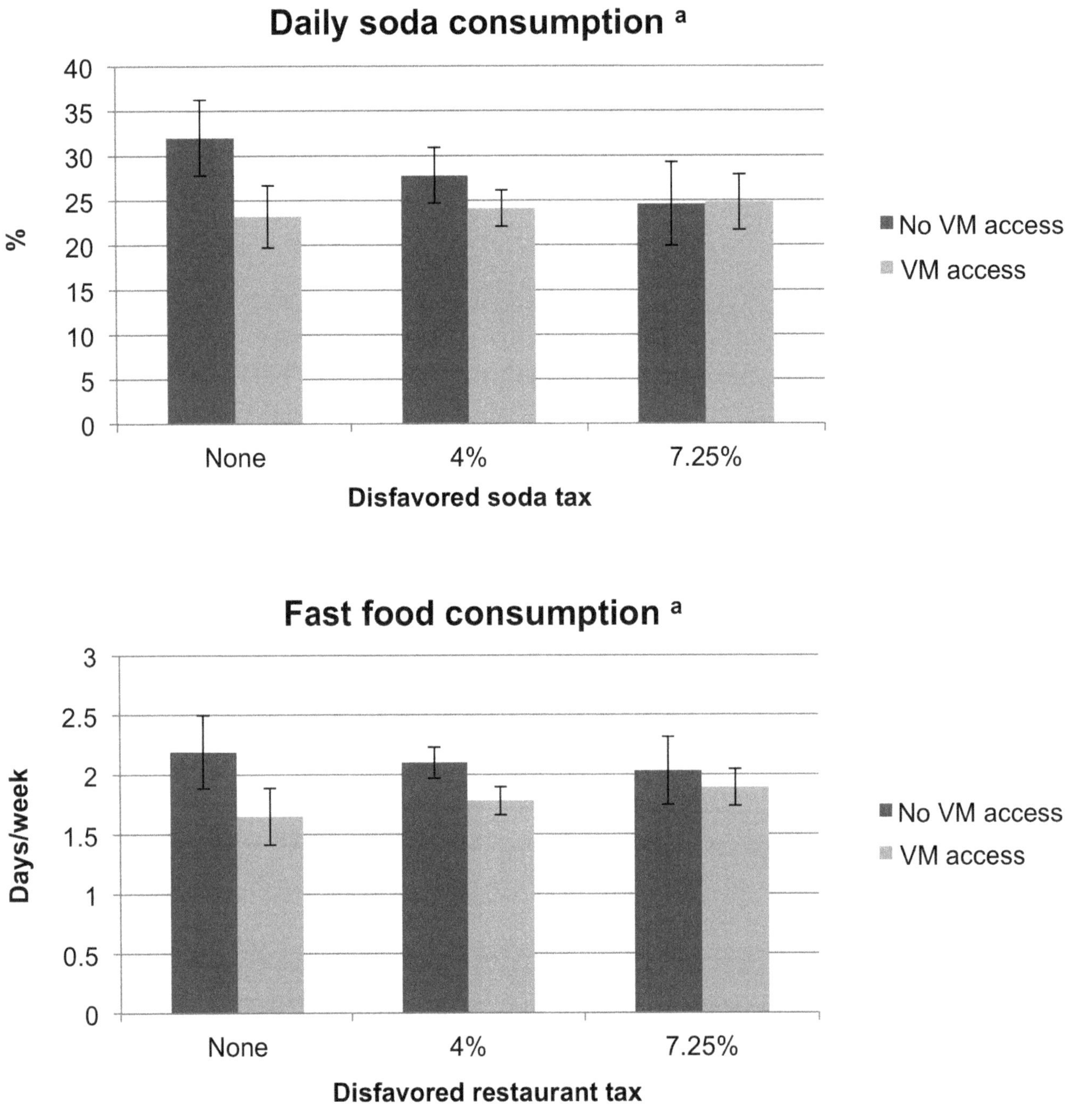

Figure 1. Prevalence of daily soda consumption and mean fast food consumption, by in-school vending machine (VM) access and state taxes. [a] As predicted by logistic and poisson models, respectively, adjusted for race/ethnicity, sex, grade, state median income, and Census region.

with state soda ban – though parameter estimates were not as precise for these outcomes.

In contrast to Table 3, the associations between vending machine access and the dependent variables did not consistently vary by most student or environmental characteristics (see Appendix S1). The exception to this was student weight loss behaviors. There was some evidence that the inverse associations noted in Table 2 were limited to students who were not actively trying to lose weight through healthy behaviors. For example, having access to vending machines was associated with 1.14 fewer servings of soda per week if students were not trying to lose weight (95% CI: -2.06, -0.22), but 0.18 more servings per week if students were trying to lose weight (95% CI: -0.55, 0.92).

Discussion

The effectiveness of removing soda and other SSBs from schools has been questioned by some [10,20,26] and advocated by others [14,37,38], in part because previous research on policies and in-school SSB access has produced a mixed bag of results [15–18,20–24]. Our objective was to explore explanations for the discrepancies by identifying student, environmental, or policy measures that

Table 3. Differences in dietary behaviors associated with in-school vending machine access and state initiatives targeting soda.

		Main effects					
		Vending machine access in school		Soda tax, restaurant tax, or in-school soda ban		Interaction	
State measure	**Dietary measure**	**AME [a]**	**95% CI**	**AME [a]**	**95% CI**	**AME [a]**	**95% CI**
Soda grocery tax [b]							
	Soda servings/week	-1.14	-1.92, -0.36	-0.13	-0.28, 0.02	0.18	0.01, 0.36
	Daily soda consumption [c]	-8.27	-12.0, -4.50	-0.94	-1.81, -0.08	1.17	0.38, 1.95
Restaurant tax [b]							
	Days of fast food/week	-0.53	-0.88, -0.18	-0.02	-0.09, 0.04	0.05	-0.02, 0.13
	Lunch outside school/home[c]	-7.47	-11.6, -3.37	-0.84	-1.61, -0.08	1.07	0.35, 1.79
In-school soda ban [d]							
	Soda servings/week	-0.64	-1.36, 0.07	0.02	-1.15, 1.19	0.35	-0.82, 1.53
	Daily soda consumption [c]	-6.23	-9.52, -2.93	-2.40	-7.93, 3.12	5.79	0.00, 11.6
	Days of fast food/week	-0.37	-0.56, -0.19	-0.19	-0.48, 0.09	0.32	-0.02, 0.66
	Lunch outside school/home [c]	-3.06	-5.71, -0.41	-2.10	-6.89, 2.69	3.22	-1.22, 7.65

[a]AME = Average marginal effect, adjusted for race/ethnicity, sex, grade, state median income, and Census region (models of in-school soda ban also adjusted for home food access.) AME represents the average difference in outcome of interest associated with presence of vending machines that sell sugar-sweetened beverages in school, the state measure of interest (soda tax, restaurant tax, or in-school soda ban); and interaction between the two.
[b]Disfavored tax (i.e., difference in tax rate relative to general tax rate for foods sold in grocery stores).
[c]Binary measure.
[d]State laws that ban the sale of soda in vending machines, school stores, and cafeterias (a la carte).

modified the association between vending machine access and overall consumption of soda, fast food, and lunch source. We found evidence that these associations were modified by three variables that each has important policy implications.

Two of these variables were other state policies related to soda consumption – taxes and laws that regulate the sale of soda in school. The unexpected inverse association between vending machine access and soda/fast food consumption was generally limited to states that did not tax soda and restaurant foods, respectively; likewise, the inverse association between vending machine access and daily consumption was limited to states that did not ban the sale of soda in school venues. These results underscore the limitations of isolated changes to the school food environment. In the absence of any other change, children have numerous sources of soda and other high-fat, high-calorie foods and beverages in most middle- and high-income countries [39]. It is unrealistic to expect a single target to have a positive impact within the obesogenic environment to which children are continuously exposed. This challenge is not unique to school nutrition policies or the U.S.; in any country and any domain, health-related or otherwise, policy resistance often occurs when policies singularly focus on specific targets without considering the broader context [40]. Unintended consequences often occur, and our results are an example of individuals possibly overcompensating for an isolated policy/environmental change and engaging in more unhealthy behavior as a result.

This study focused on only one aspect of the school food environment without considering other changes (e.g., strengthening school meal standards). This was done intentionally because our objective was to identify variables that may explain why some policy initiatives have been less successful than other. At a glance, the results may appear discouraging to those who advocate for school nutrition reform, but results should be interpreted in the context of existing literature on school nutrition policies. Studies that evaluated more comprehensive policy changes (e.g., those that required specific limits on nutrition content of competitive foods and beverages) found stronger evidence [24,25,41]. The importance of comprehensive change was exemplified by evaluations of school nutrition policy changes in Texas, where minor changes to the school food environment initially had little effect on diet because students compensated [42], but more comprehensive changes later had a positive effect [24]. Furthermore, our study did not analyze how long state policies had been in place, which has been shown to influence the impact of school-based nutrition policies [25].

We also found evidence of unintended consequences among students who were not trying to lose weight. Students who were not engaging in healthy weight loss behaviors consumed considerably more soda and fast food if they did not have access to vending machines at school. Students' healthy weight loss behaviors, in themselves, were a strong, consistent predictor of soda and fast food consumption in this study, but this association became even stronger when vending machines were not available. This raises questions of whether school environmental changes can induce behavioral change among individuals who are not otherwise motivated to lose weight. With that said, this study did not examine whether environmental changes increased students' motivation to lose weight, and this question should be explored in future research.

Future research should examine the mechanisms through which soda or fast food consumption may increase when school vending machines are not available. It is impossible to ascertain from this study whether elevated intake of soda and fast food was a direct consequence of not having vending machines. One could speculate that students who desire soda and do not have access at school simply leave campus to obtain soda elsewhere. Not only would this overcome the absence of vending machines, but it would also lead students to rely on sources that are available 7 days per week (e.g., convenience stores), which could explain why daily consumption was higher when vending machines were not available. If that were the case, it would have important implications for policies that limit students from leaving campus. Another possibility is that schools with vending machines sold other SSBs in place of soda, a trend that has been observed throughout the U.S. [19], and this led students to consume less soda by replacing it with other SSBs. These are only two possible mechanisms, and longitudinal research is needed to study this topic in greater detail.

Results should be interpreted cautiously due to other study limitations. Students were not asked which specific beverages were being sold in vending machines, so it is unknown if those with access could even purchase soda. This is a crucial distinction that should be addressed in future studies. We did not analyze intake of other SSBs because it was beyond the scope of this study, but this is a critical topic given that adolescents' SSB choices have shifted in the U.S. in recent years [6]. We did not analyze weight status either because this association may be confounded by many factors, including the possibility that schools are more likely to remove vending machines if obesity is highly prevalent. The cross-sectional design limited our ability to control for such characteristics. Associations may have been biased by unmeasured variables such as socioeconomic status (SES), a potentially important covariate given the socioeconomic disparities in obesity [43] and the food environment outside of school [26,44,45]. Finally, all student data were self-reported and may be vulnerable to measurement error [46], nor did they contain specific measures of nutrient intake. The lack of specific nutrient data makes it difficult to assess whether the associations that we observed were of a sufficient magnitude to have a public health impact. For example, a difference of 0.24 days of fast food, as presented in Table 2, may or may not have an important effect on students' health, depending on the composition of students' fast food consumption.

Conclusions

School nutrition policy research is a rapidly evolving science. As the evidence base continues to grow, it is becoming apparent that policy effects on student intake are partially determined by interactions between policies and the broader environment in which students live. This study provided another example of where small-scale changes did not appear to improve students' diet, particularly in the absence of other policies. Research suggests that comprehensive changes can have a positive effect, but small-scale changes may potentially backfire unless complemented with nutrition education and other initiatives to improve the nutritional quality of other foods and beverages within and outside of school. Policymakers must be cognizant of how minor changes can have unintended consequences, and investigators should continue to study the dynamics between within-school changes and broader policy and environmental measures.

Supporting Information

Appendix S1 Interaction between vending machine access and student weight loss, gender, race/ethnicity, and home food access. [a] AME = Average marginal effect; average difference in outcome of interest associated with presence of vending machines that sell sugar-sweetened beverages in school. [b] Adjusted for race/

ethnicity, sex, grade, state median income, Census region, and home food access.

Acknowledgments

The authors would like to gratefully acknowledge Linda Schneider; Camille Gourdet, J.D.; Tessa Adcock; and Rebecca Schermbeck for their research support provided in compiling and analyzing the laws. We also thank Dr. Nancy Brener of the CDC for providing us with the NYPANS data used in this study.

Author Contributions

Conceived and designed the experiments: DT JC. Analyzed the data: DT RV. Contributed reagents/materials/analysis tools: JC FC. Wrote the paper: DT. Critical review of manuscript: JC RV FC.

References

1. Levy DT, Friend KB, Wang YC (2011) A review of the literature on policies directed at the youth consumption of sugar sweetened beverages. Adv Nutr 2: 182S–200S.
2. Malik VS, Schulze MB, Hu FB (2006) Intake of sugar-sweetened beverages and weight gain: a systematic review. Am J Clin Nutr 84: 274–288.
3. Vartanian LR, Schwartz MB, Brownell KD (2007) Effects of soft drink consumption on nutrition and health: a systematic review and meta-analysis. Am J Public Health 97: 667–675.
4. de Ruyter JC, Olthof MR, Seidell JC, Katan MB (2012) A trial of sugar-free or sugar-sweetened beverages and body weight in children. N Engl J Med 367: 1397–1406.
5. Ebbeling CB, Feldman HA, Chomitz VR, Antonelli TA, Gortmaker SL, et al. (2012) A randomized trial of sugar-sweetened beverages and adolescent body weight. N Engl J Med 367: 1407–1416.
6. Han E, Powell LM (2013) Consumption patterns of sugar-sweetened beverages in the United States. J Acad Nutr Diet 113: 43–53.
7. Wang YC, Bleich SN, Gortmaker SL (2008) Increasing caloric contribution from sugar-sweetened beverages and 100% fruit juices among US children and adolescents, 1988-2004. Pediatrics 121: e1604–1614.
8. Reedy J, Krebs-Smith SM (2010) Dietary sources of energy, solid fats, and added sugars among children and adolescents in the United States. J Am Diet Assoc 110: 1477–1484.
9. Brownell KD, Farley T, Willett WC, Popkin BM, Chaloupka FJ, et al. (2009) The public health and economic benefits of taxing sugar-sweetened beverages. N Engl J Med 361: 1599–1605.
10. Finkelstein E, French S, Variyam JN, Haines PS (2004) Pros and cons of proposed interventions to promote healthy eating. Am J Prev Med 27: 163–171.
11. Institute of Medicine (2012) Accelerating Progress in Obesity Prevention: Solving the Weight of the Nation. Washington, DC: The National Academies Press.
12. Pomeranz JL (2012) Advanced policy options to regulate sugar-sweetened beverages to support public health. J Public Health Policy 33: 75–88.
13. Alliance for a Healthier Generation. Competitive beverage guidelines. Available: http://www.ameribev.org/nutrition-science/school-beverage-guidelines/the-guidelines/. Accessed October 1 2013.
14. Story M, Nanney MS, Schwartz MB (2009) Schools and obesity prevention: creating school environments and policies to promote healthy eating and physical activity. Milbank Q 87: 71–100.
15. Chriqui JF, Turner L, Taber DR, Chaloupka FJ (2013) Association Between District and State Policies and US Public Elementary School Competitive Food and Beverage Environments. JAMA Pediatr 167: 714–722.
16. Taber DR, Chriqui JF, Powell LM, Chaloupka FJ (2012) Banning all sugar-sweetened beverages in middle schools: reduction of in-school access and purchasing but not overall consumption. Arch Pediatr Adolesc Med 166: 256–262.
17. Terry-McElrath YM, O'Malley PM, Johnston LD (2012) Factors affecting sugar-sweetened beverage availability in competitive venues of US secondary schools. J Sch Health 82: 44–55.
18. Woodward-Lopez G, Gosliner W, Samuels SE, Craypo L, Kao J, et al. (2010) Lessons learned from evaluations of California's statewide school nutrition standards. Am J Public Health 100: 2137–2145.
19. Terry-McElrath YM, Johnston LD, O'Malley PM (2012) Trends in competitive venue beverage availability: findings from US secondary schools. Arch Pediatr Adolesc Med 166: 776–778.
20. Fletcher JM, Frisvold D, Tefft N (2010) Taxing soft drinks and restricting access to vending machines to curb child obesity. Health Aff (Millwood) 29: 1059–1066.
21. Taber DR, Stevens J, Evenson KR, Ward DS, Poole C, et al. (2011) State policies targeting junk food in schools: racial/ethnic differences in the effect of policy change on soda consumption. Am J Public Health 101: 1769–1775.
22. Terry-McElrath YM, O'Malley PM, Johnston LD (2013) School soft drink availability and consumption among U.S. secondary students. Am J Prev Med 44: 573–582.
23. Cradock AL, McHugh A, Mont-Ferguson H, Grant L, Barrett JL, et al. (2011) Effect of school district policy change on consumption of sugar-sweetened beverages among high school students, Boston, Massachusetts, 2004-2006. Prev Chronic Dis 8: A74.
24. Cullen KW, Watson K, Zakeri I (2008) Improvements in middle school student dietary intake after implementation of the Texas Public School Nutrition Policy. Am J Public Health 98: 111–117.
25. Taber DR, Chriqui JF, Perna FM, Powell LM, Chaloupka FJ (2012) Weight status among adolescents in States that govern competitive food nutrition content. Pediatrics 130: 437–444.
26. Sturm R (2008) Disparities in the food environment surrounding US middle and high schools. Public Health 122: 681–690.
27. Ellison B, Lusk JL, Davis D (2013) Looking at the label and beyond: the effects of calorie labels, health consciousness, and demographics on caloric intake in restaurants. Int J Behav Nutr Phys Act 10: 21.
28. Centers for Disease Control and Prevention. National Youth Physical Activity and Nutrition Study. Available: http://www.cdc.gov/healthyyouth/yrbs/nypans.htm. Accessed October 1 2013.
29. Cohen ML, Olson KC (1996) Legal Research in a Nutshell, 6th ed. St. Paul, MN: West Publishing Co.
30. Mersky RM, Dunn DJ (2002) Fundamentals of Legal Research, 8th ed. New York, NY: Foundation Press.
31. Chriqui JF, Chaloupka FJ, Powell LM, Eidson SS (2013) A typology of beverage taxation: multiple approaches for obesity prevention and obesity prevention-related revenue generation. J Public Health Policy 34: 403–423.
32. Chriqui JF, Eidson SS, Bates H, Kowalczyk S, Chaloupka FJ (2008) State sales tax rates for soft drinks and snacks sold through grocery stores and vending machines, 2007. Journal of Public Health Policy 29: 226–249.
33. Chriqui JF, Eidson SS, Bates H, Kowalczyk S, Chaloupka FJ (2008) State sales tax rates for soft drinks and snacks sold through grocery stores and vending machines, 2007. J Public Health Policy 29: 226–249.
34. Trust for America's Health, The Robert Wood Johnson Foundation (2010) F as in Fat: How Obesity Threatens America's Future, 2010. Washington, D.C.: Trust for America's Health.
35. National Association of State Boards of Education. State school health policy database. Available: http://nasbe.org/healthy_schools/hs/index.php. Accessed October 1 2013.
36. National Conference of State Legislatures. Childhood obesity - 2010 update of legislative policy options. Available: http://www.ncsl.org/default.aspx?tabid=22156. Accessed October 1 2013.
37. American Academy of Pediatrics (2004) Soft drinks in schools. Pediatrics 113: 152–154.
38. Institute of Medicine (2007) Nutrition Standards for Foods in Schools: Leading the Way Toward Healthier Youth. Washington, D.C.: National Academies Press.
39. Swinburn B (2009) Obesity prevention in children and adolescents. Child Adolesc Psychiatr Clin N Am 18: 209–223.
40. Ghaffarzadegan N, Lyneis J, Richardson GP (2011) How small system dynamics models can help the public policy process. Syst Dynam Rev 27: 22–44.
41. Taber DR, Chriqui JF, Chaloupka FJ (2012) Differences in nutrient intake associated with state laws regarding fat, sugar, and caloric content of competitive foods. Arch Pediatr Adolesc Med 166: 452–458.
42. Cullen KW, Watson K, Zakeri I, Ralston K (2006) Exploring changes in middle-school student lunch consumption after local school food service policy modifications. Public Health Nutr 9: 814–820.
43. Wang Y, Beydoun MA (2007) The obesity epidemic in the United States–gender, age, socioeconomic, racial/ethnic, and geographic characteristics: a systematic review and meta-regression analysis. Epidemiol Rev 29: 6–28.
44. Hilmers A, Hilmers DC, Dave J (2012) Neighborhood disparities in access to healthy foods and their effects on environmental justice. Am J Public Health 102: 1644–1654.
45. Lovasi GS, Hutson MA, Guerra M, Neckerman KM (2009) Built environments and obesity in disadvantaged populations. Epidemiol Rev 31: 7–20.
46. Livingstone MB, Robson PJ (2000) Measurement of dietary intake in children. Proc Nutr Soc 59: 279–293.

17

Evaluation of a Modified Cefsulodin-Irgasan-Novobiocin Agar for Isolation of *Yersinia* spp.

Lai Kuan Tan[1], Peck Toung Ooi[2], Elisabeth Carniel[3], Kwai Lin Thong[1]*

1 Microbiology Division, Institute of Biological Sciences, Faculty of Science, University of Malaya, Kuala Lumpur, Malaysia, **2** Department of Clinical Veterinary Studies, Faculty of Veterinary Medicine, University Putra Malaysia, Serdang, Malaysia, **3** *Yersinia* Research Unit, National Reference Laboratory and WHO Collaborating Centre for *Yersinia*, Institut Pasteur, Paris, France

Abstract

Y. enterocolitica and *Y. pseudotuberculosis* are important food borne pathogens. However, the presence of competitive microbiota makes the isolation of *Y. enterocolitica* and *Y. pseudotuberculosis* from naturally contaminated foods difficult. We attempted to evaluate the performance of a modified Cefsulodin-Irgasan-Novobiocin (CIN) agar in the differentiation of *Y. enterocolitica* from non-*Yersinia* species, particularly the natural intestinal microbiota. The modified CIN enabled the growth of *Y. enterocolitica* colonies with the same efficiency as CIN and Luria-Bertani agar. The detection limits of the modified CIN for *Y. enterocolitica* in culture medium (10 cfu/ml) and in artificially contaminated pork (10^4 cfu/ml) were also comparable to those of CIN. However, the modified CIN provided a better discrimination of *Yersinia* colonies from other bacteria exhibiting *Yersinia*-like colonies on CIN (H_2S-producing *Citrobacter freundii, C. braakii, Enterobacter cloacae, Aeromonas hydrophila, Providencia rettgeri*, and *Morganella morganii*). The modified CIN exhibited a higher recovery rate of *Y. enterocolitica* from artificially prepared bacterial cultures and naturally contaminated samples compared with CIN. Our results thus demonstrated that the use of modified CIN may be a valuable means to increase the recovery rate of food borne *Yersinia* from natural samples, which are usually contaminated by multiple types of bacteria.

Editor: Mikael Skurnik, University of Helsinki, Finland

Funding: This work was financially supported by the University of Malaya High-Impact Research Grant (reference UM.C/625/1/HIR/MOHE/02), University of Malaya Postgraduate Research Fund (PS316/2010B), MOSTI (GA013-2013), and partly by the 'Institut de Veille Sanitaire' (InVS) of France. LKT was supported by a fellowship from University of Malaya. The funders had no role in the study design, data collection and analysis, decision to publish, or preparation of the manuscript.

Competing Interests: The authors have declared that no competing interests exist.

* Email: thongkl@um.edu.my

Introduction

Yersinia are Gram-negative bacteria belonging to the family *Enterobactericeae*. Among many species of *Yersinia*, *Y. enterocolitica* and *Y. pseudotuberculosis* are food borne pathogens and are a frequent cause of human yersiniosis [1]. *Y. enterocolitica* is one of the ten most important food borne enteric pathogens in Europe and the United States [1,2]. *Y. enterocolitica* infections usually results from the consumption of contaminated food or water, and the disease tends to affect young children [1,3]. The symptoms of yersiniosis include acute gastroenteritis with fever, bloody diarrhoea, and pseudo-appendicitis, which frequently leads to unnecessary laparotomy [4]. *Y. pseudotuberculosis* infections are less frequent than *Y. enterocolitica* infections. They are more common in adults and typically cause lower right abdominal pain that resembles appendicitis and, less frequently, diarrhea [1].

The isolation of *Yersinia* is laborious and difficult because the bacteria are easily outgrown by other microorganisms [5]. Selective enrichment [6–8], post-enrichment alkaline treatment [7,9,10], and selective agar isolation [6,8] are the conventional methods for *Yersinia* isolation. The confirmation of the cultures is often accompanied by a series of biochemical tests, biotyping, serotyping, Polymerase Chain Reaction (PCR), and DNA sequencing of housekeeping genes [6,8,11]. However, the lack of a reliable and effective isolation method masks and underestimates the actual incidence of yersiniosis. The recovery of food borne *Yersinia* depends on several factors, such as (i) the amount of background microbiota present in the sample, (ii) the amount of microbiota that survives through selective enrichment and plating [5], and (iii) the amount of *Yersinia* present in the sample [12].

Several selective media have been developed for *Yersinia* isolation. The most frequently used medium is Cefsulodin-Irgasan-Novobiocin (CIN) [13]. CIN has been shown to be more specific than other conventional selective agars, such as *Salmonella-Shigella* (SS), MacConkey (MAC), Cellobiose-Arginine-Lysine (CAL), pectin agars, and other lactose-containing media, for the differentiation of *Yersinia* spp. from contaminating bacteria [14]. However, one of the weaknesses of CIN is that it fails to distinguish *Yersinia* spp. from several other mannitol-fermenting bacterial species, such as *Serratia liquefaciens*, *Enterobacter agglomerans*, *Aeromonas* spp., *Citrobacter* spp., *Providencia* spp. *Acinetobacter johnsonii, Achromobacter xylosoxidans* because all appear as a red "bull's eye" on CIN plates [14,15]. Additional biochemical tests, such as esculin, phenylalanine deaminase, arginine dihydrolase, hydrogen sulphide, urease, and lysine decarboxylase, are needed to further differentiate *Yersinia* spp. from other *Yersinia*-like bacterial species [16]. These post-isolation steps are laborious, time consuming, and costly.

Some researchers have modified the existing selective agars to improve the isolation of virulent *Y. enterocolitica*. Fukushima

Table 1. Colony morphology of *Yersinia* spp. and other bacteria on CIN and modified CIN.

Bacterial species (strain number)	Colony morphology on:		
	CIN[a] (ae[b])	Modified CIN (ae)	Modified CIN (mic[c])
Yersinia enterocolitica			
bioserotype 1A/O:6,30 (IP102)	NG[d]	NG	NG
bioserotype1A/O:5 (PC-M16-2)	Rbe	Rbe	Rbe
bioserotype 1B/O:8 (IP11105, ATCC 9610, YE036c-CY)	Rbe[e]	Rbe	Rbe
bioserotype 2/O:9 (IP383)	Rbe	Rbe	Rbe
bioserotype 3/O:1,2,3 (IP135)	Rbe	Rbe	Rbe
bioserotype 3 variant/O:3 (PC-M1-K1)	Rbe	Rbe	Rbe
bioserotype 4/O:3 (IP134)	Rbe	Rbe	Rbe
bioserotype 5/O:2,3 (IP178)	Rbe	Rbe	Rbe
Other *Yersinia* spp.			
Y. aldovae (IP6005)	Rbe	Rbe	Rbe
Y. bercovieri (IP3443)	Rbe	Rbe	Rbe
Y. frederiksenii (IP3842)	Rbe	Rbe	Rbe
Y. intermedia (IP955)	Rbe	Rbe	Rbe
Y. kristensenii (IP105)	Rbe	Rbe	Rbe
Y. mollaretii (IP33766)	Rbe	Rbe	Rbe
Y. pseudotuberculosis (IP34476)	Rbe	Rbe	Rbe
Other *Enterobacteriaceae*			
Citrobacter,			
freundii, H_2S-producing (YC-K1-3)	Rbe	Rbe + Bc[f]	Rbe + Bc
freundii, non-H_2S-producing (YC-S1-5, YC-T1-1)	Rbe	Rbe	Rbe
braakii (YC-T1-K1)	Rbe	Rbe + Bc	Rbe + Bc
koseri (YC-VG2-1)	Rbe	Rbe	Rbe
Providencia rettgeri (IC-PP2a-9, IC-PP3a-K1, IC-PP6a-10)	Rbe	Rbe + Bp	Rbe + Bp
Enterobacter cloacae (YC-I1-K1, YC-I1-K2, YC-I1-K3)	Rbe	P[g]	P
Pantoae spp. (PI-TSP30a-K1)	Rbe	Rbe	Rbe
Serratia,			
odorifera (PC-TSP36b-3)	Rbe	Rbe	Rbe
marcescens (YC-M2-11)	Rbe	Rbe	Rbe
Morganella morganii (YS-TSP7b-1)	C[h]	C + Bp	C + Bp
Salmonella,			
Paratyphi A (ATCC 9150)	NG	NG	NG
Paratyphi B (ATCC 8759)	NG	NG	NG
Paratyphi C (ATCC 9068)	NG	NG	NG
Typhimurium (ATCC 13311)	NG	NG	NG
Typhi (ATCC 6539)	NG	NG	NG
enterica (ATCC 10376)	NG	NG	NG
Escherichia coli (ATCC25922, O157:H7)	NG	NG	NG
Shigella sonnei (ATCC 11060)	NG	NG	NG
Proteus penneri (IS-TSP7b-3)	NG	NG	NG
Other Gram-Negative Bacteria			
Aeromonas hydrophila (Ae 20)	Rbe	P + Bp[i]	P + Bp
Vibrio spp. (VSP-C12-1210, VS-A29-0810)	NG	NG	NG
Pseudomonas aeruginosa (ATCC 9027)	NG	NG	NG
Gram-Positive Bacteria			

Table 1. Cont.

Bacterial species (strain number)	Colony morphology on:		
	CIN[a] (ae[b])	Modified CIN (ae)	Modified CIN (mic[c])
Enterococcus faecalis (ATCC 29212)	NG	NG	NG
Listeria monocytogenes (ATCC 7644)	NG	NG	NG
Staphylococcus aureus (ATCC 6538, MRSA 0807-1)	NG	NG	NG

[a]CIN, Cefsulodin-Irgasan-Novobiocin.
[b]ae, aerobic.
[c]mic, microaerophilic.
[d]NG, no growth.
[e]Rbe, red bull's eye.
[f]Bc, black centre.
[g]P, pink.
[h]C, colourless.
[i]Bp, brown diffusible pigment.
IP, Institut Pasteur, strain collection of the French *Yersinia* Reference laboratory.
ATCC, American Type Culture Collection.
Others, strain collection of the Laboratory of Biomedical Science and Molecular Microbiology, Institute of Graduate Studies, University of Malaya, Malaysia.

modified CIN agar by the addition of 0.1% esculin and 0.05% ferric citrate [17]. This modified medium, which is named Virulent *Yersinia enterocolitica* (VYE) agar, allows the differentiation of pathogenic *Y. enterocolitica* colonies that do not hydrolyse esculin from non-pathogenic esculin-positive colonies. However, esculin hydrolysis produces a dark-brown diffusible pigment on VYE agar that can mask esculin-negative colonies, including virulent *Y. enterocolitica* [18,19]. Furthermore, other mannitol-fermenting non-esculin-hydrolysing species cannot be distinguished from virulent *Y. enterocolitica*. Differentiation based on the size of the colonies of different bacteria on both CIN and VYE agars is also ineffective because *Y. enterocolitica* tends to grow more slowly and its colonies are smaller when in competition for space and nutrients.

Some researchers prefer to use the Statens Serum Institut (SSI) enteric medium for the detection of *Yersinia* spp. from highly contaminated samples, such as faeces, because it allows the identification of a range of enteric pathogens [20,21]. However, SSI is reported to have a lower selective effect compared with CIN agar and requires at least 3×10^6 *Yersinia* cfu/g of faeces for successful recovery [21]. This indicates that the SSI medium may provide false-negative results if the naturally occurring *Yersinia* is below the detection limit.

Chromogenic-based media have become increasingly popular in recent years for the isolation of enterobacteria. To date, three chromogenic media have been developed for the specific detection of virulent *Y. enterocolitica*: the *Y. enterocolitica* chromogenic medium (YeCM), [19] *Y. enterocolitica* agar (YECA) [18], and CHROMagar *Yersinia* (CAY) [15]. All three media allow the differentiation of virulent *Y. enterocolitica* from non-virulent strains and from other enterobacteria. However, YeCM and YECA are non-marketed media and require laborious and laboratory-made preparation. Moreover, all three media are relatively expensive, which seriously limits their routine usage. In addition, false-positive results from the chromogenic medium have been reported due to wrong colour interpretation by the user [22]. The purple, light denim blue, and light pink colours are frequently miss-interpreted as mauve and cannot be ruled out as possible presumptive colonies [22]. Furthermore, even if the chromogenic media are useful for differentiating the virulent from the non-virulent biotypes, the use of CIN is still required for the isolation step prior to plating on chromogenic media [23].

Thus, a medium that is less expensive than chromogenic media and improves the differentiation of *Yersinia* spp. from contaminating bacteria would thus be of value for routine use in microbiology laboratories. Therefore, the main objective of this study was to evaluate the performance of modified CIN agar for the differentiation of *Yersinia* spp. from other natural microbiota, such as H_2S-producing *C. freundii*, *C. braakii*, *E. cloacae*, *A. hydrophila*, and *P. rettgeri*. The plating efficiencies, detection limits, and recovery strengths of CIN and modified CIN in pure culture, artificial contaminated raw pork meat, artificially prepared bacterial mixtures, and natural contaminated samples were evaluated and compared.

Materials and Methods

Modification of CIN agar

The modified CIN agar was prepared by the addition of 1% L-arginine (Sigma, Germany), 0.8 g/L ferric ammonium citrate (BDH Prolabo, UK), 6.8 g/L sodium thiosulphate (BDH Prolabo), and 2.0 g/L DL-phenylalanine (Sigma) at pH 7.4±0.02 to the CIN Agar Base (Oxoid, UK).

Plating efficiency of CIN and modified CIN

The plating efficiencies of CIN and modified CIN agar were evaluated using the 50 bacterial strains listed in Table 1. These include *Yersinia* spp., other *Enterobacteriaceae*, selected Gram-negative and Gram-positive bacteria.

The bacterial strains retrieved from the −20°C glycerol stocks were grown on Brain Heart Infusion agar (BD, USA). *Yersinia* strains were incubated at 25°C for 24–48 h, whereas other bacteria were incubated overnight at 37°C. Using needle inoculators, fresh bacterial cultures were dotted or streaked on CIN or modified CIN agar and incubated under aerobic or microaerophilic conditions at 25°C for 24–48 h. Microaerophilic conditions were created by placing the inoculated agar plates in candle jars to facilitate the visualization of H_2S-producing bacteria [24]. The plating efficiencies on CIN and modified CIN agar were determined by screening for the presence of colonies with the expected *Yersinia* morphology [red centre with colourless translucent rim (red bull's eye)].

Limit of detections (LODs) of CIN and modified CIN for *Y. enterocolitica* strains

The LOD was determined using the method recommended by the Microbiological Methods Committee [25]. *Y. enterocolitica* was chosen as representing strain. Overnight *Y. enterocolitica* cultures were serially diluted from 10^8 to 10^1 colony forming units (cfu)/ml and spread onto CIN and modified CIN agar. The plating efficiencies were determined six times using independent cell suspension. The plates were incubated under aerobic conditions at 25°C for 24–48 h. In addition, one set of samples on modified CIN agar was incubated under microaerophilic conditions at 25°C for 24–48 h. The LOD was defined as the lowest concentration of *Y. enterocolitica* with culturable bacteria detectable in at least 50% of the replicates (as low as one colony detectable in each replicate, and at least three out of six positive replicates).

Quantification of *Y. enterocolitica* growth on CIN and modified CIN compared with that on LBA

The growth of *Y. enterocolitica* on CIN and modified CIN was compared to that on Luria-Bertani Agar (LBA)(Oxoid, USA). *Y. enterocolitica* suspension was adjusted to approximately 10^3 cfu/ml and plated on LBA, CIN, and modified CIN. The mean cfu (six replicates) of *Y. enterocolitica* on LBA, CIN, and modified CIN was calculated after incubation at 25°C for 48 h. The results were expressed as the percentages of mean cfu on CIN/LBA and on modified CIN/LBA for each incubation condition [21].

LOD and recovery rate of *Y. enterocolitica* in artificially contaminated raw pork meat on CIN and modified CIN

The effect of the natural microbiota on the recovery of *Y. enterocolitica* from a food matrix (with or without stress treatment, kept at −20°C for three weeks after bacterial spiking) was studied [25]. An artificially contaminated raw pork meat was used because yersiniosis is frequently associated with the consumption of contaminated pork products. For food matrix without stress treatment, approximately 1.5 kg of freshly purchased minced pork meat was processed immediately following spiking. Cell suspensions of *Y. enterocolitica* were serially diluted as previously described and 250 µL of each suspension was mixed with 25 g of minced meat homogenised in 24.75 mL of phosphate buffered saline (PBS, Sigma) to obtain final concentrations ranging from 10^1 to 10^8 cfu/ml. The meat suspensions were homogenised manually for 30 s and incubated at 25°C for 30 min. An aliquot of each homogenate was then plated on CIN and modified CIN agar, and the cultures were incubated under aerobic conditions at 25°C for 24–48 h. The same procedures were repeated for a set of samples on modified CIN agar incubated under microaerophilic conditions at 25°C for 24–48 h. Six replicates were performed for each bacterial concentration. The mean cfu/ml of the background microbiota in the un-inoculated pork meat (25 g of pork homogenised in 25 mL of PBS, six replicates) was determined after plating on LBA.

The LOD of *Y. enterocolitica* in the artificially contaminated pork meat was defined as the lowest concentration of culturable *Y. enterocolitica* detectable in at least 50% of the replicates (as low as one colony detectable on each replicate, and at least three out of six positive replicates) [25]. The ratio of the mean cfu of *Y. enterocolitica* to the background microbiota was also determined.

The same spiked minced meat was subjected to stress treatment by keeping the spiked food samples at −20°C for two weeks after bacterial spiking (to mimic food storage conditions) [25]. The same plating procedures were then performed. The percentage of *Y. enterocolitica* colonies recovered from the food (with and without stress treatment) was determined by the selection of representative colonies from each plate that were identified through the PCR targeting of the *Y. enterocolitica*-specific 16S rRNA and *ail* genes, as described previously [11]. The primer pairs used were Y1 (5′-AATACCGCATAACGTCTTCG-3′) and Y2 (5′-CTTCTTCTGCGAGTAACGTC-3′) for the *Y. enterocolitica*-specific 16S rRNA gene and A1 (5′–TTAATGTGTACGCTGCGAGTG-3′ and A2 (5′-GGAGTATTCATATGAAGCGTC-3′) for the *ail* gene. The PCR amplicons were purified using the MEGA-spin Agarose Gel Extraction Kit (*iNtRON* Biotechnology, Korea) and confirmed by DNA sequencing.

Determination of the recovery of *Y. enterocolitica* from artificial bacterial mixtures

Overnight cultures of *Y. enterocolitica* IP135 and bacteria exhibiting *Yersinia*-like colonies on CIN agar (H_2S-producing *C. freundii*, *C. braakii*, *A. hydrophila*, *P. rettgeri*, and *E. cloacae*) were adjusted to a concentration of 10^4 cfu/ml and mixed together. Six independent pooled bacterial suspensions were prepared, and spread on CIN and modified CIN agar, and incubated aerobically at 25°C for 24–48 h. Presumptive *Y. enterocolitica* colonies were isolated from each replicate and subjected to PCR confirmation [11] to determine the percentage of *Y. enterocolitica* on both media.

Determination of the recovery rate of *Y. enterocolitica* in naturally contaminated samples

A total of 52 rectal swabs from swine were tested for the presence of *Y. enterocolitica* using different enrichment procedures and plating on CIN and modified CIN agars (Table 2, methods 1 to 6). Briefly, all of the swab specimens were (i) directly streaked onto the selective medium (methods 1 and 2), (ii) subjected to cold enrichment (incubation at 4°C for three weeks in PBS) before being plated on CIN and modified CIN (methods 3 and 4) [8], and (iii) subjected to cold enrichment and then alkaline treatment before being plated onto the two selective media (methods 5 and 6) [7,8,9,10]. Presumptive *Y. enterocolitica* colonies were isolated and subjected to PCR confirmation [11]. In parallel to the isolation procedures, PCR detection of *Y. enterocolitica* was carried out directly on the boiled cell lysates (99°C for 5 min) of the 52 rectal swabs samples following post-cold enrichment. The isolated *Y. enterocolitica* isolates was biotyped by using biochemical tests as described by Wauters et al. [26] and serotyped by using the O-Antisera "SEIKEN" set purchased (DENKA SEIKEN Co., Ltd, Japan).

Statistical analysis

The statistical significance was calculated by the Student's t-test, Chi-square test, or Fisher's test (when appropriate) using the R software (version 2.12.2). The difference was considered significantly if $p<0.05$.

Ethics Statement

All of the rectal swab samples from swine were collected with supervision from the institution veterinarian during routine farm visits. No animal was sacrificed or injured during the sampling procedure. The sampling complied with the current guidelines for the care and use of animals and was approved by the Animal Care

Table 2. Recovery rate of *Y. enterocolitica* from the 52 naturally contaminated rectal swabs from swine.

Methods	No. of positive specimens recovered by plating (%)
Method 1 — Direct streaking onto CIN[a]	0 (0)
Method 2 — Direct streaking onto mCIN[b]	0 (0)
Method 3 — PBS[c]-CIN	0 (0)
Method 4 — PBS-mCIN	2 (3.8)
Method 5 — PBS-KOH[d]-CIN	0 (0)
Method 6 — PBS-KOH-mCIN	2 (3.8)

The prevalence of *Y. enterocolitica* determined by using a duplex PCR targeting the *Y. enterocolitica*-specific 16S rRNA and *ail* genes [11] was 2/52 (3.8%).
[a]CIN, Cefsulodin-Irgasan-Novobiocin.
[b]mCIN, modified CIN.
[c]PBS, phosphate buffered saline, a cold enrichment at 4°C for three weeks [8].
[d]KOH, post-enrichment alkaline treatment.

and Use Committee (ACUC, AUP number: T006/2013), Faculty of Veterinary Medicine, Universiti Putra Malaysia.

Results

Growth characteristics and colony morphology on CIN and modified CIN agar

The capability of bacteria to grow on CIN and modified CIN agar and the colony morphology of 50 bacterial strains were determined. Both CIN and modified CIN allowed the growth of all *Yersinia* strains tested with the exception of the non-pathogenic strain IP102 (*Y. enterocolitica* bioserotype 1A/O:6,30), which was inhibited on both media. Furthermore, all *Yersinia* colonies displayed the same characteristic red bull's eye feature (Table 1 and Figure 1, Nb 2–17). Therefore, the CIN modification did not alter the growth and colony shape of *Yersinia* strains. The *Y. enterocolitica* colonies on modified CIN were tiny (≤0.5 mm) and only exhibited the characteristic red bull's eye morphology after

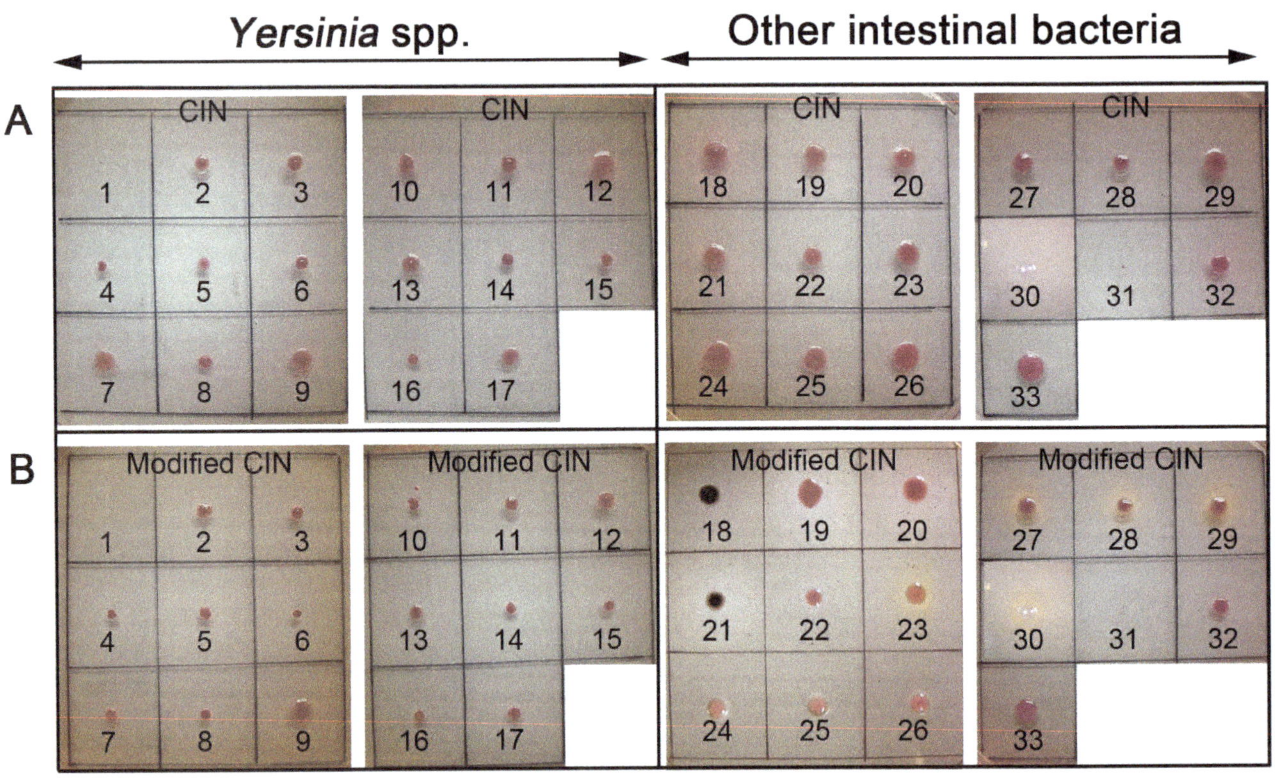

Figure 1. Bacteria on CIN (A) ***and modified CIN (B).*** 1, *Y. enterocolitica* 1A/O:6,30 (IP102); 2, *Y. enterocolitica* 1B/O:8 (IP11105); 3, *Y. enterocolitica* 2/O:9 (IP383); 4, *Y. enterocolitica* 3/O:1,2,3 (IP135); 5, *Y. enterocolitica* 4/O:3 (IP134); 6, *Y. enterocolitica* 5/O:2,3 (IP178); 7, *Y. enterocolitica* 1B/O:8 (ATCC 9610); 8, *Y. enterocolitica* 3/O:3 (PC-M1-K1); 9, *Y. enterocolitica* 1A/O:5 (PC-M16-2); 10, *Y. aldovae* (IP6005); 11, *Y. bercovieri* (IP3443); 12, *Y. frederiksenii* (IP3842); 13, *Y. intermedia* (IP955); 14, *Y. kristensenii* (IP105); 15, *Y. mollaretii* (IP33766); 16, *Y. pseudotuberculosis* (IP34476); 17, *Y. enterocolitica* 1B/O:8 (YE036c-CY); 18, *C. freundii*, H_2S-producing; 19, 20, *C. freundii*, nonxH_2S-producing; 21, *C. braakii*; 22, *C. koseri*; 23, *A. hydrophila*; 24, 25, 26, *E. cloacae*; 27, 28, 29, *P. rettgeri*; 30, *M. morganii*; 31, *Pantoae* spp.; 32, *S. odorifera*; 33, *S. marcescens*.

30 h of incubation, whereas this typical shape was visible after 24 h on CIN. This observation indicates that the modified CIN plates should not be read before 30 h.

The CIN and modified CIN exhibited the same growth inhibitory effect on various species of *Salmonella, E. coli, Shigella, Proteus, Vibrio, Pseudomonas, Enterococcus, Listeria*, and *Staphylococcus* (Table 1). The two media allowed the growth of non-H_2S-producing *C. freundii, C. koseri, S. odorifera, S. marcescens*, and *Pantoea* spp., which produced colonies with the red bull's eye morphology (Figure 1 and Table 1). Hence, the modification of CIN did not improve the differentiation of these bacteria from *Yersinia* spp.

In contrast, the modified CIN but not CIN allowed the differentiation of *Yersinia* spp. from several other *Enterobacteriaceae* and *A. hydrophila*. On the modified CIN, the colonies of *C. braakii* and H_2S-producing *C. freundii* exhibited a black centre (Figure 1, Nb 18 and 21), the *P. rettgeri* colonies were surrounded by a brown diffusible pigment (Figure 1, Nb 27–29), the *E. cloacae* colonies were light pink (Figure 1, Nb 24–26), *A. hydrophila* appeared as pink colonies surrounded by a brown pigment (Figure 1, Nb 23), and *M. morganii* formed tiny colourless colonies surrounded by a brown pigment (Figure 1, Nb 30). The modified CIN is thus more efficient than CIN for the discrimination of *Yersinia* spp. from these *Yersinia*-like bacterial species.

Changing the incubation conditions for the modified CIN had no effect on the colony morphology of the various species tested (Table 1). However, the formation of a black centre in H_2S-producing colonies could be observed under microaerophilic conditions even when their size was ≤ 1 mm, whereas the black centre appeared when the colonies were larger under aerobic conditions. Therefore, microaerophilic conditions improved the visualization of H_2S-producing bacteria.

LOD of CIN and modified CIN agar for *Y. enterocolitica* detection

The capacities of four *Y. enterocolitica* strains, which represented non-pathogenic (PC-M16-2), moderate pathogenic (IP383 and IP135), and highly pathogenic (ATCC 9610) strains, to grow on CIN and modified CIN agar were evaluated. Various cell suspensions (from 10^1 to 10^8 cfu/ml) were spread onto CIN and modified CIN agar, incubated for 24–48 h at 25°C, and then observed. In addition, one set of samples plated on modified CIN agar was incubated under microaerophilic conditions at 25°C for 24–48 h.

The LOD for all four *Y. enterocolitica* strains was 10 cfu/ml on both CIN and modified CIN under aerobic conditions (Table S1). Although the LOD for strain ATCC 9610 was slightly higher on the modified CIN under microaerophilic (10^2 cfu/ml) compared with aerobic conditions (10^1 cfu/ml), the difference in sensitivity for all four strains tested under these different conditions was not significant (Student t-test, $p>0.05$). Therefore, the use of microaerophilic conditions did not alter the growth of *Y. enterocolitica* on modified CIN.

Quantification of *Y. enterocolitica* growth on CIN and modified CIN compared with that on LBA

The ability of CIN and modified CIN to support the growth of *Y. enterocolitica*, compared with that of LBA was evaluated. The growth of four *Y. enterocolitica* strains (IP383, IP135, ATCC 9610, and PC-M16-2) on LBA, CIN, and modified CIN was quantified and is presented as percentages of the mean cfu on CIN or modified CIN versus that on LBA. Values between 80% and 120% were considered to indicate growth efficiency on CIN or modified CIN similar to that on LBA (100%) [21].

As shown in Table 3, the numbers of *Y. enterocolitica* colonies recovered on CIN, modified CIN, and LBA were similar, regardless of whether the bacteria were grown under aerobic or microaerophilic conditions (the percentages of mean colony count on CIN or modified CIN versus LBA were between 80% and 120%). Therefore, the different media and conditions allowed the growth of *Y. enterocolitica* colonies with the same efficiency.

LOD of *Y. enterocolitica* from artificially contaminated raw pork meat

The ability of CIN and modified CIN to recover *Y. enterocolitica* from a food matrix was determined using raw pork meat (with or without stress treatment, kept at −20°C, three weeks after bacterial spiking [25]) mixed with various concentrations (from 10^1 to 10^8 cfu/ml) of *Y. enterocolitica* IP135. The IP138 strain was chosen because it is of biotype 3 and this particular biotype has been frequently reported in food and animal from Asia and Southeat Asia countries with warm climate (Southern China, Malaysia, Taiwan and Thailand) [30,31,32,33]. The ratio of LOD to background microbiota was calculated by dividing the mean cfu of the LOD to the mean cfu of the un-inoculated pork meat.

The LOD of strain IP135 in both raw pork meat with and without stress treatment was 10^4 cfu/ml on both media incubated under aerobic conditions (Table S2), indicating that the modification of CIN did not impair its capability to recover *Y. enterocolitica* from the studied food matrix. The finding that this LOD was 100-fold higher than that of the bacteria grown in pure culture (Table S1, 10 cfu/ml) confirms the impact of the presence of background microbiota on the recovery of *Y. enterocolitica*. At the LOD value of 10^4 cfu/ml, the food homogenates contained a ratio of *Y. enterocolitica* to microbiota of 1:412 (Table S2), indicating that *Y. enterocolitica* colonies cannot be successfully identified in the meat sample if it is below this ratio.

For the food matrix with stress treatment (kept at −20°C for three weeks after bacterial spiking) and incubated under microaerophilic conditions, the LOD decreased to 10^3 cfu/ml on modified CIN (Table S2), which suggests that this incubation condition may slightly increase the recovery rate of *Y. enterocolitica* in food since visualization of H_2S-producing bacteria was improved.

Differentiation of *Y. enterocolitica* colonies from enterobacteria exhibiting *Yersinia*-like morphology on CIN

Suspensions containing similar concentrations (10^4 cfu/ml) of *Y. enterocolitica* (IP135) and other enterobacterial species exhibiting *Yersinia*-like colonies on CIN agar, such as H_2S-producing *C. freundii, C. braakii, E. cloacae, P. rettgeri*, and *A. hydrophila*, were plated on CIN and modified CIN to compare the number of true *Y. enterocolitica* recovered on each medium. Presumptive colonies of *Y. enterocolitica* (red bull's eye morphology) were picked and analysed by PCR for confirmation.

Only the modified CIN but not CIN allowed the differentiation of *Y. enterocolitica* (IP135) from H_2S-producing *C. freundii, C. braakii, E. cloacae, P. rettgeri*, and *A. hydrophila*. The percentages of true *Y. enterocolitica* (IP135) recovered from the bacterial mixtures were 33.3% on CIN and 60.0% on modified CIN (Table 4), and the difference was significant (Chi-square test, $p< 0.05$). Therefore, the use of modified CIN agar enhanced the differentiation of *Yersinia* colonies from those of *Yersinia*-like species.

Table 3. Growth of *Y. enterocolitica* on CIN and modified CIN under different incubation conditions compared with that on LBA (control medium).

Strains	Bioserotype	Percentage of cfu (%)			
		Aerobic		Microaerophilic	Aerobic/Microaerophilic
		CIN[a]/LBA[b]	mCIN[c]/LBA	mCIN/LBA	mCIN
PC-M16-2	1A/O:5	110.3	108.9	106.8	102.0
ATCC 9610	1B/O:8	88.5	84.3	84.3	100.0
IP383	2/O:9	109.6	101	94.5	106.9
IP135	3/O:1,2,3	96.7	82.1	82.4	99.6

[a]CIN, Cefsulodin-Irgasan-Novobiocin.
[b]LBA, Luria-Bertani agar.
[c]mCIN, modified CIN.

In artificially contaminated raw pork, the percentage of true *Y. enterocolitica* (IP135) colonies also increased from 62.3% on CIN to 72.5% on modified CIN (Table 4), however this difference was not statistically significant (Chi-square test, $p>0.05$).

Determination of the recovery of *Y. enterocolitica* from naturally contaminated samples

The efficiency of CIN and modified CIN agars for the recovery of *Y. enterocolitica* from the 52 naturally contaminated samples (rectal swabs from swine) was evaluated and compared in three ways: (i) after direct plating on the agars (methods 1 and 2); (ii) after cold enrichment followed by plating on the agars (methods 3 and 4); (iii) after cold enrichment, alkaline treatment, and plating on the agars (methods 5 and 6) (Table 2). The detection of *Y. enterocolitica* by PCR in post-PBS enrichment broths was 2/52 (3.8%). Both modified CIN and CIN did not recover any *Y. enterocolitica* from the samples using the direct plating method (methods 1 and 2). After cold enrichment (methods 3 and 4), the modified CIN allowed the recovery of *Y. enterocolitica* from all PCR-positive samples (2/52, 3.8%), while no *Y. enterocolitica* was identified on CIN (Table 2). Cold enrichment and alkaline treatment followed by plating on modified CIN (methods 5 and 6) also allowed the isolation of *Y. enterocolitica* from all PCR-positive samples (2/52, 3.8%), while no *Y. enterocolitica* was detected on CIN (Table 2). The results showed that modified CIN resulted in the detection of a larger number of positive samples than CIN for the recovery of *Y. enterocolitica* from naturally contaminated samples. The results of biotyping and serotyping indicated that all the *Y. enterocolitica* isolated were of bioserotype 3/O:3 variant (VP negative).

Discussion

Y. enterocolitica and *Y. pseudotuberculosis* are important food borne pathogens that cause human yersiniosis worldwide, and the incidence of yersiniosis is vastly underestimated. This underestimation may occur because the infection is self-limiting in most cases. The lack of a good isolation medium makes the recovery of *Yersinia* difficult. In the search for a medium that would allow a better discrimination of *Yersinia* colonies from other bacterial spp. while maintaining the selective properties of CIN, various chemical components have been added to this medium to detect three biochemical activities: phenylalanine deaminase, arginine dihydrolase, and H_2S production. According to Bergey et al. [27], *C. braakii*, H_2S-producing *C. freundii*, *E. cloacae*, *P. rettgeri*, and *A. hydrophila* can be differentiated from *Yersinia* based on their biochemical utilisation of these components.

Ferric ammonium citrate and sodium thiosulphate are substrates for H_2S production, which results in the formation of a black centre on bacterial colonies. Phenylalanine deaminase converts DL-phenylalanine in phenylpyruvate, which in the presence of iron (III) ions and citrate, forms a brown, diffusible pigment in agar around the bacterial colonies. The dihydrolysis of L-arginine produces an alkaline substrate that gives a yellow colour to bacterial colonies. The addition of these substrates did not alter the formation of the red bull's eye feature of *Yersinia* colonies, although the formation of *Y. enterocolitica* characteristic morphology was slightly delayed on modified CIN compared with

Table 4. Recovery of *Y. enterocolitica* from artificially prepared bacterial mixtures and artificially contaminated raw pork.

Experiments	Agar	Number of positive *Y. enterocolitica*		
		True[a] (%)	False[a] (%)	Total
IP135 + bacterial mixture[b]	CIN[c]	20 (33.3)	40 (66.7)	60
	Modified CIN	36 (60.0)	24 (40.0)	60
IP135 + background microbiota from raw pork	CIN	43 (62.3)	26 (37.7)	69
	Modified CIN	50 (72.5)	19 (27.5)	69

[a]True and false positive *Y. enterocolitica* colonies were determined by using a duplex PCR targeting the *Y. enterocolitica*-specific 16S rRNA and *ail* genes [11].
[b]Mixture of bacteria exhibiting *Yersinia*-like colonies on CIN agar (*C. freundii, C. braakii, E. cloacae, P. rettgeri, A. hydrophila*).
[c]CIN, Cefsulodin-Irgasan-Novobiocin.

CIN. Nevertheless, the plates could be read within 48 h (optimal incubation time for *Y. enterocolitica*) in the normal isolation step for *Yersinia* spp.

The differentiation of *Yersinia* from other mannitol-fermenting bacteria that exhibit *Yersinia*-like colonies CIN (H_2S-producing *C. freundii, C. braakii, E. cloacae, A. hydrophila*, and *P. rettgeri*) was markedly easier on modified CIN compared with CIN. These bacterial species are naturally present in feces, raw food, and other environmental samples [27]. Because H_2S-producing *C. freundii* and *C. braakii* ferment mannitol and produce H_2S, these appeared as red bull's eye colonies with a black centre on modified CIN. The capacity of *E. cloacae* and *A. hydrophila* to ferment mannitol and dihydrolyse arginine resulted in the formation of pink colonies. Furthermore, *A. hydrophila* produces phenylalanine deaminase, which generates a diffusible brown pigment around the pink colonies. Similarly, *P. rettgeri* produces a phenylalanine deaminase and therefore appeared as red bull's eye colonies with a diffusible brown pigment. The diffusible brown pigment produced will not mask the appearance of non-phenylalanine deaminase-producing bacteria because this brown pigment has a light colour that is less intense than the dark-brown pigment produced in the VYE agar [17]. Van Damme et al. [28] reported that *Y. enterocolitica* forms small white colonies and not typical red bull's eyes colonies on CIN agar in the presence of an abundant background flora [28]. Similar results were observed in this study when the colony size of *Y. enterocolitica* was ≤ 0.5 mm on CIN. The tiny white/colourless *Y. enterocolitica* colonies obtained in this case resembled *M. morganii* on CIN, causing false-negative results during colony selection. A bonus benefit obtained with the modification of CIN was that *M. morganii* appeared as colourless colonies with a diffusible brown pigment on modified CIN due to their capacity to produce phenylalanine deaminase. Based on these differential metabolic properties, it was possible to eliminate a large number of bacterial colonies prior further biochemical testing. The addition of these chemicals in the modified CIN thus reduced the workload and additional costs associated with biochemical testing by decreasing the number of colonies to be tested and enhanced the detection rate by lowering the risk of selecting non-*Yersinia* colonies.

However, the modified CIN still has the limitation of not differentiating pathogenic *Y. enterocolitica* from non-pathogenic *Yersinia* species and from non-H_2S-producing *C. freundii, C. koseri, Pantoea* spp., *S. odorifera*, and *S. marcescens*. Nevertheless, the combination usage of modified CIN with a chromogenic media, such as CHROMagar *Yersinia* [15] and YECA [18], and YeCM [19], may help eliminate non-pathogenic *Yersinia* without the need to conduct additional biochemical tests [23]. This combination usage may also reduce the false-positive results caused by wrong colour interpretations by the user [22].

A better formation of a black centre by H_2S-producing *C. freundii* and *C. braakii* colonies was observed when these were incubated under microaerophilic conditions. The reduction of sulphide to H_2S gas is an anaerobic respiration and normally occurs in the middle of bacterial colonies [29]. Tiny colonies may not provide good anaerobic conditions for the production of H_2S gas, and this phenomenon was observed in our samples (Zone A, Figure 2). The formation of a black centre could not be detected when the colonies were small and clumped together. Therefore, a longer incubation time (30 h to 48 h instead of 24 h) was required when the plates were incubated under normal (aerobic) conditions because bacteria grew bigger and fulfilled the anaerobic respiration requirement. Moreover, we observed that the formation of the brown diffusible pigment due to the phenylalanine deaminase reaction was hardly observable when the bacteria grew in clumps (Zone A) because the brown pigment diffused around the colony. Bacterial clumping may thus be a limitation of modified CIN for the visualisation of these bacteria. However, the clumped bacteria can be re-streaked on modified CIN for further identification.

The addition of chemicals did not inhibit the growth of the *Yersinia* strains tested, indicating that modified CIN has the same capacity as CIN to allow the growth of this species. It has been previously reported that CIN inhibits the growth of *Y. bercovieri* (formerly known as *Y. enterocolitica* bioserotype 3B/O:3) and some strains of *Y. pseudotuberculosis* due to the presence of cefsulodin in the medium [13,15,21,34]. Because the amount of cefsulodin was not changed in the modified CIN, we expect similar results on this medium.

In evaluating the limit of detection (LOD) and influence of background microbiota of both CIN and modified CIN media, *Y. enterocolitica* was chosen as the representating bacterium. The LOD of the modified CIN for the detection of *Y. enterocolitica* (in pure cultures or in artificially contaminated raw pork meat) was comparable to that obtained on CIN. For pure *Y. enterocolitica* cultures, the LOD was 10 cfu/ml (for all four strains tested; IP383, IP135, ATCC 9610 and PC-M16-2). For artificially contaminated raw pork meat, *Y. enterocolitica* IP135 was chosen instead of a more common biotype 4 (e.g. IP134). This is because the biotype 3 has been frequently reported in food and animals (pigs and etc.) originated/imported from Asia and Southeat Asia countries with warm climate (Southern China, Malaysia, Taiwan and Thailand) [30,31,32,33]. Whereas strains of biotype 4 are more commonly associated with humans infections in Europe and United States which is rarely reported in Southeast Asia [1,2,3,6]. Based on the results in Table 1, all pathogenic *Y. enterocolitica* strains had similar growth characteristics and colony morphology on CIN and modified CIN agar, and strains of different biotypes also had similar LODs (Table S1). Hence only one representative strain (IP135, biotype 3) was used in the spiking experiments. The biotyping and serotyping results indicated that all *Y. enterocolitica* isolates were of bioserotype 3/O:3 variant (VP negative). This supports our speculation that this particular biotype is more common and supports the choice of *Y. enterocolitica* IP135 for our medium evaluation. The LOD of IP135 for artificially contaminated pork meat increased to 10^4 cfu/ml because the presence of natural microbiota interfered with the recovery of *Y. enterocolitica*. Bacteria such as *C. freundii, C. amalonaticus, C. diversus, Hafnia alvei, Klebsiella pneumoniae, E. agglomerans, P. rettgeri,* and environmental *Yersinia* species that are naturally present in food may indeed have an inhibitory effect on the growth of *Y. enterocolitica* [34]. In a recent study conducted by Savin et al. [21], CIN was reported to be more efficient (LOD $= 3\times10^3$ cfu/g of faeces) as compared to SSI medium (LOD $= 3\times10^6$ cfu/g faeces) in isolating *Y. enterocolitica*. Therefore, we anticipate the modified CIN would be a useful medium in differentiating *Y. enterocolitica* from contaminated samples such as faeces.

Our investigation on the influence of background microbiota was done by three tests: (i) pool of bacterial mixture, (ii) artificially contaminated pork and (iii) naturally contaminated rectal swabs from swine. We observed that the *Y. enterocolitica* colonies were easily distinguished on modified CIN even when surrounded by *Yersinia*-like bacteria and background microbiota, but on CIN, it was much more difficult. The percentage of false-positive *Y. enterocolitica* recovered on CIN (66.7%) from an artificially prepared bacterial mixture can decrease to 40.0% on modified CIN, and the corresponding percentage from artificially contaminated raw pork meat can decrease from 37.7% on CIN to 27.5% on modified CIN (Table 4). At the same time, the true positive *Y. enterocolitica* isolates increased by nearly 27% and 10% on

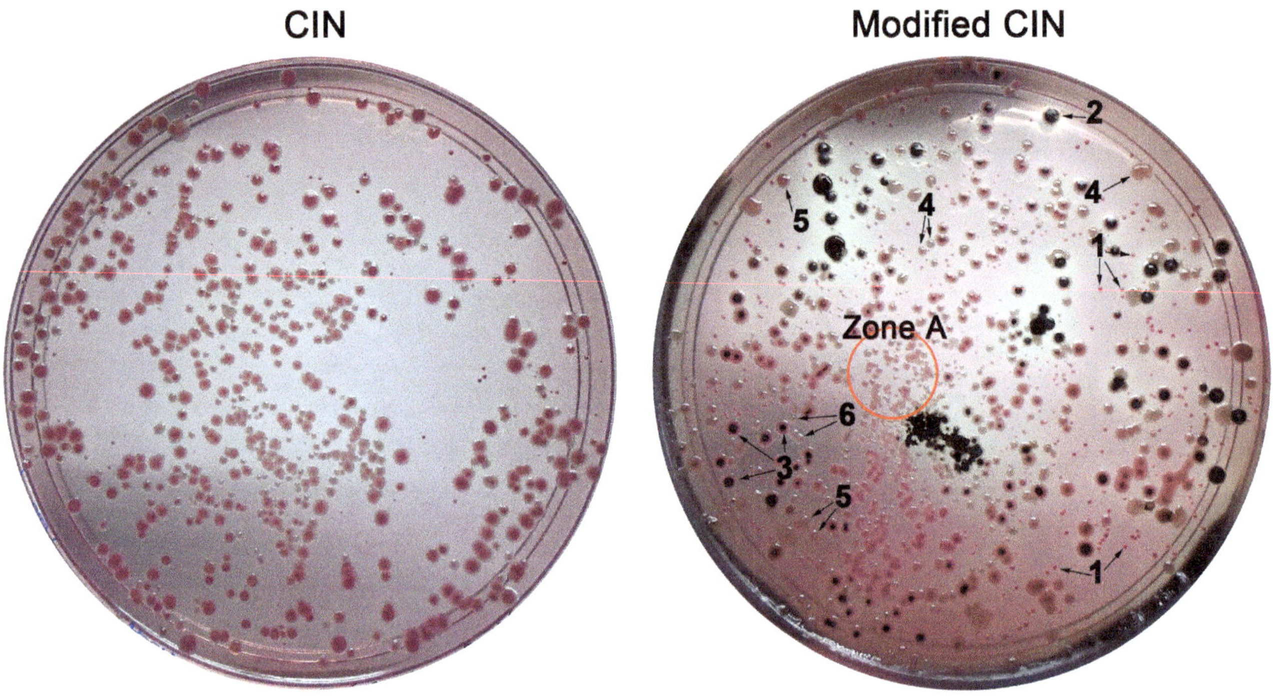

Figure 2. Colony morphology on CIN and modified CIN of artificially prepared bacterial mixtures. 1, *Y. enterocolitica* 3/O:1,2,3 (IP135); 2, *C. braakii*; 3, H_2S-producing *C. freundii*; 4, *A. hydrophila*; 5, *P. rettgeri*; 6, *E. cloacae*. Zone A shows a region of bacterial clumping in which the formation of a black centre due to H_2S production and of a brown diffusible pigment produced by a phenylalanine deaminase reaction could not be detected or could hardly be observed.

modified CIN compared to CIN in artificially prepared bacterial mixture and artificially contaminated pork, respectively (Table 4). The capability of modified CIN in reducing the number of false positive *Y. enterocolitica* isolates, especially in eliminating H_2S-producing *Citrobacter* spp., *M. morganii, P. rettgeri, A. hydrophila, E. cloacae* can shorten the processing time and reduce the workload and costs associated with biochemical assays that were reported in many studies [13,14,15,16,23,32]. Higher recovery rates from the modified CIN compared with that of CIN was further demonstrated using naturally contaminated samples (rectal swabs from swine, Table 2), indicating the modified CIN improved the recovery of *Y. enterocolitica* even on actual samples. The reason for the failure of CIN in isolating *Y. enterocolitica* from rectal specimens may due to the presence of high amount of *Yersinia*-like bacteria on CIN that caused the visualisation of the *Yersinia* difficult during plate analysis. In this study, the naturally contaminated samples were only enriched in one enrichment medium, PBS and our results indicated that a cold enrichment could help in recovering a larger number of positive samples than direct streaking method. A post-enrichment alkaline treatment showed no difference for the recovery rates of *Y. enterocolitica* (Table 2). The modification made on CIN enhanced the differentiating power of CIN while retaining the sensitivity (see results of LOD test) in isolating *Yersinia*. Hence, the modified CIN could also increase the recovery rates compared to CIN when it is used in combination with any other enrichment or isolating media that are reported to be useful in previous studies. For examples the irgarsan-ticarcillin-cholate (ITC)-CIN method [23], followed by streaking on YeCM and enrichment in peptone-sorbitol-bile (PSB) broth for 2 days [28] that are reported to be useful in isolation of pathogenic *Y. enterocolitica*.

Therefore, the use of modified CIN may significantly reduce the percentage of false-positive *Yersinia* recovered from a contaminated sample. The higher discriminatory power of the modified CIN compared with that of CIN was further demonstrated in artificially prepared bacteria mixture and naturally contaminated samples. Our results thus demonstrated that the use of modified CIN may be a valuable means to increase the recovery rate of *Yersinia* spp. from natural samples, which are usually contaminated by multiple types of bacteria.

Supporting Information

Table S1 Growth efficiency and limit of detection of CIN and modified CIN for pure cultures of *Y. enterocolitica*. [a]YE, *Yersinia enterocolitica*; [b]CIN, Cefsulodin-Irgasan-Novobiocin; [c]ae, aerobic; [d]mCIN, modified CIN; [e]mic, microaerophilic; [f]LOD, limit of detection. The underlined numbers correspond to the LOD scores for each *Y. enterocolitica* strain. The LOD is defined as the lowest cfu/ml of culturable *Y. enterocolitica* detectable in at least 50% of the replicates seeded with *Y. enterocolitica*.

Table S2 Growth efficiency and limit of detection of CIN and modified CIN for raw pork meat spiked with *Y. enterocolitica* IP135. [a]MM, microbiota in the meat sample; [b]CIN, Cefsulodin-Irgasan-Novobiocin; [c]ae, aerobic; [d]mCIN, modified CIN; [e]mic, microaerophilic; [f]LOD, limit of detection. The underlined numbers correspond to the LOD scores for each medium. The LOD is defined as the lowest cfu/ml of culturable *Y. enterocolitica* detectable in at least 50% of the replicates.

Acknowledgments

We thank the University of Malaya for the facilities. The authors would like to extend special thanks to Dr. Aziah from Makmal Kesihatan Awam Veterinar, Bandar Baru Salak Tinggi, Sepang, Malaysia for providing *Y. enterocolitica* ATCC 9610 as a positive control strain. **Funding sources**: This work was financially supported by the University of Malaya High-Impact Research Grant (reference UM.C/625/1/HIR/MOHE/02), University of Malaya Postgraduate Research Fund (PS316/2010B), MOSTI (GA013-2013), and partly by the 'Institut de Veille Sanitaire' (InVS) of France. LKT was supported by a fellowship from the University of Malaya. The funders have no role in the study design, data collection and analysis, decision to publish, or preparation of the manuscript.

Author Contributions

Conceived and designed the experiments: LKT KLT. Performed the experiments: LKT. Analyzed the data: LKT. Contributed reagents/materials/analysis tools: LKT KLT PTO EC. Wrote the paper: LKT KLT PTO EC.

References

1. European Food Safety Authority, European Centre for Disease Prevention and Control (2013) The European Union summary report on trends and sources of zoonoses, zoonotic agents and food-borne outbreaks in 2011. EFSA J 11: 3129.
2. Gould LH, Walsh KA, Vieira AR, Herman K, Williams IT, et al. (2013) Surveillance for foodborne disease outbreaks-United States, 1998–2008. MMWR 62(2): 1–34.
3. CDC (2014) Foodborne diseases active surveillance network (FoodNet): FoodNet surveillance report for 2012 (Final Report). Atlanta, Georgia: U.S. Department of Health and Human Services, CDC. Available: http://www.cdc.gov/foodnet/PDFs/2012_annual_report_508c.pdf. Accessed 20 Jun 2014.
4. Vlachaki E, Tselios K, Tsapas A, Klonizakis J (2007) *Yersinia enterocolitica* O: 3 mesenteric lymphadenopathy in an apparently healthy adult. Neth J Med 65: 311–312.
5. Schiemann DA, Olson SA (1984) Antagonism by gram-negative bacteria to growth of *Yersinia enterocolitica* in mixed cultures. Appl Environ Microbiol 48: 539–544.
6. European Food Safety Authority, European Centre for Disease Prevention and Control (2007) Monitoring and identification of human enteropathogenic *Yersinia* spp. Scientific opinion of the panel on biological hazards. EFSA J 595: 1–30.
7. Hudson JA, King NJ, Cornelius AJ, Bigwood T, Thom K, et al. (2008) Detection, isolation and enumeration of *Yersinia enterocolitica* from raw pork. Int J Food Microbiol 123: 25–31.
8. Johnson JL (1998) Isolation and identification of pathogenic *Yersinia enterocolitica* from meat and poultry products. USDA/FSIS Microbiology Laboratory Guidebook 3rd edition. pp. 1–28. Available: http://www.fsis.usda.gov/OPHS/microlab/mlgchp9.PDF. Accessed 29 Jun 2010.
9. Aulisio CC, Mehlman IJ, Sanders AC (1980) Alkali method for rapid recovery of *Yersinia enterocolitica* and *Yersinia pseudotuberculosis* from foods. Appl Environ Microbiol 39: 135–140.
10. Fukushima H (1985) Direct isolation of *Yersinia enterocolitica* and *Yersinia pseudotuberculosis* from meat. Appl Environ Microbiol 50: 710–712.
11. Wannet WJB, Reessink M, Brunings HA, Maas HME (2001) Detection of pathogenic *Yersinia enterocolitica* by a rapid and sensitive duplex PCR assay. J Clin Microbiol 39: 4483.
12. Vishnubhatla A, Oberst RD, Fung DYC, Wonglumsom W, Hays MP, et al. (2001) Evaluation of a 5′-nuclease (TaqMan) assay for the detection of virulent strains of *Yersinia enterocolitica* in raw meat and tofu samples. J Food Prot 64: 355–360.
13. Schiemann DA (1979) Synthesis of a selective agar medium for *Yersinia enterocolitica*. Can J Microbiol 25: 1298–1304.
14. Head CB, Whitty DA, Ratnam S (1982) Comparative study of selective media for recovery of *Yersinia enterocolitica*. J Clin Microbiol 16: 615–621.
15. Renaud N, Lecci L, Courcol RJ, Simonet M, Gaillot O (2013) CHROMagar *Yersinia*, a new chromogenic agar for screening of potentially pathogenic *Yersinia enterocolitica* isolates in stools. J Clin Microbiol 51: 1184–1187.
16. Weagant SD, Feng P (Jan 2001) Bacteriological Analytical Manual, Chapter 8: *Yersinia enterocolitica*. U.S. Food and Drug Administration. Available: http://www.fda.gov/Food/FoodScienceResearch/LaboratoryMethods/ucm072633.htm. Accessed 29 Jun 2010.
17. Fukushima H (1987) New selective agar medium for isolation of virulent *Yersinia enterocolitica*. J Clin Microbiol 25: 1068–1073.
18. Denis M, Houard E, Labbé A, Fondrevez M, Salvat G (2011) A selective chromogenic plate, YECA, for the detection of pathogenic *Yersinia enterocolitica*: specificity, sensitivity and capacity to detect pathogenic *Y. enterocolitica* from pig tonsils. J Pathog 2011: 1–8.
19. Weagant SD (2008) A new chromogenic agar medium for detection of potentially virulent *Yersinia enterocolitica*. J Microbiol Methods 72: 185–190.
20. Blom M, Meyer A, Gerner-Smidt P, Gaarslev K, Espersen F (1999) Evaluation of Statens Serum Institut enteric medium for detection of enteric pathogens. J Clin Microbiol 37: 2312–2316.
21. Savin C, Leclercq A, Carniel E (2012) Evaluation of a single procedure allowing the isolation of enteropathogenic *Yersinia* along with other bacterial enteropathogens from human stools. PLoS ONE 7: e41176.
22. Denys GA, Renzi PB, Koch KM, Wissel CM (2013) Three-way comparison of BBL CHROMagar MRSA II, MRSASelect, and spectra MRSA for detection of methicillin-resistant *Staphylococcus aureus* isolates in nasal surveillance cultures. J Clin Microbiol 51: 202–205.
23. Fondrevez M, Labbé A, Houard E, Fravalo P, Madec F, et al. (2010) A simplified method for detecting pathogenic *Yersinia enterocolitica* in slaughtered pig tonsils. J Microbiol Methods 83: 244–249.
24. Cheesbrough M (2006) District laboratory practice in tropical countries. Cambridge University Press. Available: http://www.nu.edu.sa/userfiles/amasad/14017630-District-Laboratory-Practice-in-Tropical-CountriesPart-2Monica-Cheesbrough.pdf. Accessed 10 Sept 2010.
25. Microbiological Methods Committee (2011) Procedure for the development and management of food microbiological methods. Part 4: Guildelines for the relative validation of indirect qualitative food microbiological methods. Food Directorate's (Health Canada's) pp. 1–12. Available: http://www.hc-sc.gc.ca/food-aliment. Accessed 23 Apr 2012.
26. Wauters G, Kandolo K, Janssens M (1987) Revised biogrouping scheme of *Yersinia enterocolitica*. Contrib Microbiol Immunol 9: 14–21.
27. Bergey DH, Breed RS, Hitchens AP, Murray E (1948) Bergey's Manual of Determinative Bacteriology. Williams & Wilkins. 964 p.
28. Van Damme I, Berkvens D, Botteldoorn N, Dierick K, Wits J, et al. (2013) Evaluation of the ISO 10273: 2003 method for the isolation of human pathogenic *Yersinia enterocolitica* from pig carcasses and minced meat. Food Microbiol 36: 170–175.
29. Stilinovic B, Hrenovic J (2009) Plate method for counting the proteolytic sulphide-producing bacteria. Acta Bot Croat 68: 57–66.
30. Liang J, Wang X, Xiao Y, Cui Z, Xia S, et al. (2012) Prevalence of *Yersinia enterocolitica* in pigs slaughtered in chinese abattoirs. Appl Environl Microbiol 78: 2949–2956.
31. Wang X, Cui Z, Jin D, Tang L, Xia S, et al. (2009) Distribution of pathogenic *Yersinia enterocolitica* in China. Eur J Clin Microbiol Infect Dis 28: 1237–1244.
32. Zheng XB, Xie C (1996) Note: isolation, characterization and epidemiology of *Yersinia enterocolitica* from humans and animals. J Appl Microbiol 81: 681–684.
33. Tan LK, Ooi PT, Thong KL (2014) Prevalence of *Yersinia enterocolitica* from food and pigs in selected states of Malaysia. Food Control 35: 94–100.
34. Fukushima H, Gomyoda M (1986) Inhibition of *Yersinia enterocolitica* serotype O3 by natural microflora of pork. Appl Environ Microbiol 51: 990–994.

18

Oral Administration of Royal Jelly Restores Tear Secretion Capacity in Rat Blink-Suppressed Dry Eye Model by Modulating Lacrimal Gland Function

Toshihiro Imada[1], Shigeru Nakamura[1]*, Naoki Kitamura[2], Izumi Shibuya[2], Kazuo Tsubota[1]

1 Department of Ophthalmology, Keio University School of Medicine, Tokyo, Japan, **2** Department of Veterinary Physiology, Faculty of Agriculture, Tottori University, Tottori, Japan

Abstract

Tears are secreted from the lacrimal gland (LG), a dysfunction in which induces dry eye, resulting in ocular discomfort and visual impairment. Honey bee products are used as a nutritional source in daily life and medicine; however, little is known about their effects on dry eye. The aim of the present study was to investigate the effects of honey bee products on tear secretion capacity in dry eye. We selected raw honey, propolis, royal jelly (RJ), pollen, or larva from commercially available honey bee products. Tear secretion capacity was evaluated following the oral administration of each honey bee product in a rat blink-suppressed dry eye model. Changes in tear secretion, LG ATP content, and LG mitochondrial levels were measured. RJ restored the tear secretion capacity and decrease in LG ATP content and mitochondrial levels to the largest extent. Royal jelly can be used as a preventative intervention for dry eye by managing tear secretion capacity in the LG.

Editor: Michele Madigan, Save Sight Institute, Australia

Funding: This work was supported by a Yamada research grant from Yamada Bee company, Inc.

Competing Interests: The authors have declared that no competing interests exist.

* Email: vdtwork@gmail.com

Introduction

The ocular surface, comprising the cornea and conjunctiva, is covered by a thin layer of an aqueous tear film secreted from the lacrimal gland (LG). The role of tear fluid is to provide a proper environment to maintain homeostasis for the ocular surface [1]. The tear film acts as the first defense system against environmental microbes, desiccation, and foreign bodies and also smooths the refractive surface of the transparent cornea [2]. Dry eye disease is a multifactorial disorder characterized by the status of the tear film, results in ocular discomfort and visual impairment [3], and has become a major public health issue in industrial societies that have many of the risk factors for this disease, including the use of digital devices (computers, tablets, and smart phones) [4]. The incidence of dry eye was previously showed to be particularly high in workers that stare at the screens of technological devices [5,6]. We previously demonstrated that a chronic reduction in tear production was induced by extended computer use in both human and animal studies, and suggested that LG hypofunction may be a critical mechanism in digital device-induced dry eye [7]. The function of the LG also has been shown to decrease with aging, a known potent risk factor for dry eye [8,9]. Therefore, the discovery and development of novel preventative interventions that could maintain healthy LG function may have considerable clinical implications. However, temporal tear replacement therapy, the frequent application of artificial tear eye drops, has long been used in the basis management of dry eye [10].

Beekeeping products have been deeply rooted in the lives of different people and cultures worldwide for thousands of years as a nutritional source and medicine. The main products of beekeeping are honey, royal jelly, propolis, pollen, and bee larva produced or collected by Apidae. These products exhibit a wide range of biological effects, including antibacterial [11,12], antiviral [13], anti-inflammatory [14,15], and/or antiallergenic actions [16,17]. Honey eye drops have been used in corneal wound therapy as a traditional medicine [18] in the ophthalmic field and propolis was shown to protect against neuronal damage in the retina [19]. However little is known about the effects of honey bee products on tear secretion capacity in dry eye.

In the present study, we assessed the potential usefulness of orally applied honey bee products as a preventative intervention in dry eye associated with the excessive use of digital devices. We used a blink-suppressed dry eye model: persistent strain by swing treatment in combination with exposure to an evaporative environment, which induces disordered tear dynamics, decreased blink frequency, and LG dysfunction. This dry eye model was established based on the concept that the long-lasting use of technological devices is associated with a marked reduction in the frequency of blinking while gazing at the screen and awkward postures in a dry environment [7].

Materials and Methods

Animals

Female 8-weeks-old Sprague-Dawley rats (CLEA Japan, Japan) were used in this study. All animals were quarantined and acclimatized for 1 week prior to the experiments under the following general conditions: room temperature of 23±2°C, relative humidity of 60±10%, alternating 12-hour light-dark cycle (8 AM to 8 PM), and water and food *ad libitum*. All animals were used according to the Association of Research and Vision in Ophthalmology (ARVO) statement for the Use of Animals in Ophthalmic and Vision Research. The protocol for this study was approved by the Ethics Committee on Animal Research of the Keio University School of Medicine (Approval No. 11008-2).

Honey bee products

Raw honey, an ethanolic extract of propolis, the lyophilized powder of RJ, pollen granules, and the lyophilized powder of larva were used. The detailed information of each honey bee products used in this study is described in Table S1. All honey bee products were supplied by Yamada Bee Company, Inc. (Okayama, Japan).

Protein secretion from isolated LGs

Rats were euthanized by excess pentobarbital administration and their LG were rapidly dissected. LG digested by collagenase type 3 (Worthington, USA) was incubated in saline solution (140 mM NaCl, 5 mM KCl, 2 mM $CaCl_2$, 1 mM $MgCl_2$, 10 mM HEPES, 10 mM dextrose [pH 7.4]) with each honey bee product. Carbachol (CCH), a cholinergic stimulus, was used as a positive control. The protein concentration in the medium was measured using the Bradford reagent (Sigma-Aldrich, USA) with bovine serum albumin (BSA) as the standard. The protein secretion rate was calculated as a percentage of that the before stimulation. 5 rats were used in each group.

Rat blink-suppressed dry eye model

The model and methodology used to simulate VDT has been described previously [7,20,21]. In brief, a series of treatments were performed under dry conditions, with a room temperature of 23±2°C, relative humidity of 25±5%, and constant air flow at 2 to 4 m/s produced by an electric fan. Each rat was placed on a swing for 7.5 hours per day between 9 AM and 5 PM. A photograph of the rat blink-suppressed model was shown in figure S1. This series of treatment, procedure to simulate VDT in rat, was repeated for 5 days for screening of honey bee products and 10days for the RJ evaluation. Each honey bee product was dissolved in distilled water at 240 mg/ml (honey), 40 mg/ml (pollen, larva, and propolis), and 60 mg/ml (RJ) and was repeatedly administered orally each 1 ml to rats once a day. Distilled water was used as vehicle control. To screen honey bee products at the effective dose for health benefits, the dosage of each honey bee product was chosen by reference to previous reports [14,22,23]. Lacrimal function was evaluated on day 11. For each experiment using rat blink-suppressed dry eye model, 6 to 18 rats were used in each group.

Tear secretion. We used a modified Schirmer test on rat eyes to measurement tear fluid secretion under topical anesthesia by 0.4% oxybuprocaine hydrochloride solution (Santen Pharmaceutical, Japan) [24]. A phenol red thread (Zone-Quick; Showa Yakuhin kako, Japan) was placed on the temporal side of the upper eyelid margin for 1 minute. The length of the moistened area from the edge was measured within 1 mm.

Corneal fluorescein staining. Changes in the corneal surface were determined by the application of a fluorescein solution under a blue-free barrier filter [25], and corneal staining of the area was graded according to previously described criteria [20].

Histopathological examination. The fixed LG in 10% formalin was embedded in paraffin and sectioned. Sections were subjected to HE staining or immunostaining. The acinar cell density of each section was determined by quantifying the nuclear number in three randomly selected areas (2500 μm^2).

Vesicle-associated membrane protein 8 (VAMP8) was immnostained to evaluate the occupied pattern of secretory vesicles (SVs) in the acinar cells of specimens. VAMP8 was previously shown to be enriched on the membranes of zymogen granules [26]. The primary antibody used for immunostaining was a rabbit monoclonal antibody against VAMP8 (Abcam, UK). Nuclear staining was performed by treating specimens with hematoxylin.

Mitochondrial function. The homogenized LG was examined to measure ATP levels and mitochondrial content. ATP levels were determined according to the instructions for the ATP Bioluminescence Assay Kit CLS 2 (Roche Molecular Biochemicals, Germany). Mitochondrial content was measured by using the fluorescence dye, Mitotracker green FM (Molecular Probes, USA) and Hoechst 33342 (Dojin Chemical, Japan). These measurements were performed on a Synergy 4 plate reader (Biotek Company, USA). The mitochondrial membrane potential of the LG was visualized by staining with Mitotracker red (Invitrogen), a membrane potential-dependent fluorescence dye.

Western blot. Total protein extracts from the LG were separated by polyacrylamide gel electrophoresis, transferred to PVDF membranes using a dry blotting system (V20-SDB, SCIE-PLAS, UK), and incubated with antibodies. Immunolabeled proteins were detected using Pierce Western blotting Substrate Plus (Thermo SCIENTIFIC, Germany) and a Lumino-image analyzer (LAS-4000, FujiFilm, Japan). All bands were normalized to β-actin. The primary antibodies used for Western blotting were as follows; AMP-activated protein kinase [AMPK (Cell Signaling, Japan), Phospho-AMPK (Cell Signaling)], and β-actin (Sigma Aldrich). 6rats were used in each group.

Intracellular calcium ion concentration ($[Ca^{2+}]i$) measurements

The LG digested by collagenase type 3 was filtered through a 100 μm nylon mesh (Cell Strainer, BD Biosciences, Japan) to isolate LG acinar cells. Acinar cells were loaded with fura-2/AM (Invitrogen, USA), the fluorescent Ca^{2+} indicator, and transferred to round coverslips. Coverslips were then mounted on a chamber fixed on the stage of an inverted fluorescence microscope (IX71, Olympus, Japan). Acinar cells were continuously perfused with diverse experimental solutions through polyethylene tubes connected to a peristaltic pump (Minipulse 3, Gilson, USA) at flow rate of 0.8 ml per minutes.

Royal jelly (100, 300, and 500 μg/ml), CCH (10 μM; Tokyo Kasei Kougyo, Japan), and 10-hydroxy-2-decenoic acid (500 μg/ml; 10-HDE, Cayman, USA) were diluted to the desired concentrations with saline solution and used as stimulants. AG1478 (10 μM; Wako, Japan), Atropine sulfate (1 μM; Nacalai, Japan), U73122 (1 μM; Sigma, Japan), and cyclopiazonic acid (10 μM; CPA, Sigma, Japan) were appropriately prepared in saline solution before use. Changes in $[Ca^{2+}]i$ were measured by dual excitation microfluorometry using a digital image analyzer (Aqua Cosmos/Ratio, Hamamatsu Photonics, Japan). The fluorescence signal was detected using UV objective lens (UApo 20×3/340, Olympus), and the emission passing through a band pass filter (500±10 nm) was detected by a cooled CCD camera (ORCAER, Hamamatsu Photonics, Japan). Data acquisition was performed at a sampling frequency of 0.2 Hz throughout the experiments using Aqua Cosmos software (Hamamatsu Photonics). The fluorescence intensity of each pixel was measured and digitalized at the excitation wavelengths of 340 and 380 nm by the analyzing software (Aqua Cosmos). For each experiment, 10 to 53 acinar cells were used in each group.

Statistical analysis

The Student's *t*-test was used to compare the two groups and Dunnett's test was used for multiple comparisons. Differences between the measured variables were considered significant if the resultant *P* value was 0.05 or less.

Results

Effects of honey bee products on tear secretion capacity

Figure 1 shows the effects of the screened honey bee products on tear secretion capacity. In the dry eye model, which corresponded to that of our previous study [7], tear secretion was significantly less in the vehicle group than in the normal group. The prevention of a reduction in tear secretion was significantly more prominent in the RJ and propolis group than in the vehicle group (Fig 1A). In the other products (honey, pollen, and larva) and vehicle, significant decreases were observed (Fig 1A).

Protein secretion from LG acinar cells were significantly increased by the RJ and CCH stimulation. The stimulation of protein secretion was not observed with the other products (Fig 1B).

Evaluation of the rat blink-suppressed dry eye model

A significant difference was not observed in body weight gain among any dose of RJ and vehicle groups (Fig 2A). Tear secretion was significantly less from 5 days to 11 days than the initial value in the vehicle group.

RJ dose-dependently suppressed the reduction in tear secretion. This suppression was significantly stronger with 300 and 3000 mg/kg RJ than with the vehicle at all time points throughout the experiment (Fig2B, left). Figure 2B right shows representative photographs of tear secretion patterns measured by the modified Schirmer test. The wetted length on the thread showed by a red discolored area was shorter in vehicle eyes than in RJ eyes.

We performed corneal epithelial fluorescein staining on 300 mg/kg RJ at day 11 to investigate whether the effects of RJ on tear secretion altered corneal epithelial damage in the dry eye condition. The grade of corneal epithelial fluorescein staining was significantly higher in the vehicle than the initial value. The intake of RJ maintained the graded score at the same level as the initial value and the graded score was significantly less than that of the vehicle. Representative SPK patterns restored by RJ are shown in Figure 2C.

Alteration in LG morphology

Figure 2D shows a representative microphotograph of the LG stained by HE (upper) and secretory vesicle-occupied pattern by VAMP8 immunostaining (lower) in the dry eye condition. In the vehicle group, the cytoplasm of acinar cells was occupied by more enlarged acini with expanded cytoplasm than that of the normal group. Aciner cell density was significant reduced in the vehicle than in the normal value of the dry eye condition. RJ maintained the aciner cell density as the same level as the normal value, and the value was significantly higher than that of vehicle (Fig. 2D, bar chart).

VAMP8 was primary localized near the apical membrane in the normal state, while it was distributed diffusely in the entire cytoplasm of acinar cells in the vehicle group. VAMP8 was localized to the proximity of the apical membranes in the RJ group and its distribution was identical to that found in the normal state. These results suggest that acinar cells were enlarged by the accumulation of secretory vesicles and returned to the normal state by the intake of RJ in this dry eye model.

Alteration in mitochondrial function in the LG

ATP levels were significantly lower in the vehicle group than in the normal group. The intake of RJ significantly restored the decrease in ATP levels in the vehicle group (Fig 3A). Mitochondrial content was significantly lower in the vehicle group than in the normal group. Mitochondrial content was restored signifi-

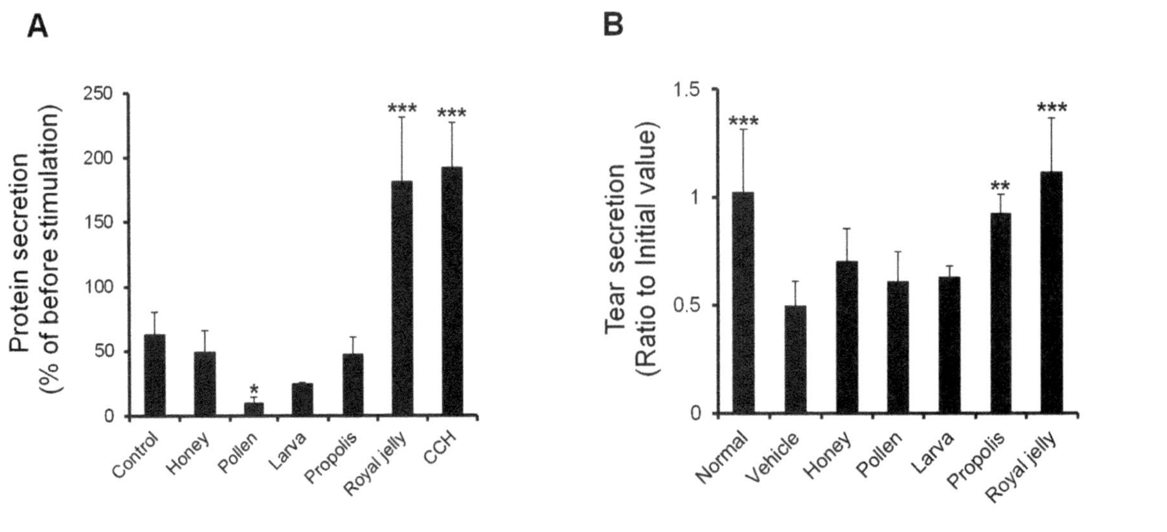

Figure 1. Evaluation of various honey bee products. A: Effect of various honey bee products on tear secretion in a rat blink-suppressed dry eye model. The oral administration doses of honey, pollen, larva, propolis, and RJ were 1200, 200, 200, 200, and 300 mg/kg, respectively (n = 5 rats). B: Protein secretion rate from normal LG after stimulation by various honey bee products. The LG was stimulated with 500 μg/ml of each honey bee product (n = 5 LG). All data represent the mean ± SD. *$P<0.05$, **$P<0.01$, ***$P<0.001$ versus the vehicle.

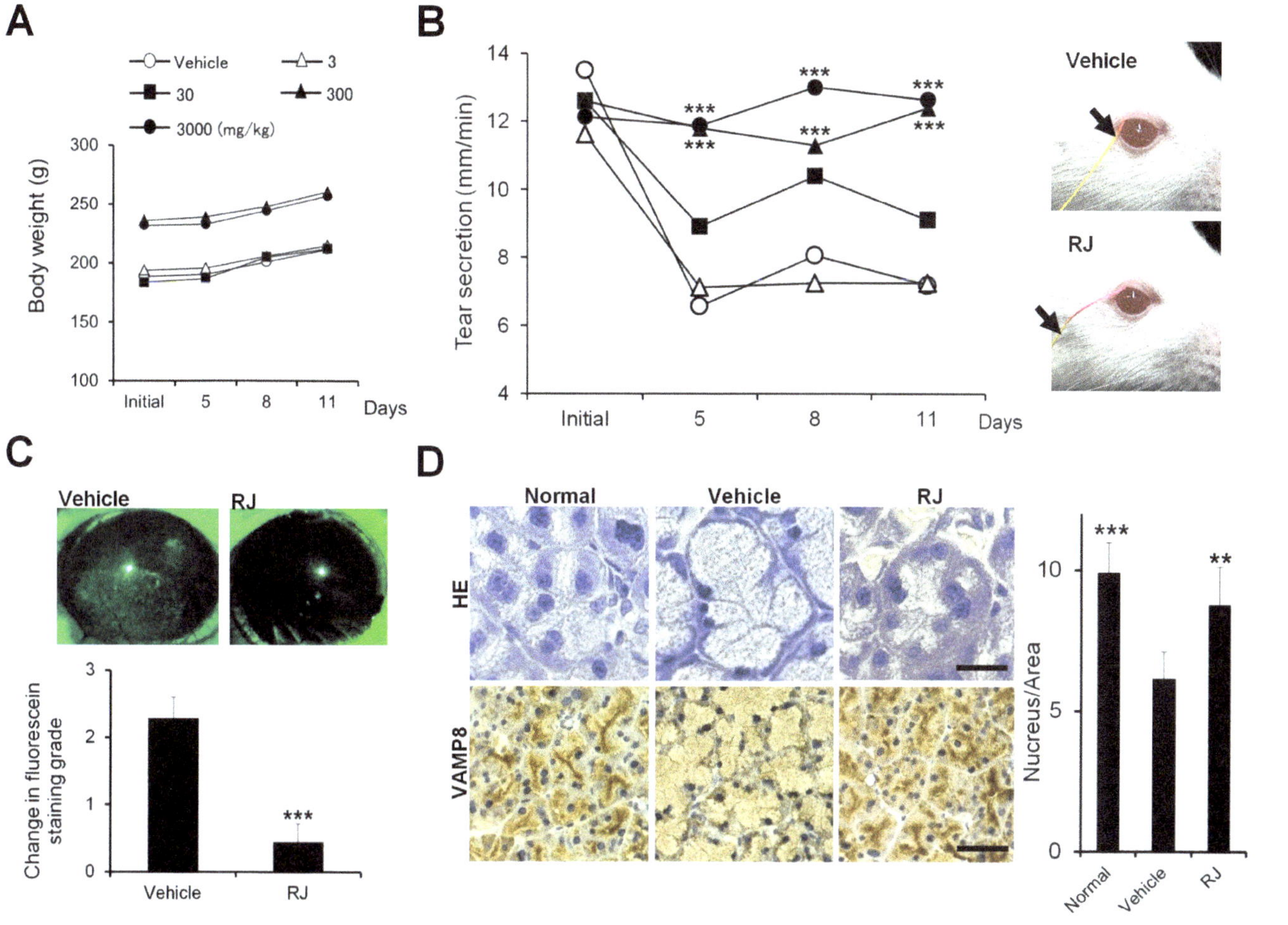

Figure 2. Royal jelly restored tear secretion in a rat blink-suppressed dry eye model. A: Changes in body weight. B: Changes in tear secretion (Left). (n = 10 rats) Representative photographs of tear secretion patterns measured by a cotton thread (Right). The arrow shows the wetted length by tear secretion. C: Effect of RJ on corneal surface damage. Changes in the grading score (lower, n = 9 rats), Typical pattern of staining (Upper). Punctate staining appeared in the whole area of cornea surface with the vehicle treatment. D: Histopathological changes in the LG. HE staining (Left upper). VAMP8 immunostaining (Left lower). Scale bar, 20 μm (HE) or 50 μm (VAMP8). Acinar cell size (Right, n = 6 LG). All data represent the mean ± SD. $^{**}P<0.01$, $^{***}P<0.001$ versus the vehicle.

cantly more in the RJ group than in the vehicle group (Fig 3B). Figure 3B right shows a representative image of mitochondrial activity detected by staining with a membrane potential-dependent fluorescein probe. The accumulation of fluorescein probe in acinar cells was less in the vehicle group than in the normal group. The accumulation of the probe was observed in the entire cytoplasm of acinar cells in the RJ group. These results suggest that mitochondrial activity in the LG was restored by the intake of RJ in the dry eye condition.

Effect of RJ on AMPK phosphorylation in the LG

The oral intake of RJ induced a significant increase in AMPK phosphorylation after 3 and 6 hours, and this increase returned to initial levels after 24 hours (Figure 3C).

Effect of RJ on LG [Ca^{2+}]i mobilization

RJ dose-dependently induced an increase in [Ca^{2+}]i (Fig 4A). To investigate the calcium signaling pathway involved in this elevation, the effects of possible factors found in RJ were examined [27,28,29]. An elevation in [Ca^{2+}]i was not detected in 10-HDE (Fig 4B). No significant change was observed in the [Ca^{2+}]i elevation by RJ with or without AG1478, an epidermal growth factor receptor (EGFR) antagonist (Fig 4C). The effects of muscarinic acetylcholine pathway inhibitors on the [Ca^{2+}]i elevation by RJ were shown in Figure 4D. The acetylcholine receptor antagonist atropine abolished the [Ca^{2+}]i elevation. U73122 and CPA, potent inhibitors of PLC or ER-Ca^{2+}-ATPase respectively, significantly suppressed the [Ca^{2+}]i elevation by RJ. No significant differences were observed between the inhibitory effects of these agents on the responses to RJ and CCH.

The RJ-induced [Ca^{2+}]i elevation was compared to that of raw RJ material, in order to eliminate the possibility that the activity was due to preparation process from raw material. No difference in the [Ca^{2+}]i elevation was observed between the raw RJ and RJ (Fig S3). These result demonstrated that [Ca^{2+}]i elevation by RJ was via active ingredients formed by Apis.

Discussion

To verify the potential nutritional benefits of commercially available honey bee products in the prevention of dry eye, we screened the effects of each product on tear secretion capacity in this study.

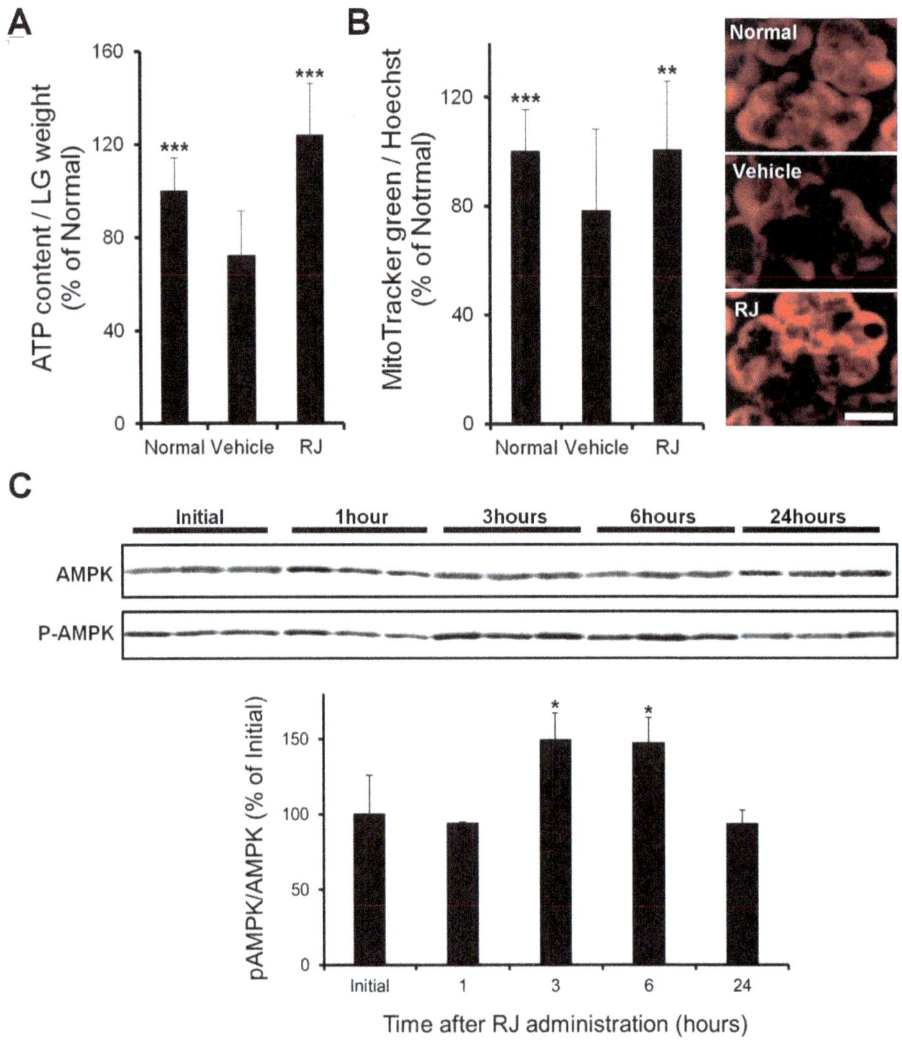

Figure 3. Effect of royal jelly on lacrimal gland function. A: ATP levels. B: Mitochondria content (Left). Imaging of the mitochondrial membrane potential (Right). Scale bar, 20 μm. (n = 12–18 LG) C: AMPK activity in a normal lacrimal gland after the oral administration of RJ (n = 6 LG). All data represent the mean ± SD. * $P<0.05$, ** $P<0.01$, *** $P<0.001$, versus the vehicle (ATP and mitochondria) or initial (AMPK).

Protein secretion from the LG, a critical function for tear secretion, was only evoked by RJ and the decrease in tear secretion *in vivo* in the dry eye model was restored by RJ and propolis at a dosage sufficient for human health benefits. In addition, the intake of RJ suppressed corneal epithelial damage, which is considered as one of the clinical manifestations changes on the ocular surface in dry eye. These results indicate that RJ restored dry eye symptoms by directly acting on the LG and may represent a very potent nutritional treatment for the prevention of dry eye compared with the honey bee products screened.

The formation of tear fluid by the LG is thought to be achieved by a combination of transepithelial water flow generated by an osmotic gradient and protein secretion from intracellular vesicles by exocytotic release in acinar cells [30].

The activation of multiple water channels and ion transporters were previously shown to be involved in the facilitation of a transepithelial osmotic gradient [31,32]. The process of secretory vesicle-mediated exocytosis comprises a chain of complex mechanisms involving intracellular trafficking and fusion with the plasma membrane to release their contents into the extracellular space [33]. These secretory processes require ATP as an energy source to produce protein rich aqueous fluid from LG cells while tearing [34,35]. We previously demonstrated that the stressful condition used in this dry eye model, an immobilized rat on a swing board in the presence of a continuous desiccated air blower, causes a decrease in tear secretion capacity accompanied an increased volume of secretory vesicles and loss of the intracellular cell structure, which indicates a dysfunction in the secretory system [7]. Exposure to stress is known to exacerbate the energy status of various organs, resulting in the loss of mitochondrial function [36,37,38]. In the present study, we showed a decrease in ATP levels and mitochondria content in the LG, in addition to lacrimal dysfunction. Thus, our results suggest that the reduction in the energy status in the LG is critical in the impairment of tear secretion capacity in the dry eye condition

Most cellular ATP is generated from mitochondrial oxidative phosphorylation. To maintain cellular ATP levels, $[Ca^{2+}]i$ levels play a critical role in the control of ATP synthesis by activating

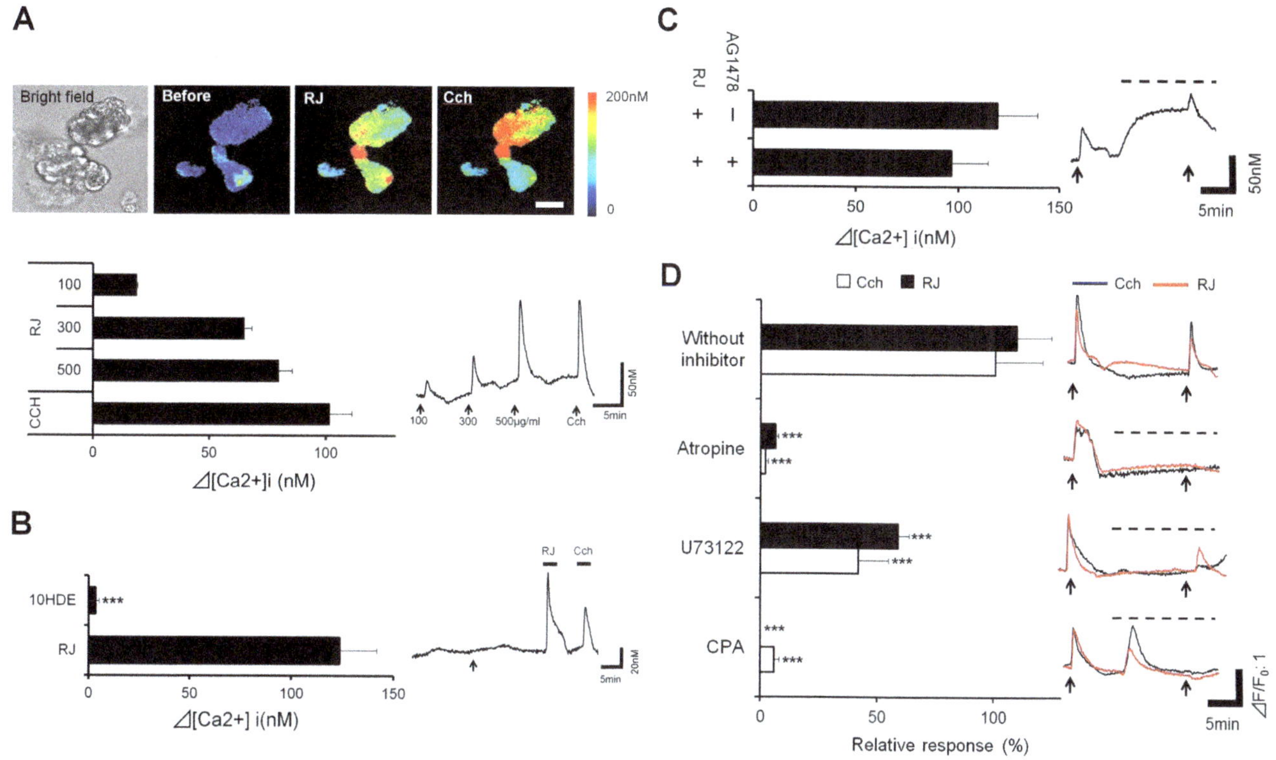

Figure 4. Effect of royal jelly on lacrimal gland acinar [Ca^{2+}]i mobilization. A: Changes in [Ca^{2+}]i in normal lacrimal acinar cells. Pseudo colored images of [Ca^{2+}]i (Upper). Scale bar, 50 μm. The bar graph shows the summarized data of the amplitudes of [Ca^{2+}]i responses. (n = 13 acini) B: Effect of 10-HDE (Left, n = 14 acini). The typical response to 10HDE (Right). C: Effect of AG1478 (n = 10 acini). D: Effect of muscarinic acetylcholine pathway inhibitors (Left, n = 22–53 acini). Responses to the stimulation with or without inhibitors (Right). The arrow indicates the time at which RJ or CCH was applied to the cells. Dotted line over the trace indicated the presence of each inhibitor. Relative responses were calculated as a percentage of the decrease in the RJ-induced [Ca^{2+}]i response with the application of an inhibitor relative to the stimulation seen with RJ alone in each acinus. All data represent the mean ± SE. ***P<0.001 versus RJ (Fig 4C) or without an inhibitor (Fig 4D).

oxidative phosphorylation-related enzymes in mitochondria [39]. Adenosine monophosphate-activated protein kinase (AMPK), a key regulator of mitochondrial biogenesis and energy production pathways, is activated by Ca^{2+}/calmodulin-dependent protein kinase kinase-β in response to an increase in the cytosolic-free calcium levels [40]. Our results demonstrated that the oral administration of RJ enhanced tear secretion capacity associated with an increased level of ATP, mitochondria, and phosphorylation of AMPK in the LG. In addition, stimulation with RJ on LG acinar cells evoked [Ca^{2+}]i in a dose-dependent manner. However the mobilization of [Ca^{2+}]i in LG acinar cells is believed to directly stimulate tear fluid secretion by activating ion transporters and exocytosis, and the elevated period and level in tear secretion stimulated by the intake of RJ in the normal rat was insufficient to compensate for decreased tear secretion in the dry eye condition (Fig S2).

Several substances that could potentially promote to maintain cellular ATP levels via increase in cytosolic Ca^{2+} are found in RJ. Acetylcholine, a major neurotransmitter involved in tear secretion, was found of 1 mg/g in RJ [27] and increases intracellular Ca^{2+} levels by activating muscarinic receptors. 10-hydroxy-2-decenoic acid is a unique fatty acid found in RJ that induces the entry of extracellular Ca^{2+} by activating Ca^{2+} -permeable nonselective cation channels [28]. Royalactin, a specific protein drives queen development in honeybees, acts through EGFR to increase [Ca^{2+}]i [29].

Our results showed that 10-HDE did not stimulate [Ca^{2+}]i, and a muscarinic receptor inhibitor, but not EGFR abolished RJ-induced [Ca^{2+}]i mobilization. Furthermore, RJ-induced [Ca^{2+}]i mobilization was suppressed by inhibitors of PLC and ER-Ca^{2+}-ATPase, which are essential enzymes involved in the muscarinic signal transduction pathway [41]. These results demonstrated, for the first time, to the best of our knowledge, that RJ mobilizes [Ca^{2+}]i through the muscarinic signal transduction pathway and suggest that preserving the energy status via this pathway is a potential mechanism by which RJ restores tear secretion capacity. To further identify and characterize the active components of RJ on tear secretion capacity, a separation and purification technique such as bioassay-guided fractionation with chemical structure analysis is needed.

In conclusion, this study is the first to demonstrate that orally administrated RJ restores tear secretion capacity in dry eye. This effect was assumed to be associated with the LG energy status through modulation of the calcium signaling pathway stimulated by RJ. Since the safety of RJ is well-known, further clinical studies on the prevention or treatment by RJ with a focus on information technology-associated dry eye will contribute to establish new therapeutic interventions for this disease.

Supporting Information

Figure S1 Photograph of the rat blink-suppressed dry eye model. Electric fan (A), swing (B). In addition to being placed on the swing, the rats were exposed to constant low humidity air flow aimed at the face, produced by an electric fan.

Figure S2 Changes in tear secretion after RJ was administered orally to normal rats. The dose of the oral administration was 3000 mg/kg RJ. Data represent the mean ± SD for 6 rats. *P* values versus the vehicle.

Figure S3 Changes in [Ca^{2+}]i elevation by raw RJ. The acini were stimulated by 500 µg/ml of raw RJ. (n = 18–24 acini) Data represent the mean ± SE.

Acknowledgments

The authors thank Sachiko Shimoda and Kohei Yoshimoto for their technical assistance.

Author Contributions

Conceived and designed the experiments: TI SN KT. Performed the experiments: TI. Analyzed the data: TI SN. Wrote the paper: TI SN NK IS KT.

References

1. Mathers WD (2000) Why the eye becomes dry: a cornea and lacrimal gland feedback model. CLAO J 26: 159–165.
2. Mishima S (1965) Some physiological aspects of the precorneal tear film. Arch Ophthalmol 73: 233–241.
3. Lemp MA (2008) Advances in understanding and managing dry eye disease. Am J Ophthalmol 146: 350–356.
4. World Health Organization (1987) Visual display terminals and workers' health. Offset publications. 99 WHO.
5. Tsubota K, Nakamori K (1993) Dry eyes and video display terminals. N Engl J Med 328: 584.
6. Uchino M, Schaumberg DA, Dogru M, Uchino Y, Fukagawa K, et al. (2008) Prevalence of dry eye disease among Japanese visual display terminal users. Ophthalmology 115: 1982–1988.
7. Nakamura S, Kinoshita S, Yokoi N, Ogawa Y, Shibuya M, et al. (2010) Lacrimal hypofunction as a new mechanism of dry eye in visual display terminal users. PLoS One 5: e11119.
8. Schaumberg DA, Dana R, Buring JE, Sullivan DA (2009) Prevalence of dry eye disease among US men: estimates from the Physicians' Health Studies. Arch Ophthalmol 127: 763–768.
9. Schaumberg DA, Sullivan DA, Buring JE, Dana MR (2003) Prevalence of dry eye syndrome among US women. Am J Ophthalmol 136: 318–326.
10. Friedman NJ (2010) Impact of dry eye disease and treatment on quality of life. Curr Opin Ophthalmol 21: 310–316.
11. Zainol MI, Mohd Yusoff K, Mohd Yusof MY (2013) Antibacterial activity of selected Malaysian honey. BMC Complement Altern Med. 13: 129.
12. Souza RM, de Souza MC, Patitucci ML, Silva JF (2007) Evaluation of antioxidant and antimicrobial activities and characterization of bioactive components of two Brazilian propolis samples using a pKa-guided fractionation. Z Naturforsch C. 62: 801–807.
13. Shimizu T, Hino A, Tsutsumi A, Park YK, Watanabe W, et al. (2008) Anti-influenza virus activity of propolis in vitro and its efficacy against influenza infection in mice. Antivir Chem Chemother. 19: 7–13.
14. Pagliarone AC, Missima F, Orsatti CL, Bachiega TF, Sforcin JM (2009) Propolis effect on Th1/Th2 cytokines production by acutely stressed mice. J Ethnopharmacol. 125: 230–233.
15. Karaca T, Simsek N, Uslu S, Kalkan Y, Can I, et al. (2012) The effect of royal jelly on CD3(+), CD5(+), CD45(+) T-cell and CD68(+) cell distribution in the colon of rats with acetic acid-induced colitis. Allergol Immunopathol (Madr). 40: 357–361.
16. Okamoto I, Taniguchi Y, Kunikata T, Kohno K, Iwaki K, et al. (2003) Major royal jelly protein 3 modulates immune responses in vitro and in vivo. Life Sci. 73: 2029–2045.
17. Nakamura R, Nakamura R, Watanabe K, Oka K, Ohta S, et al. (2010) Effects of propolis from different areas on mast cell degranulation and identification of the effective components in propolis. Int Immunopharmacol 10: 1107–1112.
18. Mansour AM (2002) Epithelial corneal oedema treated with honey. Clin Experiment Ophthalmol 30: 149–150.
19. Inokuchi Y, Shimazawa M, Nakajima Y, Suemori S, Mishima S, et al. (2006) Brazilian green propolis protects against retinal damage in vitro and in vivo. Evid Based Complement Alternat Med. 3: 71–77.
20. Nakamura S, Shibuya M, Nakashima H, Imagawa T, Uehara M, et al. (2005) D-beta-hydroxybutyrate protects against corneal epithelial disorders in a rat dry eye model with jogging board. Invest Ophthalmol Vis Sci. 46: 2379–2387.
21. Nakamura S, Shibuya M, Nakashima H, Hisamura R, Masuda N, et al. (2007) Involvement of oxidative stress on corneal epithelial alterations in a blink-suppressed dry eye. Invest Ophthalmol Vis Sci. 48: 1552–1558.
22. Takaki-Doi S, Hashimoto K, Yamamura M, Kamei C (2009) Antihypertensive activities of royal jelly protein hydrolysate and its fractions in spontaneously hypertensive rats. Acta Med Okayama 63: 57–64.
23. Bogdanov S, Jurendic T, Sieber R, Gallmann P (2008) Honey for nutrition and health: a review. J Am Coll Nutr. 27: 677–689.
24. Sakamoto R, Bennett ES, Henry VA, Paragina S, Narumi T, et al. (1993) The phenol red thread tear test: a cross-cultural study. Invest Ophthalmol Vis Sci. 34: 3510–3514.
25. Koh S, Watanabe H, Hosohata J, Hori Y, Hibino S, et al. (2003) Diagnosing dry eye using a blue-free barrier filter. Am J Ophthalmol 136: 513–519.
26. Wang CC, Shi H, Guo K, Ng CP, Li J, et al. (2007) VAMP8/endobrevin as a general vesicular SNARE for regulated exocytosis of the exocrine system. Mol Biol Cell 18: 1056–1063.
27. Wei W, Wei M, Kang X, Deng H, Lu Z (2009) A novel method developed for acetylcholine detection in royal jelly by using capillary electrophoresis coupled with electrogenerated chemiluminescence based on a simple reaction. Electrophoresis 30: 1949–1952.
28. Terada Y, Narukawa M, Watanabe T (2011) Specific hydroxy fatty acids in royal jelly activate TRPA1. J Agric Food Chem 59: 2627–2635.
29. Kamakura M (2011) Royalactin induces queen differentiation in honeybees. Nature 473: 478–483.
30. Dartt DA (2009) Neural regulation of lacrimal gland secretory processes: relevance in dry eye diseases. Prog Retin Eye Res 28: 155–177.
31. Saito Y, Ozawa T, Nishiyama A (1987) Acetylcholine-induced Na+ influx in the mouse lacrimal gland acinar cells: demonstration of multiple Na+ transport mechanisms by intracellular Na+ activity measurements. J Membr Biol 98: 135–144.
32. Mircheff AK (1989) Lacrimal fluid and electrolyte secretion: a review. Curr Eye Res 8: 607–617.
33. Wu K, Jerdeva GV, da Costa SR, Sou E, Schechter JE, et al. (2006) Molecular mechanisms of lacrimal acinar secretory vesicle exocytosis. Exp Eye Res 83: 84–96.
34. Wood RL, Mircheff AK (1986) Apical and basal-lateral Na/K-ATPase in rat lacrimal gland acinar cells. Invest Ophthalmol Vis Sci. 27: 1293–1296.
35. Hamm Alvarez SF (1998) Molecular motors and their role in membrane traffic. Adv Drug Deliv Rev. 29: 229–242.
36. Garcia Bueno B, Caso JR, Perez Nievas BG, Lorenzo P, Leza JC (2007) Effects of peroxisome proliferator-activated receptor gamma agonists on brain glucose and glutamate transporters after stress in rats. Neuropsychopharmacology 32: 1251–1260.
37. Wang X, Liu X, Kong R, Zhan R, Wang X, et al. (2009) NGFI-B targets mitochondria and induces cardiomyocyte apoptosis in restraint-stressed rats by mediating energy metabolism disorder. Cell Stress Chaperones 14: 639–648.
38. Israeli E, Hershcovici T, Berenshtein E, Zannineli G, Wengrower D, et al. (2008) The effect of restraint stress on the normal colon and on intestinal inflammation in a model of experimental colitis. Dig Dis Sci 53: 88–94.
39. Glancy B, Balaban RS (2012) Role of mitochondrial Ca2+ in the regulation of cellular energetics. Biochemistry 51: 2959–2973.
40. Hardie DG, Ross FA, Hawley SA (2012) AMPK: a nutrient and energy sensor that maintains energy homeostasis. Nat Rev Mol Cell Biol. 13: 251–262.
41. Clapham DE (2007) Calcium signaling. Cell 131: 1047–1058.

19

Antibacterial Compounds of Canadian Honeys Target Bacterial Cell Wall Inducing Phenotype Changes, Growth Inhibition and Cell Lysis That Resemble Action of β-Lactam Antibiotics

Katrina Brudzynski*, Calvin Sjaarda

Bee-Biomedicals Inc., Drug Discovery and Development Department, St. Catharines, Ontario, Canada

Abstract

Honeys show a desirable broad spectrum activity against Gram-positive and negative bacteria making antibacterial activity an intrinsic property of honey and a desirable source for new drug development. The cellular targets and underlying mechanism of action of honey antibacterial compounds remain largely unknown. To facilitate the target discovery, we employed a method of phenotypic profiling by directly comparing morphological changes in *Escherichia coli* induced by honeys to that of ampicillin, the cell wall-active β-lactam of known mechanism of action. Firstly, we demonstrated the purity of tested honeys from potential β-lactam contaminations using quantitative LC-ESI-MS. Exposure of log-phase *E. coli* to honey or ampicillin resulted in time- and concentration-dependent changes in bacterial cell shape with the appearance of filamentous phenotypes at sub-inhibitory concentrations and spheroplasts at the MBC. Cell wall destruction by both agents, clearly visible on microscopic micrographs, was accompanied by increased permeability of the lipopolysaccharide outer membrane as indicated by fluorescence-activated cell sorting (FACS). More than 90% *E. coli* exposed to honey or ampicillin became permeable to propidium iodide. Consistently with the FACS results, both honey-treated and ampicillin-treated *E. coli* cells released lipopolysaccharide endotoxins at comparable levels, which were significantly higher than controls ($p < 0.0001$). *E. coli* cells transformed with the ampicillin-resistance gene (β–lactamase) remained sensitive to honey, displayed the same level of cytotoxicity, cell shape changes and endotoxin release as ampicillin-sensitive cells. As expected, β–lactamase protected the host cell from antibacterial action of ampicillin. Thus, both honey and ampicillin induced similar structural changes to the cell wall and LPS and that this ability underlies antibacterial activities of both agents. Since the cell wall is critical for cell growth and survival, honey active compounds would be highly applicable for therapeutic purposes while differences in the mode of action between honey and ampicillin may provide clinical advantage in eradicating β-lactam-resistant pathogens.

Editor: Raymond Schuch, Rockefeller University, United States of America

Funding: Bee-Biomedicals Inc. provided support in the form of salaries for authors KB and CS but did not have any additional role in the study design, data collection and analysis, decision to publish, or preparation of the manuscript.

Competing Interests: KB and CS are employees of Bee-Biomedicals Inc. There are no patents, products in development or marketed products to declare.

* Email: beebio@sympatico.ca

Introduction

Research into antibacterial properties of honey and compounds involved in this activity provided a significant opportunity to discover potential novel lead compounds for the development of antibacterial therapy. Both raw and sterilized (pasteurized or irradiated) honeys showed a desirable broad spectrum activity against Gram-positive and Gram-negative bacteria [1], including medically important pathogens such as *Burkholderia cepacia* [2], *Pseudomonas aeruginosa* [3,4], *Salmonella enterica, Serratia marcescens, Escherichia coli, Klebsiella pneumoniae* [5], *Staphylococcus aureus, Salmonella typhymurium, Shigella sonnei* [6] and *Streptococcus pyogenes* [7]. Moreover, several multidrug-resistant bacteria, including methicillin-resistant *Staphylococcus aureus* (MRSA) and vancomycin-resistant *Enterococci* (VRE) showed susceptibility to honey action [8,9]. Studies on activity-associated biomarkers revealed that hydrogen peroxide and methylglyoxal significantly contribute to honey antibacterial activity [10–13]. However, neither action of hydrogen peroxide nor methylglyoxal could account for the total antibacterial activity of honey, since their removal did not completely abrogate honey cytotoxicity [6,11,14].

It is undeniable fact that almost all honeys exert at least bacteriostatic activities independently of their botanical or geographical origins making antibacterial activity an intrinsic property of honey and a desirable source for new drug development. We hypothesized that these putative, antibacterial molecule(s) must have been able to recognize and damage cellular targets that are crucial for bacterial viability. Therefore, we aimed at discovery of targets for these compounds and underlying mechanism of action in order to facilitate progress in elucidating the basis for honey antibacterial activity. In our target- based approach, we employed a method of phenotypic profiling [15] by directly comparing morphological changes in *Escherichia coli* evoked by honeys to those evoked by antibiotics of known mechanism of action. We have chosen in this study ampicillin, a cell wall-active β-lactam, as a drug model.

The cellular target of β-lactam is the peptidoglycan (PG) that surrounds on the outside the plasma membrane of bacterium and is linked to the lipopolysaccharide layer of outer membrane in Gram-negative bacteria. PG is the mesh-like polymer of β-(1, 4) linked *N*-acetylglucosamine and *N*-acetylmuramic acid crosslinked by short three to five amino acid stem peptides. PG synthesis requires penicillin-binding proteins (PBPs) that functions as DD-transpeptidases (DD-TPases) to crosslink the peptides to glycan chains, polymerized by glycotransferases (GTases) [16,17]. A concerted action of several *E. coli* PBPs is required for a formation of PG sacculus and the characteristic rod shape. In general, the activities of PBP1A, PBP1B have been shown to be associated with the cell elongation while PBP2 and PBP3 are responsible for maintaining the rod-shape structure and a septation during cell division, respectively [16–19]. β-Lactams covalently bind PBPs (DD-TPases) thereby inhibiting transpeptidation, the final stage of peptidoglycan synthesis. β-Lactams binding to PBPs result in a series of well-defined, characteristic morphological changes: inactivation of PBP2 lead to formation of spherical cells, inhibition of PBP3 results in formation of long filaments while inactivation of PBP 1A and 1B results in rapid cell lysis [16–19,20,21].We hypothesized that these well characterized morphological changes caused by β-lactams could serve as a reference point to compare with changes evoked by honey components. This phenotypic profiling in conjunctions with comparative analyses of the growth rate and cell viability of different phenotypes could provide an important clue as to the cellular targets recognized by honey antibacterial molecule(s). The target identification is an important starting point allowing and guiding our future discovery of active compounds and their mode of action.

Results

1. A comparison of *E. coli* susceptibility to honey and ampicillin

The *E. coli* growth inhibition and time-kill kinetics evoked by exposure to honeys and ampicillin were analyzed using broth microdilution assay and a standard plate count. The MIC_{90}, MBC_{100} values are summarized in Table 1. Each reported value is based on twelve to fifteen replicates from three independent experiments.

2. A comparison of functional dynamics of ampicillin and honey on *E. coli*

Growth inhibition and bactericidal action of β-lactams depends on the bacterial growth phase and correlates with generation time [22]. To compare the growth dynamics and viability of *E. coli* exposed to honey, the lag-phase cultures were either directly challenged with honey and ampicillin (Fig. 1A, B, and C) or were first incubated to reach the exponential phase (0.2 A_{595}nm) before adding these two agents (Fig. 1D). In both cases, the cultures were treated with honeys at concentrations ranging from 50% to 3.125% (w/v) and ampicillin (1.25 μg/ml to 0.31 μg/ml).

Starting from the lag-phase, growth curves of *E. coli* (10^6 CFU/ml) showed a latent period of about 2 h during which an increase in absorbance was observed in all tested samples; in untreated, honey-treated and ampicillin-treated cultures (Fig.1A, B and C). The reduction of growth by honey and ampicillin occurred immediately *after* the cells entered the early exponential phase and started to divide, suggesting that honey targeted events related to initiation of growth and cell division.

Honeys at and above their 1xMICs (6.25% v/v) were inhibitory for the entire 18 h of incubation (Fig.1A and B). Similarly, ampicillin at concentrations >0.625 μg/ml completely blocked *E. coli* growth (Fig.1C). No viable cells were observed in the standard plate count when samples from incubation wells were plated onto agar plates. In contrast, sub-inhibitory honey concentrations (3.12% (w/v) and 1.5% (w/v)), were unable to kill the cells but were capable to reduce the growth (Fig.1A, B, C, lag-phase and D, log-phase *E. coli*).

Application of honeys into the log-phase *E. coli* cultures caused the reduction of growth in all treated samples in the first 20 to 30 min that correspond to one generation time (Fig. 1D). Thereafter, the increase in absorbance indicated the gradual loss of honeys' inhibitory efficiencies. Honeys at concentrations 12.5% (w/v) (H208) and 25%w/v (H210) caused a reduction of viable cells by 2 to $3log_{10}$, respectively, within 1 to 2 h incubation time (Fig. 1D). The $>5log_{10}$ reduction of bacterial counts required 2 to 4x lag-phase MICs, corresponding to log-phase MICs 25% and 50%w/v for honey H208 and H210, respectively (Fig. 1E and F).

These results suggested that honey effects on *E. coli* were dependent on the MIC/MBC, bacterial growth phase and incubation time (the duration of exposure of *E. coli* to honey). The picture that emerges from these results indicates that the initial rapid decline in bacterial counts in both lag-phase and log-phase cultures resulted from the successful binding of honey antibacterial components to its target. Loss of bactericidal potency occurred when the concentration of unbound antibacterial component fell below the MBC level (25% (w/v) and 50% (w/v) for H208 and H210, respectively, for log-phase cultures). Although the bactericidal activity was lost, honeys continued to be inhibitory (Fig. 1D). Thus, honey antibacterial effects were concentration-dependent; when the effective concentrations of honey antibacterial compounds decreased below the MBC/MIC levels, the cell viability and growth were not longer affected and *E. coli* proliferation resumed.

On the other hand, exposure of log-phase *E. coli* to ampicillin in concentrations ranging from 10 μg/ml to 0.31 μg/ml caused a complete growth inhibition at the MIC/MBC 0.625 μg/ml (Fig. 1C and D) and bacterial death. No viable cells were observed in a standard plate count.

Table 1. Susceptibility of *E. coli* to honeys.

	Buckwheat Honey H208	Wildflower Honey H210	Ampicillin
MIC	6.25% (w/v)	6.25% (w/v)	0.625 μg/ml
MBC	6.25% (w/v)	12.5% (w/v)	0.625 μg/ml

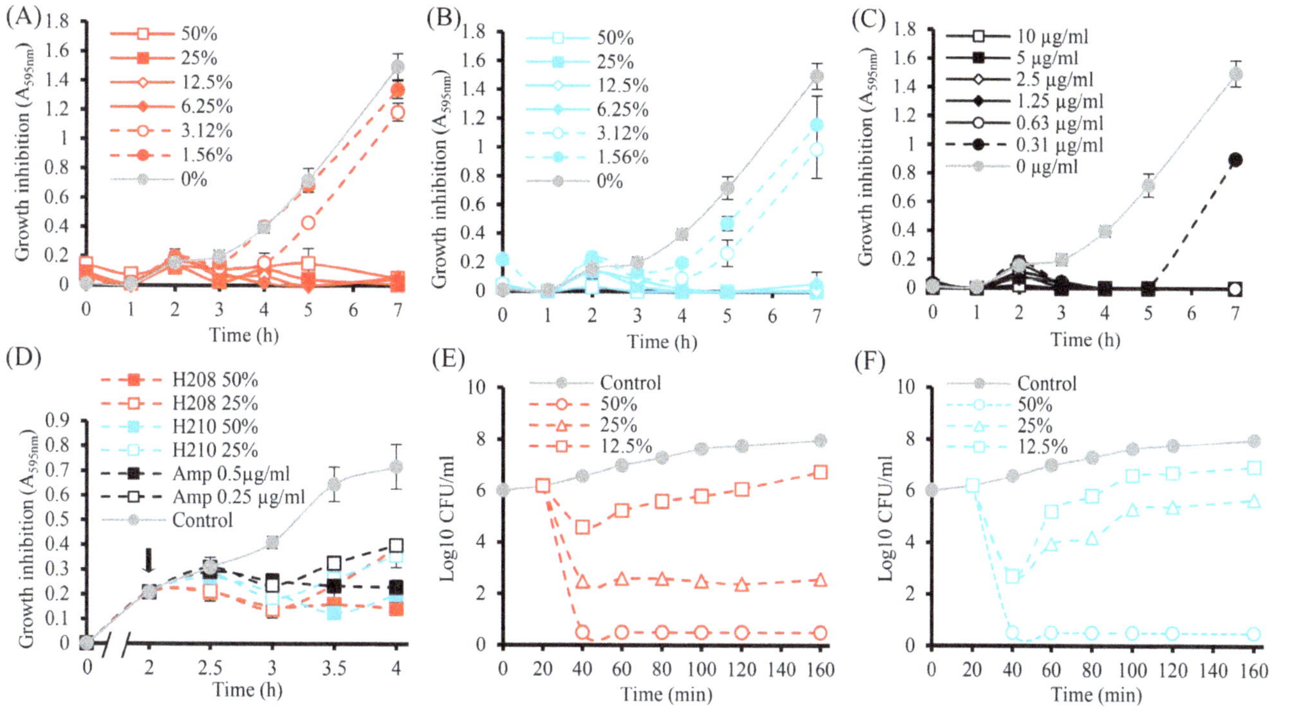

Figure 1. Kinetics of growth inhibition of lag-phase and log-phase *E. coli* exposed to honeys and ampicillin (A,B,C) and (D), respectively, and time-kill kinetics (E, F). The arrow indicates the application time of honeys or ampicillin into log-phase *E. coli*. In A to D, each point represents the mean ± standard deviation (n = 9), in E and F (n = 4).

The results indicated that both honey and ampicillin recognized and interfered with the cellular targets of *E. coli* cell that were important for sustained growth and multiplications. The observed differences in rates of bacterial killing in the lag versus log-phase cultures and differences in bactericidal potency between honey and ampicillin suggested that the bactericidal effects of both agents might results from independent killing modes.

3. A comparison of morphological dynamics in *E. coli* induced by honey and ampicillin

The ampicillin mode of action involves inhibition of PG synthesis that, in turn, changes the structural integrity of the cell wall resulting in characteristic morphological alterations. We confirmed ampicillin effects on *E. coli* morphology at concentrations used in our growth inhibition and time-kill kinetics. The addition of 0.3-2.5 µg/ml ampicillin to the log-phase *E. coli* cultures resulted in a dose-dependent phenotype changes (Fig.2). Increased filamentation was observed at ampicillin concentration of 0.31 µg/ml, the filament lysis and formation of spheroplasts was visible at 0.62 µg/ml, while spheroplast phenotypes were predominate forms at concentration of 1.25 µg/ml to 2.5 µg/ml (Fig. 2).

To investigate whether honey could alter cell morphology in a similar manner, samples taken at regular time intervals from incubation wells, during incubation of honeys with log-phase *E. coli,* were simultaneously analyzed for their morphology, growth inhibition and time-kill kinetics. Firstly, the initiation of growth of *E. coli* cells from the lag phase was seen as the transition from coccoidal forms of the stationary phase to the typical 2–4 µm short rods of normal, growing *E. coli* (Fig.3A and B). Addition of honey during initiation of growth (after 2h incubation) correlated with the formation of a heterogeneous population of phenotypes consisting of rods, filaments and spheroidal cells (Fig. 3C). The decreased number of cells observed on microscopic micrographs during the first hour after honey application to the culture, was consistent with a rapid decline of cell viability observed in time-kill

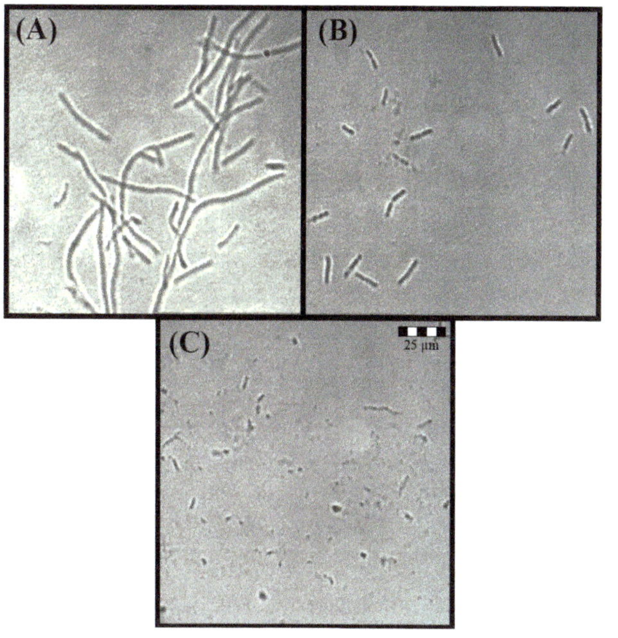

Figure 2. Concentration-dependent changes in *E. coli* phenotype after treatment with ampicillin. Ampicillin concentrations: (A) 0. 31 µg/ml, (B) 0.625 µg/ml and (C) 1.25 µg/ml. The size-scale is the same for all micrographs in the figure, obtained under the same 400x magnification.

kinetics (Fig. 3D and E and Fig. 1E and F). From the initial heterogeneous cell population, the cells that survived consisted of longer rods and filaments, indicative of the inhibition of septation and cell division (Fig. 3D and E). After 18 h incubation, spheroplasts of different sizes, mini cells and cell debris were the main components observed in honey-treated samples (Fig.3F-H). The appearance of these phenotypes correlated with the >5log$_{10}$ reduction of bacterial counts by honey H208 at the MBC as shown in Fig. 1 E and F.

These results indicated that, similarly to ampcillin, honey action affected the cell wall structure that is responsible for *E. coli* cell shape. As in the case of ampicillin, the changes were dose-dependent and related to the appearance of the filamentous phenotypes at sub-inhibitory concentrations and spheroplast formation at the MBC (Fig.4). Morphological similarities between *E. coli* spheroplasts formed by ampicillin and honey-treatment were also supported by the SEM images (Fig.5). Importantly, spheroplasts generated by honey-treatment were prone to lysis (Fig. 5).

The altered *E. coli* morphology critically affected *E. coli* growth and cell viability as indicated in the functional assays (Fig. 1). Thus, it became clearly revealed that honey compounds targeted the cell wall of *E. coli* causing structural changes and that the cell wall damaging effect constituted the mechanism underlying the antibacterial effects of honey and ampicillin.

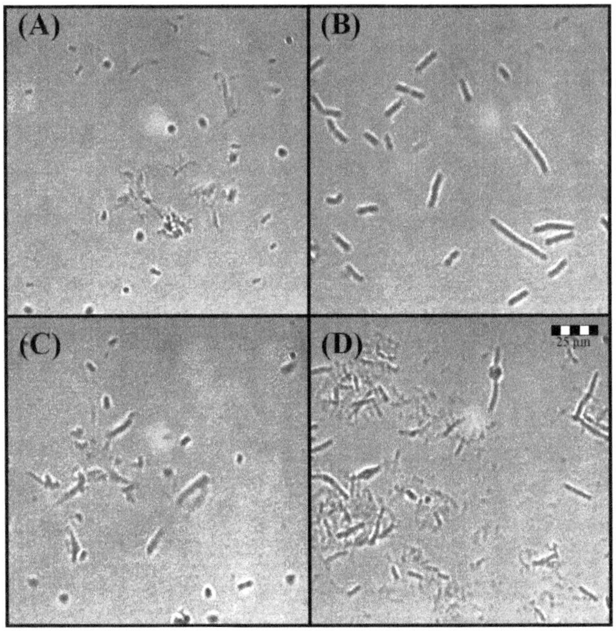

Figure 4. Concentration-dependent *E. coli* cell lysis induced by honey (A and C) and ampicillin (B and D) at sub-inhibitory (A and B) and inhibitory concentrations (C and D). The size-scale is the same for all micrographs in the figure, obtained under the same 400x magnification.

4. A comparison of effects of honey and ampicillin on a permeability of *E. coli* outer membrane

Lipopolysaccharide (LPS) of outer membrane in Gram-negative bacteria is a permeability barrier. LPS is cross-bridged to the peptidoglycan of the cell wall [23] and the loss of the cell wall integrity induced by ampicillin affects also the LPS integrity [23,24]. To compare the changes in LPS permeability induced by honey and ampicillin in a quantitative way, we used forward and side scatter measurements of fluorescence-activated cell sorting

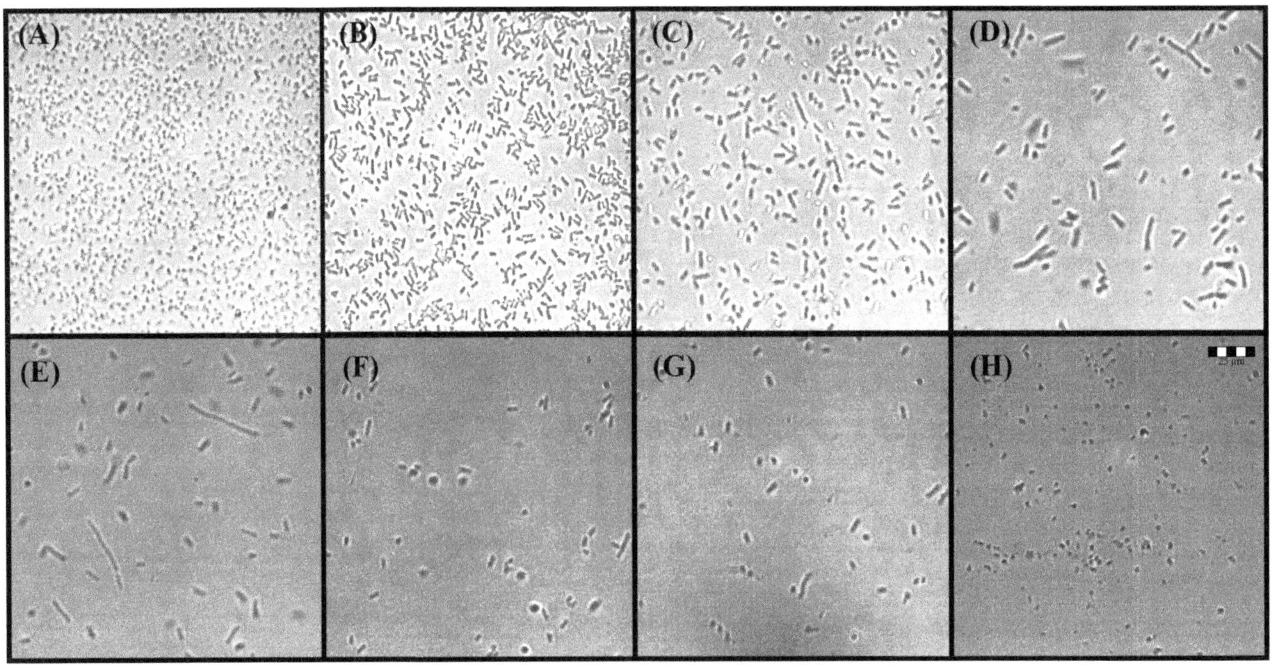

Figure 3. Time-dependent phenotypic changes observed after application of honey to log phase *E. coli* cultures. The changes paralleled the growth kinetics shown in Fig. 1D. (A) lag phase *E. coli* culture, (B) log phase *E. coli* culture at the time of honey application, (C) *E. coli* phenotypes after 30 min incubation with honey H208 (12.5% v/v), (D). *E. coli* phenotypes observed after 1 h incubation with honey H210 (12.5% v/v), (F) and (G) *E. coli* spheroplasts formed after 2 h incubation with honey H208 and H210 at 50% v/v, (H) spheroplasts observed after 18 h incubation, lag phase. The size-scale is the same for all micrographs in the figure, obtained under the same 400x magnification.

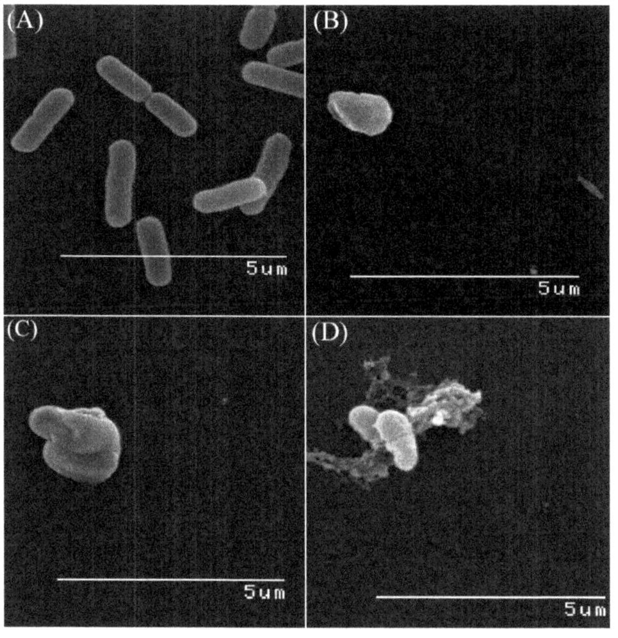

Figure 5. SEM of *E.coli* spheroplasts generated by ampicillin and honey-treatments. Log-phase *E. coli* cells were treated with bactericidal concentrations of ampicillin (2.5 µg/ml) and honey H208 (25% w/v) for 3 hr at 37°C. Cells were harvested and glutaraldehyde-fixed (see Materials and Methods). (A). *E. coli* control, (B). *E. coli* cels after treatment with ampicillin and (C). *E. coli* cell after treatment with honey and (D) honey-induced spheroplast lysis.

using two nucleic acid-specific stains; membrane-permeable Syto9 and membrane-impermeable propidium iodide (PI).

After 3 h exposure of log-phase *E. coli* cultures to honey or ampicillin, the stained cells were sorted into four distinct *E. coli* subpopulations: PI- positive (dead cells), Syto-positive (live cells), Syto9/PI double positive cells as injured, cells and Syto9/PI double negative cells that may include cell debris. The FACS results showed that the distribution of fluorescence was striking comparable between *E. coli* exposed to honey or ampicillin (Fig.6). At sub-inhibitory concentrations, both agents caused a marked increase in double-stained PI/Syto9 cells. The percent of these injured cells ranged from 95.5% to 78.6% for honeys (at concentrations of 25% and 12.5% w/w) and ampicillin (at concentration 1.25 ug/ml), respectively (Fig. 6). Thus, both ampicillin and honey actions inflicted severe damages to the *E. coli* LPS with comparable efficacies.

Unexpectedly, exposure of log phase *E. coli* to bactericidal concentrations of honeys produced 59% to 41% of Syto9–positive (live cells), respectively, and only limited amounts of injured cells (26% to 7. 8%), respectively, while no PI-positive (dead) cells were visible (Fig. 6). Despite the presence of over 50% of Syto9-positive, live cells, these cell populations did not grow well when plated on the agar plates: honey H210 at concentration of 25% w/v showed $2\log_{10}$ CFU/ml reduction of viable cells, while honey H208 at the concentration of 25% w/v reduced viable cells by $>4\log_{10}$ CFU/ml with no colony observed at the concentration of 50%w/v of both honeys (Fig. 1E). Under microscope, they presented themselves as spheroidal forms and mini cells (Fig. 4H). The spheroidal forms devoid of peptidoglycan layer (spheroplasts) and mini cell populations are often suggested to represent the antibiotic-tolerant state of viable but nonculturable cells (VBNC) [25–28] and persisters cells [29], respectively. These morphological forms are known, protective phenotypes of *E. coli* observed under stressful conditions [25,26,29]. Whether the spheroidal forms represent VBNC requires further studies to clarify the apparent discrepancy between the plate count and flow cytometry results.

The results of FACS showed that sub-inhibitory concentrations of honey and ampicillin drastically increased the LPS permeability allowing a penetration of PI into the cell. The LPS disintegration caused by honey action was yet another, previously unknown phenomenon.

5. A comparison of endotoxin release from *E. coli* induced by honey and ampicillin

The LPS disintegration in *E. coli* induced by ampicillin is accompanied by a simultaneous release of high levels of endotoxins [23,24]. We asked whether LPS release would also be observed following *E. coli* exposure to honey. The log-phase cells were incubated for 3 h with honeys H210 and H208 at concentrations ranging from 25% to 6.25% w/v, respectively and with ampicillin at concentrations 0.625 µg/ml to 2.5 µg/ml. Free endotoxin levels in cell supernatants were quantified using a chromogenic Limulus amebocyte lysate (LAL assay) using a constructed standard curve with linearity of $R^2 = 0.9912$. The endotoxin levels released from *E. coli* were significantly higher in honey and ampicillin-treated groups than in untreated *E. coli* controls ($p<0.0001$) (Fig.7).

To generate an additional, negative control for endotoxin release, we transformed *E. coli* with plasmid-encoded ampicillin-resistance gene coding for β-lactamase, to create a model of β-lactam resistance. Firstly, we evaluated the susceptibility of *amp*-resistant *E. coli* to honey antibacterial compounds. As expected, the growth of *amp*-resistant *E. coli* (EA) was not affected by the presence of ampicillin in the culture media (Fig.8). The insensitivity of EA to ampicillin was also reflected by the lack of phenotype changes in the presence of this antibiotic (Fig. 9). In contrast, honeys inhibited the growth of EA with the same efficacy as ampicillin-sensitive cells (Fig.8). The honeys MIC_{90} 6.25%w/v against lag-phase EA was not different from those of ampicillin-sensitive *E. coli* (Fig.8 and Table 1). The cell wall lysis induced by honey was clearly evident in both *amp*-resistant and sensitive *E. coli* (Fig.9). It became apparent that the destruction of bacterial cell wall by honey and ampicilln occurred by independent modes of action; the presence of β-lactamase gene did not change *E. coli* susceptibility to honey.

Next, we investigated the effects of ampicillin resistance on the level of endotoxin release. When *amp*-resistant (EA) and *amp*–sensitive *E. coli* (Ec) were exposed to honeys, the levels of endotoxin liberated were essentially identical (Fig. 7, bars Ec H208, Ec H210, EA H208, and EA H210, differences n.s.). However, the amount of endotoxin release from honey-treated groups was significantly higher from that of untreated controls (honey-treated groups versus controls Ec and EA), $t[50] = 8.99$, $p<0.0001$). Moreover, amicillin-resistance had no effects on honey-induced endotoxin release. In contrast, ampicillin treatment of *amp*-resistant *E. coli* did not increase endotoxin release over the levels observed in control cells (Fig. 7, control groups Ec and EA versus EA AMP did not significantly differ ($t[9] = 2.1$, n.s.) and no morphological changes were observed (Fig. 9). At the same time, ampicillin caused significantly higher amounts of endotoxin release from ampicillin-sensitive than ampicillin-resistant cells (Fig. 6, the bars Ec AMP vs. bars EA AMP, compared jointly, t-test, $t [22] = 21.9$, $p<0.0001$) (Fig. 7).

Thus, endotoxin release from the LPS of ampicillin–sensitive *E. coli* by honey was similar to that of ampicillin but the modes of actions were different. The ampicillin-resistance gene provided

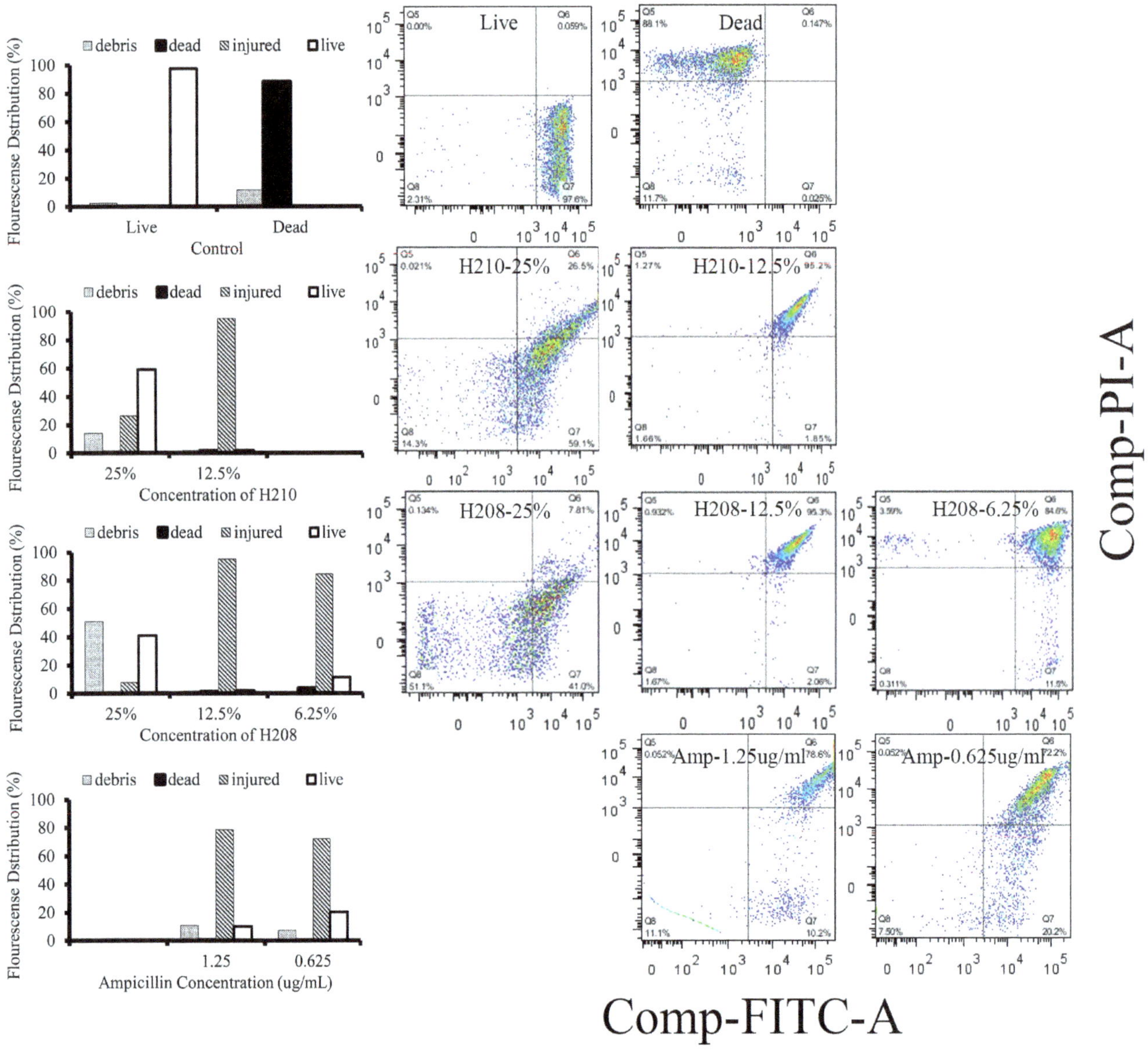

Figure 6. Effects of ampicillin and honey treatments of log-phase *E. coli* on lipopolysaccharide membrane permeability using fluorescence-activated flow cytometry. The distribution of *E. coli* populations in each of the four quadrants was quantified by the forward scatter of green fluorescence of Syto9 (as FITC-A) versus side scatter of red fluorescence of PI. The left panel shows the percentage of dead (PI positive), live (Syto9-positive) and PI/Syto9-double positive, injured cells after *E. coli* treatment with honeys H210, H208 and ampicillin.

"protection" against ampicillin action on the cell wall and LPS. The differences in susceptibility patterns against *amp*-resistant *E. coli* between honey and ampicillin may be of clinical significance in the treatment of β-lactam-resistant *E. coli*.

6. Quantitative analysis of potential β-lactam contaminations in tested honeys

To analyze a potential contamination of honey with β-lactam antibiotics, honey samples were extracted with ethyl acetate, purified using SPE procedures and analyzed using LC-ESI-MS. The total ion chromatogram and mass spectrum of ampicillin standard (C16H19N3O4S, molecular weight 349.41) gave a main mass ion $[M-H]^-$ m/z 348.1 at retention time (RT) 11.9 min (Fig. 10). This mass ion was used to screen honeys for antibiotic traces. Honeys spiked with amplicillin at 250 ng/ml, 500 ng/ml and 1000 ng/ml served as internal standards and produced the mean peak area linearity of $R^2 = 0.907$. The LC-ESI-MS method was sensitive to detect nanogram quantities of ampicillin in spiked honeys, but no traces of antibiotic were found in non-spiked honeys H208 and H210 (Fig. 10). Thus, the results showed that the membrane damaging and bacteriolytic effects of H208 and H210 did not result from the potential presence of β-lactam traces.

Discussion

The method of phenotypic profiling combined with functional and morphological analyses of *E. coli* exposed to honey and ampicillin allowed uncovering previously unknown targets for honey compounds and allowed understanding the antibacterial effects they produced. Targeting of the cell wall and the lipopolysaccharide outer membrane by honey compounds is

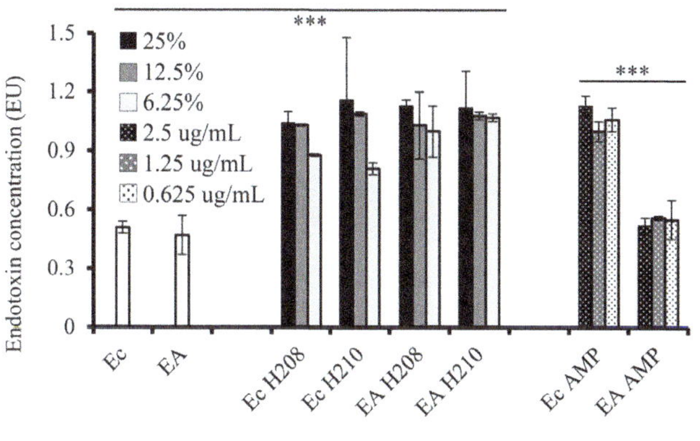

Figure 7. Endotoxin release from ampicillin-sensitive and ampicillin-resistant *E. coli* cells after exposure to different concentrations of honey and ampicillin. (EA: ampicillin-resistant *E. col*, Ec-*E. coli*). The bars represent the mean ± standard deviation (n = 4). See text for statistical results. *** - p<0.0001.

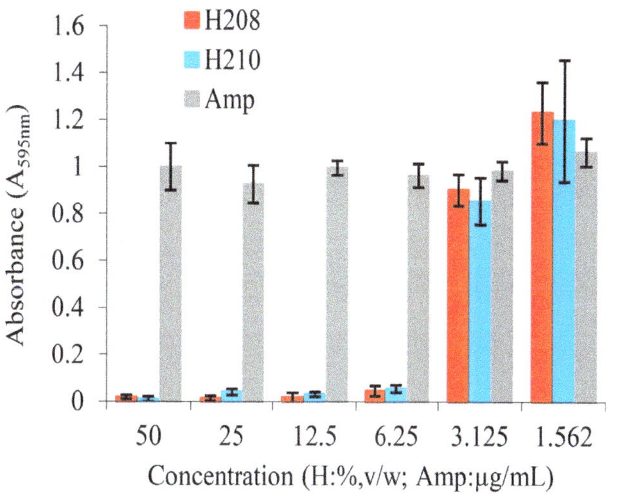

Figure 8. Susceptibility of ampicillin-resistant *E. coli* to honey and ampicillin. The bars represent the mean ± standard deviation (n = 9).

arguably the most important finding of this study. The cell wall peptidoglycan is vital for maintaining cell shape and for sustaining bacterial growth and reproduction [23,30,31,37,38]. We showed here that honey, similarly to ampicillin, caused cell shape changes that resulted from the loss of cell wall integrity. Using SEM and an image-based microscopy in combination with functional assays we have shown that exposure of *E. coli* to honey disrupted the cell wall and caused morphological changes that included filamentation, filament lysis, formation of spheroplasts and ultimately, cell lysis. The suite of phenotypic changes matched a specific action of ampicillin on the cell wall. Moreover, the cell shape changes occurred in time- and concentrations-dependent manner and correlated with the honey MIC and MBCs. The new phenotypes became visible immediately upon initiation of *E. coli* growth in the presence of honey and were followed by growth cessation and a rapid decrease in viable cell counts. Thus, targeting the cell wall and its damage by honey compounds was accountable for honey antibacterial effects. These findings advance our understanding of the reasons behind honey antibacterial activity.

The mechanism of antibacterial activity of ampicillin is linked to an inhibition of cell wall synthesis by a direct binding to penicillin-binding protein, PBP1A, and inactivating its transpeptidase activity [16,20,21]. High concentrations of ampicillin and other β-lactam antibiotics usually inactivate transpeptidase activity in all PBPs. This generates spheroplast phenotype with up-regulated expression of genes involved in spheroplast lysis [35,36]. Rapid autolysis ensues. At sub-inhibitory concentrations however, activity of PBP2 responsible for cell elongation might be preserved and produce filamentous phenotype [20,32–34]. Similarly, we have shown here that honey-induced formation of spheroidal forms occurred at the MBC during the first 20 to 30 min after honey application to log-phase *E. co*li culture, that is, during one generation time. The drastic reduction of cell viability (up to $5\log_{10}$ CFU/ml) indicated that injury done to *E. coli* cells was critical and beyond recovery. Scanning electron microscopy clearly showed spheroplast lysis. Despite the overlapping phenotypic changes and functional outcomes induced by honey and ampicillin, the mode of honey action on cell wall remains unknown. Whether cell shape changes caused by honey were the results of inhibition of the cell wall synthesis or the results of a direct physical injury to the cell wall integrity have to be further investigated.

The exposure of *E. coli* to honey and ampicillin also affected structural integrity of lipopolysaccharide (LPS) of outer membrane that regulates the cell permeability. The outer membrane is impermeable to large molecules and hydrophobic compounds. However, fluorescence-activated cell sorting (FACS) showed that over 90% of honey-treated *E. coli* became permeable to propidium iodide suggesting that the LPS barrier was compromised. Although the increase in membrane permeability to nucleic acid dyes of bacterial cell exposed to β-lactam antibiotics has been previously described [40,41], the LPS destruction by honey is a

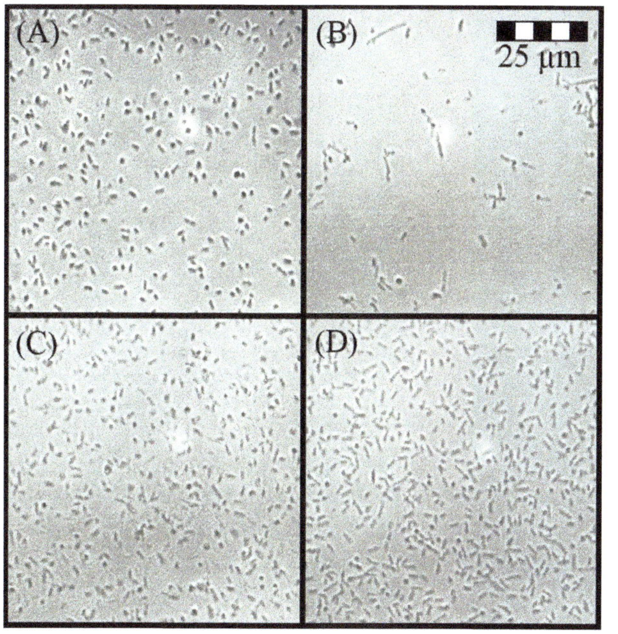

Figure 9. Morphological changes in ampicillin-resistant *E. coli* after exposure to honey or ampicillin. Ampicillin-resistant *E. coli* before (A) and after treatment with honey, H210, 25%w/v, (B) and ampicillin-resistant *E. coli* before (C) and after treatment with 2.5 ug/ml of ampicillin (D). The size-scale is the same for all micrographs in the figure, obtained under the same 400x magnification.

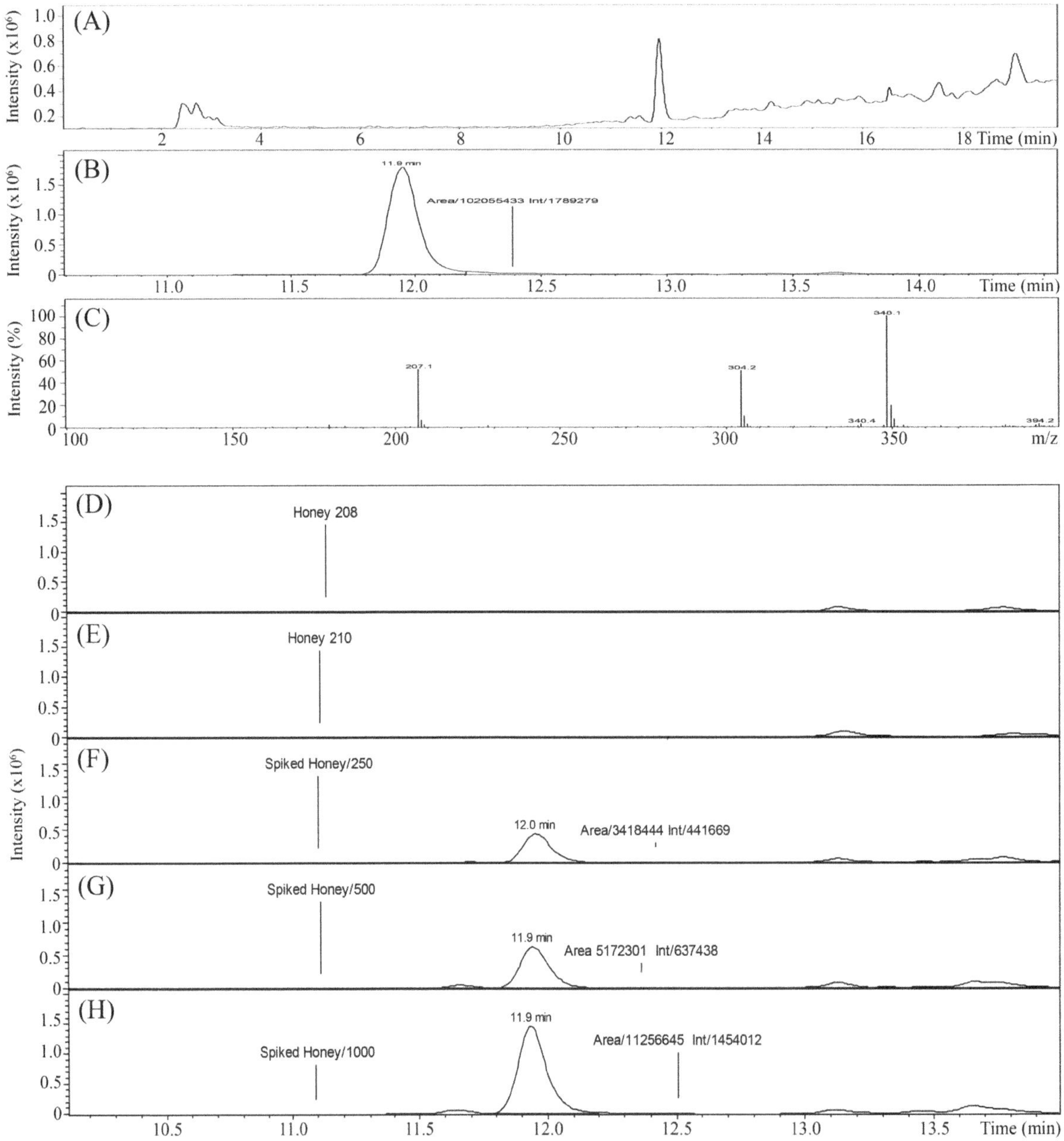

Figure 10. Total Ion Current (TIC) and MS full-scan analysis of ampicillin standard obtained from LC/ESI/MS in negative mode. The *m/z* 348.1 eluting at RT 11.9 min was used for quantitation of antibiotic traces in honeys H208 and H210. Honey H208 spiked with amplicillin at 250 ng, ml, 500 ng/ml and 1000 ng/ml served as internal standards.

new, previously unknown phenomenon.

Consistent with FACS results, honey-treated cells released LPS endotoxins at the levels comparable to that of ampicillin-treated cells but significantly higher than that of untreated *E. coli* as measured using Limulus Amoebocyte Lysate (LAL) assay. Endotoxins are LPS constituents of the outer membrane of cell wall of gram-negative bacteria and their toxicity is associated with the Lipid A which cross-bridge the outer membrane with peptidoglycan layer [23]. Cell lysis caused by exposure of Gram-negative bacteria to β-lactam antibiotics increases release of endotoxins [42]. We have shown here that honey-induced cell wall damage was also associated with endotoxin release. Since cell lysis requires both cell wall and LPS disintegration, this provided additional strong support that the cell wall and lipopolysaccharide of outer membrane were targets for honey action. Disruption of these targets was responsible for the antibacterial effects of honey.

Although honey and ampicillin targeted *E. coli*'s cell wall and induced overlapping changes in phenotype, suppression of cell division and reduction of cell viability, the modes of their actions were likely different. In our ampicillin-resistance model of *E. coli* transformed with plasmid containing ampicillin-resistance gene, β-lactamase production prevented cytotoxic effects of ampicillin and endotoxin release but did not affect *E. coli* sensitivity to honey antibacterial effects.

To the best of our knowledge, there are no reports that identify bacterial cell wall as a specific cellular target for honey compounds. The cell wall and LPS are "new targets" that have been suspected but not yet definitively established. The cell lysis, specifically of Gram-negative bacteria, has been recently observed in studies aiming at elucidation of molecule(s) responsible for bactericidal effects in honey of *Leptospermum spp* (manuka honey) [14,39]. In *Pseudomonas aeruginosa,* manuka honey induced phenotype changes, growth inhibition and cell lysis [39,43]. On genetic level, it affected cell survival by reducing the expression of three microcolony-forming genes [43]. Specifically, the reduced expression of *oprF* gene, seen after 60 min incubation of *P. aeruginosa* with manuka honey, suggested that the gene was a target for this honey. It has been further postulated that the possible reduction of protein product of the *oprF* gene, localized to outer membrane, might cause a significant stress and facilitates its disruption [43]. In contrast to manuka honey, we have shown in this study that buckwheat and wildflower honeys induced a rapid, concentration and time-dependent disruption of the cell wall, reducing bacterial counts by >5log10 CFU/ml within the first 30 min of honey application to bacterial cultures. The differences in killing kinetics and efficiency may suggest that manuka and Canadian honeys did not target the same structures, and that these targets might be located at different cellular compartments.

From this study, Canadian honeys have emerged as an antibacterial agent active against the bacterial cell wall. Since the cell wall plays a fundamental role in the cell growth and survival, the compounds responsible for the cell wall damaging effects would be highly applicable for therapeutic purposes. Moreover, differences in their mode of action from ampicillin may be advantageous in eradicating β-lactam-resistant strains.

Materials and Methods

Honeys

Honeys were donated by Canadian beekeepers and consisted of mixed buckwheat honey (H208) (fagopyrum/solidago/brassica) and wildflower honey (H210) (rhamnaceae/ligustrum/trifolium) as indicated by melissopalynology. The honeys were collected during 2012/13 season.

Bacterial strains and growth cultures

Standard strains of *Escherichia coli* (ATCC 14948) purchased from Thermo Fisher Scientific Remel Products (Lenexa, KS 66215) were grown in Mueller-Hinton Broth (MHB) (Difco Laboratories) overnight in a shaking water bath at 37°C. Overnight cultures were diluted with broth to the equivalent of the 0.5 McFarland standard.

Broth microdilution assay and determination of the MIC

The susceptibility of *Escherichia coli* (10^6 CFU/ml) to honeys or ampicillin (sodium salt) was analyzed by the broth microdilution assay in a 96 well microtitre plate format using serial, two- fold dilution, as previously described [9]. Bacterial growth was monitored at A_{595} nm using the Synergy HT multidetection microplate reader (Synergy HT, Bio-Tek Instruments, Winooski, VT, USA). The MIC was established to be the concentration of honey or ampicillin that reduced bacterial growth by 90% in comparison to a control, untreated culture, after 18 h incubation with shaking at 37°C. Statistical analysis and dose response curves were obtained using K4 software provided by Synergy HT (Bio-Tek Instruments, Winooski, VT, USA).

General experimental design

E. coli culture (10^6 CFU/ml in 110 μl) were grown in 96-well plates until they reach log phase (A_{595}nm 0.2-0.3) at which point honeys or ampicillin was added in triplicate to separate wells at 1xMIC and 0.5x MIC concentrations. At indicated time intervals, the aliquots were taken for incubation wells to examine (a) growth inhibition kinetics (b) total viable counts by the standard plate count, (c) morphological changes and (d) for flow cytometry. The total incubation time was 18 hr at 37°C.

Time-kill kinetics

After bacterial cultures reached exponential growth, the inhibitory action and killing rate were measured simultaneously at every 20 to 30 min for 2 h and at the end 18 h incubation. The generation time of 20 min for *E. coli* (ATCC 14948) has been established experimentally under conditions used in our laboratory. In a separate experiment, log phase cultures of *E. coli* were first diluted with warm MHB to obtain 10^6 CFU/ml (using 0.5 McFarland standard), placed in 96-well microplates (100 μl/well) to which honeys or ampicillin were added at 1xMIC or 0.5x MIC. The inhibitory action and killing rate were measured every 20 min using microplate reader. The killing curves were constructed by withdrawing 10 μl aliquots from wells containing inoculum (assay control) and experimental wells. The 10 μl aliquots were serially 10-fold diluted with sterile water to obtain cell density ranging from 10^4 to 10^2 CFU/ml and then a 10 μl and 100 μl aliquot from each dilution were plated onto Mueller-Hinton agar (MHA) plates. Since the kinetic results did not differ between 20 min and 30 min of incubation times, we combined the data obtained from these two sets of experiments (6 separate experiments, n = 18).

After 18 hr incubation at 37°C, the viable cells were enumerated. The MBC endpoint was determined as the minimum concentration of glycoproteins at which 99.9% of the initial inoculum was eradicated and at which only one or no colonies could be seen on MHA.

Cell morphology examination by light microscopy

To examine phenotype changes in *E. coli* induced by honey or ampicillin at different growth phases, 10 μl samples were removed from the experimental and control wells at each time interval at log-phase and at stationary phase (18 hr incubation) from the 96 well plates. The samples were examined on glass slides at 400 x magnifications under light microscope (Zeiss, Axiolab, Germany). Images were viewed and photographed using the digital camera and built-in software (Singer Instruments MSM 400, Somerset, UK).

Scanning electron microscopy

A log-phase *E. coli* (100 μl, ~10^8 CFU/ml) was treated with ampicillin (2.5 μg/ml) or honey H208 (25%w/v) for 3 hr, at 37°C. Cells were harvested by centrifugation (1000×g, 3 min), washed 3 times with filtered-sterilized 0.1 M Tris-buffered saline (TBS, pH 7.3) to remove culture medium, re-suspended in 500 μl of 2.5% glutaraldehyde in 0.1 M TBS (EM grade, Sigma-Aldrich) and incubated for 30 min at room temperature. Cells were washed with 0.1 M TBS and re-suspeded in 100 μl of 0.1 M TBS. Samples (50 ul) were placed on a on a poly-L-lysine coated glass coverslip and left for 60 minutes at room temperature. The samples were dehydrated (2×2 min) in a graded ethanol (70%, 95% and 100%), critical point dried and then sputter coated with gold. The samples were examined using a Hitachi S-530 scanning electron microscope operating at 20 kV. Images were captured using Quartz PCI version 8 software.

Table 2. Condition for ampicillin quantification in unspiked and spiked honeys using LC-ESI-MS.

Time (min)	Solvent A (%)	Solvent B (%)
0.00	95	5
2.00	95	5
12.00	20	80
15.00	10	90
20.00	10	90

Column: Eclipse XDB-C18/4.6×75 mm/3.5u.
Flow: 0.250 ml/min.
Solvent A: water with 0.1% formic acid.
Solvent B: acetonitrile with 0.1% formic acid.

Sample preparation for flow cytometry

The Live/Dead BacLight Bacterial Viability and Counting Kit (L34856, Invitrogen) has been used to evaluate *E. coli* cells viability after their exposure to honey and ampicillin. This kit contains two nucleic acid-specific dyes: Syto9 is membrane-permeable, will stain all cells and can be detected by green fluorescence, and propidium iodide (PI) which is membrane-impermeable, stains cells with damaged membranes and gives red fluorescence. "Log phase" cultures were obtained from time-kill experiments, and were tested after 2 h incubation from the time of honey application to the exponentially growing cells. "Lag phase" cultures resulted from 18 h incubation of lag phase *E. coli* with honey and ampicillin. Both log phase and lag phase *E. coli* cells were treated with honeys H208 and H210 at 1xMIC and 0.5xMIC or ampicillin at concentrations 2.5, 1.25, 0.625 and 0.31 μg/ml. Cultures from the time-kill experiments were collected from 8 replicate wells of 96-well microplates into separate eppendorf tubes, harvested by centrifugation (1,000 *g* for 3 min) washed three times with filtered-sterilized 0.1 M Tris-buffered saline (TBS, pH 7.3) to remove culture medium, resuspended in 300 μl of TBS and double- stained with Syto9 (5 μl final concentration) and PI (30 μl final concentration). Untreated lag phase and log phase cultures were stained only with Syto (live cells) and isopropanol-killed cells were labeled with PI only (dead cells). Samples were incubated at room temperature in the dark for 20 min. After staining, cells were fixed in 100% ethanol overnight at 4°C. Prior flow cytometry, cells were centrifuged and resuspended in TBS.

Flow cytometric analysis

Untreated *E. coli* cells of intact membranes stained with Syto9 were used as a positive control of live cells, while *E. coli* cells killed with 70% isopropyl alcohol and stained with PI comprised a positive control of dead cells. These cells were used to gate the sorting of the stained cells into four distinct *E. coli* subpopulations: PI- positive (dead cells), Syto-positive (live cells), Syto9/PI double positive cells as injured, dying cells and Syto9/PI double negative cells that may include cell debris. Unstained control *E. coli* culture was also used to compensate for unspecific sorting. The quantitation of cell viability was based on the ratio of green fluorescence of Syto 9 (live cells) to red fluorescence of PI (dead cells) using Live/Dead BacLight Kit (Invitrogen).

The cell populations upon staining with Syto9 and PI were analyzed on a multi-laser flow cytometer BD LSR II (Becton Dickinson, San Jose, CA, USA) by forward and side scatter measurements using fluorescein isothiocyanate filter (green fluorescence) and propidium iodide channels (red fluorescence). BD FACS software was used for data acquisition and analysis. Both fluorescence emission signals were compensated to adjust for overlapping emission signals from the two fluorophores. Microsphere beads (6 um in diameter) were used in the flow cytometry acquision.

Construction of ampicillin resistant *E. coli*

One hundred μl of an overnight *E. coli* culture was inoculated into 10 ml of Luria Broth (LB: 1% tryptone, 1% NaCl, 0.5% yeast extract) and grown to an OD_{600} of 0.1. The cells were cooled on ice for 10 min, centrifuged (1500 *g*, 5 min, 4°C) and suspended in 10 mL of TBS (Sigma) containing 50 mM $CaCl_2$. The suspension was removed in aliquots of 100 μL and pUC19 (New England Biolabs) was added to a final concentration of 4 μg/mL. The cells were incubated on ice for 30 min, heat shocked (42°C, 45 sec) and returned to the ice for 2 min. Nine hundred μL of LB was added to the cells before a 60 min incubation at 37°C with shaking at 250 rpm. The *E.coli* suspension (0.1 mL) was spread on LB plates (2% agar) containing 100 μg/mL ampicillin and grown overnight. Transformants containing the plasmid, identified as growing colonies, were selected and sub-cultured on LB with 100 μg/mL ampicillin.

Endotoxin release from *E. coli* after treatment with honey and ampicillin

Sterile, pyrogen-free plasticware and water was used for these assays.

The log-phase *E. coli* cultures ($\sim 10^8$ CFU/ml) were incubated with two-fold serially diluted honeys H208 and H210 (25% (w/v) to 6.25% (w/v)) and ampicillin at concentrations 2.5 μg/ml to 0.625 μg/ml (in triplicate) at 37°C for 3 hr in 96-well plates. Cells were harvested by centrifugation (3000×g for 10 min). Samples of cell supernatants were four-times diluted with pyrogen-free water and free endotoxin levels were quantified using a chromogenic Limulus amebocyte lysate (LAL) assay according to the manufacturer instructions (Pierce^R LAL chromogenic endotoxin quantitation kit, Pierce Biotechnology, Rockford, IL, USA). The standard curve was constructed according to manufacturer instruction.

LC-ESI-MS

To determine potential presence of residues of ampicillin in honey, honey samples (5 g) was dissolved in 5 ml sterile, Mili-Q water by vortexing and extracted with 5 ml of ethyl acetate. After centrifugation at 3200 rpm for 5 min, the upper organic layer was collected. The extraction was repeated three times and collected organic layers were dried down with N_2 flow at 50°C. The extract was reconstituted into 5 ml of sterile, Mili-Q water and purified by solid-phase extraction. Honeys were spiked with amplicillin (stock solution 5 mg/ml) to obtain the final concentration of 250 ng/ml, 500 ng/ml and 1000 ng/ml. The presence of ampicillin in unspiked honeys and spiked honeys were quantified by liquid chromatography coupled to electrospray ionization mass spectrometry (LC-ESI-MS) operating in negative mode (Table 2). Ampicillin was used as a standard. The method was validated by achieving reproducible, quantitative results.

Statistical analysis

All data were presented as mean values ± SD. Groups were compared with unpaired t-test using Graph Pad InStat version 3.00, GraphPad Software Inc., San Diego California USA. The data were tested for normality of distribution and they passed the test. Differences between means were considered to be significant at $p<0.05$.

Acknowledgments

We thank Liang Hong (Department of Immunology, McMaster University) for flow cytometry analyses; beekeepers, Mikhail Kutsyy and Margarita and Valeri Spirichin for donating honey samples. We thank Dr. Teper for melissopalyonological analysis of honeys (Research Institute of Pomology and Floriculture, Poland) and Bob Temkin (Electron Microscopy, Department of Biological Sciences, University of Toronto), for SEM analysis.

Author Contributions

Conceived and designed the experiments: KB CS. Performed the experiments: KB CS. Analyzed the data: KB CS. Contributed reagents/materials/analysis tools: KB CS. Contributed to the writing of the manuscript: KB CS.

References

1. Lusby PE, Coombes A, Wilkinson JM (2002) Honey: a potent agent for wound healing? J Wound Ostomy Continence Nurs. 29(6): 295–300.
2. Cooper RA, Wigley P, Burton N (2000) Susceptibility of multiresistant strains of *Burkholderia cepacia* to honey. Lett Appl Microbiol 31: 20–24.
3. Cooper RA, Halas E, Molan PC (2002) The efficacy of honey in inhibiting strains of *Pseudomonas aeruginosa* from infected burns. J Burn Care Rehabil. 23(6): 366–70.
4. Wilkinson JM, Cavanagh HM (2005) Antibacterial activity of 13 honeys against *Escherichia coli* and *Pseudomonas aeruginosa*. J Med Food, 8: 100–103.
5. Lusby PE, Coombes AL, Wilkinson JM (2005) Bactericidal activity of different honeys against pathogenic bacteria. Arch Med Res. 2005, 36(5): 464–7.
6. Taormina PJ, Niemra BA, Bauchat LR (2001) Inhibitory activity of honey against foodborne pathogens as influenced by the presence of hydrogen peroxide and level of antioxidant power. Int J Food Microbiol 69: 217–225.
7. Maddocks SE, Lopez MS, Rowlands RS, Cooper RA (2012) Manuka honey inhibits the development of Streptococcus pyogenes biofilms and causes reduced expression of two fibronectin binding proteins. Microbiol 158: 781–790.
8. Cooper RA, Molan PC, Harding KG (2002) The sensitivity to honey of Gram-positive cocci of clinical significance isolated from wounds. J Appl Microbiol 93: 857–863.
9. Brudzynski K Lannigan R (2012) Mechanism of honey bacteriostatic action against MRSA and VRE involves hydroxyl radicals generated from honey's hydrogen peroxide. Front Microbiol 3: 36.
10. White JW, Subers MH, Schepartz AL (1963) The identification of inhibine, the antibacterial factor in honey, as hydrogen peroxide and its origin in a honey glucose-oxidase system. Biochem Biophys Acta 73: 57–70.
11. Brudzynski K (2006) Effect of hydrogen peroxide on antibacterial activities of Canadian honeys. Can J Microbiol 52: 1228–1237.
12. Adams JC, Boult CH, Deadman BJ, Farr JM, Grainger MNC, et al. (2008) Isolation by HPLC and characterization of the bioactive fraction of New Zealand manuka (*Leptospermum scoparium*) honey. Carbohydr Res 343: 651–659.
13. Mavric E, Wittmann S, Barth G, Henle T (2008). Identification and quantification of methylglyoxal as the dominant antibacterial constituent of Manuka (*Leptospermum scoparium*) honey from New Zealand. Mol Nutr Food Res 52: 483–489.
14. Jenkins R, Burton N, Cooper R (2011) Manuka honey inhibits cell division in methicillin-resistant *Staphylococcus aureus*. J Antimicrob Chemother 66: 2536–2542.
15. Peach KC, Bray WM, Winslow D, Linington PT, Linington RG (2013) Mechanism of action-based classification of antibiotics using high-content bacterial image analysis. Mol Biol Syst 9: 1837.
16. Typas A, Banzhaf M, Cross CA, Volimer W (2012) From the regulation of peptidoglycan synthesis to bacterial growth and morphology. Nat Rev Microbiol 10: 123–136.
17. Waxman DJ, Strominger JL (1983) Penicillin-binding proteins and the mechanism of action of β-lactam antibiotics. Ann Rev Biochem 52: 825–69.
18. Spratt BG (1975) Distinct penicillin-binding proteins involved in the division, elongation and shape of *Escherichia coli*. Proc Natl Acad Sci USA 72: 2999–3003.
19. Spratt BG (1983) Penicillin-binding proteins and the future of β-lactam antibiotics. J Gen Microbiol 129: 1247–1260.
20. Kitano K, Tomasz A (1979) Triggering of autolytic cell wall degradation in *Escherichia coli* by beta-lactam antibiotics. Antimicrob Agents Chemother 16: 838–848.
21. Yao Z, Kahne D, Kishony R (2012) Distinct single cell morphological dynamics under beta-lactam antibiotics. Mol Cell 48: 705–712.
22. Tuomanen E, Cozens R, Tosch W, Zak O, Tomasz A (1986) The rate of killing of *Escherichia coli* by β-lactams antiobiotics is strictly proportional to the rate of bacterial growth. J Gen Microbiol 132: 1297–304.
23. Silhavy TJ, Kahne D, Walker S (2010) The bacterial cell envelope. Cold Spring Harb Perspect Biol. 2:a000414.
24. Evans EM, Pollack M (1993) Effect of antibiotic class and concnetration on the release of lipopolysacchride from E. coli. J Infec Dis 167: 1336–1343.
25. Khan MMT, Pyle BH, Camper AK (2010) Specific and rapid enumeration of viable but nonculturable and viable-culturable Grma-negative bacteria by using flow cytometry. Appl Environ Microbiol 76: 5088–5096.
26. Oliver JD (2010) Recent findings on the viable but nonculturable state in pathogenic bacteria. FEMS Microbiol Rev 34: 415–425.
27. Tuomanen E (1986) Phenotypic tolerance: The search for β-lactam antibiotics that kill nongrowing bacteria. *Clin Infect Dis* 8(3): S279–S291.
28. Roostalu J, Jõers A, Luidalepp H, Kaldalu N, Tenson T (2008) Cell division in *Escherichia coli* cultures monitored at single cell resolution. BMC Microbiol 8: e68.
29. Balaban NQ, Merrin J, Chait R, Kowalic L, Leibler S (2004) Bacterial persistence as a phenotypic switch. Science 305: 1622–1625.
30. Chung HS, Yao Z, Goehring NW, Kishony R, Beckwith J, Kahne D (2009) Rapid beta-lactam-induced lysis requires successful assembly of the cell division machinery. Proc Natl Acad Sci USA 106: 21872–7.
31. Young K (2006) The selective value of bacterial shape. Microbiol Mol Biol Rev 70: 660–703.
32. Martinez OV, Gratzner HG, Malinin TI, Ingram M (1982) The effect of some β-lactam antibiotic on *Escherichia coli* studied by flow cytometry. Cytometry 6: 129–133.
33. Bayles KW (2000) The bactericidal action of penicillin: new clues to an unsolved mystery. Trends Microbiol. 8: 274–278.
34. Young K (2007) Reforming L-forms: The need of part of wall after all? J Bacteriol. 189: 6509–6511.
35. Kaldalu N, Mei R, Lewis K (2004) Killing by ampicillin and ofloxacin induces overlapping changes in *Escherichia coli* transcription profile. Antimicrob Agents Chemoth 48: 890–896.
36. Young KD (2008) Why spherical *Escherichia coli* dies: the inside story. J Bacteriol 190: 1497–1498.
37. Lederberg J (1956) Bacterial protoplasts induced by penicillin. Proc Natl Acad Sci USA 42: 574–577.
38. Osborn MJ, Rothfield L (2007) Cell shape determination in *Escherichia coli*. Curr Opin Microbiol 10: 606–610.
39. Henriques AF, Jenkins R, Burton N, Cooper R (2011) The effect of manuka honey on the structure of *Pseudomonas aeruginosa*. Eur J Clin Microbiol Infect Dis 30: 167–171.
40. Gant VA, Warnes G, Phillips I, Savidge GF (1993) The application of flow cytometry to the study of bacterial responses to antibiotics. J. Med. Microbiol 39:147–154.
41. Roth B, Poot M, Yue S, Millard PJ (1997) Bacterial viability and antibiotic susceptibility testing with Sytox Green nucleic acid stain. Appl. Environ. Microbiol 63: 2421–2431.
42. Prins JM, van Deventer SJH, Kuijper EJ, Speelman P (1994) Clinical relevance of antibiotic-induced endotoxin release. Antimicrob Agents Chemother 38: 1211–1218.
43. Roberts AEL, Maddocks SE, Cooper RA (2012) Manuka honey is bactericidal against *Pseudomonas aeruginosa* and results in differential expression of *oprF* and *algD*. Microbiol 158: 3006–13.

20

Selectively Adsorptive Extraction of Phenylarsonic Acids in Chicken Tissue by Carboxymethyl α-Cyclodextrin Immobilized Fe_3O_4 Magnetic Nanoparticles Followed Ultra Performance Liquid Chromatography Coupled Tandem Mass Spectrometry Detection

Jing Jia[2], Wei Zhang[1,3], Jing Wang[1,3], Peilong Wang[1,3]*, Ruohua Zhu[2]*

1 Key Laboratory of Agrifood Safety and Quality, Ministry of Agriculture, Beijing, P.R. China, **2** Department of Chemistry, Capital Normal University, Beijing, China, **3** Institute of Quality Standards and Testing Technology for Agriculture Products, China Agricultural Academy of Science, Beijing, P.R. China

Abstract

Carboxymethyl α-cyclodextrin immobilized Fe_3O_4 magnetic nanoparticles (CM-α-CD-Fe_3O_4) were synthesized for the selectively adsorptive extraction of five phenylarsonic acids including *p*-amino phenylarsonic acid, *p*-nitro phenylarsonic acid, *p*-hydroxy phenylarsonic acid, *p*-acylamino phenylarsonic acid and *p*-hydroxy-3-nitro phenylarsonic acid in chicken tissue. Using ultra performance liquid chromatography coupled with tandem mass spectrometry (UPLC-MS/MS), a highly sensitive analytical method was proposed for the determination of five phenylarsonic acids. It was shown that CM-α-CD-Fe_3O_4 could extract the five phenylarsonic acids in complex chicken tissue samples with high extraction efficiency. Under the optimal conditions, a high enrichment factor, ranging from 349 to 606 fold, was obtained. The limits of detection (LODs) (at a signal-to-noise ratio of 3) were in the range of 0.05–0.11 μg/kg for the five phenylarsonic acids. The proposed method was applied for the determination of five target phenylarsonic acids in chicken muscle and liver samples. Recoveries for the spiked samples with 0.2 μg/kg, 2.0 μg/kg and 20 μg/kg of each phenylarsonic acids were in the range of 77.2%–110.2%, with a relative standard deviation (RSD) of less than 12.5%.

Editor: Bing Xu, Brandeis University, United States of America

Funding: The authors would like to thank the NSFC (No. 31201832), Special Fund for Agro-scientific Research in the Public Interest (No. 201203094), and National International cooperation program (No. 2012DFA31140) for financially supporting this research. The funders had no role in study design, data collection and analysis, decision to publish, or preparation of the manuscript.

Competing Interests: The authors have declared that no competing interests exist.

* Email: wplcon99@163.com (PW); zhurh@mail.cnu.edu.cn (RZ)

Introduction

4-Hydroxy-3-nitrobenzenearsonic acid, also known as roxarsone (ROX), has been used since 1944 as a feed additive in the poultry industry to promote growth and to control coccidiosis, a parasitic disease that infects the intestinal tract of poultry [1]. Besides ROX, some other organic arsenic compounds, including p-amino phenylarsonic acid (p-APAA), p-nitro phenylarsonic acid (p-NPAA), p-hydroxy phenylarsonic acid (p-HPAA) and p-acylamino phenylarsonic acid (AAPAA) (**Fig. 1**) have been successively employed for the same purposes. Their slight structural difference, i. e. different substituent groups on the aromatic ring, results in different growth-promoting and disease-controlling effects [2]. Phenylarsonic acids have been approved as feed additives by many countries at levels of 25–50 mg/kg [3]. Recent studies showed that phenylarsonic acids in the environment might be converted into elemental arsenic and other inorganic arsenic compounds, which are known to be strongly carcinogenic [4]. Some countries in EU strictly control the use of phenylarsonic acid additives, while in the U.S., Tyson Foods, the country's largest poultry producer, stopped the use of arsenic compounds in 2004. After the release of 2011 FDA report of elevated inorganic arsenic in the livers of chickens treated with ROX, Pfizer Animal Health, the US manufacturer of ROX, quickly suspended ROX sales [5]. In order to monitor the residues of phenylarsonic acid in animal products, it is of great significance to establish a convenient, sensitive and reliable method to analyze the organic arsenic in samples [6].

Several analytical methods for the determination of phenylarsonic acids in the environment have been reported, including liquid chromatography (LC) coupled to atomic absorption spectroscopy (AAS) [7], atomic emission spectroscopy (AES) [8] or atomic fluorescence spectrometry (AFS) [9] as well as gas chromatography-mass spectrometry (GC-MS) [10], capillary electrophoresis (CE) coupled to ultraviolet and visible light detector [11] or inductively coupled plasma-mass spectrometry (ICP-MS) [12]. LC has been demonstrated to be the most effective method in arsenic separation, and ICP-MS can provide low

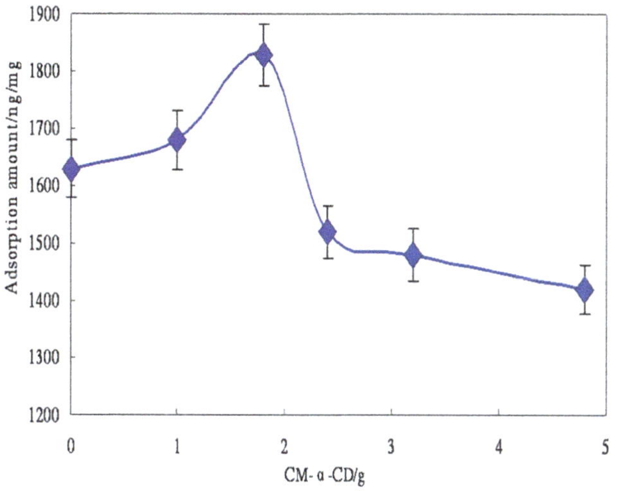

Figure 1. Effect of CM-α-CD amount used in modification on the adsorption efficiency of phenylarsonic acids (ROX). (n = 3, with RSD<6.5%).

detection limit. Therefore, LC-ICP-MS is one of the most powerful research means for analysis of organic arsenic in complex samples [2,13]. The LC-MS/MS is a powerful separation and detection platform in multi residues analysis. Pergantis et al [14] have developed a stable method for determination of 5 phenylarsonic acids including ROX, p-APAA, p-NPAA, AAPAA, p-HPAA and other organic arenics using LC-MS/MS in positive ionization mode. The LODs of the developed method achieved sub ng/g level, whereas the analytical time was too long. Furthermore, compared with other arsenic speciation methods, the LC-MS/MS could provide more structural information of the phenylarsonic acids.

After feeding, nearly all phenylarsonic acids are excreted unchanged to the environment through the disposal of poultry litter, so the residues in animal tissues are very low [15,16]. Some studies indicated that the approved conditions of use mandate a 5-day withdrawal period from the medicated feed before animals are slaughtered, and limits are in place for total residues of combined arsenic (As) in meat from ROX treated animals [0.5 mg kg^{-1} As in muscle tissue and eggs, and 2 mg kg^{-1} As in liver and kidney] [17]. To further lower the detection limits of phenylarsonic acids in complex biological samples, nano-materials have been used to selectively extract and concentrate arsenic compounds. The most commonly used nano-materials for the adsorption of arsenic compounds include goethite [18], titania [19], iron oxide [20,21], Fe_3O_4 nanoparticles [22,23] or modified Fe_3O_4 nanoparticles [24]. Among these nano-materials, Fe_3O_4 nanoparticles are well suited for arsenic analysis due to the following advantages. First, they can be easily isolated from solutions by applying an external magnetic field [25], which ensures simplified sample adsorption and elution processes. Second, Fe_3O_4 nanoparticles have been demonstrated to have higher affinity toward arsenic element than other nano-materials, resulting in higher arsenic extraction efficiency. Fe_3O_4 magnetic nanoparticles have been used for removing inorganic arsenic ions in water sample. For example, Fe_3O_4 nanoparticles dispersed in chelating resins or coated with adequate chelating agents have been used for the removal of a wide range of metal ions from wastewater, overall displaying higher adsorption capacity than traditional materials [26–29]. More recently, β-CD coated Fe_3O_4 nanoparticles have been successfully applied for the removal of methylene blue and copper ions [30,31]. It is found that the cavity of cyclodextrin and its surface hydroxyl group can impart better binding capability and chemical stability to the magnetic particle [32].

In this work, a highly sensitive determination method was established to monitor five phenylarsonic acids in chicken tissues. In our first attempt, it was found that the adsorption of phenylarsonic acids by Fe_3O_4 magnetic nanoparticles was not as good as inorganic arsenic compounds. It was then decided to use CM-α-CD to couple on the surface of Fe_3O_4 providing CD cavities to fit the benzene rings in the structures of phenylarsonic acid compounds. In addition, hydrogen bonding and electrostatic interactions between hydroxyl/carboxyl groups of modified CM-α-CD and amino/nitro of phenyl arsenic acids were also increased. The adsorption properties of modified Fe_3O_4 magnetic nanoparticles to phenylarsonic acids were studied, and the interactions between nanoparticles and phenylarsonic acids were examined. The synthesized materials were successfully applied in the sample clean-up and pre-concentration of phenylarsonic acids in chicken muscle and liver samples, which were subsequently separated and detected by UPLC-MS/MS.

Materials and Methods

Apparatus

ICP-MS (Agilent7500Ce, USA) was used to study the adsorption properties of synthesized material for phenylarsonic acids. The optimum operation parameters of ICP-MS were selected by tuning. The power was 1550W, the flow rates of cooling air, auxiliary air and carrier were 15.0 L/min, 1.0 L/min and 1.12 L/min, respectively. The sample rate of ascension by using peristaltic pump was set as 1.0 mL/min. The integration time for arsenic was 0.3 s/isotope. The operating parameters of UPLC-MS/MS (Waters Xevo TQ, USA) were as follows: capillary voltage = 2.8 kv, desolvation temperature = 450°C, desolvation gas flow rate = 600 L/Hr. The mobile phase was a mixture of acetonitrile (solvent A) and water containing 0.1% formic acid (solvent B) at a flow rate of 0.3 mL/min. All chromatographic separations were carried out in linear gradient mode as follows. In the first minute, solvent A was maintained at 98% (v/v). Solvent B quickly dropped to 30% from 1 to 3 min, followed by dramatic increase back to 98% from 3 to 5 min. MS parameters of UPLC-MS/MS are showed in **Table 1**.

The closed microwave digestion system (CEM MARS, American) was used to digest samples for the determination of the total arsenic in the crude samples. The homogenizer (IKA, Germany) was applied to sample pretreatment and rocking hammock bed was from Zhicheng, Shanghai, China.

Standard solutions and reagents

Five phenylarsonic acids (98%) were obtained from the Chinese Academy of Agricultural Sciences. The standard stock solutions were prepared by dissolving each arsenic species in pure water at an arsenic concentration equivalent to that of 1 mg/mL phenylarsonic acids and stored at 4°C in the dark.

Reagents for preparing magnetic nanoparticles: $FeCl_2 \cdot 4H_2O$ and $FeCl_3 \cdot 6H_2O$ (analytical reagent grade) were purchased from Tianjin Guangfu Fine Chemical Research Institute. Sodium chloroacetate (98%) was bought from Alfa Aesar. α-cyclodextrin (98%) was purchased from Beijing Dilang Biochemical Technology Co., Ltd., China. Other reagents including methanol, ethanol, acetone, toluene, formic acid and sodium hydroxide were of analytical reagent grade and all bought from Beijing Chemical

Table 1. Analytical parameters of MS/MS.

Compounds	Molecular weight	Precursor Ion (m/z)	Product Ion (m/z)	Cone voltage (V)	Collision voltage (V)
p-APAA	217	218	92	27	21
			109	27	16
p-HPAA	218	219	110	28	18
			201	28	13
p-NPAA	247	248	202	30	18
			230	30	14
AAPAA	260	261	244	29	14
ROX	263	264	246	33	14

Plant. The water used throughout the experiment was purified using a Milli-Q water purification system (Millipore, Germany).

Preparation of CM-α-CD stabilized magnetic nanoparticles

Synthesis of CM-α-CD. CM-α-CD was prepared according to the following procedures. α-CD (3.55 mmoL) and NaOH (90.2 mmoL) were first dissolved into 20 ml water. The solution was then heated at 90°C for 5 min, followed by the addition of 74.6 mmoL sodium chloroacetate. The solution was heated for 3 h at 90°C under stirring. Once cooled to room temperature, the pH of the solution was adjusted to 6–7 by hydrochloric acid. The nearly neutral solution obtained was then poured into about 500 mL methanol. CM-α-CD was precipitated out as white solids, which was filtered and washed with methanol for a few times and then dried under vacuum for 3 d at 50°C and 0.085 MPa. The melting point of the CM-α-CD product was about 245.5°C as determined by micro melting point apparatus.

Synthesis of Fe_3O_4 nanoparticles. Fe_3O_4 magnetic nanoparticles were prepared according to the conventional co-precipitation method [33]. A mixture of 2.0 g $FeCl_2{\cdot}4H_2O$ and 5.2 g $FeCl_3{\cdot}6H_2O$ was added into a 500 mL conical flask containing 200 ml 0.05 M HCl. After dissolution of the solids, 250 ml 0.75 M NaOH solution was poured into the flask under a blanket of N_2. The mixture was stirred for another 2 h at 80°C. The Fe_3O_4 nanoparticles were then obtained in the form of black precipitates, which were separated with a magnet and washed subsequently by water (3 times) and ethanol (twice). It should be noted that both the HCl and NaOH solutions were degassed by a sonicator for 20 min before use.

CM-α-CD modified Fe_3O_4 nanoparticles (CM-α-CD-Fe_3O_4). The Fe_3O_4 nanoparticles prepared in the previous step were added into 60 ml PBS buffer solution (pH = 6.6) containing 1.6 g of CM-α-CD. The suspension was sonicated for 3 min and then stirred for 3 h at 80°C. After cooling to room temperature, the nanoparticles were washed several times by PBS buffer solution to remove excess CM-α-CD. The CM-α-CD modified Fe_3O_4 nanoparticles were then dried at 80°C in a vacuum oven.

Adsorption procedure

Static adsorption. In a 10 mL centrifuge tube, 5 mg CM-α-CD-Fe_3O_4 nanoparticles were mixed with 8 mL standard solution of phenylarsenic acid with a given concentration. The centrifuge tube was placed on a rocking hammock bed at a rate of 270 rpm. After equilibrating for 30 min, the magnetic nanoparticles were separated from the solution with external magnetic field. The nanoparticles were rinsed twice with ethanol and dried in N_2. To desorb target compounds, 1.0 mL pure water was added to the nanoparticles followed by equilibration for 10 min. The aqueous solution containing target compounds was filtered through a 0.22 μm Poly (ether sulfones) (PES) syringe filter and analyzed by ICP-MS. Standard phenylarsenic acid solutions of other concentrations were analyzed in the same way.

Dynamic adsorption. In a 10 mL centrifuge tube, 5 mg CM-α-CD-Fe_3O_4 nanoparticles were mixed with 8 mL standard solution of phenylarsenic acid with a given concentration. A number of centrifuge tubes were prepared in this manner for a given concentration of standard. The centrifuge tubes were placed on an orbital shaker at a rate of 270 r/min. At different time points, one tube was removed and the magnetic nanoparticles contained in the tube were separated from the solution with external magnetic field. The following washing, desorption and ICP-MS analysis procedures were the same as those in the static adsorption step. Standard phenylarsenic acid solutions of other concentrations were analyzed in the same way.

Sample analysis

Chicken tissues including meat and liver were bought from a supermarket in Beijing. Chicken meat and chicken liver samples were pulverized and freeze-dried for 24 h. The freeze-dried sample was homogenized by grinding and frozen until analysis. In a 50 mL centrifuge tube, 5.0 g freeze-dried chicken tissue sample and 10 mL ethanol were added. The extraction was repeated twice, each lasting 30 min. The combined extracts were equilibrated with 5 mg CM-α-CD-Fe_3O_4 nanoparticles for 10 min. Then the magnetic nanoparticles which adsorbed target analytes were separated under external magnetic field, the analytes adsorbed on the nanoparticles were then desorbed with 2 mL deionized water. The aqueous solution containing target compounds was filtered through a 0.22 μm PES syringe filter and analyzed by UPLC-MS-MS.

Determination of total arsenic

The total amount of arsenic in chicken tissue samples was determined by microwave digestion ICP-MS according to reference [34]. Each digestion can containing 0.5 g chicken tissues samples was added 5 mL 65% nitric acid. Stages digestion method by controlling temperature was used. The obtained digestion solution was diluted until the concentration of nitric acid fell below 5% and then subjected to ICP-MS analysis.

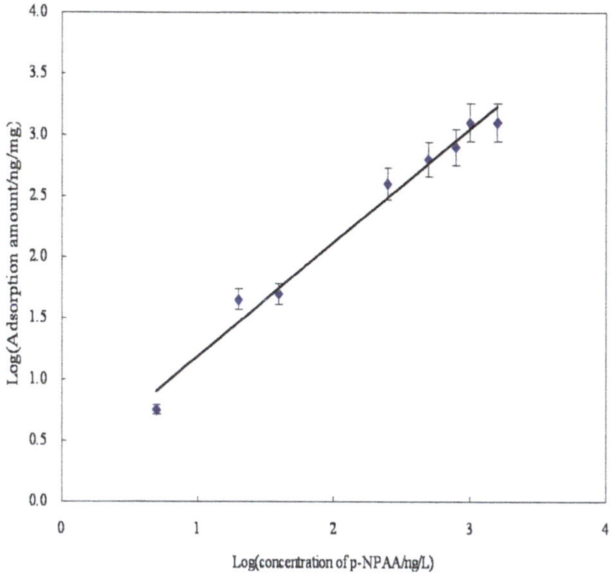

Figure 2. Recovery of different concentrations of phenylarsonic acids (ROX). (n = 3, with RSD<5.0%).

Results and Discussion

Optimization of adsorption efficiency

For optimal adsorption efficiency, the amounts of CM-α-CD for the modification of Fe_3O_4 nanoparticles were varied in six dosages of 0.8, 1.6, 2.4, 3.2, and 4.8 g to obtain 450 mL of Fe_3O_4 suspension as described in section 2.3.2. The adsorption was carried out by equilibrating 5 mg CM-α-CD-Fe_3O_4 in 8 mL ROX standard solution at a concentration of 1 μg/L. The adsorption efficiency was then determined by ICP-MS. As shown in **Fig. 1**, the highest adsorption efficiency corresponds to 1.6 g CM-α-CD. **Fig. 2** shows the adsorption behaviors of ROX at different concentrations by CM-α-CD-Fe_3O_4. The amount of

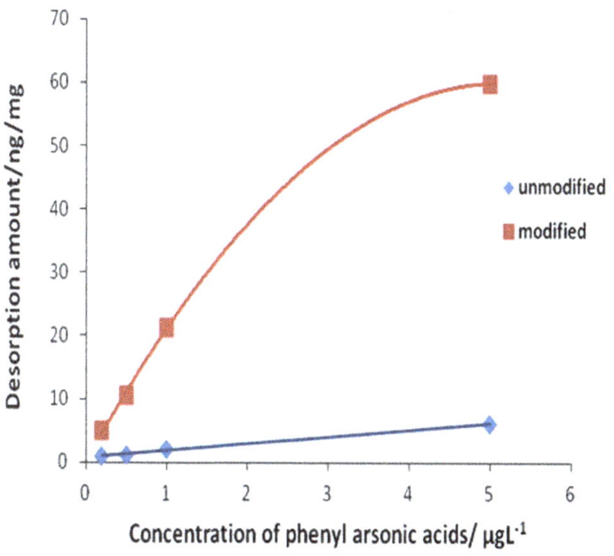

Fig. 3 Comparison of Fe3O4 nanoparticles (blue diamond) and CM-a-CD-Fe3O4 nanoparticles for adsorption of ROX (red square).

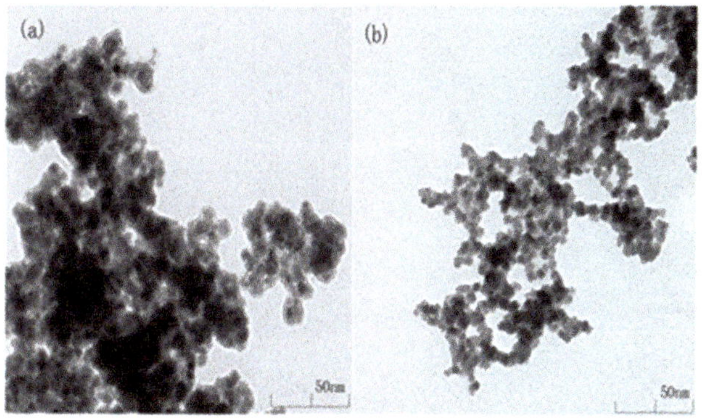

Figure 4. TEM images of magnetic Fe_3O_4 nanoparticles (a) and CM-α-CD-Fe_3O_4 nanoparticles (b).

adsorbed ROX is linear over a large concentration range of ROX. To verify the important role of CM-α-CD in the adsorption of phenylarsonic acid, the adsorption efficiencies of modified and unmodified Fe_3O_4 nanoparticles for p-NPAA were compared. As shown in **Fig. 3**, modified material was obviously superior to unmodified material.

Characterization of magnetic CM-α-CD-Fe_3O_4

The transmission electron microscope (TEM), fourier transform infrared spectrometry (FTIR) and thermo gravimetric analyzer (TGA) were used to characterized the magnetic nanoparticles. The TEM images of Fe_3O_4 and CM-α-CD-Fe_3O_4 nanoparticles are shown in **Fig. 4 (a)** and **Fig. 4 (b)**, respectively. Unmodified Fe_3O_4 nanoparticles, approximately 10 nm in diameter, trend to aggregate because of size effect of Fe_3O_4 nanoparticles. On the other hand, CM-α-CD-Fe_3O_4 nanoparticles shown in **Fig. 4 (b)** are much better dispersed in an aqueous solution with diameters of about 5 nm, because the Fe_3O_4 nanoparticles were modified with CM-α-CD and the surface of Fe_3O_4 nanoparticles was protected by CM-α-CD. It can be observed in **Fig. 4 (b)** that the composite of modified nanoparticles was more compacted and displayed roughly spherical shapes.

The FTIR spectrums of Fe_3O_4, CM-α-CD and CM-α-CD-Fe_3O_4 nanoparticles respectively were scanned (See Fig. S1). In all three samples, a strong characteristic O-H absorption band at

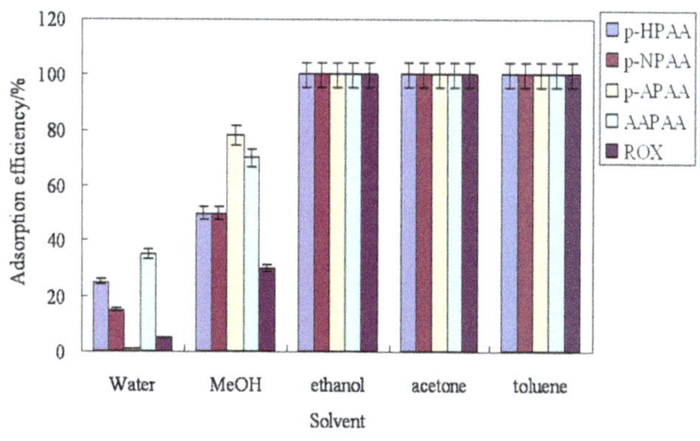

Figure 5. Effect of adsorption solvent on the adsorption efficiency of five phenylarsonic acids. The concentration of each phenylarsonic acids was 50 ng/mL. Adsorption time was 30 min. 5 mg adsorbent was used. (n = 3, with RSD<4.5%).

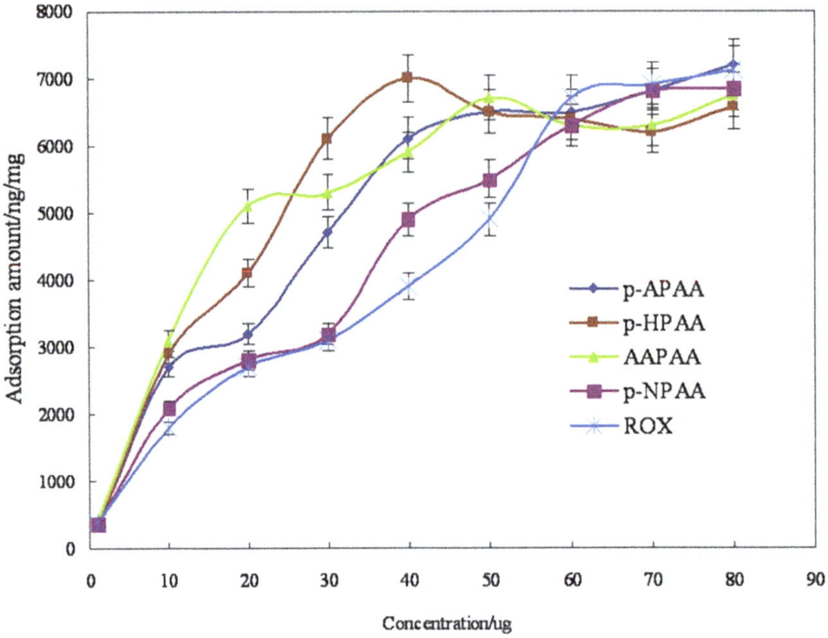

Figure 6. Adsorption saturation curve of CM-α-CD-Fe_3O_4 nanoparticles to five phenylarsonic acids. 5 mg adsorbent was used for each solution. Adsorption time was 30 min. Desorption was in water for 10 min. (n = 3, with RSD<5.7%).

around 3400 cm^{-1} is clearly visible. There is a strong Fe-O absorption peak at 580 cm^{-1} for both Fe_3O_4 and CM-α-CD-Fe_3O_4, suggesting the intactness of the Fe-O bond during the modification process. Compared with the innate Fe_3O_4 nanoparticles, new characteristic peaks at 1100 and 2900 cm^{-1} appeared in the spectrum of CM-α-CD- Fe_3O_4 nanoparticles, corresponding to C-O-C and C-H groups of CM-α-CD, which are also visible in the spectrum of pure CM-α-CD. This confirms the success of the modification of CM-α-CD to Fe_3O_4 nanoparticles.

The amount of CM-α-CD grafted on the surface of Fe_3O_4 and the number of CM-α-CD molecules immobilized on a single Fe_3O_4 nanoparticle can be estimated from the TGA results. It is known that CM-α-CD decomposes completely above 600°C.The TGA curves of Fe_3O_4 and CM- α-CD-Fe_3O_4 exhibit two steps of weight loss. In both cases, the first step can be attributed to the loss of residual water.The amounts of CM-α-CD coated on the surface of Fe_3O_4, calculated on the basis of the second-step loss, are 5.3% and 9.6% for Fe_3O_4 nanoparticles and CM-α-CD-Fe_3O_4 nanoparticles, respectively. The increase of the weight loss can be ascribed to CM-α-CD grafted on Fe_3O_4 nanoparticles (about 43 mg/g). According to Y. P. Wu [35], the number of CM-α-CD molecules immobilized on a single Fe_3O_4 can be calculated in equation (1):

$$N = \frac{4 \times (W_{CD} - W_{Fe_3O_4}) \times N_A \rho \pi R^3}{3 \times M_{CD} \times (1 - W_{CD}) \times 10^{21}} \tag{1}$$

where N is the number of CM-α-CD molecules immobilized on each Fe_3O_4, R is the mean radius of CM-α-CD-Fe_3O_4 (5.0 nm based on the TEM results), ρ is the density of the nanoparticle (4.8 g/cm^3), N_A is Avogadro's number, W_{CD} and W_{Fe3O4} are the weight losses of the CM-α-CD-Fe_3O_4 and Fe_3O_4 respectively, M_{CD} is the molar mass of CM-α-CD immobilized on CM-α-CD-Fe_3O_4. The calculated number of CM-α-CD molecules immobilized on each CM-α-CD-Fe_3O_4 is about 70.

Selection of adsorption solvent

The solvent for phenylarsonic acid solutions is an important factor affecting the adsorption efficiency. Five candidate solvents, i.e., water, methanol, ethanol, acetone and toluene, were compared (Fig. 5). The adsorption efficiency of all target arsenic species could reach 100% in ethanol, acetone and toluene. Ethanol was selected as the solvent in the following experiments

Table 2. Enrichment factors of CM-α-CD-Fe_3O_4 for 0.1 μg/L of each phenylarsonic acids in toluene solvent.

Phenylarsonic acids	Theory concentration (μg/L)	Experimental concentration (μg/L)	Enrichment factor	Enrichment Efficiency (%)
p-APAA	50.0	41.4	414	82.8
AAPAA	50.0	42.6	426	85.2
ROX	50.0	58.1	581	116.2
p-HPAA	50.0	60.6	606	121.2
p-NPAA	50.0	34.9	349	69.8

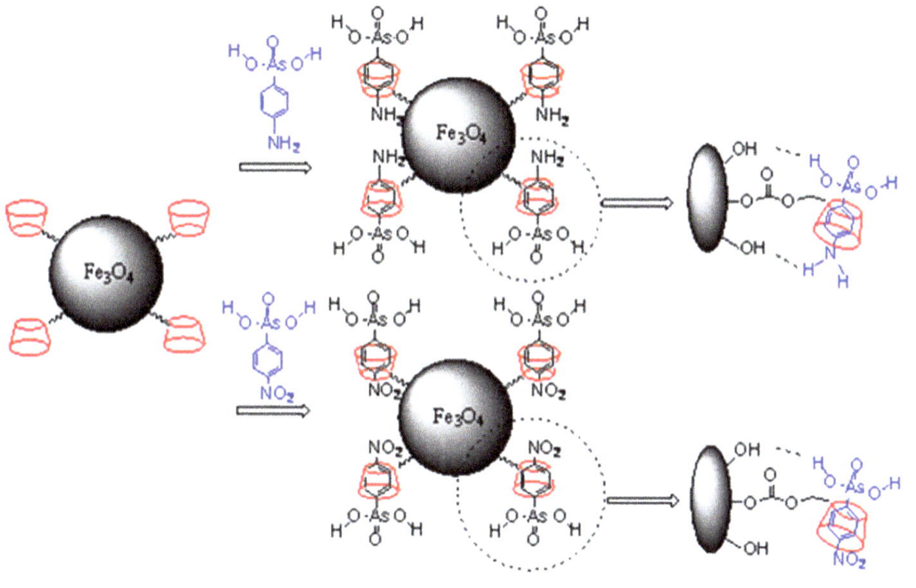

Figure 7. The likely interactions between CM-α-CD-Fe_3O_4 and the acids p-APAA and p-NPAA.

due to the relatively low toxicity. In water and methanol, the adsorption efficiencies of the five target compounds are very poor, which might be because of the water and methanol possess higher polarity than ethanol, acetone and toluene.

Static adsorption

Saturation of adsorption. The adsorption saturation curve is shown in **Fig. 6**. The point of saturation was reached at 40 μg for p-HPAA, p-APAA, and AAPAA, whereas it was 60 μg for p-NPAA and ROX, corresponding to about 0.2 μmol of each phenylarsonic acid.

The amount of CM-α-CD coated on the surface of Fe_3O_4 could be estimated from the saturation of adsorption. Since one phenylarsonic acid molecule was supposed to fit one CD cavity, there should be approximately equal amount of CD and phenylarsonic acid. Thus, the amount of CM-α-CD might be calculated through its molecular mass of 1029 according to equation (2). The estimated amount of grafted CM-α-CD was about 41.2 mg/g, which was similar to 43 mg/g calculated by TGA in 3.2.3.

$$m_{\mathrm{CM-a-CD}} = \frac{\mathrm{n_{saturated}} \times M_{\mathrm{CM-a-CD}}}{m_{\mathrm{adsorbent}}} \quad (2)$$

Enrichment factors of low concentration. The lowest concentrations of phenylarsonic acids that could be absorbed by CM-α-CD-Fe_3O_4 as well as enrichment factors were investigated. Ultimately, the enrichment factors of p-APAA, AAPAA, ROX, p-HPAA and p-NPAA were 414, 426, 581, 606 and 349 (theoretical enrichment factor was 500) at the concentration of 0.1 μg/L. Enrichment efficiency was 69.8%-121.2% and experimental results are shown in **Table 2**.

Dynamic adsorption

Optimization of adsorption time and desorption time. The water was selected as desorption solvent. The adsorption efficiency was optimized by varying the adsorption time in the range of 1–40 min with all other parameters held constant. The adsorption efficiency increased with the adsorption time from 1 to 30 min followed by a plateau. The rate of adsorption was so high that 5 min was enough to adsorb the target compounds. Similarly, desorption efficiency was optimized by varying desorption time in the range of 1–10 min. The desorption efficiency increased with desorption time till 10 min, at which point it plateaued. Therefore, 10 min was selected as desorption time and desorption efficiency was achieved above 75%.

The tolerance of coexisting inorganic ions and organic analogues. By fixing the concentration of each phenylarsonic acids at 50 μg/L and 12 coexisting inorganic ions including Mn^{2+}, Cu^{2+}, K^{+}, Zn^{2+}, Ba^{2+}, Fe^{3+}, Mg^{2+}, Ca^{2+}, Pb^{2+}, Cr^{3+}, Cd^{2+}, and

Table 3. Concentration (μg/L) of coexisting analogues when tolerance factor less than 5%.

	phenol	benzoic acid	p-hydroxbenzoic acid	m-hydroxbenzoic acid
AAPAA	500	500	500	500
p-HPAA	500	250	250	250
p-NPAA	50	500	50	250
p-APAA	>500	500	500	250
ROX	250	500	500	250

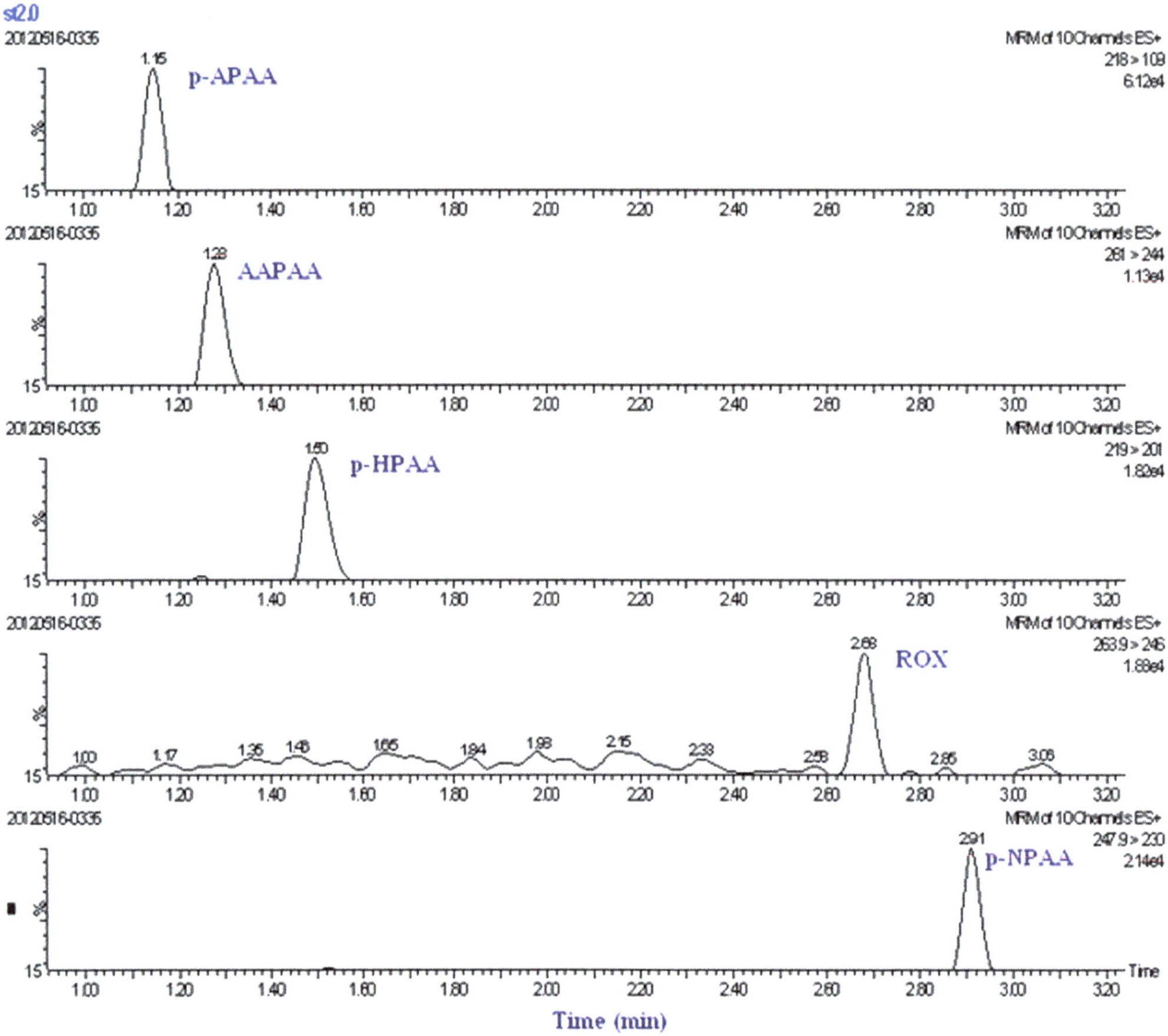

Figure 8. MRM chromatogram of five arsenical compounds standards at 2.0 μg/L.

Sn^{2+} at concentrations of 500, 5000, and 50000 μg/L for each inorganic ions respectively, interference of inorganic ions on the adsorption of phenylarsonic acids was studied. No significant interferences were observed under the optimum conditions described above in the presence of inorganic ions as high as 50000 μg/L. The influence of four organic analogues including phenol, benzoic acid, p-hydroxbenzoic and m-hydroxbenzoic acid at concentrations of 50, 250 and 500 μg/L for each organic

Table 4. Analytical performance data with UPLC-MS/MS.

Compounds	Linear range (μg/L)	Linear equation	R^2	LOD (μg/kg)
p-APAA	0.2–10.0	y = 7305.3x+2211.7	0.9952	0.05
AAPAA	0.2–10.0	y = 2287.2x+398.63	1.0000	0.05
p-HPAA	0.2–10.0	y = 5739.4x+935.79	0.9984	0.10
ROX	0.2–10.0	y = 3249.2x-144.89	1.0000	0.10
p-NPAA	0.2–10.0	y = 1712.3x-87.287	0.9988	0.11

x: the concentration of five phenylarsonic acids, y: peak area. LOD = 3 S/N of blank chicken tissues sample.

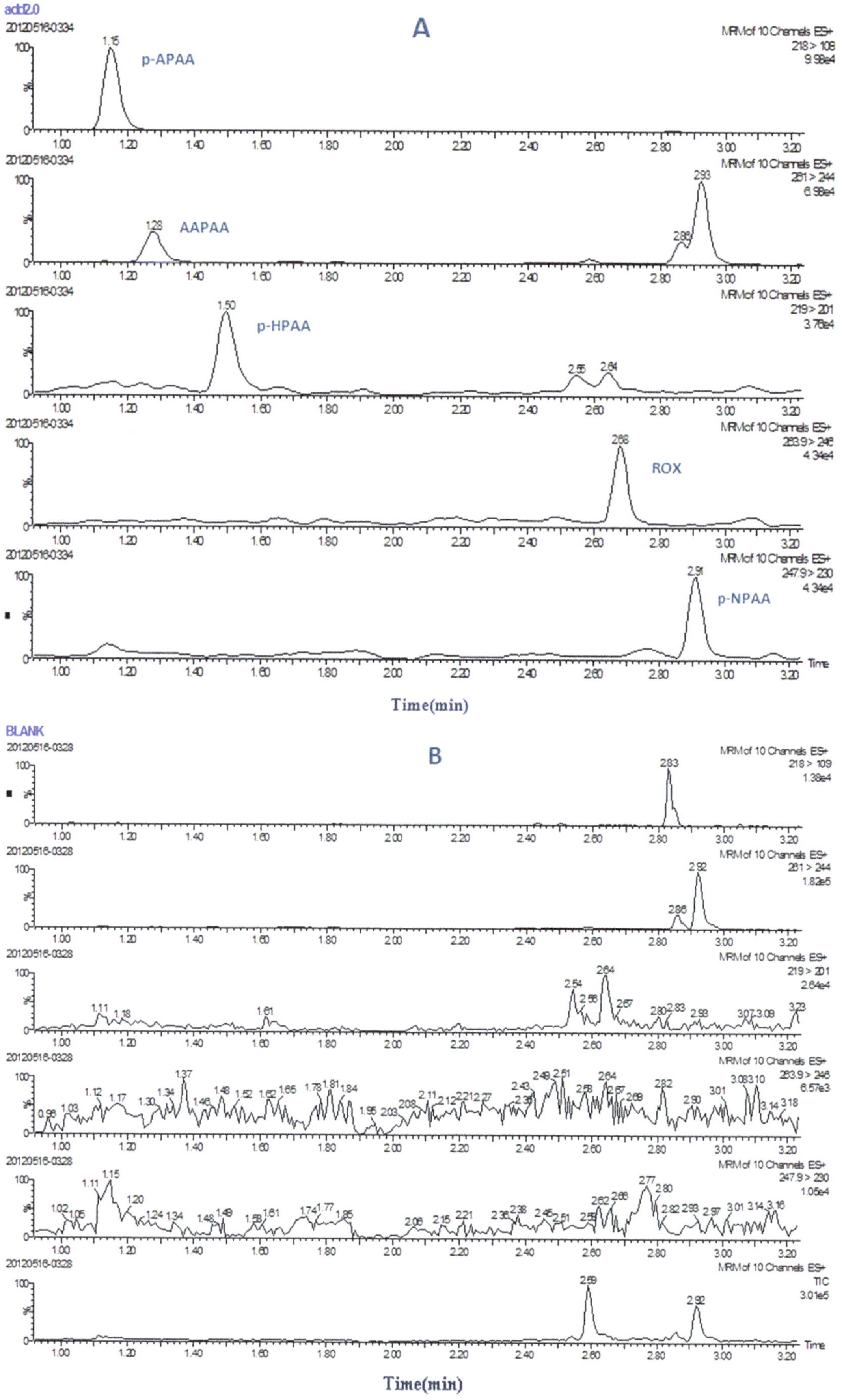

Figure 9. MRM chromatogram of spiked chicken meat (2.0 μg/kg) (A) and blank (B).

Table 5. Recoveries of spiked arsenics in chicken liver and muscle sample (n = 5).

Compounds	Chicken liver			Chicken meat		
	Added (μg/kg)	Recovery (%)	RSD (%)	Added (μg/kg)	Recovery (%)	RSD (%)
p-APAA	0.2	80.7	5.0	0.2	87.3	8.0
	2.0	89.5	6.7	2.0	86.1	7.6
	20	87.7	4.2	20	101.8	5.2
p-HPAA	0.2	94.3	4.9	0.2	77.2	9.1
	2.0	97.9	6.6	2.0	95.1	5.1
	20	93.7	12.5	20	79.9	5.2
p-NPAA	0.2	102.2	4.7	0.2	91.8	7.6
	2.0	110.2	5.4	2.0	98.8	5.7
	20	99.0	10.8	20	102.8	6.3
AAPAA	0.2	82.4	4.4	0.2	83.7	12.1
	2.0	82.6	5.4	2.0	82.6	8.1
	20	78.3	2.0	20	79.6	8.5
ROX	0.2	93.4	2.9	0.2	96.9	10.1
	2.0	104.2	7.3	2.0	104.2	6.4
	20	106.1	4.8	20	108.7	5.2

analogues respectively on the adsorption of target arsenic species was investigated. As shown in **Table 3**, the allowed concentrations of coexisting analogues were about 500 μg/L or 250 μg/L with a tolerance factor of less than 5%. However, p-NPAA was an exception. The tolerance concentration of p-hydroxybenzoic acid was only 50 μg/L. Possible explanation is shown in **Fig. 7**. Despite other interactions, the hydrogen bonding between hydroxyl on the surface of CM-α-CD-Fe_3O_4 and amino groups of p-APAA and AAPAA was very strong but there was hardly any hydrogen bonding between the hydroxyl and nitro of p-NPAA. In any case, phenylarsonic acid could form inclusion complex with α-CD and therefore the arsenate, hydroxyl or amino group were forced closer to the magnetic particles, leading to stronger interactions between the modified material and phenylarsonic acids. Both selectivity and adsorption efficiency were improved compared to that of Fe_3O_4 nanoparticles without modification.

Analytical performance

Optimization of UPLC-MS-MS chromatograph separation condition. A mixture of five arsenic compound standards, each at a concentration of 2.0 μg/L, was successfully separated and analyzed by UPLC-MS/MS in less than 3 min on a C18 column. Under the optimal separation conditions, baseline separation was achieved for every arsenic compound. The multi-reaction monitoring (MRM) chromatograms of arsenic compounds are shown in **Fig. 8**.

Optimization of sample pretreatment condition. To extract phenylarsonic acids from chicken tissue samples, different extraction methods (including ultrasonic extraction, microwave extraction), extraction time (10, 20, 30, 40, 50 and 60 min) and extraction solvents (methanol, ethanol and toluene) were studied. The optimal recovery was above 75% with the ultrasonic extraction method and toluene as the extraction solvent. The proper extraction time was found to be 30 min and extraction should be conducted twice.

Method evaluation

The developed method was validated by determining the linearity and LOD of arsenic species listed in **Table 4**. A linear response can be seen in the concentration range of 0.20–10 μg/L (enrichment factor 2.5), with the R^2 ranging from 0.9951 to 1.0000. The repeatability study was performed for each of the phenylarsonic acids under the optimal conditions. The LOD of each phenylarsonic acid was estimated by analyzing blank samples spiked at 0.2 μg/kg of each target analytes and they were determined as the lowest concentrations of the analyte for which signal-to-noise ratios were 3 respectively. The resultant repeatabilities expressed as RSD varied from 0.85% to 4.49%. These results show that the method has a high sensitivity and good repeatability.

Sample analysis

The phenylarsonic acid in tissue was stored with the prototype compound. So the sample preparation of real tissue samples is same as the spiked samples [17]. In order to validate the suitability of the developed method, the method was applied to analyze spiked chicken tissue samples. For comparison, the total arsenic in these samples was also determined.

In the samples of chicken meat and liver, 0.2, 2 and 20 μg/kg of each phenylarsonic acids were spiked, respectively. The recoveries of five phenylarsonic acids in chicken tissue samples, as shown in **Table 5**, fell in the ranges of 77.2%–110.2%, with a RSD less than 12.5%. The chromatograms of spiked chicken meat sample (2.0 μg/kg) and blank chicken meat sample are shown in **Fig. 9**. To confirm the selectivity of CM-α-CD-Fe_3O_4, five phenylarsonic acids were spiked individually in each sample at 0.2 μg/kg and determined by ICP-MS. Recoveries were in the range of 81.5%–119.2% which agreed with the UPLC-MS/MS results. This shows that the CM-α-CD-Fe_3O_4 nanoparticles have high selectivity for phenylarsonic acid and can be used for sample clean-up. Combining CM-α-CD-Fe_3O_4 nanoparticles clean-up procedure with UPLC-MS-MS technique would potentially result in practical application in the analysis of trace phenyl arsenic acids.

Conclusions

In this work, CM-α-CD-Fe_3O_4 nanoparticles were synthesized to selectively extract and enrich phenylarsonic acids. CM-α-CD-Fe_3O_4 nanoparticles exhibited excellent selectivity and adsorption efficiency for five phenylarsonic acids because of the size selectivity of α-CD and the affinity of Fe_3O_4 to arsenic. In the sub ppb level of phenylarsonic acids, the enrichment factor was higher than 400 and the extraction efficiency higher than 70%. Coupled with UPLC-MS/MS, a fast, selective and convenient analytical method for the determination of phenylarsonic acid was developed. Comparing with published method [14], the developed method showed satisfactory sensitivity due to the selectively adsorption of CM-α-CD-Fe_3O_4 nanoparticles for phenylarsonic acids in complex sample matrix.

Supporting Information

Figure S1 FTIR spectra of Fe_3O_4 magnetic nanoparticles (a), CM-α-CD (b) and CM-α- CD- Fe_3O_4 (c).

Author Contributions

Conceived and designed the experiments: PW RZ. Performed the experiments: JJ. Analyzed the data: JW PW. Contributed reagents/materials/analysis tools: WZ PW. Contributed to the writing of the manuscript: PW RZ.

References

1. Jaafar J (2001) Separation of phenylarsonic compounds by ion-pairing reversed phase-high performance liquid chromatography. Jurnal Teknologi C UTM 35: 71–83.
2. Wang PL, Zhao GL, Tian J, Su XO (2010) High-performance liquid chromatography-inductively coupled plasma mass spectrometry based method for the determination of organic arsenic feed additives and speciation of anionic arsenics in animal feed. J. Agric. Food Chem 58(9): 5263–70.
3. Chiou PW, Chen KL, Yu B (1997) Effects of roxarsone on performance, toxicity, tissue accumulation and residue of eggs and excreta in laying hens. J. Sci. Food Agric 74(2): 229–236.
4. Bartel M, Ebert F, Leffers L (2011) Toxicological characterization of the inorganic and organic arsenic metabolite thio-DMA(V) in cultured human lung cells. J. Toxicol 2011: 1–9.
5. FDA (2011) Study 275. 30 Arsenic speciation in broiler chickens. a) Summary Final Report. b) Amendments to final report. c) Analyst's report. d) Statistician's Report.
6. Thirunavukkarasu OS, Viraraghavan T, Subramanian KS, Tanjore S (2002) Organic arsenic removal from drinking water. Urban Water 4: 415–21.
7. Samanta G, Chowdhury TR, Mandal BK, Biswas BK, Chowdhury UK, et al. (1999) Flow Injection Hydride Generation Atomic Absorption Spectrometry for Determination of Arsenic in Water and Biological Samples from Arsenic-Affected Districts of West Bengal, India, and Bangladesh. Microchemical J 62(1): 174–91.
8. Ma MS, Le XC, Hu B, Jiang ZC (2000) High performance liquid chromatography with hydride generation atomic fluorescence detection for rapid urinary arsenic speciation. J. Ana. Sci 16: 89–96.
9. Liu JJ, Yu HX, Song HB, Qiu J, Sun FM, et al. (2008) Simultaneous determination of *p*-arsanilic acid and roxarsone in feed by liquid chromatography-hydride generation online coupled with atomic fluorescence spectrometry. J. Environ. Monit 10: 975–8.
10. Roerdink AR, Aldstadt JH (2004) Sensitive method for the determination of roxarsone using solid-phase microextraction with multi-detector gas chromatography. J. Chromatogr. A 1057 (1-2): 177–83.
11. Li P, Hu B (2011) Sensitive determination of phenylarsenic compounds based on a dual preconcentration method with capillary electrophoresis/UV detection. J. Chromatogr. A 1218 (29): 4779–87.
12. Rosal CG, Momplaisir GM, Heithmar EM (2005) Roxarsone and transformation products in chicken manure: determination by capillary electrophoresis-inductively coupled plasma-mass spectrometry. Electrophoresis 26(7-8) 1606–14.
13. Bednar AJ, Garbarino JR, Burkhardt MR, Ranville JF, Wildeman TR (2004) Field and laboratory arsenic speciation methods and their application to natural-water analysis. Water Res 38 (2): 355–64.
14. Pergantis SA, Winnik W, Betowski D (1997) Determination of ten organoarsenic compounds using microbore high-performance liquid chromatography coupled with electrospray mass spectrometry-mass spectrometry. J. Anal. At. Spectrom 12: 531–6
15. Chen SL, Yeh SJ, Yang MH, Lin TH (1995) Trace element concentration and arsenic speciation in the well water of a Taiwan area with endemic Blackfoot disease. Biol. Trace Elem. Res 48 (3): 263–74.
16. Kuehnelt D, Goessler W (2003) Organometallic compounds in the environment, ed. P. J. Craig, John Wiley & Sons Ltd., Chichester, pp. 223–75.
17. Conklin SD, Shockey N, Kubachka K, Howard KD, Carson MC (2012) Development of an ion chromatography-inductively coupled plasma-mass spectrometry method to determine inorganic arsenic in liver from chickens treated with roxarsone. J. Agric. Food Chem. 60(37): 9394–404.
18. Chen WR, Huang CH (2012) Surface adsorption of organoarsenic roxarsone and arsanilic acid on iron and aluminum oxides. J. Hazard. Mater 227–228: 378–85.
19. Mao XJ, Chen BB, Hu B (2011) Titania immobilized polypropylene hollow fiber as a disposable coating for stir bar sorptive extraction–high performance liquid chromatography–inductively coupled plasma mass spectrometry speciation of arsenic in chicken tissues. J.Chromatogr.A 1218 (1):1–9.
20. Mayo JT, Yavuz C, Yean S, Cong L, Shipley H, et al. (2007) The effect of nanocrystalline magnetite size on arsenic removal. Sci.Technol. Adv. Mater 8(1-2):71–5.
21. Akin I, Arslan G, Tor A, Ersoz M, Cengeloglu Y (2012) Arsenic(V) removal from underground water by magnetic nanoparticles synthesized from waste red mud. J. Hazard. Mater 235–236: 62–8.
22. Li RX, Liu SM (2011) Preparation and characterization of cross-linked β-cyclodextrin polymer/Fe_3O_4 composite nanoparticles with core-shell structures. Chin. Chem. Lett 22 (2): 217–20.
23. Kan XW, Zhao Q, Shao DL, Geng ZR, Wang ZL, et al. (2010) Preparation and Recognition Properties of Bovine Hemoglobin Magnetic Molecularly Imprinted Polymers. J. Phys. Chem. B 114 (11): 3999–4004.
24. Liu ZG, Zhang FS, Sasai R (2010) Arsenate removal from water using Fe_3O_4-loaded activated carbon prepared from waste biomass. Chem. Eng. J. 160 (1): 57–62.
25. Badruddoza AZM, Hidajat K, Uddin MS (2010) Synthesis and characterization of β-cyclodextrin-conjugated magnetic nanoparticles and their uses as solid-phase artificial chaperones in refolding of carbonic anhydrase bovine. J. Colloid. Interface Sci 346 (2): 337–46.
26. Zhang CC, Li X, Pang JX (2001) Synthesis and adsorption properties of magnetic resin microbeads with amine and mercaptan as chelating groups. J. Appl. Polym. Sci 82 (7) 1587–92.
27. Atia AA, Donia AM, El-Enein SA, Yousif AM (2007) Effect of Chain Length of Aliphatic Amines Immobilized on a Magnetic Glycidyl Methacrylate Resin towards the Uptake Behavior of Hg(II) from Aqueous Solutions. Sep. Sci. Technol. 42 (2): 403–20.
28. Atia AA, Donia AM, Yousif AM (2008) Removal of some hazardous heavy metals from aqueous solution using magnetic chelating resin with iminodiacetate functionality. Sep. Purif. Technol 61 (3): 348–57.
29. Mohan D, Pittman CU (2007) Arsenic removal from water/wastewater using adsorbents—A critical review. J. Hazard. Mater 142 (1-2): 1–53.
30. Badruddoza AZM, Hazel GSS, Hidajat K, Uddin MS (2010) Synthesis of carboxymethyl-β-cyclodextrin conjugated magnetic nano-adsorbent for removal of methylene blue. Colloids Surf. A 367 (1-3): 85–95.
31. Badruddoza AZM, Tay ASH, Tan PY, Hidajat K, Uddin MS (2011) Carboxymethyl-β-cyclodextrin conjugated magnetic nanoparticles as nano-adsorbents for removal of copper ions: Synthesis and adsorption studies. J. Hazard. Mater.185 (2-3): 1177–86.
32. Zhi J, Tian XL, Zhao W, Shen JB, Tong B, et al. (2008) Self-assembled film based on carboxymethyl-β-cyclodextrin and diazoresin and its binding properties for methylene blue. J. Colloid. Interface Sci. 319 (1): 270–6.
33. Wu W, He QG, Jiang CZ (2008) Magnetic Iron Oxide Nanoparticles: Synthesis and Surface Functionalization Strategies. Nanoscale Res. Lett 3(11): 397–415.
34. Krachler M, Radner H, Irgolic KJ (1996) Microwave digestion methods for the determination of trace elements in brain and liver samples by inductively coupled plasma mass spectrometry. Fresenius' Journal of Analytical Chemistry 355(2): 120–8.
35. Wu YP, Zuo F, Zheng ZH, Ding XB, Peng YX (2009) A Novel Approach to Molecular Recognition Surface of Magnetic Nanoparticles Based on Host–Guest Effect. Nanoscale Res. Lett. 4 (7): 738–47.

Three Months of High-Fructose Feeding Fails to Induce Excessive Weight Gain or Leptin Resistance in Mice

Erik J. Tillman[1¤], **Donald A. Morgan**[2], **Kamal Rahmouni**[2], **Steven J. Swoap**[1*]

1 Department of Biology, Williams College, Williamstown, Massachusetts, United States of America, **2** Department of Pharmacology, University of Iowa Carver College of Medicine, Iowa City, Iowa, United States of America

Abstract

High-fructose diets have been implicated in obesity via impairment of leptin signaling in humans and rodents. We investigated whether fructose-induced leptin resistance in mice could be used to study the metabolic consequences of fructose consumption in humans, particularly in children and adolescents. Male C57Bl/6 mice were weaned to a randomly assigned diet: high fructose, high sucrose, high fat, or control (sugar-free, low-fat). Mice were maintained on their diets for at least 14 weeks. While fructose-fed mice regularly consumed more kcal and expended more energy, there was no difference in body weight compared to control by the end of the study. Additionally, after 14 weeks, both fructose-fed and control mice displayed similar leptin sensitivity. Fructose-feeding also did not change circulating glucose, triglycerides, or free fatty acids. Though fructose has been linked to obesity in several animal models, our data fail to support a role for fructose intake through food lasting 3 months in altering of body weight and leptin signaling in mice. The lack of impact of fructose in the food of growing mice on either body weight or leptin sensitivity over this time frame was surprising, and important information for researchers interested in fructose and body weight regulation.

Editor: Julie A. Chowen, Hosptial Infantil Universitario Niño Jesús, CIBEROBN, Spain

Funding: KR is supported by funds from the National Institutes of Health (HL084207) and American Heart Association (14EIA18860041). SJS is supported by funds from the National Institutes of Health (R15AG37959-1). The funders had no role in study design, data collection and analysis, decision to publish, or preparation of the manuscript.

Competing Interests: The authors have declared that no competing interests exist.

* Email: sswoap@williams.edu

¤ Current address: Department of Biology, Massachusetts Institute of Technology, Cambridge, Massachusetts, United States of America

Introduction

Concurrent with the rise in obesity in the United States since 1980, there has been a rise in food manufacturers' use of high fructose corn syrup as a low-cost sweetening ingredient, as well as an increase in total national sugar consumption through both food additives and sweetened beverages [1–3]. This observation has led to recent research into the consequences of over-consuming sugars, with a particular focus on fructose [4,5]. Consumption of calorically sweetened beverages is correlated with childhood and adolescent obesity, increased abdominal adiposity, dyslipidemia, and elevated blood pressure [6–8]. In addition, fructose in particular causes decreased insulin sensitivity with elevated insulin levels [9].

Fructose has been suggested to be an obesogen [5,10]. The consumption of dietary fructose in humans leads to significantly lower circulating glucose levels and higher triglyceride levels postprandially than dietary glucose, and the activity of the anorexigenic hormone leptin depends on levels of circulating glucose [11]. Therefore, one mechanism by which fructose may cause obesity is by failing to elevate glucose levels in the blood to the same levels as other dietary sweeteners after a meal, thereby failing to elicit the same leptin-mediated anorexia. Supporting its putative role in regulation of caloric intake, it is thought that fructose does not cause the satiety that is observed with other carbohydrates [12,13]. Such a hypothesis is supported by recent work showing that glucose, but not fructose, ingestion reduces activation of the appetite-sensing region of the brain in humans and induces a network response consistent with satiety [14].

In particular, fructose is known to alter leptin sensitivity in rats [15]. Leptin is a canonical regulator of energy balance through its signaling in the arcuate nucleus of the hypothalamus, as well as other structures throughout the brain [11,16–18]. Leptin reflects the general adiposity of an individual as it is secreted primarily by adipose tissue [19]. Leptin is anorexigenic, and as such, is part of a negative feedback system that decreases appetite as fat stores grow [16,20,21]. Deregulation of this system leads to obesity through several known mechanisms [22–25].

Fructose feeding has been implicated in the development of leptin resistance and obesity in numerous studies using rodents [15,26]. Consumption of high fructose corn syrup administered in drinking water leads to obesity marked by increased body weight, body fat, and circulating triglycerides in rats [10]. Also in rats, the administration of a diet high in fructose diminishes leptin sensitivity and makes the animals susceptible to obesity, confirmed through increased weight gain when transferred to a high fat diet [15]. Rats on a high-fat, high-fructose diet that are switched to a high-fat, fructose-free diet become resensitized to leptin, centrally and peripherally, indicating that any induced leptin sensitivity is reversible simply by dietary changes [27]. Additionally, a sustained fructose diet led to oxidative stress, glucose intolerance, and insulin resistance in rats [28]. Together, these studies support the deleterious effects of dietary fructose in rodents.

Because of the numerous genetically modified strains available, mice represent a good model for studying genetic and nutritional interactions in obesity. We hypothesized that fructose feeding in young mice weaned directly to a diet containing high fructose would recapitulate the studies previously described in rats [15,26,29,30]. Surprisingly, however, we found that 14 weeks of high fructose feeding in young C57Bl/6 mice did not negatively affect either their final body weight or sensitivity to leptin.

Materials and Methods

Animals – experiment #1

Pregnant C57Bl/6H females were purchased from Harlan and housed at Williams College, Williamstown, MA. Upon delivery, litters were housed with mothers for 3 weeks. 38 males were weaned from their mothers, and moved to individual housing at 23°C on a 12:12-hour light-dark cycle and placed on one of two randomly assigned experimental diets. Control mice (n = 19) were allowed free access to a fructose-free diet (Harlan Teklad, TD.05075). This diet consisted of 5.2% fat (by weight) obtained from lard, 60% carbohydrates from corn starch, and 18.3% protein (mostly casein), with a caloric content of 3.6 kcal/g. The experimental group (n = 19) was given free access to a 60% fructose diet (Harlan Teklad, TD.89247), which is identical to the fructose-free diet with the exception that fructose was the carbohydrate, and not corn starch. Food intake was measured five times weekly and body weight twice weekly for 14 weeks in the hour before the onset of the dark phase. All procedures and experimental protocols were approved by the Williams College Animal Care and Use Committee.

Animals – experiment #2

Male C57Bl/6J mice were purchased from The Jackson Laboratory and housed at the University of Iowa College of Medicine, Iowa City, Iowa. Upon delivery, mice were group housed (3 or 4 per cage) at 22–24°C on a 12:12-hour light-dark cycle, and placed onto one of four randomly assigned experimental diets purchased from Research Diets Inc.: control diet (Catalog #D12450K: 12% of calories from fat, 67% carbohydrates, 21% protein, 3.9 kcal/g: n = 48), high fat diet (Catalog #D12451: 45% of calories from fat, 35% carbohydrates, 20% protein, 4.7 kcal/g: n = 56), a high sucrose diet (Catalog #D02022703: 60% of calories from sucrose, 13% fat, 27% protein, 3.9 kcal/g: n = 82), and a high fructose diet (Catalog #D02022704: 60% of calories from fructose, 13% fat, 27% protein, 3.9 kcal/g: n = 64). Body weight was measured once weekly for 20 weeks. This experiment was approved by the University of Iowa Animal Research Committee.

Metabolic Rate Measurements

In weeks 2, 9, and 14 of high-fructose or control feeding of experiment #1, seven animals from each feeding group were housed for indirect calorimetry. The same seven animals were used each time metabolic rate was measured. To measure metabolic rate, mice were housed in standard, clear, polycarbonate mouse cages (volume approximately 7L) fitted with an airtight seal on the top, and inflow and outflow ports for air exchange. Room air was dried with calcium sulfate and pumped into the cage at a regulated flow rate of 250–350 mL min^{-1}. Outflow from the cage was pulled through an O_2 analyzer (S-3A/II; AEI Technologies, Naperville, IL) and subsequently a CO_2 analyzer (CD-3A; AEI Technologies) at a rate of 140 mL min^{-1}. Up to 3 cages were serially sampled, with an empty cage serving as a reference. The outflow from each cage was sampled once every 8 minutes. Ambient pressure and temperature were concurrently measured electronically (APR-1 and C10T, Data Sciences International, St. Paul, MN). Data from gas sensors were digitized and recorded using LabVIEW 8 (National Instruments, Austin, TX), while ambient pressure and temperature data were recorded using Dataquest A.R.T. 3.01 acquisition and analysis software (Data Sciences International, St, Paul, MN).

Leptin Responsiveness

Recombinant murine leptin (R & D Systems), reconstituted in 20 mM Tris-HCl, pH 8, was administered to randomly chosen mice from experiment #1 after 14 weeks of either high-fructose (n = 9) or control (n = 10) diet intraperitoneally (I.P.) at a dose of 5 mg/kg of body weight, in a total volume of 0.1–0.2 ml. As vehicle control, 20 mM Tris-HCl, pH 8, was injected I.P. in the remainder of the high-fructose-fed (n = 10) or control-fed (n = 9) mice. Injections took place in the hour before the start of the dark phase. Food intake was recorded 6, 24, and 48 hours after injections.

Plasma Analysis

At least 7 days after mice were tested for leptin sensitivity, while still on their respective diets, and one hour before the start of the dark phase, mice were sacrificed under isofluorane anesthesia and blood was collected by cardiac puncture. Plasma was isolated by microcentrifugation and immediately frozen at −80°C. Plasma non-esterified fatty acids were measured using the NEFA HR(2) colorimetric assay (Wako) following the microtiter procedure on a 96 well plate. Plasma triglyceride and glucose levels were measured using the LiquiColor Triglyceride assay and the LiquiColor Glucose assay (Stanbio).

Data Analysis

Data are reported as mean ± standard error of the mean. Body weight averages and daily food intake for mice across feeding groups in experiment #1 were compared using a 2 (Treatment) × 14 (Week) ANOVA followed by a Bonferroni post hoc analysis. Total food consumption was compared using a non-paired T-test. Metabolic rate was compared across feeding groups using a 2 (Treatment) × 3 (Week) ANOVA followed by a Bonferroni post hoc analysis. Average food intake following leptin or saline injection was compared using an ANOVA followed by a Bonferroni post hoc analysis. Body weights for experiment #2 were compared across feeding groups using a 4 (Treatment) × 14 (Week) ANOVA followed by a Bonferroni post hoc analysis. For all tests, the significance threshold was $p<0.05$.

Results

Fructose feeding increases food intake and metabolic rate without increasing body weight

At the beginning of experiment #1, the body weight of the male C57Bl/6H mice did not differ between the two groups (Control: 17.6±0.5 g, High fructose: 17.5±0.4 g). Statistical analysis revealed a significant main effect of time and diet, as well as a significant interaction. Analysis of the simple main effects indicated differences between high-fructose and control fed mice for weeks 2–8 ($p<0.05$; Figure 1A). After 14 weeks, mice on the high-fructose diet (26.1±0.4 g) did not have body weights that significantly differed from mice on the control diet (26.2±0.5 g) (Figure 1A).

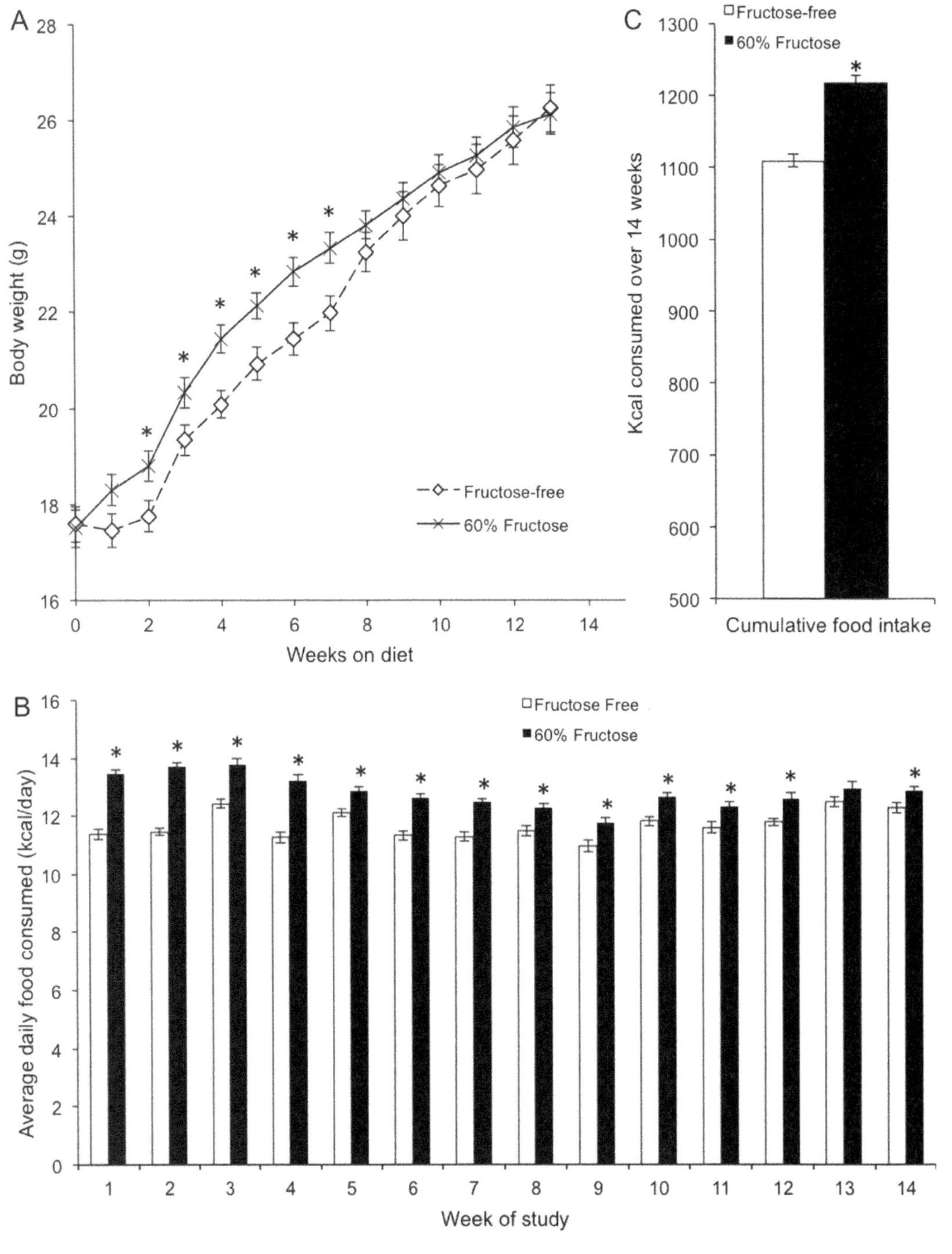

Figure 1. High-fructose-feeding does not increase body weight despite increased caloric intake. A) Transient changes in body weight in response to a high fructose diet. Fructose-fed mice were significantly heavier than control-fed mice from weeks 2–7 (*$p<0.05$). From 8 weeks to 14 weeks on their respective diets, there was no statistical difference in body weight between control-fed (n = 19) and fructose-fed (n = 19) mice. B) Fructose-fed mice consumed more food on average daily than control-fed mice for all weeks except week 13 (*$p<0.05$). C) Elevated cumulative caloric intake of fructose-fed mice. Over the course of the 14 weeks, fructose-fed mice consumed more total kcal than control-fed mice (*$p<0.05$).

The high-fructose fed mice consumed significantly more calories than control fed mice (Figure 1B). Statistical analysis revealed a significant main effect of time and diet, as well as a significant interaction. Analysis of the simple main effects indicated differences between high-fructose and control fed mice for all weeks except week 13 ($p<0.05$; Figure 1B). During week 2, for example, the control-fed mice consumed 80.3±1.0 kcal, significantly less ($p<0.05$) than 96.0±1.0 kcal consumed by the fructose-fed mice. By the end of the 14 weeks (Figure 1C), mice on the high-fructose diet had consumed 1218.9±9.3 kcal cumulatively, significantly more than mice on the control diet (1109.6±8.6 kcal).

Energy expenditure was estimated at three time points (week 2, week 9, and week 14) during the feeding experiment from 24-hour O_2 consumption and CO_2 production measurements. The respiratory exchange ratio was approximately 1.1–1.2 for both groups, and did not change with time (data not shown). Figure 2A shows metabolic differences between mice on the high-fructose diet and mice on the control diet during week 9. During both the dark phase and the light phase, fructose-fed mice consumed more O_2 than their control-fed counterparts. This difference appeared greater in the dark phase (Figure 2B). Assuming the mice were oxidizing 100% carbohydrates, which is a reasonable assumption given the measured RER, the fructose-fed mice had a daily expenditure of 10.6±0.9 kcal/day during week 9, while the control-diet mice had a significantly lower expenditure at 8.4±0.4 kcal/day. It is notable that the metabolic rate of both groups of mice was lower than the caloric intake over the same time period (Figure 1B). When compared across weeks over the course of the study, we found this difference in caloric expenditure between the feeding groups was present in weeks 2, and 9, but not week 14 (Figure 2B).

Fructose feeding does not change leptin sensitivity in mice

Despite the lack of difference in body weight between the two groups, we tested whether the fructose feeding could still induce changes in leptin sensitivity. Caloric intake (Figure 3) was measured for the two days prior to injection of either vehicle or leptin, and a 24-hour average caloric intake was calculated for mice in each feeding group. Control-fed mice consumed 12.6±0.3 kcal/day, and fructose-fed mice consumed 12.9±0.2 kcal/day during the two days prior to injection. Leptin-treated mice consumed significantly less food compared to vehicle injection after 6 hours for both control-fed (4.7±0.6 kcal vs. 6.1±0.2 kcal; $p<0.05$) and fructose-fed (5.5±0.3 kcal vs. 6.8±0.5 kcal; $p=0.050$) mice. After 24 hours, mice consuming the control diet still had a significantly lower cumulative caloric intake in response to the leptin injection compared to vehicle injection (10.1±0.9 kcal vs. 13.4±0.4 kcal; $p<0.05$) but leptin administration to fructose-fed mice led only to a downward trend in caloric intake in the 24 hours post-injection compared to vehicle injection (12.9±0.8 kcal vs. 15.0±0.9 kcal; $p=0.053$). Caloric intake in the second 24-hour interval after leptin injection was not different from vehicle injection for either control-fed (11.7±0.4 kcal vs. 11.9±0.3 kcal) or fructose-fed mice (13.1±0.5 kcal vs. 13.2±0.4 kcal).

Fructose feeding does not alter circulating glucose, NEFAs, or triglycerides

Mice from both feeding groups were sacrificed 1 hour prior to the onset of the dark phase, and plasma was isolated. Plasma glucose, free fatty acid, and triglyceride levels were unchanged by the diet (Table 1).

Absence of fructose-induced weight gain is not substrain specific

It has become apparent that different strains of mice can respond differently to varying environmental conditions [31,32]. Further, even the same strain purchased from different vendors (i.e. different substrains) can exhibit different phenotypes or drug sensitivities [33–35]. While C57BL/6 mice from Harlan were used for experiment #1 (C57Bl/6H), C57Bl/6 mice from Jackson labs was used in experiment #2 (C57Bl/6J). Here, mice that were the same age as in experiment #1 were fed one of four diets: 1) control, 2) high fat (45%), 3) 60% sucrose, which is a 30% fructose diet, and 4) 60% fructose. This substrain of mice (C57Bl/6J) gained significantly more weight than any of the other three groups when fed a high fat diet (Figure 4). The high fat diet had a greater caloric density at 4.7 kcal/gram of food than any of the other diets which each had a caloric density of 3.9 kcal/gram of food. Mice on either the 60% sucrose or 60% fructose did not exhibit any difference in body weight from control-fed mice until the 11th week of treatment, when the body weights of the fructose group became significantly less than the 60% sucrose group or the normal chow (Figure 4). An additional 6 weeks, for a total of 20 weeks on these diets, produced no change in the relationship between body weights for any of the groups (high fat = 37.2±0.7, 60% sucrose = 30.8±0.4, 60% fructose = 28.9±0.5, control = 32.1±0.3 g). These data support the conclusion that in mice, fructose feeding does not induce excess weight gain over a span from 3–4.5 months, and prolonged exposure to a high-fructose diet can lead to a lower body weight.

Discussion

After 14 weeks on a diet in which 60% of caloric intake through food was fructose, developing male mice failed to exhibit elevated body weight compared to control mice fed a diet lacking fructose (Figure 1 and 4). This was shown at two different institutions using C57Bl/6 mice from two different vendors (Harlan and Jackson Labs). In fact, the only long term weight gains seen in the C57Bl/6 mice were those on a high fat diet (Figure 4). Additionally, our results fail to support the hypothesis that fructose feeding for 3 months desensitizes mice to exogenous, systemically administered leptin. Indeed both control- and fructose-fed mice decreased caloric intake after leptin treatment, consistent with maintained leptin sensitivity despite a high-fructose diet. In response to fructose feeding for 3 months, we observed no changes in circulating non-esterified fatty acids, blood glucose, or blood triglycerides.

Based on previous studies in rodents, we had expected to see a drastic difference in body weight, leptin sensitivity, circulating triglycerides and circulating glucose between the feeding groups of mice [10,13,15,26,29,36–39,51]. There are at least three possibilities that could explain the lack of obesity in the mice on the high-fructose diet in the current study. First, many previous studies examining the effects of fructose consumption in rodents have utilized rats, which may differ in their metabolic response to fructose from the mice used in the current study. As mice have a much greater surface area to volume ratio than rats, the higher mass-specific metabolic rate of mice might allow for greater tolerance to fructose consumption as the fructose may be oxidized to CO_2 and H_2O to a greater extent in mice than rats, without the deleterious effects of fructose metabolites shuttled into VLDL (very low density lipoprotein) synthesis. However, it is important to note that wild-caught spiny mice actually lose weight on a 50% sucrose diet (25% of calories from fructose) that was associated with hepatomegaly, elevated VLDL, and β-cell hypertrophy [37]. Similarly, it was recently reported that mice on a high-fructose diet develop hepatic steatosis [40]. Among different strains of rats, there is variation in the phenotypic response to a high-fructose or sucrose diet. Some strains of rats gain weight on a high fructose diet [10,15,38,39], some have no change in weight [26,29], and one strain loses weight [39]. We found here that one substrain of mice (C57Bl/6H) on a high-fructose diet experienced a transient increase in body weight during development while a second substrain (C57Bl/6J) on a high-fructose diet failed to grow at the same rate as compared to siblings on a normal diet after 11 weeks of exposure.

A second reason for the lack of response to fructose may be age-dependent. In this experiment, we wished to test the effects of a

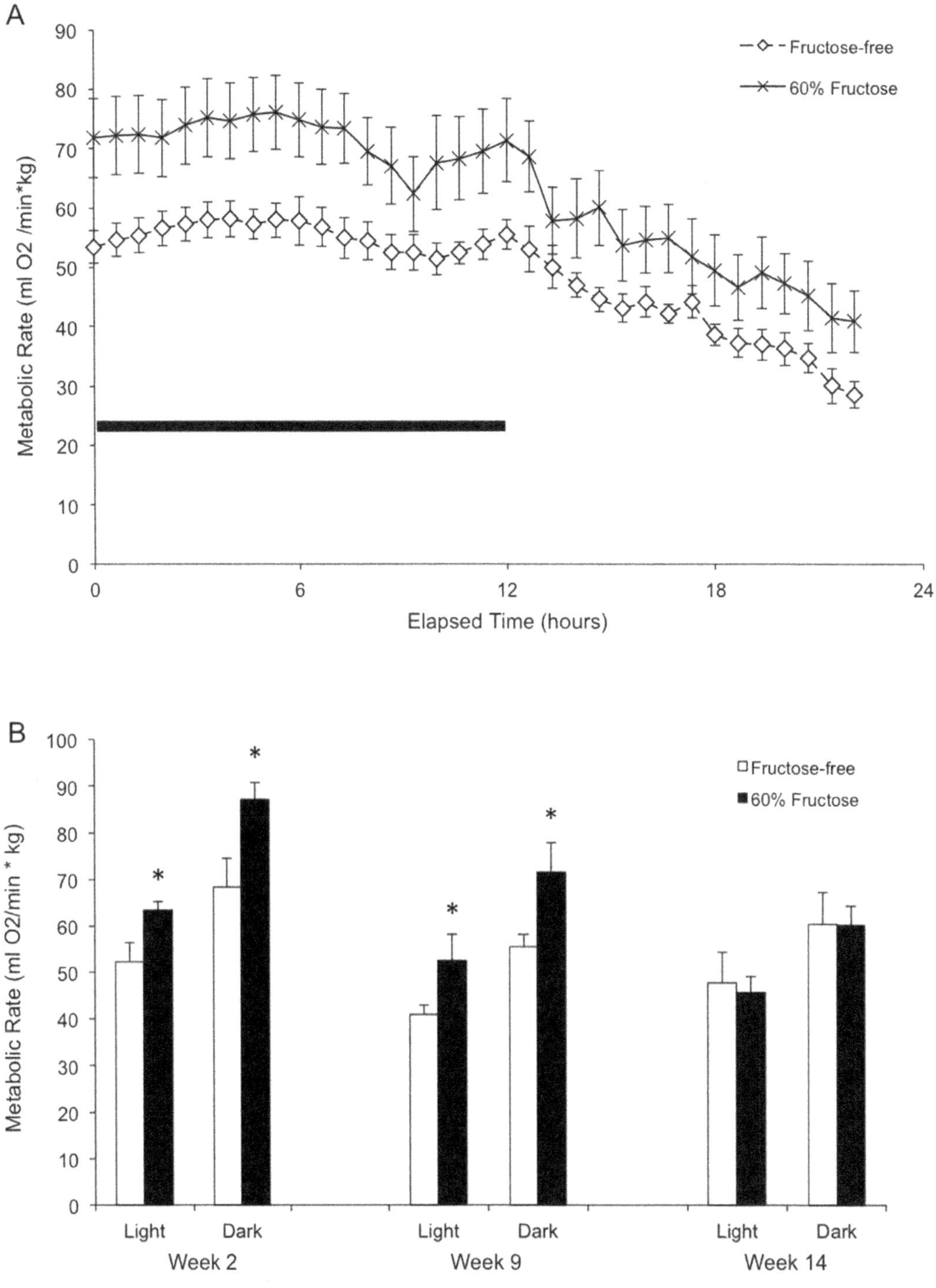

Figure 2. Differences in metabolic rate across feeding groups. A) Representative comparison of metabolic rates between high-fructose-fed (n = 7) and control-fed (n = 7) mice, week 9. Each data point represents a condensed 40-minute average for all the mice in that feeding group. The dark (active) phase—denoted by the black bar—spans hours 0–12, and the light (inactive) phase, hours 12–23. B) Average light- and dark-phase metabolic rates throughout the study. In weeks 2 and 9, fructose-fed mice (n = 7) had elevated metabolic rates compared to control-fed mice (n = 7). This difference was not present in week 14 (*- $p<0.05$ vs. control diet for indicated week).

high-fructose diet on the adolescent/young adult mouse, as fructose consumption appears to have an impact on adolescent humans [6,41,42]. The mice were weaned directly onto a high-fructose diet. In those studies that have utilized mice to examine the physiological changes induced by fructose consumption, they have done so using adult mice. It may be that the elevated mass-specific metabolic rate during maturation of the mouse in the current study was able to fully oxidize the fructose. However, multiple studies using fructose consumption in mice have observed increased adiposity or insulin resistance [43–45]. It is important to point out that those studies delivered fructose in liquid form as opposed to the current study, which delivered fructose in the food.

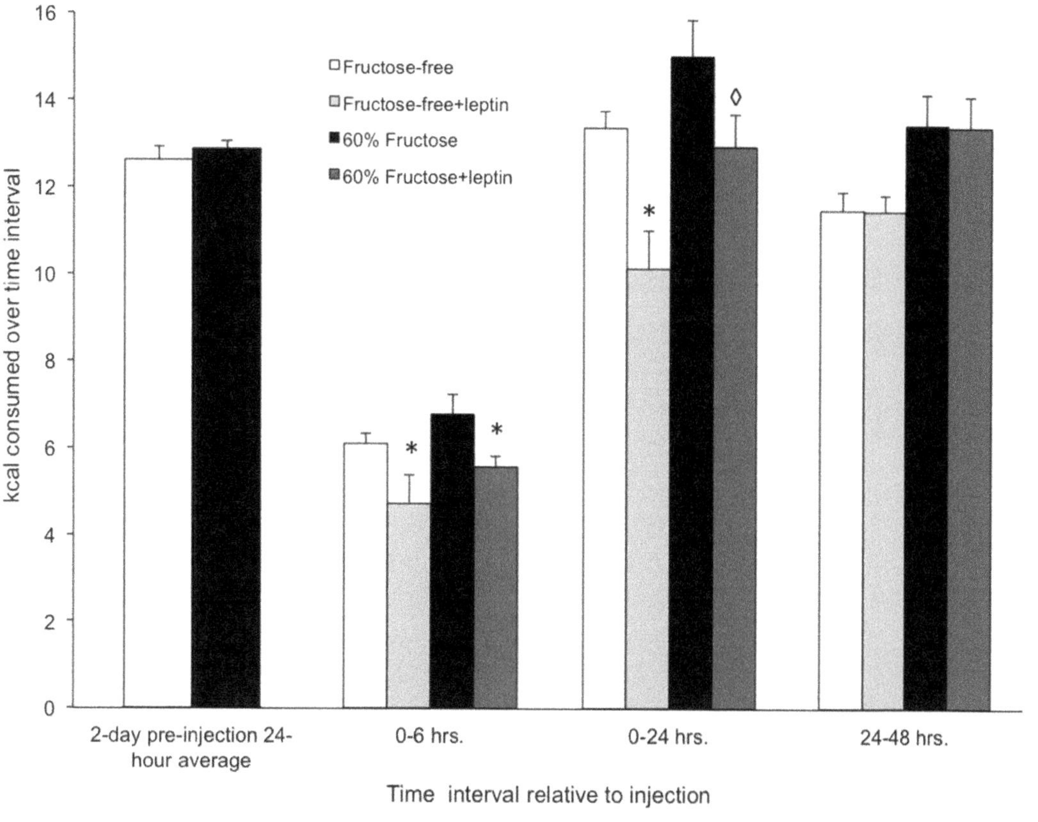

Figure 3. Persistence of leptin sensitivity in fructose-fed mice. Leptin injection leads to decreased food intake in both control-fed and fructose-fed mice compared to injection of vehicle over 6 and 24 hours, and returns to normal after 24 hours (*$p<0.05$ vs. the same diet and same time point with injection of vehicle; ◊$p=0.053$ vs. 60% fructose). The first time point is a 24-hour average of the two days prior to the injection. Later time points are total caloric intake over indicated time interval after injection.

While we did not measure adiposity or insulin sensitivity in the current study, we found that circulating fats were normal in fructose-fed mice. Given that fats in the blood are associated with insulin resistance, and fasting blood glucose was normal in these mice, it may be that fructose-fed mice in this study were not insulin resistant, in contrast to the above-mentioned studies [43–45]. This leads to the third possible explanation of the lack of observed effect– the different modes of fructose delivery. Whereas Bocarsly et al. [10] administered different sugars in aqueous solution as a supplement to standard chow, we opted to deliver fructose in food rather than in liquid to better control and monitor caloric intake. Their study found that high fructose corn syrup supplementation led to obesity in mice, characterized by increased body weight, elevated circulating triglycerides, and increased adiposity. We reasoned that fructose would lead to a positive energy balance independent of mode of delivery, though it remains possible that in mice, only aqueous fructose elicits an obesogenic response. This very different response in mice to either fed fructose (no long lasting effects of fructose consumption) or given fructose in liquid (significant long lasting effects of fructose consumption) is extremely important to highlight, and requires further detailed examination.

While we saw no overall difference in energy balance between the feeding groups at the study's conclusion, we observed that mice on the high fructose diet consumed more calories early in the study, accompanied by an elevated metabolic rate, and increased growth as mice compared to the control fed mice. Such an increase is supported by previous studies correlating fructose consumption with increased food intake, via the rapid early steps in fructose metabolism causing—through multiple biochemical steps—to lower malonyl-CoA in the hypothalamus [46]. Between weeks 2 and 7 in experiment #1, the fructose-fed mice gained weight faster than the control-fed mice, possibly due to faster acclimation to the sweeter food as compared to the unsweetened

Table 1. Fed plasma glucose, triglyceride, and free fatty acid concentrations.

	Control diet	High fructose diet
[Glucose] (mg/dL)	81.4±8.2	81.0±5.4
[Triglycerides] (mg/dL)	23.6±3.9	20.0±1.4
[NEFA] (mM)	0.42±0.05	0.36±0.04

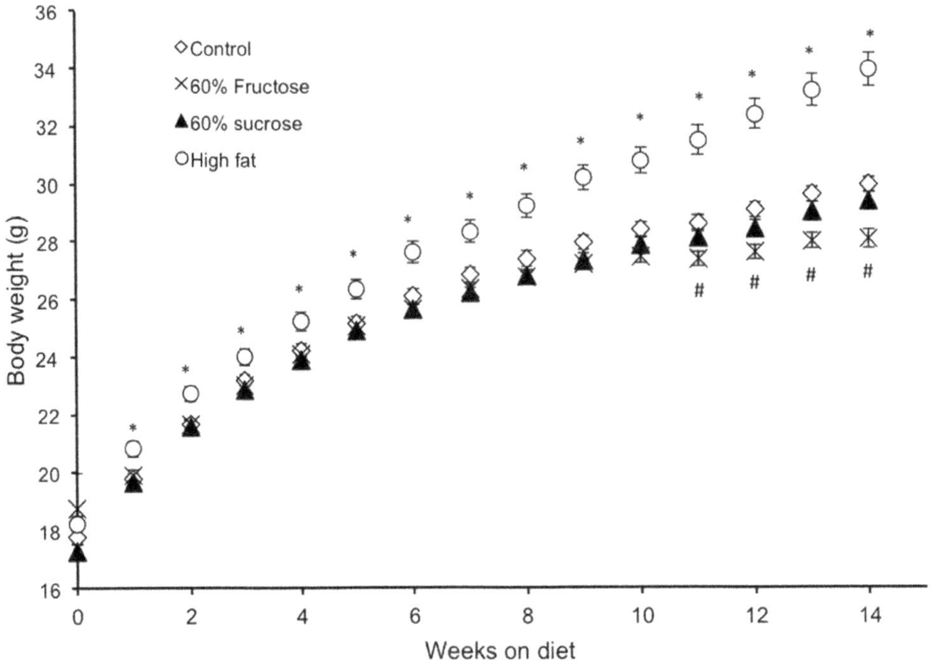

Figure 4. High-fat-feeding, but not high-fructose-feeding, increases body weight in C57Bl/6J mice. Male C57Bl/6J mice were fed a high fat (n = 56), high sucrose (n = 82), high fructose (n = 64), or control (n = 48) diet. The body weight of only the high-fat fed mice was significantly different from control-fed mice throughout the duration of the experiment (*$p<0.05$ vs. control diet and vs. high fructose diet and vs. high sucrose diet; #$p<0.05$ vs. control diet and vs. high sucrose diet).

control food fed to the control mice. Because the difference in body weight disappears after 8 weeks through the end of the study, there must be either an equal shift towards negative energy balance in the fructose fed mice, or a corresponding positive shift in energy balance in the control fed mice. Because caloric intake in the control mice did not increase over the course of the study, we would predict energy expenditure in the fructose fed mice to increase. A metabolic increase has not been reported previously in response to fructose feeding. Indeed, it was recently reported that mice fed a high-fructose diet actually have a lower metabolic rate than mice fed a control diet [51]. However, our data suggest that such an increase in metabolic rate plays a role in the maintenance of energy balance between the groups: high fructose fed mice ate more and had a higher metabolic rate. Such a phenomenon may be behaviorally driven, in that the sweetness of the food increases consumption, which consequently increases digestion and measured metabolic rate [47], though it is also possible that fructose consumption increases metabolic rate independent of the elevated metabolic rate associated with increased food intake. In addition, many hormones regulate diet-induced thermogenesis as well as cold-induced thermogenesis in mice [48]. Further research is warranted to examine the circulating levels of these hormones throughout exposure of mice to a high fructose diet. It should be noted, however, that the faster weight gain in fructose-fed mice was not observed in experiment #2.

At the conclusion of experiment #1, we observed no change in leptin sensitivity resulting from fructose feeding, in contrast to previous studies conducted in rats [15]. Fructose-induced leptin resistance had been observed accompanying increased triglycerides, which Shapiro et al. posited decreased the permeability of the blood-brain barrier (BBB) to leptin [49]. However, recent evidence suggests that the ability of leptin to cross the blood brain barrier is not impaired in fructose-fed rats [30]. Three months of fructose feeding failed to induce leptin resistance, changes in circulating glucose, or changes in circulating triglycerides/free fatty acids. As stated above, two studies have found increased insulin resistance in high-fructose fed mice [40,43,45], and one has shown decreased glucose tolerance [51]. The fructose-fed mice in the current study were not diabetic (Table 1), exhibited a normal body weight, and had normal circulating fats in the blood after 14 weeks on the diet. Because obesity can deregulate leptin signaling, an attractive explanation for our results is that a high-fructose diet in mice fails to cause obesity, and therefore no leptin resistance would be expected. A high fructose diet can lead to an increase in visceral adiposity with no change in body weight that might influence leptin or insulin sensitivity [51]. However, leptin resistance and obesity do not always go hand-in-hand; leptin resistance can occur in the absence of obesity. Despite the lack of effect of dietary fructose on obesity in these mice, we tested leptin sensitivity in fructose-fed mice and found they displayed normal sensitivity to leptin. It is possible that 3 months is not long enough to evoke changes in leptin sensitivity. Given the lack of effect on body weight after 4.5 months on a high fructose diet, the duration of a high-fructose diet may need to be considerably longer to induce obesity or leptin resistance. Similarly, it may be that our study started too late for such diet-induced phenotypic variation to manifest in mice, and perhaps the mothers should have been fed either high-fructose or control food while nursing, or during the course of their sexual maturation, as parental nutrition is known to play a role in epigenetic patterning of offspring [50].

Author Contributions

Conceived and designed the experiments: SJS EJT KR. Performed the experiments: EJT DAM. Analyzed the data: EJT SJS DAM KR. Contributed reagents/materials/analysis tools: SJS KR. Wrote the paper: EJT SJS.

References

1. Bray GA, Nielsen SJ, Popkin BM (2004) Consumption of high-fructose corn syrup in beverages may play a role in the epidemic of obesity. American Journal of Clinical Nutrition 79: 537–543.
2. Bray GA (2010) Soft drink consumption and obesity: it is all about fructose. Current Opinion in Lipidology 21: 51–57.
3. Duffey KJ, Popkin BM (2007) Shifts in patterns and consumption of beverages between 1965 and 2002. Obesity (Silver Spring) 15: 2739–2747.
4. Tappy L, Le KA (2010) Metabolic effects of fructose and the worldwide increase in obesity. Physiol Rev 90: 23–46.
5. Havel PJ (2005) Dietary fructose: Implications for dysregulation of energy homeostasis and lipid/carbohydrate metabolism. Nutrition Reviews 63: 133–157.
6. Denova-Gutierrez E, Jimenez-Aguilar A, Halley-Castillo E, Huitron-Bravo G, Talavera JO, et al. (2008) Association between sweetened beverage consumption and body mass index, proportion of body fat and body fat distribution in Mexican adolescents. Ann Nutr Metab 53: 245–251.
7. Bremer AA, Auinger P, Byrd RS (2009) Relationship between insulin resistance-associated metabolic parameters and anthropometric measurements with sugar-sweetened beverage intake and physical activity levels in US adolescents: findings from the 1999–2004 National Health and Nutrition Examination Survey. Arch Pediatr Adolesc Med 163: 328–335.
8. Ludwig DS, Peterson KE, Gortmaker SL (2001) Relation between consumption of sugar-sweetened drinks and childhood obesity: a prospective, observational analysis. Lancet 357: 505–508.
9. Stanhope KL, Schwarz JM, Keim NL, Griffen SC, Bremer AA, et al. (2009) Consuming fructose-sweetened, not glucose-sweetened, beverages increases visceral adiposity and lipids and decreases insulin sensitivity in overweight/obese humans. Journal of Clinical Investigation 119: 1322–1334.
10. Bocarsly ME, Powell ES, Avena NM, Hoebel BG (2010) High-fructose corn syrup causes characteristics of obesity in rats: increased body weight, body fat and triglyceride levels. Pharmacol Biochem Behav 97: 101–106.
11. Ma X, Zubcevic L, Ashcroft FM (2008) Glucose regulates the effects of leptin on hypothalamic POMC neurons. Proceedings of the National Academy of Sciences 105: 9811–9816.
12. Cha SH, Wolfgang M, Tokutake Y, Chohnan S, Lane MD (2008) Differential effects of central fructose and glucose on hypothalamic malonyl-CoA and food intake. Proceedings of the National Academy of Sciences of the United States of America 105: 16871–16875.
13. Schaefer EJ, Gleason JA, Dansinger ML (2009) Dietary Fructose and Glucose Differentially Affect Lipid and Glucose Homeostasis. Journal of Nutrition 139: S1257–S1262.
14. Page KA, Chan O, Arora J, Belfort-Deaguiar R, Dzuira J, et al. (2013) Effects of fructose vs glucose on regional cerebral blood flow in brain regions involved with appetite and reward pathways. JAMA 309: 63–70.
15. Shapiro A, Mu W, Roncal C, Cheng KY, Johnson RJ, et al. (2008) Fructose-induced leptin resistance exacerbates weight gain in response to subsequent high-fat feeding. Am J Physiol Regul Integr Comp Physiol 295: R1370–1375.
16. Balthasar N, Coppari R, McMinn J, Liu SM, Lee CE, et al. (2004) Leptin receptor signaling in POMC neurons is required for normal body weight homeostasis. Neuron 42: 983–991.
17. Cowley MA, Smart JL, Rubinstein M, Cerdan MG, Diano S, et al. (2001) Leptin activates anorexigenic POMC neurons through a neural network in the arcuate nucleus. Nature 411: 480–484.
18. Sahu A (2003) Leptin signaling in the hypothalamus: emphasis on energy homeostasis and leptin resistance. Frontiers in Neuroendocrinology 24: 225–253.
19. Friedman JM, Halaas JL (1998) Leptin and the regulation of body weight in mammals. Nature 395: 763–770.
20. Erickson JC, Hollopeter G, Palmiter RD (1996) Attenuation of the obesity syndrome of ob/ob mice by the loss of neuropeptide Y. Science 274: 1704–1707.
21. Ernst MB, Wunderlich CM, Hess S, Paehler M, Mesaros A, et al. (2009) Enhanced Stat3 Activation in POMC Neurons Provokes Negative Feedback Inhibition of Leptin and Insulin Signaling in Obesity. Journal of Neuroscience 29: 11582–11593.
22. El-Haschimi K, Pierroz DD, Hileman SM, Bjorbaek C, Flier JS (2000) Two defects contribute to hypothalamic leptin resistance in mice with diet-induced obesity. Journal of Clinical Investigation 105: 1827–1832.
23. Lin S, Thomas TC, Storlien LH, Huang XF (2000) Development of high fat diet-induced obesity and leptin resistance in C57Bl/6J mice. International Journal of Obesity 24: 639–646.
24. VanHeek M, Compton DS, France CF, Tedesco RP, Fawzi AB, et al. (1997) Diet-induced obese mice develop peripheral, but not central, resistance to leptin. Journal of Clinical Investigation 99: 385–390.
25. Zhang Y, Scarpace PJ (2006) The role of leptin in leptin resistance and obesity. Physiology & Behavior 88: 249–256.
26. Huang BW, Chiang MT, Yao HT, Chiang W (2004) The effect of high-fat and high-fructose diets on glucose tolerance and plasma lipid and leptin levels in rats. Diabetes Obesity & Metabolism 6: 120–126.
27. Shapiro A, Tumer N, Gao Y, Cheng KY, Scarpace PJ (2011) Prevention and reversal of diet-induced leptin resistance with a sugar-free diet despite high fat content. Br J Nutr 106: 390–397.
28. Cummings BP, Stanhope KL, Graham JL, Evans JL, Baskin DG, et al. (2010) Dietary fructose accelerates the development of diabetes in UCD-T2DM rats: amelioration by the antioxidant, alpha-lipoic acid. Am J Physiol Regul Integr Comp Physiol 298: R1343–1350.
29. D'Angelo G, Elmarakby AA, Pollock DM, Stepp DW (2005) Fructose Feeding Increases Insulin Resistance but Not Blood Pressure in Sprague-Dawley Rats. Hypertension 46: 806–811.
30. Haring SJ, Harris RB (2011) The relation between dietary fructose, dietary fat and leptin responsiveness in rats. Physiol Behav 104: 914–922.
31. Meyer C, Elvert R, Scherag A, Ehrhardt N, Gailus-Durner V, et al. (2007) Power matters in closing the phenotyping gap. Naturwissenschaften 94: 401–406.
32. Rikke BA, Yerg JE, Battaglia ME, Nagy TR, Allison DB, et al. (2003) Strain variation in the response of body temperature to dietary restriction. Mechanisms of Ageing and Development 124: 663–678.
33. Bryant CD, Zhang NN, Sokoloff G, Fanselow MS, Ennes HS, et al. (2008) Behavioral Differences among C57BL/6 Substrains: Implications for Transgenic and Knockout Studies. Journal of Neurogenetics 22: 315–331.
34. Chang H-YS, Mitzner W, Watson J (2012) Variation in Airway Responsiveness of Male C57BL/6 Mice from 5 Vendors. Journal of the American Association for Laboratory Animal Science 51: 401–406.
35. Müller CJ, Gröticke I, Hoffmann K, Schughart K, Löscher W (2009) Differences in sensitivity to the convulsant pilocarpine in substrains and sublines of C57BL/6 mice. Genes, Brain and Behavior 8: 481–492.
36. Juergens H, Haass W, Thoene-Reineke C, Castaneda T, Spranger J, et al. (2003) Ad libitum consumption of fructose or soft drinks increases body fat mass in mice. Obesity Research 11: A19–A20.
37. Shafrir E (2000) Overnutrition in spiny mice (Acomys cahirinus): β-cell expansion leading to rupture and overt diabetes on fat-rich diet and protective energy-wasting elevation in thyroid hormone on sucrose-rich diet. Diabetes/Metabolism Research and Reviews 16: 94–105.
38. Michaelis OE, Ellwood KC, Judge JM, Schoene NW, Hansen CT (1984) Effect of dietary sucrose on the SHR/N-corpulent rat: a new model for insulin-independent diabetes. The American Journal of Clinical Nutrition 39: 612–618.
39. Schemmel RA, Teague RJ, Bray GA (1982) Obesity in Osborne-Mendel and S 5B/Pl rats: effects of sucrose solutions, castration, and treatment with estradiol or insulin. American Journal of Physiology - Regulatory, Integrative and Comparative Physiology 243: R347–R353.
40. Ushio M, Nishio Y, Sekine O, Nagai Y, Maeno Y, et al. (2013) Ezetimibe prevents hepatic steatosis induced by a high-fat but not a high-fructose diet. American Journal of Physiology - Endocrinology And Metabolism 305: E293–E304.
41. Harrington S (2008) The role of sugar-sweetened beverage consumption in adolescent obesity: a review of the literature. J Sch Nurs 24: 3–12.
42. Le KA, Faeh D, Stettler R, Ith M, Kreis R, et al. (2006) A 4-wk high-fructose diet alters lipid metabolism without affecting insulin sensitivity or ectopic lipids in healthy humans. American Journal of Clinical Nutrition 84: 1374–1379.
43. Ishimoto T, Lanaspa MA, Le MT, Garcia GE, Diggle CP, et al. (2012) Opposing effects of fructokinase C and A isoforms on fructose-induced metabolic syndrome in mice. Proc Natl Acad Sci U S A 109: 4320–4325.
44. Jurgens H, Haass W, Castaneda TR, Schurmann A, Koebnick C, et al. (2005) Consuming fructose-sweetened beverages increases body adiposity in mice. Obesity Research 13: 1146–1156.
45. Beigy M, Vakili S, Berijani S, Aminizade M, Ahmadi-Dastgerdi M, et al. (2013) Alternate-day fasting diet improves fructose-induced insulin resistance in mice. J Anim Physiol Anim Nutr (Berl).
46. Lane MD, Cha SH (2009) Effect of glucose and fructose on food intake via malonyl-CoA signaling in the brain. Biochemical and Biophysical Research Communications 382: 1–5.
47. Welle S, Lilavivat U, Campbell RG (1981) Thermic effect of feeding in man: increased plasma norepinephrine levels following glucose but not protein or fat consumption. Metabolism-Clinical and Experimental 30: 953–958.
48. Gordon CJ (2012) Thermal physiology of laboratory mice: Defining thermoneutrality. Journal of Thermal Biology 37: 654–685.
49. Banks WA, Coon AB, Robinson SM, Moinuddin A, Shultz JM, et al. (2004) Triglycerides induce leptin resistance at the blood-brain barrier. Diabetes 53: 1253–1260.
50. Attig L, Gabory A, Junien C (2010) Nutritional developmental epigenomics: immediate and long-lasting effects. Proc Nutr Soc 69: 221–231.
51. DeBosch BJ, Chen Z, Finck BN, Chi M, Moley KH (2013) Glucose transporter-8 (GLUT8) mediates glucose intolerance and dyslipidemia in high-fructose diet-fed male mice. Mol Endocrinol 27: 1887–1896.

Differential Acute Postprandial Effects of Processed Meat and Isocaloric Vegan Meals on the Gastrointestinal Hormone Response in Subjects Suffering from Type 2 Diabetes and Healthy Controls

Lenka Belinova[1,2]*, Hana Kahleova[1], Hana Malinska[1], Ondrej Topolcan[3], Jindra Vrzalova[3], Olena Oliyarnyk[1], Ludmila Kazdova[1], Martin Hill[4], Terezie Pelikanova[1]

1 Institute for Clinical and Experimental Medicine, Prague, Czech Republic, **2** First Faculty of Medicine, Charles University, Prague, Czech Republic, **3** University Hospital in Pilsen, Pilsen, Czech Republic, **4** Institute of Endocrinology, Prague, Czech Republic

Abstract

Background: The intake of meat, particularly processed meat, is a dietary risk factor for diabetes. Meat intake impairs insulin sensitivity and leads to increased oxidative stress. However, its effect on postprandial gastrointestinal hormone (GIH) secretion is unclear. We aimed to investigate the acute effects of two standardized isocaloric meals: a processed hamburger meat meal rich in protein and saturated fat (M-meal) and a vegan meal rich in carbohydrates (V-meal). We hypothesized that the meat meal would lead to abnormal postprandial increases in plasma lipids and oxidative stress markers and impaired GIH responses.

Methods: In a randomized crossover study, 50 patients suffering from type 2 diabetes (T2D) and 50 healthy subjects underwent two 3-h meal tolerance tests. For statistical analyses, repeated-measures ANOVA was performed.

Results: The M-meal resulted in a higher postprandial increase in lipids in both groups ($p<0.001$) and persistent postprandial hyperinsulinemia in patients with diabetes ($p<0.001$). The plasma glucose levels were significantly higher after the V-meal only at the peak level. The plasma concentrations of glucose-dependent insulinotropic peptide (GIP), peptide tyrosine-tyrosine (PYY) and pancreatic polypeptide (PP) were higher ($p<0.05$, $p<0.001$, $p<0.001$, respectively) and the ghrelin concentration was lower ($p<0.001$) after the M-meal in healthy subjects. In contrast, the concentrations of GIP, PYY and PP were significantly lower after the M-meal in T2D patients ($p<0.001$). Compared with the V-meal, the M-meal was associated with a larger increase in lipoperoxidation in T2D patients ($p<0.05$).

Conclusion/Interpretation: Our results suggest that the diet composition and the energy content, rather than the carbohydrate count, should be important considerations for dietary management and demonstrate that processed meat consumption is accompanied by impaired GIH responses and increased oxidative stress marker levels in diabetic patients.

Trial Registration: ClinicalTrials.gov NCT01572402

Editor: Stephen L. Atkin, Weill Cornell Medical College Qatar, Qatar

Funding: This study was supported by: the grant project NT/11238-4 from the Ministry of Health, Czech Republic, and the Grant Agency of Charles University GAUK, Project No. 702312. The funders had no role in study design, data collection and analysis, decision to publish, or preparation of the manuscript.

Competing Interests: The authors have declared that no competing interests exist.

* Email: bell@ikem.cz

Introduction

The current guidelines for the treatment of diabetic patients focus primarily on carbohydrate counts [1]. However, the postprandial metabolic response is likely also modified by the contents of other macronutrients in meals and by gastrointestinal hormone (GIH) release.

Dietary saturated fat is known to impair insulin sensitivity and to enhance hepatic glucose production [2]. Studies of patients suffering from diabetes have revealed that dietary fat delays gastric emptying, leading to a lag in glucose absorption [3,4]. On the other hand, studies suggest that in patients suffering from diabetes, higher fat meals acutely increase the glucose concentration and the requirement for insulin compared with meals containing similar

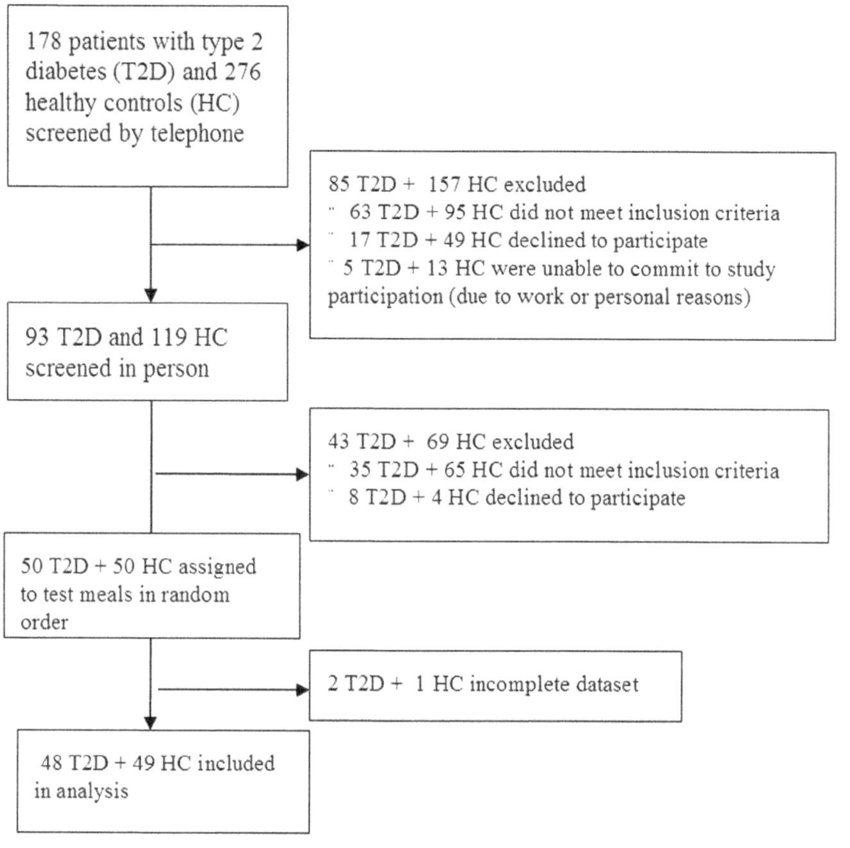

Figure 1. Enrollment of the participants and completion of the study.

carbohydrate but lower fat contents [5]. Additionally, addition of protein energy to a meal likely increases the postprandial glucose level [6].

Epidemiological studies suggest a positive association between high consumption of total and red meat and incident T2D [7,8]. Subjects who consumed any processed meats (salted fish and frankfurters) were 38% more likely to develop diabetes [9]. Previous studies support the concept that increased oxidative stress may play an important role in T2D manifestation [10]. Dietary fat quality has been proposed to be a critical factor. Several studies have suggested that a high intake of saturated fatty acids naturally present in meat contributes to the risk of glucose intolerance [11,12]. In an intervention study, humans suffering from metabolic syndrome who were consuming a high saturated fatty-acid diet displayed higher oxidative stress markers postprandially [13,14].

In contrast, some intervention trials demonstrated a greater improvement in insulin sensitivity, glycemic control and a reduction in oxidative stress markers in T2D patients consuming a vegetarian diet compared with those consuming a traditional diabetes diet [15,16]. The aim of our study was to determine the acute effects of meat and plant-based meals on postprandial GIH secretion. Thus, we designed this randomized crossover study to evaluate the acute (a time span of hours) postprandial response to two standardized meals containing the same caloric content but a different nutritional content: a processed meat (hamburger) meal rich in protein and saturated fat and a plant-based meal rich in carbohydrates. The objective of our study was to examine whether the acute intake of different types of isocaloric meals consumed in amounts typical of normal eating (food intake representative of real life) would be associated with different postprandial changes in glucose, lipid, immunoreactive insulin (IRI), GIH and oxidative stress marker levels in patients with T2D compared with healthy subjects. We investigated the hypothesis that a processed meat meal would lead to an abnormal postprandial increase in the levels of plasma lipids and oxidative stress markers and impaired GIH responses in T2D patients. Our results should contribute knowledge relevant to the dietary management of diabetic patients.

Methods and Materials

1. Study subjects and design

The protocol for this trial and supporting CONSORT checklist are available as supporting information; see Checklist S1 and Trial protocol S1 and S2. The study used a prospectively randomized crossover design and included a group of 50 patients suffering from T2D and 50 healthy controls. Their characteristics are presented in Table 1. The mean age was 55; about half of the subjects were men; and the mean duration of diabetes among the T2D patients was 9.8 years. Written informed consent was obtained from all participants prior to enrollment in the study; the study protocol, informed consent, and patient information were reviewed and approved by the Ethics Committee of the Thomayer Hospital and Institute for Clinical and Experimental Medicine in Prague, Czech Republic on November 9, 2011. On January 5, 2012 we started the telephone screening of potential participants. Subjects were screened in person and enrolled into the study between April 3, 2012 and April 20, 2012. The first patient entered the intervention phase on April 10, 2012 and the last completed on May 5, 2012. There was no follow-up phase. The study flowchart is presented in Figure 1. Of the 178 patients with T2D and 276 healthy controls, who were screened, 50 participants of both groups were included and randomized, 2 participants with T2D and 1 healthy subject did not complete the trial. The reasons for study participant exclusion are given in Figure 1. Registration on ClinicalTrials.gov was initiated on April 3, 2012 (Identifier: http://clinicaltrials.gov/show/NCT01572402). The authors authors confirm that all ongoing and related trials for this intervention are registered.

2. Inclusion and exclusion criteria

The inclusion criteria were men and women aged between 30–70 years with a body mass index (BMI) between 27–50 kg/m^2. Patients diagnosed with T2D had been treated with diet and/or oral hypoglycemic agents (metformin and/or sulfonylureas) for at least one year. Healthy volunteers exhibiting normal glucose tolerance and without metabolic syndrome or diagnosed diabetes among first-line relatives were included. Subjects exhibiting renal, liver or thyroid disease, drug abuse, including alcoholism, and pregnant or breastfeeding women were excluded.

3. Study procedure

All measurements were performed on an outpatient basis after a 10- to 12-h overnight fast with only tap water allowed ad libitum. The diabetic patients did not take any of their diabetes medication the evening or the morning before the assessments. The postprandial state was measured after intake of a standard breakfast – one of two isocaloric test meals in a random order consisting of either a processed meat burger meal (a fastfood burger: cooked-pork seasoned meat in a wheat bun with sesame seeds, tomato, cheddar-type cheese, lettuce, spicy sauce, onion) or a plant-based burger meal (a couscous burger: boiled couscous, baked with onion, garlic, plant oil, spices, oat-flakes in a wheat bun with sesame seeds). For each intervention visit, the meals were delivered fresh from the manufacturer. The study nurses generated the random sequence of the meals and assigned participants to the interventions in one-week intervals. The participants ate the meals under the nurse's control in the laboratory. Neither the study staff nor the participants were blinded to the content of the meals. The compositions of the meals are presented in Table 2.

The plasma concentrations of glucose, immunoreactive insulin, C-peptide, triglycerides (TG), free fatty acids (FFA), oxidative stress markers and GIH were measured during the fasting state (time 0) and then 30, 60, 120 and 180 min after the meal. In this single-center study the samples were collected in the Laboratory of Clinical Pathophysiology in Institute for Clinical and Experimental Medicine.

4. Analytic methods

4.1 Metabolic parameters. Plasma glucose was analyzed via the glucose-oxidase method using a Beckman Analyzer (Beckman Instruments Inc., Fullerton, CA, USA). Serum immunoreactive insulin and C-peptide concentrations were determined using Insulin and C-peptide IRMA kits (Immunotech, Prague, Czech Republic), respectively. Plasma lipid concentrations were measured via enzymatic methods (Roche, Basel, Switzerland).

4.2 Gastrointestinal and appetite hormones. Protease and dipeptidyl peptidase-4 inhibitors were added to two samples at each time point. The concentrations of glucagon-like peptide –1 (GLP-1), gastric inhibitory peptide (GIP), pancreatic polypeptide (PP), peptide YY (PYY), leptin and ghrelin were determined via multiplex immunoanalyses based on xMAP technology using a MILLIPLEX MAP Human Gut Hormone Panel (Millipore, Billerica, MA, USA) and a Luminex 100 IS analyzer (Luminex Corporation, Austin, TX, USA) [17]. The assay sensitivities, expressed as the minimum detectable concentrations reported in the instructions for use by the manufacturer, are (in pg/mL): ghrelin 1.8; leptin 157.2; GIP 0.2; GLP-1 5.2; PP 2.4; and PYY 8.4. For our measurements, the sensitivity was set as the value of the lowest standard concentration: ghrelin 13.7; GIP 2.7; GLP-1 13.7; and PP 13.7. For other analytes, there were no values below the corresponding calibration range.

4.3 Oxidative stress markers. The levels of lipid peroxidation were determined via a home-made method using thiobarbituric acid reactive substances (TBARS) [18]. The activity of superoxide dismutase (SOD) was analyzed using a SOD assay kit (Sigma-Aldrich, St Louis, MO, USA). The serum level of ascorbic acid was measured via a home-made method [19]. The level of reduced glutathione in whole blood was determined using a glutathione HPLC diagnostic kit (Chromsystems, Munich, Germany).

Table 1. General characteristics of the Diabetic and Control Population.

Characteristics	Patients with T2D (n = 50)	Healthy Controls (n = 50)
Age – years	56±6	54±8
Male – No. (%)	23 (46)	23 (46)
Female – No.(%)	27 (54)	27 (54)
Smokers – No. (%)	11 (22)	7 (14)
Weight – kg	96.5±17	71±11
BMI – kg.m^{-2}	33.3±5.6	24.4±2.5
Waist – cm	107±13.0	85±8.0
Hips – cm	115±12.0	98±5.0
HbA1c (DCCT) – %	7.0±3.2	5.6±2.4
HbA1c (IFCC) – mmol/mol	53.7±12.0	37.3±2.7
Fasting glucose level – mmol/l	8.0±3.1	5±0.44
Duration of diabetes – years	9.8±6.3	

Data are means ± SD.

Table 2. Composition of the test meals.

Meal	Hamburger (M - meal)	Vegan burger (V - meal)
Total weight (g)	150	235
Energy content (kCal/kJ)	455/1904	456/1907
Carbohydrates (g) (%)	31 (27%)	60 (52%)
Proteins (g) (%)	24 (21%)	13 (11%)
Lipids (g) (%)	26 (52%)	19 (37%)
Saturated fatty acids (g)	*10*	*6*
Monounsaturated fatty acids (g)	*7*	*5*
Polyunsaturated fatty acids (g)	*9*	*8*
Fiber (g)	5	8

5. Statistical analyses

For statistical analysis, repeated-measures ANOVA was performed. An estimate of the number of subjects that we recruited was carried out using a power analysis of repeated measurements via PASS 2005 statistical software (Number Cruncher Statistical Systems, Kaysville, UT, USA). The power analysis was completed for the most important variables and the number of subjects should provide the power >0.8 for all these variables. The factors of subject, group, meal and time were included in the analyses. The interactions between meal and time (meal×time) were calculated for each variable. ANOVA was followed by least significant difference (LSD) multiple comparisons post-hoc analysis. The original dependent variable was subjected to a power transformation to obtain constant variance and a symmetric distribution of the data and residuals [20]. The data are presented as the means with 95% CI. We have checked the carry-over effect using the model including the factor "sequence" and we have not found any significance of this factor for any dependent variables.

Results

1. Glucose, C-peptide, insulin and lipid responses

The plasma concentrations of glucose, IRI, C-peptide and lipids during the fasting state and their postprandial profiles are illustrated in Fig. 2. All of these measured parameters were significantly higher in the T2D patients than in healthy controls at nearly every time point. The fasting concentrations did not differ before the M- and V-meals in both groups. In both the diabetic and healthy subjects, the postprandial plasma levels of glucose were significantly higher after the V-meal at only one time point – at peak blood glucose level, after 30 min in healthy subjects and 60 min in patients with T2D. The two different meals induced relatively similar glucose responses in both groups when the time-course is considered. Although the M-meal resulted in a significantly lower IRI and C-peptide response than the V-meal in healthy subjects, these levels decreased more slowly, and after 180 min the IRI after the M-meal was significantly higher in both groups of subjects. In the T2D patients, the postprandial increases in IRI and C-peptide were not significantly different after both diets, and the peak of the IRI curve was considerably postponed. After the M-meal, hyperinsulinemia persisted longer in both groups. The plasma concentration of triglycerides inversely correlated to the plasma concentration of free fatty acids. The M-meal resulted in a significantly higher postprandial increase in triglycerides and a further decrease in free fatty acids in both groups, and these differences were more pronounced among the patients with T2D.

2. GIHs

The basal concentrations of nearly all of the GIHs were significantly increased in the T2D patients compared with the healthy controls. There was a considerable difference in the GIH response after ingestion of the M-meal compared with the V-meal in both healthy subjects and the T2D patients (Fig. 3). The V-meal resulted in a significantly higher GIH response than the M-meal but only among the T2D patients. In healthy subjects, the postprandial GIH levels were significantly lower after the V-meal than after the M-meal. The largest difference was detected in the postprandial concentrations of PP and PYY. In the T2D patients, the postprandial concentrations of GLP-1, GIP and PYY were significantly higher after the V-meal. The largest difference between the two meals was detected in the postprandial secretion of GLP-1, both with respect to quantity and dynamics.

3. Appetite hormones

The concentrations of ghrelin and leptin differed significantly between the T2D patients and the healthy controls throughout the entire meal assessment (Fig. 3). In the fasting state, the plasma concentration of ghrelin was 56% lower in the diabetic subjects ($p<0.001$), and the plasma concentration of leptin was 150% higher than the healthy controls ($p<0.001$). The plasma concentration of ghrelin was significantly lower and that of leptin was significantly higher in the T2D patients throughout the entire meal assessment, with no difference between the two isocaloric diets. The physiological postprandial suppression of ghrelin secretion was less pronounced in the diabetic subjects than in the healthy controls, and there was a rapid decrease in the ghrelin level beyond the first 60 min after consumption, and the postprandial decrease was significantly larger after the M-meal among healthy controls ($p<0.001$).

We have added a subanalysis by adding a "baseline ghrelin" factor to the model. The baseline ghrelin was the most important factor when included in the model with $F = 187$, $p<0.0001$. It means that the higher the baseline level of ghrelin is, the larger the drop. The difference between the two meals remained significant with $F = 19.43$, $p<0.001$.

4. Oxidative stress parameters

The fasting concentrations of all of the oxidative stress markers differed between the groups. (Fig. 4). In the T2D patients,

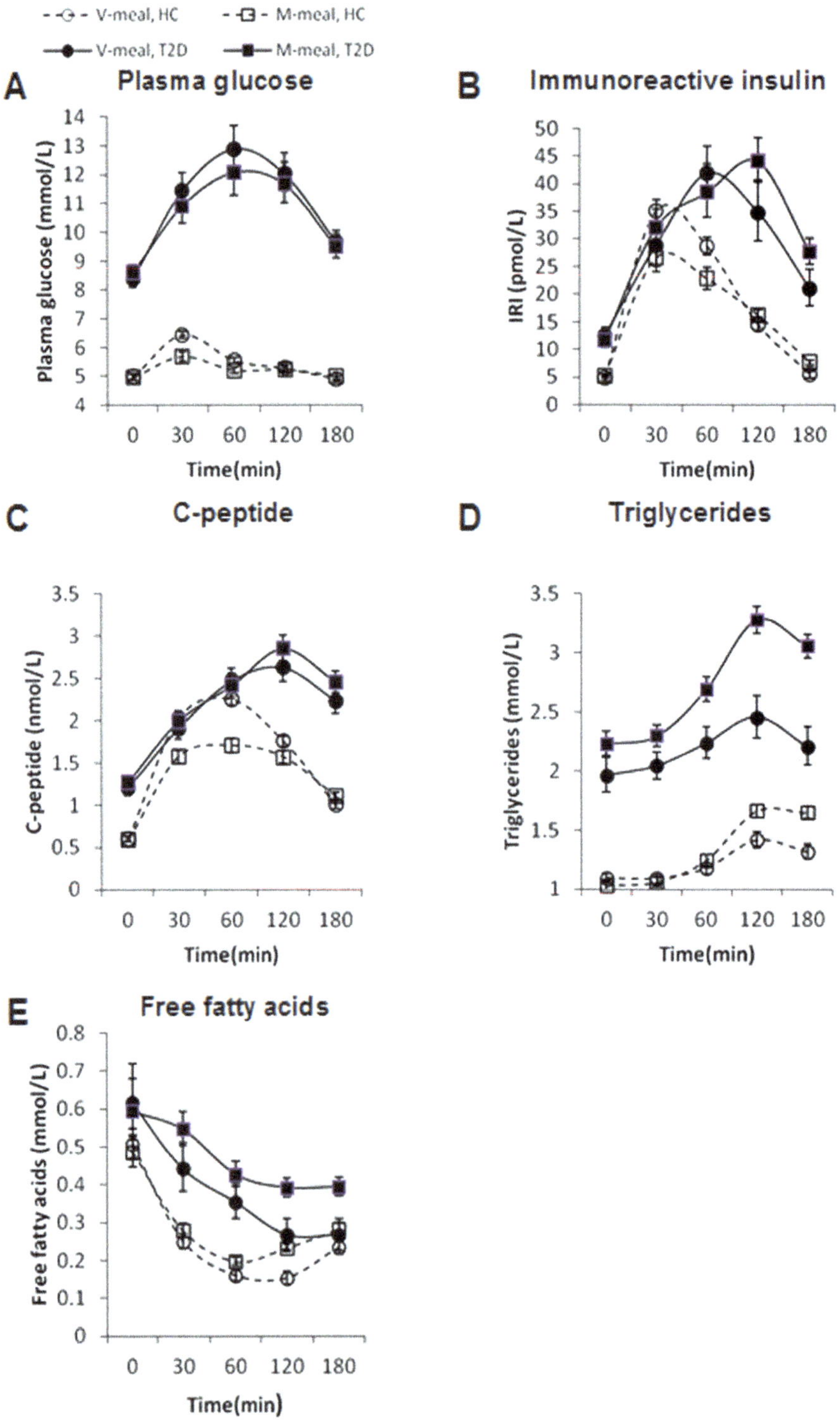

Figure 2. Postprandial changes in plasma concentrations of glucose, immunoreactive insulin, C-peptide, triglycerides and free fatty acids in patients with diabetes (T2D, full line) (n = 48) and healthy controls (HC, dashed line) (n = 49) after ingestion of the V-meal (circles) and the M-meal (squares). Data are expressed as mean with 95%CI. Repeated-measures ANOVA was performed. **A: Plasma glucose: Healthy controls:** Factors diet: $p = 0.0001$; time: $p < 0.0001$; interaction diet × time: $p = 0.0001$; **T2D:** diet: $p = 0.3767$; time: $p < 0.0001$; interaction diet × time: $p = 0.708$. **B: Immunoreactive insulin: Healthy controls:** Factors diet: $p = 0.9156$; time: $p < 0.0001$; interaction diet × time: $p < 0.0001$; **T2D:** diet: $p = 0.1084$; time: $p < 0.0001$; interaction diet × time: $p = 0.098$. **C:** C-peptide: **Healthy controls:** Factors diet: $p < 0.0001$; time: $p < 0.0001$; interaction diet × time: $p < 0.0001$; **T2D:** diet: $p = 0.0713$; time: $p < 0.0001$; diet × time: $p = 0.6615$. **D: Triglycerides: Healthy controls:** Factors diet: $p = 0.0001$; time: $p < 0.0001$; interaction diet × time: $p < 0.0001$; **T2D:** diet: $p < 0.0001$; time: $p < 0.0001$; interaction diet × time: $p = 0.0192$. **E: Free fatty acids: Healthy controls:** Factors diet: $p < 0.0001$; time: $p < 0.0001$; interaction diet × time: $p = 0.0003$; **T2D:** diet: $p < 0.0001$; time: $p < 0.0001$; interaction diet × time: $p = 0.058$.

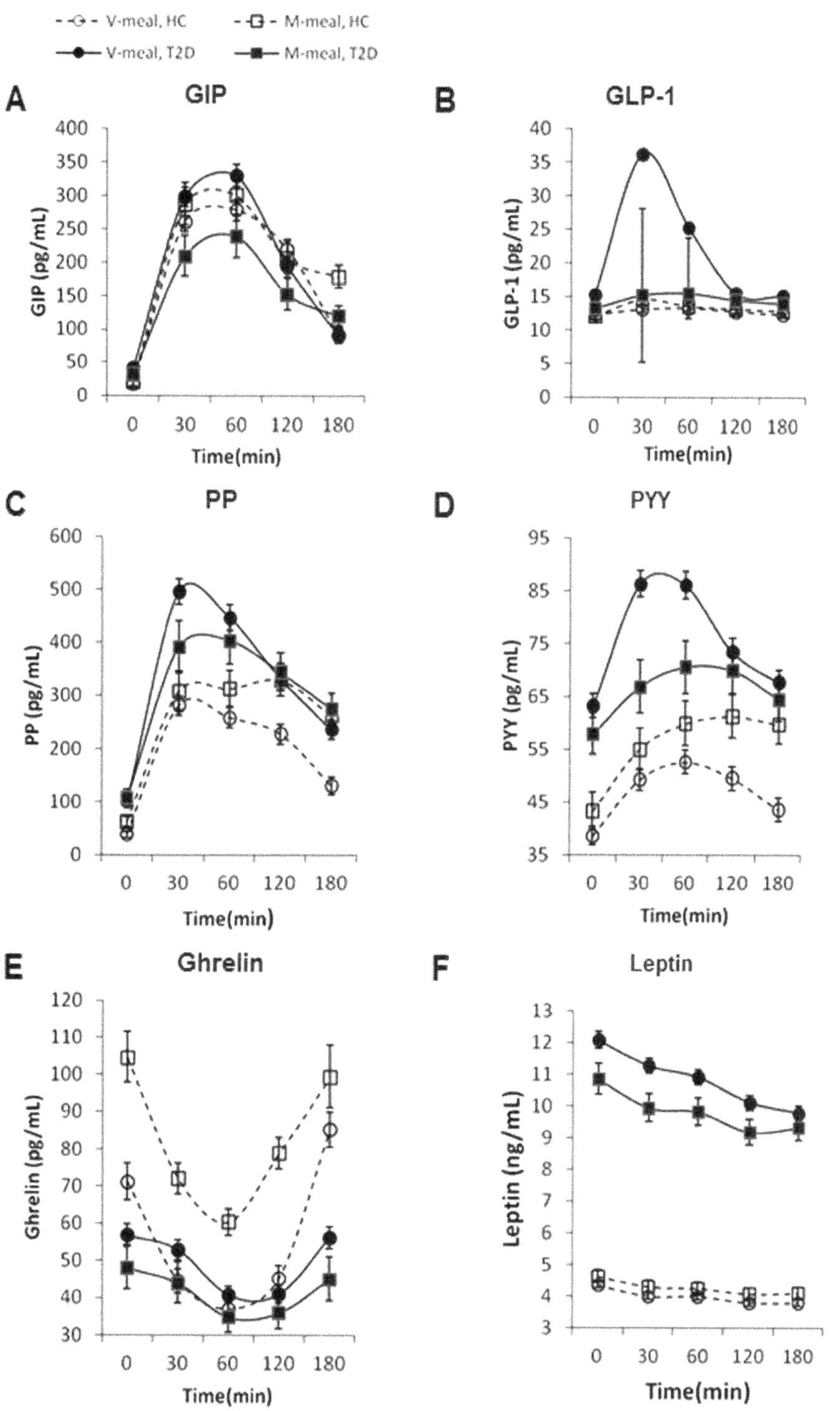

Figure 3. Postprandial changes in plasma concentrations of gastrointestinal and appetite hormones in patients with diabetes (T2D, full line) (n = 48) and healthy controls (HC, dashed line) (n = 49) after ingestion of the V-meal (circles) and the M-meal (squares). Data are expressed as mean with 95%CI. Repeated-measures ANOVA was performed. **A: GLP-1: Healthy controls:** Factors diet: $p = 0.1072$; time: $p < 0.0001$; interaction diet × time: $p = 0.2731$; **T2D:** diet: $p < 0.0001$; time: $p < 0.0001$; interaction diet × time: $p < 0.0001$. **B: GIP: Healthy controls:** Factors diet: $p = 0.0128$; time: $p < 0.0001$; interaction diet × time: $p = 0.0001$; **T2D:** diet: $p = 0.0005$; time: $p < 0.0001$; interaction diet × time: $p < 0.0001$. **C: PP: Healthy controls:** Factors diet: $p < 0.0001$; time: $p < 0.0001$; interaction diet × time: $p = 0.0016$; **T2D:** diet: $p = 0.5702$; time: $p < 0.0001$; interaction diet × time: $p = 0.0124$. **D: PYY: Healthy controls:** Factors diet: $p < 0.0001$; time: $p < 0.0001$; interaction diet × time: $p = 0.0768$; **T2D:** diet: $p < 0.0001$; time: $p < 0.0001$; interaction diet × time: $p = 0.004$. **E: Ghrelin: Healthy controls:** Factors diet: $p < 0.0001$; time: $p < 0.0001$; interaction diet × time: $p = 0.0004$; **T2D:** diet: $p = 0.0002$; time: $p < 0.0001$; interaction diet × time: $p = 0.9519$. **F: Leptin: Healthy controls:** Factors diet: $p = 0.0019$; time: $p < 0.0001$; intraction diet × time: $p = 0.9983$; **T2D:** diet: $p < 0.0001$; time: $p < 0.0001$; interaction diet × time: $p = 0.4988$.

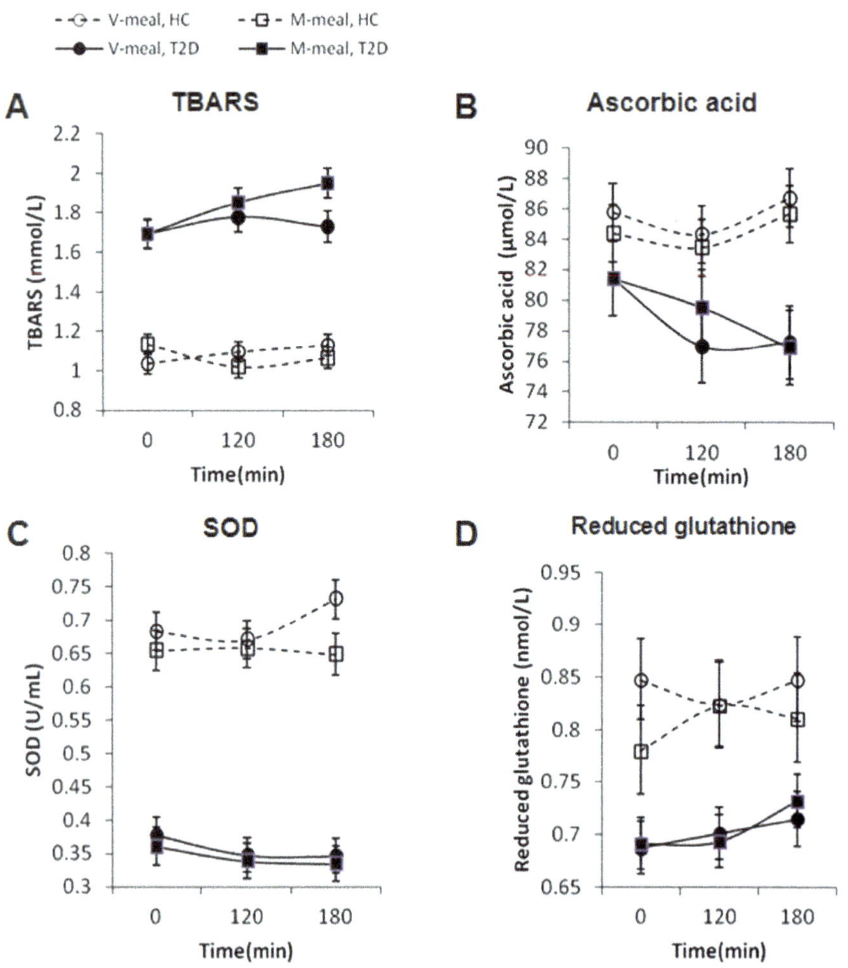

Figure 4. Postprandial changes in plasma concentrations of oxidative stress markers in patients with diabetes (T2D, full line) (n = 45) and healthy controls (HC, dashed line) (n = 49) after ingestion of the V-meal (circles) and the M-meal (squares). Data are expressed as mean with 95% CI. Repeated-measures ANOVA was performed. **A: TBARS: Healthy controls:** Factors diet: $p = 0.5952$; time: $p = 0.5647$; interaction diet × time: $p = 0.0405$; **T2D:** diet: $p = 0.0317$; time: $p = 0.0138$; interaction diet × time: $p = 0.113$. **B: Ascorbic acid: Healthy controls:** Factors diet: $p = 0.3292$; time: $p = 0.2324$; interaction diet × time: $p = 0.9802$; **T2D:** diet: $p = 0.6016$; time: $p = 0.0378$; interaction diet × time: $p = 0.6626$. **C: Superoxide dismutase**: **Healthy controls:** Factors diet: $p = 0.0171$; time: $p = 0.4608$; interaction diet × time: $p = 0.2388$; **T2D:** diet: $p = 0.4312$; time: $p = 0.2792$; interaction diet × time: $p = 0.9834$. **D: Reduced glutathione: Healthy controls:** Factors diet: $p = 0.1504$; time: $p = 0.8466$; interaction diet × time: $p = 0.5018$; **T2D:** diet: $p = 0.7654$; time: $p = 0.1475$; interaction diet × time: $p = 0.7935$.

compared with the control subjects, the levels of TBARS, a measure of lipoperoxidation, were increased by 67% ($p<0.001$), while the levels of ascorbic acid, reduced glutathione and SOD activity were decreased by 5%, 13% and 48%, respectively ($p< 0.001$).

During the postprandial phase, consumption of the M-meal was associated with a significantly greater increase in the TBARS levels in diabetic patients than that of the V-meal. In the healthy controls, no postprandial dynamics of the TBARS levels were detected. The SOD activity in the healthy controls was significantly increased after the V-meal compared with the M-meal. There was no significant change in the plasma concentration of SOD during the postprandial phase in diabetic subjects after either meal. The plasma concentrations of reduced glutathione and ascorbic acid did not change significantly in either patients with diabetes or healthy subjects after either meal.

Discussion

1. Postprandial changes in the plasma concentrations of glucose, lipids and insulin

Our results suggest that after two isocaloric meals containing different carbohydrate contents (M- and V-meals), the postprandial plasma glucose levels during the first 180 min after meal ingestion differed significantly only with respect to the peak glucose levels. Some human studies suggest that other macronutrients can modify the postprandial insulin demand and the glycemic response and therefore exert an additional impact on the postprandial increase in the glucose levels, as shown in healthy subjects [21] as well as patients suffering from T1D [6] or T2D [22].

Concerning the lipid levels, the significantly higher postprandial increase in the triglyceride levels and the smaller decrease in the free fatty acid levels detected in both groups after the M-meal is not surprising. Free fatty acids are known to impair insulin sensitivity and to enhance hepatic glucose production [2].

Decreases in the levels of these components leads to improvements in insulin sensitivity and glucose tolerance based on intervention studies [23].

We initially detected significantly lower IRI and C-peptide responses after the M-meal than the V-meal in healthy subjects. However, these levels decreasing more slowly, and after 180 min, the level of IRI was significantly higher in both groups after the M-meal. This result indicates that after the M-meal, hyperinsulinemia persisted longer in both groups.

This finding is in accordance with a glucose clamp study of non-diabetic human subjects indicating that increases in the FFA levels lead to insulin resistance within several hours [24]. Several studies confirmed that meals containing higher protein and/or fat contents exert an additional impact on the postprandial insulin demand and the increase in the glucose levels. In patients suffering from type 1 diabetes, high-fat meals containing identical carbohydrate and protein contents required a larger dose of insulin than low-fat meals [5]. Furthermore, addition of protein increases the insulin demand [6].

2. Postprandial changes in the plasma concentrations of GIHs and appetite hormones

Carbohydrate, fat and protein in the lumen of the gut have been demonstrated to stimulate the secretion of a broad range of GIHs [25].

The incretin effect, the postprandial augmentation of insulin secretion by gut hormones, has been primarily associated with the secretion and insulinotropic effect of two GIHs – GIP and GLP-1. The incretin effect is thought to mediate approximately 50–70% of the overall insulin response after a mixed meal or glucose ingestion in healthy subjects [26,27].

It is well understood that in patients with diabetes, the incretin effect is diminished secondarily [28,29], and this result appears to be due to impaired beta cell sensitivity [30].

The mechanisms underlying the loss of incretin activity remain incompletely understood, but several hypotheses have been proposed, including hyperglycemia- and hyperlipidemia-associated receptor desensitization [31,32].

Studies that have examined the GIP and GLP-1 responses after meals differing with respect to caloric and macronutrient content report inconsistent results regarding the contribution of meal composition to the stimulation of these hormones. One study reported a higher GIP response after a mixed meal than after an oral glucose load [33]. Another study demonstrated that fat preferentially stimulated GIP secretion, whereas carbohydrates stimulated GLP-1 secretion, both regardless of the diabetes status [34]. Dietary protein exerted a variable effect on incretin release [35,36].

Our results suggest that the intake of each type of isocaloric meal consumed in amounts typical of normal eating was associated with different postprandial changes in the GIP and GLP-1 plasma levels. In the T2D patients, the V-meal resulted in a larger release of GLP-1 and GIP than the M-meal. This result is in accordance with a study suggesting that the GLP-1 response after fat intake is impaired in T2D patients [37]. In contrast, in healthy individuals, the GLP-1 and GIP responses after ingestion of the V-meal were smaller than after the M-meal.

Our data suggest that carbohydrates appear to represent the strongest activator of GLP-1 and GIP secretion among T2D patients, whereas healthy subjects display higher GLP-1, GIP, PYY and PP responses to the mixed meal containing higher fat and protein contents.

In our study, we demonstrated increased basal and postprandial levels of GIP and GLP-1 in the T2D patients compared with the healthy subjects. This finding is in accordance with a study that evaluated the GLP-1 secretion levels and indicated relatively unchanged or even elevated secretion in response to oral nutrition intake in subjects suffering from diabetes [38].

Additionally, a recent meta-analysis revealed that T2D patients do not exhibit reduced GLP-1 secretion in response to an OGTT or a meal test [39]. With respect to GIP secretion, most studies quantifying GIP secretion reported that the GIP levels are normal or even higher in T2D subjects compared with healthy controls [40]. However, reductions in the GLP-1 levels were found in patients suffering from a long disease duration and poor compensation [41]. A recent meta-analysis revealed a negative influence of HbA1c levels on plasma GLP-1 responses [39].

Other gastrointestinal peptides play a role in the regulation of energy intake, appetite and overall energy homeostasis in humans. They are secreted by different cells in the intestine and from the pancreas, and their release is modulated by food ingestion.

PYY is co-secreted predominantly from the endocrine L cells in the ileum together with GLP-1. PYY plays an important regulatory role in GIT function [42].

PP is secreted from endocrine cells in the pancreas. Both PYY and PP, when infused intravenously, reduce appetite and energy intake in healthy humans [43]. They are secreted in response to all three macronutrients, with fat being the most potent stimulus. In healthy humans, it was shown that the presence of fat in the small intestine induced stimulation of PYY and PP in a manner dependent on fat digestion and the presence of free fatty acids [44]. This finding is in accordance with our results; in healthy subjects, we detected significantly greater secretion of PYY and PP after ingestion of the M-meal compared with the V-meal.

The course of PYY secretion consisted of two phases. The initial rise in the PYY level is likely due to a link to the proximal small intestine, and the continuous rise reflects the direct contact of lipids with the distal small intestine [45]. This result was not detected in our diabetic group of patients; their postprandial response with respect to both peptides was significantly higher after the V-meal. Similarly, a previous study suggested that both insulin resistance and abnormal glucose metabolism impaired the PYY response to fat intake [37]. To the best of our knowledge, this is the first report of the different secretory responses of PP after both isocaloric meals in T2D patients compared with healthy controls.

Ghrelin stimulates appetite and food intake and is secreted in the stomach. In healthy individuals, the ghrelin plasma concentrations increase during fasting and are suppressed by meal intake [46], likely via postprandial hyperinsulinemia [47,48].

We detected postprandial suppression of ghrelin secretion during the first 60 min after meal ingestion. The postprandial decrease depended significantly on the baseline level of ghrelin, which means that the higher the baseline level of ghrelin is, the larger the drop. Furthermore, it was significantly greater after the M-meal in healthy subjects. This finding is in accordance with a study that demonstrates that fat digestion is required for the suppression of ghrelin [44]. The related changes in ghrelin could be deemed positive with respect to the meat meal. We detected lower fasting and postprandial plasma concentrations of ghrelin and a diminished postprandial suppression of ghrelin secretion in the T2D patients, with no difference between the two meals in time.

3. Postprandial changes in the plasma concentrations of oxidative stress markers

The postprandial state, characterized by hyperglycemia and hyperlipidemia, is associated with increased oxidative stress in patients suffering from diabetes [49]. In our group of T2D patients, we detected significantly higher fasting concentrations of all oxidative stress markers and significantly lower concentrations of blood antioxidants. Previous studies support the concept that increased oxidative stress may play an important role in T2D manifestation [10]. Dietary fat quality has been proposed to be a critical factor. Several studies have suggested that a high intake of saturated fatty acids naturally present in meat contributes to the risk of glucose intolerance [11,12]. Based on an intervention study, humans suffering from metabolic syndrome who were consuming a high saturated fatty acid diet displayed higher levels of oxidative stress markers postprandially [13,14]. We found that in diabetic patients during the postprandial phase, the processed meat meal was associated with a significantly greater increase in the products of oxidative damage, namely TBARS, compared with the plant based meal. This finding could also be due to the method of cooking at a high temperature. It has been reported that most of the lipid-peroxidation products ingested from popular foods are derived from meat products and high-fat processed foods such as red meats cooked at high temperatures [50]. Another study has shown that adding antioxidants to hamburger meat could significantly reduce the formation of lipid-peroxidation products during cooking [51].

4. Strengths and limitations of the study

The strength of our study was that we took a physiological approach to measure the postprandial state. We selected two simple isocaloric meals at amounts corresponding to those ingested during a typical meal. The M-meal was rich in both saturated fat and protein; thus, we cannot separate the effect of each macronutrient.

This study also had several limitations. First, the T2D patients exhibited a significantly higher body weight and BMI compared with the control subjects, and these differences may have affected some of the responses reported. The object of our study was to compare the effect of the two different meals within each group (patients with T2D and healthy subjects). In healthy subjects, no effect of adiposity on the postprandial GIP and GLP-1 levels has been reported [52]. The effect of obesity on other GIHs is unclear. In this study, we primarily aimed to compare the two meals rather than the two groups of subjects.

Finally, the 3-h study duration might be insufficient for complete absorption of the nutrients, and this limitation may have led to an underestimation of the measured parameters.

Conclusions

In conclusion, according to our hypothesis, our results suggest that a processed meat meal is accompanied by an impaired GIH response and increased oxidative stress marker levels in diabetic patients. Our results revealed comparable glycemic responses to isocaloric meals containing different carbohydrate contents, despite the distinct peak glucose concentrations. This finding illustrates that the diet composition and the energy content, rather than the carbohydrate count or the glycemic load, should be important considerations for the dietary management of diabetes.

Acknowledgments

We thank Thomas O'Hearn for great help with text corrections and we thank our nurses for their technical assistance and care provided to the study participants.

Author Contributions

Conceived and designed the experiments: LB HK HM TP. Performed the experiments: HM OO OT JV LK. Analyzed the data: LB HK HM MH TP. Contributed reagents/materials/analysis tools: LB HK HM LK OO JV OT. Contributed to the writing of the manuscript: LB HK HM TP.

References

1. American Diabetes Association (2013) Standards of medical care in diabetes-2013. Diabetes Care: 36 Suppl 1: S11–66.
2. Savage DB, Petersen KF, Shulman GI (2007) Disordered lipid metabolism and the pathogenesis of insulin resistance. Physiol Rev 87: 507–20.
3. Lodefalk M, Aman J, Bang P (2008) Effects of fat supplementation on glycaemic response and gastric emptying in adolescents with Type 1 diabetes. Diabet Med: 1030–5. doi:10.1111/j.1464-5491.2008.02530.
4. Gentilcore D, Chaikomin R, Jones KL, Russo A, Feinle-Bisset C, et al. (2006) Effects of fat on gastric emptying of and the glycemic, insulin, and incretin responses to a carbohydrate meal in type 2 diabetes. J Clin Endocrinol Metab 91: 2062–7.
5. Wolpert HA, Atakov-Castillo A, Smith SA, Steil GM (2013) Dietary fat acutely increases glucose concentrations and insulin requirements in patients with type 1 diabetes: implications for carbohydrate-based bolus dose calculation and intensive diabetes management. Diabetes Care 36: 810–6.
6. Peters AL, Davidson MB (1993) Protein and fat effects on glucose responses and insulin requirements in subjects with insulin-dependent diabetes mellitus. Am J Clin Nutr 58: 555–60.
7. Aune D, Ursin G, Veierød MB (2009) Meat consumption and the risk of type 2 diabetes: a systematic review and meta-analysis of cohort studies. Diabetologia 52: 2277–87.
8. Pan A1, Sun Q, Bernstein AM, Schulze MB, Manson JE, et al. (2011) Red meat consumption and risk of type 2 diabetes: 3 cohorts of US adults and an updated meta-analysis. Am J Clin Nutr 94: 1088–96.
9. Pan A1, Sun Q, Bernstein AM, Schulze MB, Manson JE, et al. (2008) Meats, processed meats, obesity, weight gain and occurrence of diabetes among adults: findings from Adventist Health Studies. Ann Nutr Metab 52: 96–104.
10. Ceriello A, Motz E (2004) Is oxidative stress the pathogenic mechanism underlying insulin resistance, diabetes, and cardiovascular disease? The common soil hypothesis revisited. Arterioscler Thromb Vasc Biol 24: 816–23.
11. Feskens EJ, Virtanen SM, Räsänen L, Tuomilehto J, Stengård J, et al. (1995) Dietary factors determining diabetes and impaired glucose tolerance. A 20-year follow-up of the Finnish and Dutch cohorts of the Seven Countries Study. Diabetes Care 18: 1104–12.
12. Maron DJ, Fair JM, Haskell WL (1991) Saturated fat intake and insulin resistance in men with coronary artery disease. The Stanford Coronary Risk Intervention Project Investigators and Staff Circulation 84: 2020–7.
13. Perez-Martinez P1, Garcia-Quintana JM, Yubero-Serrano EM, Tasset-Cuevas I, Tunez I, et al. (2010) Postprandial oxidative stress is modified by dietary fat: evidence from a human intervention study. Clin Sci (Lond) 15: 251–61.
14. Cardona F, Túnez I, Tasset I, Montilla P, Collantes E, et al. (2008) Fat overload aggravates oxidative stress in patients with the metabolic syndrome. Eur J Clin Invest 38: 510–5.
15. Barnard ND1, Katcher HI, Jenkins DJ, Cohen J, Turner-McGrievy G (2009) Vegetarian and vegan diets in type 2 diabetes management. Nutr Rev 67: 255–63.
16. Kahleova H, Matoulek M, Malinska H, Oliyarnik O, Kazdova L, et al. (2011) Vegetarian diet improves insulin resistance and oxidative stress markers more than conventional diet in subjects with Type 2 diabetes. Diabet Med 28: 549–59.
17. Kellar KL, Iannone MA (2002) Multiplexed microsphere-based flow cytometric assays. Exp Hematol 30: 1227–37.
18. Yokode M1, Kita T, Kikawa Y, Ogorochi T, Narumiya S, et al. (1988) Stimulated arachidonate metabolism during foam cell transformation of mouse peritoneal macrophages with oxidized low density lipoprotein. J. Clin Invest 81: 720–9.

19. Nakagawa K, Kanno H, Miura Y (1997) Detection and analyses of ascorbyl radical in cerebrospinal fluid and serum of acute lymphoblastic leukemia. Anal Biochem 254: 31–5.
20. Meloun M, Hill M, Militký J, Kupka K (2000) Transformation in the PC-aided biochemical data analysis. Clin Chem Lab Med 38: 553–9.
21. Nuttall FQ, Gannon MC, Wald JL, Ahmed M (1985) Plasma glucose and insulin profiles in normal subjects ingesting diets of varying carbohydrate, fat and protein content. J Am Coll Nutr 4: 437–50.
22. Estrich D, Ravnik A, Schlierf G, Fukayama G, Kinsell L, et al. (1967) Effects of Co-ingestion of fat and protein upon carbohydrate-induced hyperglycemia. Diabetes 16: 232–7.
23. Bajaj M, Suraamornkul S, Kashyap S, Cusi K, Mandarino L, et al. (2004) Sustained reduction in plasma free fatty acid concentration improves insulin action without altering plasma adipocytokine levels in subjects with strong family history of type 2 diabetes. J Clin Endocrinol Metab 89: 4649–55.
24. Gormsen LC, Nielsen C, Jessen N, Jørgensen JO, Møller N (2011) Time-course effects of physiological free fatty acid surges on insulin sensitivity in humans. Acta Physiol 201: 349–56.
25. Tolhurst G, Reimann F, Gribble FM (2012) Intestinal sensing of nutrients. Handb Exp Pharmacol 209: 309–35.
26. Creutzfeld W (1979) The incretin concept today. Diabetologia 16: 75–85.
27. Nauck MA, Homberger E, Siegel EG, Allen RC, Eaton RP, et al. (1986) Incretin effects of increasing glucose loads in man calculated from venous insulin and C-peptide responses. J Clin Endocrinol Metab 63: 492–8.
28. Nauck M, Stöckmann F, Ebert R, Creutzfeldt W, et al. (1986) Reduced incretin effect in type 2 (non-insulin-dependent) diabetes. Diabetologia 29: 46–52.
29. Knop FK, Vilsbøll T, Højberg PV, Larsen S, Madsbad S, et al. (2007) Reduced incretin effect in type 2 diabetes: cause or consequence of the diabetic state? Diabetes 56: 1951–9.
30. Kjems LL, Holst JJ, Vølund A, Madsbad S (2003) The influence of GLP-1 on glucose-stimulated insulin secretion: effects on beta-cell sensitivity in type 2 and nondiabetic subjects. Diabetes 52: 380–6.
31. Xu G1, Kaneto H, Laybutt DR, Duvivier-Kali VF, Trivedi N, et al. (2007) Downregulation of GLP-1 and GIP receptor expression by hyperglycemia: possible contribution to impaired incretin effects in diabetes. Diabetes 56: 1551–8.
32. Kang ZF1, Deng Y, Zhou Y, Fan RR, Chan JC, et al. (2013) Pharmacological reduction of NEFA restores the efficacy of incretin-based therapies through GLP-1 receptor signalling in the beta cell in mouse models of diabetes. Diabetologia 56: 423–33.
33. Vollmer K1, Holst JJ, Baller B, Ellrichmann M, Nauck MA, et al. (2008) Predictors of incretin concentrations in subjects with normal, impaired and diabetic glucose tolerance. Diabetes 57: 678–87.
34. Rijkelijkhuizen JM1, McQuarrie K, Girman CJ, Stein PP, Mari A, et al. (2010) Effects of meal size and composition on incretin, alpha-cell, and beta-cell responses. Metabolism 59: 502–11.
35. Carr RD1, Larsen MO, Winzell MS, Jelic K, Lindgren O, et al. (2008) Incretin and islet hormonal responses to fat and protein ingestion in healthy men. Am J Physiol Endocrinol Metab 295: E779–84.
36. Carrel G1, Egli L, Tran C, Schneiter P, Giusti V, et al. (2011) Contributions of fat and protein to the incretin effect of a mixed meal. Am J Clin Nutr 94: 997–1003.
37. Fernández-García JC1, Murri M, Coin-Aragüez L, Alcaide J, El Bekay R, et al. (2014) GLP-1 and peptide YY secretory response after fat load is impaired by insulin resistance, impaired fasting glucose and type 2 diabetes in morbidly obese subjects. Clin Endocrinol (Oxf) 80: 671–6.
38. Meier JJ, Nauck MA (2010) Is the diminished incretin effect in type 2 diabetes just an epi-phenomenon of impaired beta-cell function? Diabetes 59: 1117–25.
39. Calanna S1, Christensen M, Holst JJ, Laferrère B, Gluud LL, et al. (2013) Secretion of glucagon-like peptide-1 in patients with type 2 diabetes mellitus: systematic review and meta-analyses of clinical studies. Diabetologia 56: 965–72.
40. Cernea S (2011) The role of incretin therapy at different stages of diabetes. Rev Diabet Stud Fall 8: 323–38.
41. Vilsbøll T, Krarup T, Deacon CF, Madsbad S, Holst JJ (2001) Reduced postprandial concentrations of intact biologically active glucagon-like peptide 1 in type 2 diabetic patients. Diabetes 50: 609–13.
42. Kim BJ1, Carlson OD, Jang HJ, Elahi D, Berry C, et al. (2005) Peptide YY is secreted after oral glucose administration in a gender-specific manner. J Clin Endocrinol Metab 90: 6665–71.
43. Batterham RL1, Le Roux CW, Cohen MA, Park AJ, Ellis SM, et al. (2003) Pancreatic polypeptide reduces appetite and food intake in humans. J Clin Endocrinol Metab 88: 3989–92.
44. Feinle-Bisset C1, Patterson M, Ghatei MA, Bloom SR, Horowitz M (2005) Fat digestion is required for suppression of ghrelin and stimulation of peptide YY and pancreatic polypeptide secretion by intraduodenal lipid. Am J Physiol Endocrinol Metab 289: E948–53.
45. Adrian TE, Ferri GL, Bacarese-Hamilton AJ, Fuessl HS, Polak JM, et al. (1985) Human distribution and release of a putative new gut hormone, peptide YY. Gastroenterology 89: 1070–7.
46. Wren AM1, Small CJ, Ward HL, Murphy KG, Dakin CL, et al. (2000) The novel hypothalamic peptide ghrelin stimulates food intake and growth hormone secretion. Endocrinology 141: 4325–8.
47. Blom WA, Stafleu A, de Graaf C, Kok FJ, Schaafsma G, et al. (2005) Ghrelin response to carbohydrate-enriched breakfast is related to insulin. Am J Clin Nutr 81: 367–75.
48. Hagemann D1, Holst JJ, Gethmann A, Banasch M, Schmidt WE, et al. (2007) Glucagon-like peptide 1 (GLP-1) suppresses ghrelin levels in humans via increased insulin secretion. Regul Pept 143: 64–8.
49. Ceriello A, Esposito K, Testa R, Bonfigli AR, Marra M, et al. (2011) The possible protective role of glucagon-like peptide 1 on endothelium during the meal and evidence for an "endothelial resistance" to glucagon-like peptide 1 in diabetes. Diabetes Care 34: 697–702.
50. Goldberg T1, Cai W, Peppa M, Dardaine V, Baliga BS, et al. (2004) Advanced glycoxidation end products in commonly consumed foods. J Am Diet Assoc 104: 1287–91.
51. Li Z1, Henning SM, Zhang Y, Zerlin A, Li L, et al. (2010) Antioxidant-rich spice added to hamburger meat during cooking results in reduced meat, plasma, and urine malondialdehyde concentrations. Am J Clin Nutr 91: 1180–4.
52. Runchey SS, Valsta LM, Schwarz Y, Wang C, Song X, et al. (2013) Effect of low- and high-glycemic load on circulating incretins in a randomized clinical trial. Metabolism 62: 188–95.

23

Traditional vs Modern: Role of Breed Type in Determining Enteric Methane Emissions from Cattle Grazing as Part of Contrasting Grassland-Based Systems

Mariecia D. Fraser*, Hannah R. Fleming, Jon M. Moorby

Institute of Biological, Environmental and Rural Sciences, Aberystwyth University, Aberystwyth, Ceredigion, United Kingdom

Abstract

Ruminant livestock turn forages and poor-quality feeds into human edible products, but enteric methane (CH_4) emissions from ruminants are a significant contributor to greenhouse gases (GHGs) and hence to climate change. Despite the predominance of pasture-based beef production systems in many parts of Europe there are little data available regarding enteric CH_4 emissions from free-ranging grazing cattle. It is possible that differences in physiology or behaviour could influence comparative emissions intensities for traditional and modern breed types depending on the nutritional characteristics of the herbage grazed. This study investigated the role of breed type in influencing CH_4 emissions from growing beef steers managed on contrasting grasslands typical of intensive (lowland) and extensive (upland) production systems. Using the SF_6 dilution technique CH_4 emissions were estimated for a modern, fast-growing crossbred (Limousin cross) and a smaller and hardier native breed (Welsh Black) when grazing lowland perennial ryegrass (high nutritional density, low sward heterogeneity) and semi-improved upland pasture (low/medium nutritional density, high sward heterogeneity). Live-weight gain was substantially lower for steers on the upland system compared to the lowland system (0.31 vs. 1.04 kg d^{-1}; s.e.d. = 0.085 kg d^{-1}; $P<0.001$), leading to significant differences in estimated dry matter intakes (8.0 vs. 11.1 kg DM d^{-1} for upland and lowland respectively; s.e.d. = 0.68 kg DM d^{-1}; $P<0.001$). While emissions per unit feed intake were similar for the lowland and upland systems, CH_4 emissions per unit of live-weight gain (LWG) were substantially higher when the steers grazed the poorer quality hill pasture (760 vs 214 g kg^{-1} LWG; s.e.d. = 133.5 g kg^{-1} LWG; $P<0.001$). Overall any effects of breed type were relatively small relative to the combined influence of pasture type and location.

Editor: Bernhard Kaltenboeck, Auburn University, United States of America

Funding: This work was collectively funded by the UK Department for Environment, Food and Rural Affairs, the Scottish Government, the Northern Ireland Department for Agriculture and Rural development, and the Welsh Government, as part of the UK's Agricultural GHG Research Platform (www.ghgplatform.org.uk). The funders had no role in study design, data collection and analysis, decision to publish, or preparation of the manuscript.

Competing Interests: The authors have declared that no competing interests exist.

* Email: mariecia.fraser@aber.ac.uk

Introduction

The world faces unprecedented challenges with regards to food security for future populations [1]. Ruminant livestock turn forages and poor-quality feeds into human edible products, but there is an inevitable environmental cost in terms of excretion of pollutants [2–4]. Methane (CH_4) is a significant contributor to greenhouse gases (GHGs) and hence to climate change. Agriculture is the source of about 38% of total UK emissions of CH_4, and of this about 85% comes from livestock enteric sources (mostly ruminants). While beef makes up around 20% of the total meat produced and consumed in the UK, beef cattle account for 27% of the GHG emissions from UK livestock species [3]. Larger, faster-growing animals should theoretically partition relatively more feed nutrients into production and excrete less polluting products during their lifetime, and therefore be more efficient in terms of quantity of product produced. Consequently, the output of polluting excretion products on a per unit product basis should be less for modern cattle breeds than traditional British cattle breeds, which are generally smaller and slower-maturing. However, the latter have frequently been bred under conditions that required them to be hardy and able to survive in exposed conditions on nutritionally poor vegetation [5]. Thus it is possible that physiological or behavioural differences may result in them utilising low-quality native pasture more efficiently than modern breeds. There is also a perception that such breeds have an important role to play in terms of maintaining cultural landscapes [5].

While management-intensive grazing offers potential for more efficient utilisation of grazed forage crops and more efficient conversion of forage into meat and milk [6], within the UK only 12% of meat from cattle is produced in intensive systems [3]. Instead, beef production is predominantly found in areas where physical and climatic challenges limit management options. Over 42% of utilised agricultural land in the UK carries the EU designation of Less Favoured Area (LFA). Among the many factors influencing CH_4 emissions from ruminants are quantity of feed intake and quality of the diet, with CH_4 production rising as feed intake increases and as dietary fibre concentrations increase [7]. Consequently emissions would be expected to be lower per unit intake from animals consuming the type of poorer-quality extensively-managed pastures characteristic of farming systems in marginal environments compared to those grazing higher quality cultivated lowland swards, but this has not been directly quantified. Experimental work to date with beef cattle has focussed on the impact of altering feed components within housed systems [8–17], and there is a dearth of corresponding data for animals at pasture. The relatively few data which have been collected relate to intensively managed swards [18–20] or forage species largely unrepresentative of Western European grasslands [6,21,22]. The current study addressed this deficiency, and tested for the first time the role of breed type in influencing CH_4 emissions from growing beef cattle when pastured on contrasting pasture types representative of intensive (lowland) and extensive (upland) grazing systems.

Methods

Ethics statement

The work described was conducted in accordance with the requirements of the UK Animals (Scientific Procedures) Act 1986 and with the approval of the Aberystwyth University Animal Welfare and Ethical Review Board. The conditions under which the animals were studied were designed to be as similar as possible to those used in commercial livestock production systems, and all stock were assessed daily for health and well-being. The research was conducted on one of IBERS' own research farms (lowland site) and on land leased from the Welsh Government specifically for this research (upland site). All pastures were managed in accordance with EU standards of good agricultural and environmental condition (GAECs).

Experimental design

Enteric CH_4 emission values were established for steers of contrasting breed types: a modern, fast-growing cross ((dairy × Belgian Blue) × Limousin) (LimX) and a smaller and hardier traditional breed (purebred Welsh Black) (WB). Separate experimental runs were carried out with animals grazing contrasting pasture types: 1) a lowland monoculture of perennial ryegrass (high nutritional density, low sward heterogeneity), and 2) a semi-improved hill pasture (low/medium nutritional density, high sward heterogeneity).

At the lowland site a total of 4.2 ha of monoculture perennial ryegrass was grazed on a rotational basis. The plots were located 140 m a.s.l. near Aberystwyth, Ceredigion (52°25′43.76″N, 4° 4′9.76″W), and had been sown with perennial ryegrass (cv Premium) in the summer of 2009. The plots were fertilised with 27:4:4 (N:P:K) compound fertiliser at a rate of 185 kg ha^{-1} in mid-May 2012, shortly before the start of the experiment.

The upland site grazed consisted of a mosaic of several community types, and was located within the Cambrian Mountains (52°24′5.81′′N, 3°44′0.81′′W), between 525 and 550 m a.s.l. A botanical survey of the 16 ha enclosure was carried out immediately prior to grazing. Around a third of the total area was recorded as being made up of large patches of semi-improved pasture interspersed to varying degrees with *Juncus effusus*. The predominant grass species present within those areas that had been re-seeded decades previously were *Agrostis* spp., *Festuca* spp, *Anthoxanthum odoratum* and *Lolium perenne*. Forbs, mainly *Trifolium repens* and *Cerastium arvense,* were a minor component, accounting for <5% of the sward. At one time these areas had received annual applications of inorganic fertilizer, but no fertiliser had been applied in the two years immediately preceding the experiment. The remaining two-thirds of vegetation within the enclosure consisted of patches of Blanket Bog Priority Habitat, Purple Moorgrass and Rush Pastures Priority Habitat [23], and dense *J. squarrosus*. When grazing the hill pasture the animals had access to the entire enclosure for the duration of the experiment.

Groups of steers born March – May 2011 were selected for each experimental run based on uniformity of age, body condition score (BCS) [24] and within-breed live weight (n = 9 steers per breed/system combination). All animals were drenched with an anthelmintic prior to the start of grazing. The lowland ryegrass experimental run commenced on 28 June 2012, and the hill sward experimental run on 23 July 2012. The later start at the upland site reflected the three-week or so delay in the start of the growing season and subsequent timing of peak growth at this location relative to the coastal lowland site. Each experimental run consisted of three phases: an adaptation phase, a performance measurement phase, and a CH_4 measurement phase. Following turnout onto the experimental pastures the animals were given at least two weeks to adapt to the site and pasture before data collection began. There then followed a six-week performance measurement period during which live weight was recorded weekly in order to establish individual growth rates. During a subsequent two-week CH_4 measurement period associated enteric emissions of CH_4 were then estimated. The animals at each site grazed together as a single group to ensure that opportunities for selective grazing were similar for the two breeds when grazing the heterogeneous hill sward.

Sward measurements

Sward height and biomass data were collected weekly to monitor herbage availability. Sward height was measured at each site using a sward stick (50 measurements per plot) [25]. At each measurement location the height of the first touch of grass/forb vegetative growth was recorded. Herbage biomass samples were collected by cutting the material along a 1 m rule to ground level at 10 random locations across each site using electric shears (ryegrass; 2 cuts per location) or a hedge-trimmer (hill sward; 1 cut per location). In order to reflect availability of preferred vegetation, sampling on the hill sward was restricted to areas when the cattle had been observed as grazing; generally the patches of semi-improved pasture. Following weighing of the fresh cut material a representative sub-sample was oven dried (100°C) to constant weight to determine dry matter (DM) content. The remaining herbage from each sampling location was bulked into a single weekly sample per site. A sub-sample of this bulked material was subsequently freeze-dried and milled to pass through a 1 mm sieve prior to chemical analysis. Ash was measured by igniting samples in a muffle furnace at 550°C for 16 h, and gross energy (GE) was determined by adiabatic bomb calorimetry (Gallenkamp autobomb; Sanyo Gallenkamp PLC, Loughborough UK). Total nitrogen (TN) concentrations were determined using a Leco FP 428 nitrogen analyser (Leco Corporation, St. Joseph, MI, USA), and expressed as crude protein (CP) (TN × 6.25). Water-soluble carbohydrate (WSC) concentrations were measured by an automated anthrone technique [26]. Neutral-detergent fibre (NDF) and acid-detergent fibre (ADF) were determined using the method of Van Soest *et al.* [27], adapted for the Gerhardt Fibrecap detergent system (FOSS UK Ltd, Warrington, UK). Digestibility of organic matter in the DM (DOMD) was determined using the two-stage pepsin-cellulase *in-vitro* method described by Jones & Hayward [28].

Animal measurements

The live weights and BCS of the animals were recorded once weekly throughout each grazing session. Incremental live-weight gains were calculated and averaged across the performance measurements period on an individual animal basis. Assessments of BCS were made using a scale from 1 to 5 [24], with quarter scores as intermediate points along the scale.

Enteric CH_4 emissions were estimated using the sulphur hexafluoride (SF_6) tracer technique as described by Muñoz *et al.* [29]. A brass permeation tube with known SF_6 release rate was inserted *per os* into the reticulo-rumen of each steer prior to turn-out onto the experimental pastures. The release rates of the permeation tubes used averaged 4.773 mg d^{-1}. Breath was sampled from each steer via an inlet mounted on a halter and located above the nose. All animals were allowed at least a week to adapt to wearing the equipment prior to sample collection. Within the collection period samples were collected for 4 d for each animal during two consecutive weeks. Animals were fitted with a 1.7 l collection canister, previously evacuated to>90 kPa pressure and fitted with a capillary tube previously prepared to provide gaseous collection at a rate of between 0.35 and 0.45 ml min^{-1}. The time between changing collection canisters was as close to 24 h as possible. In order to record ambient CH_4 and SF_6 concentrations two additional canisters were placed close to each grazing area, but away from the animals. These were replaced every 24 h as for each animal collection canister. After each 24 h collection period, the residual vacuum pressure was recorded for each canister. The canisters were then pressurised with nitrogen to approximately 50 kPa prior to analysis by gas chromatography within 48 hrs. Methane and SF_6 concentrations were quantified using a gas chromatograph (Clarus 560; PerkinElmer, Cambridge, UK) fitted with a flame ionisation detector and an electron capture detector. The sample inlet was connected to a 1 ml sample loop via a valve, which at the initiation of each analytical run delivered the sample via a T connection to two packed stainless steel columns: 1.219 m × 3.175 mm OD × 2 mm ID 80/100 Porapak N for CH_4 analysis, and 1.829 m × 3.175 mm OD × 2 mm ID 45/60 molecular sieve 5A, for SF_6 analysis (both columns sourced from Sigma-Aldrich Company Ltd, Gillingham, Dorset, UK). The carrier gas was oxygen-free nitrogen with a flow rate of 40 ml min^{-1}, split between the two columns; air and hydrogen were supplied to the flame ionisation detector at the rates of 450 ml min^{-1} and 45 ml min^{-1} respectively. The oven temperature was a constant 70°C, and the heater temperature on both detectors was set at 250°C. Total run time was 1.30 min. Calibration curves for quantification were prepared using standard gas mixtures in nitrogen (Scott-Marin, Inc, Riverside CA, USA): 1) 10.25 ppmv CH_4 (±1% NIST) and 9.43 pptv SF_6 (±10% NIST); 2) 102.9 ppmv CH_4 (±1% NIST) and 146 pptv SF_6 (±5% NIST); and 3) 307 ppmv (±1% NIST) and 295 pptv SF_6 (±5% NIST). A fourth standard mixture (51.3 ppmv CH_4, ±1% NIST, and 81.8 pptv SF_6, ±5% NIST) was used as a quality assurance standard during sample analysis runs.

Methane emissions (g d^{-1}) from each individual animal were calculated from the measured SF_6 and CH_4 concentrations sampled by the canisters (SF_6C and CH_4C respectively), background concentrations of SF_6 and CH_4 (SF_6B and CH_4B respectively) and the release rate of SF_6 (SF_6R, in g d^{-1}) from individual permeation tubes determined before the start of the experiment according to Equation 1.

$$CH_4 = \left(CH_4C - CH_4B\right) / \left(SF_6C - SF_6B\right) \times SF_6R \times \left(\text{molecular weight } CH_4 / \text{molecular weight } SF_6\right) \quad (1)$$

Climatic conditions

During the CH_4 sampling periods at each site wind speed was measured using a yacht anemometer (Type 454; Schiltknecht Messtechnik AG, Gossau, Switzerland) fixed approximately 1.5 m from ground level and connected to a battery powered datalogger (MSR 145; MSR Electronics GmbH, Seuzach, Switzerland) that also recorded atmospheric pressure, temperature and relative humidity at 30 second intervals. The datalogger was housed in a standard Stevenson screen located at the edge of the experimental plots. Data relating to measured rainfall were obtained from the meteorological station nearest to each experimental site.

Data analysis

The effect of breed type and production systems on animal performance was investigated with individual animal as the experimental unit. Feed intake was estimated by calculating metabolisable energy (ME) requirements for measured live-weight gain using AFRC [30] equations. The GE density of CH_4 used was 55.65 MJ kg^{-1}, and feed GE density was as analysed in samples collected (17.53 and 18.65 MJ kg^{-1} DM for lowland and upland pastures respectively). The metabolisability of feed GE at maintenance (qm) was calculated from sward sample ME values, with forage ME being calculated as 2.34+0.0111 × DOMD [30]. Energy requirements for maintenance and growth were estimated from mean live weight and live-weight change respectively, with mean scaling factors (C2) of 1.15 and 1.0 for LimX and WB cattle respectively, to account for differences in the maturing age of the breeds [30]. The DM intake required to supply ME requirements was calculated using predicted feed ME density.

Data relating to live weight, BCS, growth and CH_4 emissions were analysed using analysis of variance with a treatment structure of breed type (WB, LimX) × system (Lowland, Upland). In this context 'system' was used as a collective term for the combination of factors relating to sward, climate and terrain which potentially influenced the nutritional demands and grazing behaviour of the animals at each site. One LimX steer on the lowland system had to be excluded from the study on behavioural grounds, and two LimX steers on the upland systems had to be excluded on health grounds. These animals were treated as missing values in the analysis. Tier 1 [31] equivalent emission factors (EFs) (kg y^{-1}) were calculated as: CH_4 (g d^{-1}) x 365.

Results

Climatic conditions

Mean temperatures recorded during the CH_4 collection period at the lowland site were considerably higher those recorded at the upland site, while average wind speeds recorded were broadly similar, with an identical range (Table 1). Mean relative humidity was lower at the lowland site than at the upland site, with similar ranges. Based on data from the nearest meteorological stations to the two sites, rainfall was estimated to be substantially higher at the upland site across the experimental periods (193 vs 104 mm respectively). Differences in atmospheric pressure between the two sites reflected the differences in altitude.

Sward characteristics

The mean sward surface height of the grazed ryegrass sward across the 8 weeks of data recording was 12 cm (s.e. = 0.9 cm), with the corresponding mean herbage biomass 1570 kg ha^{-1} (s.e. = 117 kg ha^{-1}). The mean sward surface height of the grassy (i.e. non-*Juncus*) areas of the hill sward was 16 cm (s.e. = 2.2 cm), and the mean herbage biomass for these areas was 2740 kg ha^{-1} (s.e. = 281 kg ha^{-1}). These results indicate that performance

Table 1. Meteorological data recorded during the methane data collection periods. Values are means (minimum – maximum).

	Lowland	Upland
Temperature (°C)	14.2 (5.8–18.0)	6.9 (2.3–11.1)
Wind speed (km h^{-1})	8 (0–44)	11 (0–44)
Atmospheric pressure (kPa)	99.8 (98.1–101.6)	94.4 (92.1–96.0)
Relative humidity (%)	87 (60–99)	94 (66–100)

would be limited by the quality rather than the quantity of herbage available, particularly at the upland site.

The herbage cut from the upland site was characterised by having lower CP and WSC concentrations relative to the material collected from the lowland site, and a lower DOMD (Table 2). The high ash concentration for the ryegrass cut from the lowland site likely reflects the higher than average rainfall during the summer of 2012 [32] and associated soil contamination during cutting.

Animal performance

In keeping with what would be expected for a native breed type, the WB steers were smaller than the LimX steers at the start of data recording at both sites (Table 3). The BCS of the two breeds was similar however (grand mean = 2.5).

Pasture type had a highly significant effect on live-weight gain (s.e.d. = 0.08 kg d^{-1}; $P<0.001$), which was just over 1 kg d^{-1} when grazing the lowland ryegrass sward, but less than 0.35 kg d^{-1} when grazing the hill sward (Fig. 1). Overall the growth rates for the two breed types were similar, and there were no breed type × pasture type interaction effects. There was a trend towards estimated DM intakes being influenced by breed type, but once again the results obtained were more strongly influenced by system type, with the steers grazed on the upland site estimated to consume substantially less forage than those grazed on the lowland site (Table 2).

Methane production

When the effects of breed type and system were analysed, CH_4 yield was significantly lower for animals on the upland system (Table 3). Neither breed type nor system influenced the amount of CH_4 emitted per unit of feed consumed. Likewise, the yield of CH_4 energy per unit GE intake (Y_m) was similar for both systems, with the grand mean 6.0%. Emissions intensities (CH_4 emitted per unit weight gain) were significantly lower for steers on the lowland system (s.e.d. = 133 g kg^{-1} live-weight gain; $P<0.001$) compared to the upland system (Fig. 2). There was also considerably more between-animal variation recorded for steers of both breed types on the upland compared to the lowland system.

Discussion

Improvements in production efficiency have the potential to decrease the carbon footprint of livestock product [3]. Increasing the proportion of concentrates in the diet generally reduces CH_4 emissions, both as a proportion of energy intake and when expressed per unit of meat or milk output [33]. Dawson [34] compared the carbon footprint of a long-keep steer system (in which cattle were offered grazed grass in the summer and grass silage in the winter) with that of an intensive bull system (in which bulls were housed throughout their lives and offered concentrates *ad libitum*), and showed that the carbon footprint of the bulls expressed as CO_2e per kg carcass weight was approximately half that of the steers. The challenge to grass-based livestock systems is therefore to strive for levels of animal performance that are comparable to those associated with intensive cereal-based systems.

Comparative performance of different breed types under lowland and upland conditions

There was no effect of breed type on the performance figures recorded for either production system. In previous years the hill enclosure had been mixed grazed by sheep and suckler cows during the summer months as part of commercial farm operations, and as such the swards were expected to support productive stock. Despite the expectation that selective grazing of the improved

Table 2. Chemical composition of swards available to steers on contrasting beef production systems (where Lowland = rotational grazing of monoculture perennial ryegrass, Upland = extensive grazing of a diverse hill sward).

	Lowland	Upland
DM (g kg^{-1})	221 (17.0)	203 (16.0)
Ash	119 (16.1)	33 (1.6)
CP	148 (6.7)	120 (5.2)
WSC	126 (9.8)	94 (6.4)
NDF	508 (17.8)	677 (5.8)
ADF	283 (11.1)	363 (8.6)
DOMD	591 (8.9)	502 (5.0)
GE (MJ kg^{-1} DM)	17.5 (0.40)	18.7 (0.35)

Values are means (with standard errors) of eight weekly samplings across the measurement period at each site. All values g kg^{-1} DM unless otherwise stated.

Table 3. Effects of breed type and production system on animal performance and methane (CH_4) emissions of beef steers (where WB = Welsh Black, LimX = Limousin cross; Lowland = rotational grazing of monoculture perennial ryegrass, Upland = extensive grazing of a diverse hill sward).

	Lowland		Upland			*F* prob.[2]	
	WB	LIM	WB	LIM	s.e.d.	Breed	System
Start weight (kg)	386	458	410	467	12.7	<0.001	ns
BCS at start	2.5	2.4	2.4	2.4	0.08	ns	ns
Estimated DM intake (kg d^{-1})	10.3	11.8	7.7	8.2	0.67	0.05	<0.001
CH_4 (g d^{-1})	216	217	173	190	10.4	ns	<0.001
EF[1] (kg $year^{-1}$)	79	79	63	69	3.8	ns	<0.001
CH_4/DM intake (g kg^{-1})	21.0	18.7	22.9	23.4	1.33	ns	<0.01
CH_4-E/GE intake (%)	6.7	6.0	6.8	7.0	0.41	ns	<0.05

[1]Calculated for comparison with IPCC [31] Tier 1 default values; [2]F probability; ns = non-significant, $P>0.1$; there were no significant interaction effects.
Where BSC = body condition score; EF = Emission Factor; GE = gross energy.

areas within the enclosure would raise the nutritional value of the diets consumed relative to the average for the sward as a whole, the growth rates achieved by both breeds during the current study were low and not dissimilar to those previously recorded for yearling cattle when grazing another site in the area that was entirely dominated by the native hill grass species *Molinia caerulea* [35]. Likewise the growth rates are considerably lower than the figure of 0.64 kg d^{-1} recently reported for dairy-cross steers grazing botanically diverse upland pasture at a lower altitude in Northern Ireland [36]. It would therefore seem that withdrawal of fertiliser inputs had already had a deleterious effect on the species composition and therefore the nutritional quality of the sward despite ryegrass and white clover still being in evidence [37]. In the longer term, further reductions in the competitive ability of the sown species would be expected. At the same time, ceasing applications of inorganic fertiliser would be expected to reduce net nitrous oxide emissions from the production system. Further research is required to build on these baseline data and simultaneously test the impact of such management practices on carbon and nitrogen capture and loss in order to assess overall system efficiency.

During the current experiment voluntary feed intake was estimated by back calculation based on the predicted energy requirements of the stock to achieve the performance recorded and the corresponding nutritional value of the sward being consumed. However, a range of factors may have influenced the demands of the animals. In particular the exposed nature of the upland site would have placed additional burdens on the animals. Climatic conditions (temperature, rainfall, windspeed etc) are not taken into account by the AFRC [30] energy requirement calculations. The thermoneutral zone of cattle is generally considered to be greater than that of other livestock [38], although it is affected by coat depth, coat conditions (wet, muddy etc) and wind speed [39]. Even though the lower critical temperature for beef cattle is estimated to be about −21°C in still dry conditions [38], energy requirements increase to support metabolic heat production in wet beef cattle at temperatures as high as 15°C [40]. At the same time, high wind speeds coupled with the animals being frequently wet from rainfall, particularly at the upland site, may have altered grazing behavior and led to reductions in grazing time as the animals sought shelter.

When estimating intake qm was calculated using predicted ME values of sward samples. While the sward samples were taken from patches preferentially grazed by the cattle, they will not have reflected within-patch selection of particular sward components which may have led to the diet consumed having a higher digestibility than the average of the sward on offer. Furthermore, *in vitro* digestibility estimations based on enzyme preparation do not leave any scope for possible interaction between microbial species in the rumen and the modification of this by the diet of the host animal [41]. This will have likely led to the calculated figures overestimating actual feed intake. This would mean that the estimates of CH_4 yield from feeds and Y_m are lower than the true values, and may be altered to some extent if actual DM and GE intakes were known. Despite this, the values of Y_m measured in this study are similar to those reported by other studies for grazing cattle [42–44]. Alternative marker-based methods of estimating feed intake such as the *n*-alkane technique [45] also have limitations, particularly when used in situations where it is difficult to obtain a representative sample of the diets selected from a heterogeneous sward. Another approach to measuring intake and CH_4 emissions is housing the animals in respiration chambers and offering them cut forage. However, crucially this significantly reduces any environmental effects on productive and excretion

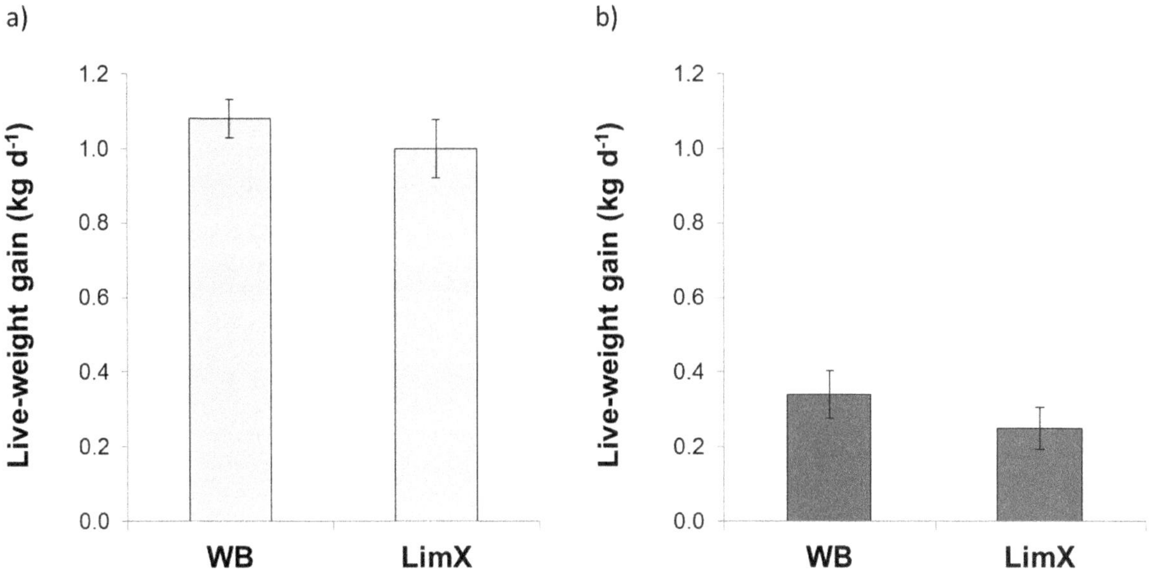

Figure 1. Effect of breed type on growth rates of steers grazing on a) lowland ryegrass, and b) semi-improved hill pasture. (Where WB = Welsh Black and LimX = Limousin cross; values plotted are mean±standard errors).

outputs, and prevents the animals from exhibiting normal grazing behaviour. Therefore, it was felt that the methods employed in this study were most appropriate to obtain the data collected, and any deviation of estimates from absolute values are likely to be small while relative differences are comparatively precise.

Comparative enteric emissions under lowland and upland conditions

There are previous reports of CH_4 emissions differing on different forage types [18], and CH_4 emissions per unit carcass gain have been shown to decrease as pasture quality improves [46]. Consequently it is not surprising that the emissions per kg live-weight gain from the cattle grazing the poorer quality pasture within the upland system are higher. While differences between pastures types are confounded with environmental conditions within the present study, the values recorded are representative of the grazing system as a whole. Zero-grazing of the different swards would have allowed the influence of climatic conditions to be controlled, but crucially the role of foraging strategy in influencing emissions would also have been negated. Selective feeding can lead to the nutritive value of a diet consumed by animals grazing heterogeneous swards being substantially higher than the average for the sward as a whole. Furthermore, it was possible that breed differences in the composition of the diet selected by the steers

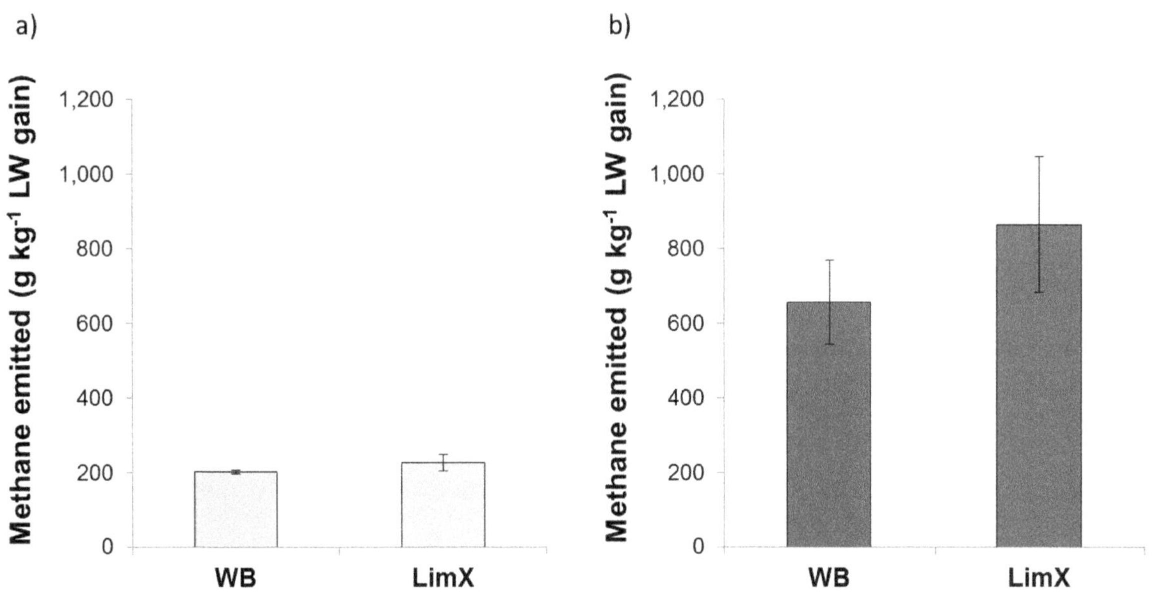

Figure 2. Effect of breed type on methane emissions per kilogram of live-weight (LW) gain for steers grazing on a) lowland ryegrass, and b) semi-improved hill pasture. (Where WB = Welsh Black and LimX = Limousin cross; values plotted are mean±standard errors).

grazing the hill pasture could be reflected in differing CH_4 emissions. The overall similarity in emissions for the two breeds would however suggest that there were no substantial differences in the diets chosen, in keeping with the findings of previous research on breed differences in cattle grazing preferences [5,47]. Although the WB steers were smaller than the LimX steers they are a comparatively large native breed. Previous calculations estimating potential CH_4 emissions from suckler cows with calves at foot suggested that CH_4 emissions per kilogram of calf weight gain would be higher for smaller Belted Galloway cattle compared to Limousin-crosses [48]. This difference in predicted relative performance of a traditional breed was due to lower absolute weight gains by the Belted Galloway calves, despite them having higher proportional gains per kilogram initial weight.

The current UK National GHG Inventory largely reports emissions from agriculture to the United Nations Framework on Climate Change using the most simplified approach to accounting (i.e. Tier 1 methodology). This methodology uses generic assumptions and factors about livestock management to estimate GHG emissions, and relies on default EFs published by the IPCC [31]. The EF quoted by the IPCC for non-dairy cattle in Western Europe is 48 kg $head^{-1}$ yr^{-1}, and is applicable to bulls, calves and growing steers or heifers. The equivalent EFs calculated from the current experimental work are higher than this, although it must be noted that the values reported here are representative of values achieved under summer grazing only rather than the production system as a whole. The inclusion of grain-based diets within the winter feeding phase could reduce the overall emission burden [34]. The values obtained provide a valuable contribution towards the development of the necessary evidence base for the UK and other countries with similar temperate grassland systems of beef production to move to the more complex Tier 2 and Tier 3 approaches for reporting livestock emissions.

Wider implications

Many upland areas can, with appropriate nutrient inputs, sustain moderate levels of animal performance and although the carbon footprint per kilogram of carcass will be higher relative to lowland intensive systems, there are benefits both for human health and for food security from grass-based meat production [49], particularly when forage from areas unsuitable for cultivation are turned into human-edible products. Furthermore, the vegetation communities found in the hill and uplands support a variety of ecosystem services, such as biodiversity and landscape character, which are frequently dependent upon livestock farming. The UK, European and worldwide importance of the associated habitats in terms of nature conservation is recognised under legislation such as the EU Habitat and Bird Directives. The management of priority habitats such as those included within the hill enclosure used during the current experiment are frequent targeted by options within higher level agri-environment schemes. However, the results from the current study confirm that the associated conservation strategies designed to enhance biodiversity result in increased GHG emissions per unit of product due to the poorer quality of the vegetation consumed. Thus they make an important addition to the evidence base for future policies relating to Areas of Natural Constraint (ANC); the new designation due to replace LFA shortly. Further multi-disciplinary research is required to quantify and explore the trade-off between biodiversity and other ecosystem benefits and GHG emissions arising from grazing of semi-natural vegetation communities. This is of particular relevance to situations where incentives are being used to encourage the re-introduction of grazing to abandoned or under-utilised pasture. While CH_4 emission intensities would be expected to be relatively high in the first instance, these may lower as grazing rejuvenates the pasture and related changes in plant morphology or species balance within the sward lead to an improvement in nutritional value.

Although dietary strategies such as supplementation with fat, higher starch diets, use of monensin, exogenous enzymes and direct-fed microbials are being evaluated as potential means of reducing enteric CH_4 emissions [50], options for deploying such strategies are limited in extensive grazing systems. Further research is also required to develop and test alternative or modified strategies for manipulating rumen microbial populations as a means of reducing CH_4 from free-ranging grazing animals.

Conclusions

The current study was the first to quantify enteric CH_4 emissions for free-ranging beef cattle pastured on these common grassland types. It has shown that CH_4 emission intensities for growing steers at pasture are more strongly influence by production system than breed type, and established that emissions per unit of live-weight gain are substantially higher for animals grazed extensively on semi-improved hill pasture than animals grazing lowland ryegrass swards. Breed had comparatively little impact on the results obtained, and any numerical differences observed are likely to be caused by differences in feed intake. The data generated will strengthen the comparatively limited evidence base for future policy development regarding climate change mitigation and adaptation strategies within pastoral livestock systems.

Acknowledgments

Thanks go to John Davies and Vince Theobald for assistance with plot preparation and animal handling, and to Jim Vale for carrying out the sward survey on the hill sward. John Williams (ADAS) provided rainfall data for the Pwllpeiran site. Forage analyses were carried out by the Analytical Chemistry Group at IBERS.

Author Contributions

Conceived and designed the experiments: MDF JMM. Performed the experiments: MDF HRF JMM. Analyzed the data: MDF JMM. Contributed to the writing of the manuscript: MDF JMM.

References

1. Godfray HCJ, Beddington JR, Crute IR, Haddad L, Lawrence D, et al. (2010) Food security: the challenge of feeding 9 billion people. Science 327: 812–818.
2. O'Mara FP (2011) The significance of livestock as a contributor to global greenhouse gas emissions today and in the near future. Animal Feed Science and Technology 166–67: 7–15.
3. Gill M, Smith P, Wilkinson JM (2009) Mitigating climate change: the role of domestic livestock. Animal 4: 323–333.
4. Lassey KR (2008) Livestock methane emission and its perspective in the global methane cycle. Australian Journal of Experimental Agriculture 48: 114–118.
5. Rook AJ, Dumont B, Isselstein J, Osoro K, WallisDeVries MF, et al. (2004) Matching type of livestock to desired biodiversity outcomes in pastures - a review. Biological Conservation 119: 137–150.
6. DeRamus HA, Clement TC, Giampola DD, Dickison PC (2003) Methane emissions of beef cattle on forages: Efficiency of grazing management systems. Journal of Environmental Quality 32: 269–277.
7. Dijkstra J, Oenema O, Bannink A (2011) Dietary strategies to reducing N excretion from cattle: implications for methane emissions. Current Opinion in Environmental Sustainability 3: 414–422.
8. Hales KE, Cole NA, MacDonald JC (2012) Effects of corn processing method and dietary inclusion of wet distillers grains with solubles on energy metabolism,

carbon-nitrogen balance, and methane emissions of cattle. Journal of Animal Science 90: 3174–3185.

9. Doreau M, van der Werf HMG, Micol D, Dubroeucq H, Agabriel J, et al. (2011) Enteric methane production and greenhouse gases balance of diets differing in concentrate in the fattening phase of a beef production system. Journal of Animal Science 89: 2518–2528.
10. Cooprider KL, Mitloehner FM, Famula TR, Kebreab E, Zhao Y, et al. (2011) Feedlot efficiency implications on greenhouse gas emissions and sustainability. Journal of Animal Science 89: 2643–2656.
11. McGeough EJ, O'Kiely P, Hart KJ, Moloney AP, Boland TM, et al. (2010) Methane emissions, feed intake, performance, digestibility, and rumen fermentation of finishing beef cattle offered whole-crop wheat silages differing in grain content. Journal of Animal Science 88: 2703–2716.
12. McGeough EJ, O'Kiely P, Foley PA, Hart KJ, Boland TM, et al. (2010) Methane emissions, feed intake, and performance of finishing beef cattle offered maize silages harvested at 4 different stages of maturity. Journal of Animal Science 88: 1479–1491.
13. McGinn SM, Chung YH, Beauchemin KA, Iwaasa AD, Grainger C (2009) Use of corn distillers' dried grains to reduce enteric methane loss from beef cattle. Canadian Journal of Animal Science 89: 409–413.
14. Beauchemin KA, McGinn SM, Petit HV (2007) Methane abatement strategies for cattle: Lipid supplementation of diets. Canadian Journal of Animal Science 87: 431–440.
15. Beauchemin KA, McGinn SM (2006) Methane emissions from beef cattle: Effects of fumaric acid, essential oil, and canola oil. Journal of Animal Science 84: 1489–1496.
16. Beauchemin KA, McGinn SM (2006) Enteric methane emissions from growing beef cattle as affected by diet and level of intake. Canadian Journal of Animal Science 86: 401–408.
17. Huenerberg M, McGinn SM, Beauchemin KA, Okine EK, Harstad OM, et al. (2013) Effect of dried distillers grains plus solubles on enteric methane emissions and nitrogen excretion from growing beef cattle. Journal of Animal Science 91: 2846–2857.
18. Chaves AV, Thompson LC, Iwaasa AD, Scott SL, Olson ME, et al. (2006) Effect of pasture type (alfalfa vs. grass) on methane and carbon dioxide production by yearling beef heifers. Canadian Journal of Animal Science 86: 409–418.
19. Jones FM, Phillips FA, Naylor T, Mercer NB (2011) Methane emissions from grazing Angus beef cows selected for divergent residual feed intake. Animal Feed Science and Technology 166–67: 302–307.
20. Laubach J, Kelliher FM, Knight TW, Clark H, Molano G, et al. (2008) Methane emissions from beef cattle - a comparison of paddock-and animal-scale measurements. Australian Journal of Experimental Agriculture 48: 132–137.
21. Pavao-Zuckerman MA, Waller JC, Ingle T, Fribourg HA (1999) Methane emissions of beef cattle grazing tall fescue pastures at three levels of endophyte infestation. Journal of Environmental Quality 28: 1963–1969.
22. Chung YH, Mc Geough EJ, Acharya S, McAllister TA, McGinn SM, et al. (2013) Enteric methane emission, diet digestibility, and nitrogen excretion from beef heifers fed sainfoin or alfalfa. Journal of Animal Science 91: 4861–4874.
23. Carey PD, Barnett CL, Greensdale PD, Garbutt RA, Warman EA, et al. (2002) A comparison of the ecological quality of land between an English agri-environment scheme and the countryside as a whole. Biological Conservation 108: 183–197.
24. Lowman BG, Scott NA, Somerville SH (1976) Condition scoring of cattle. Rev Ed Bulletin, East of Scotland College of Agriculture, No.6.
25. Barthram GT (1986) Experimental techniques: the HFRO sward stick. Biannual Report, Hill Farming Research Organisation, 1984–85: 29–30.
26. Thomas TA (1977) An automated procedure for the determination of soluble carbohydrates in herbage. Journal of the Science of Food and Agriculture 28: 639–642.
27. Van Soest PJ, Robertson JB, Lewis BA (1991) Methods for dietary fibre, neutral detergent fibre and nonstarch polysaccharides in relation to animal nutrition. Journal of Dairy Science 74: 3583–3597.
28. Jones DIH, Hayward MV (1975) The effect of pepsin pretreatment of herbage on the predition of dry matter digestibility from solubility in fungal cellulase solution. Journal of Science Food and Agriculture 26: 711–718.
29. Muñoz C, Yan T, Wills DA, Murray S, Gordon AW (2012) Comparison of the sulfur hexafluoride tracer and respiration chamber techniques for estimating methane emissions and correction for rectum methane output from dairy cows. Journal of Dairy Science 95: 3139–3148.
30. AFRC (1993) Energy and protein requirements of ruminants. An advisory manual prepared by the AFRC Technical Committee on Responses to Nutrients. Wallingford, UK: CAB International.
31. IPCC (2006) Emissions from livestock and manure management, chapter 10. In: Guidelines for National Greenhouse Gas Inventories, Vol 4, Prepared by the National Greenhouse Gas Inventories Programme (eds Eggleston HS, Buendia L, Miwa K, Ngara T, Tanabe K), 10.7–10.84. IGES, Japan.
32. Met Office (2012) Meteorological Office Climate Report 2012: Regional values - summer. Avbailable: http://www.metoffice.gov.uk/climate/uk/2012/summer/averages.html.
33. Martin C, Morgavi DP, Doreau M (2008) Methane mitigation in ruminants: from microbe to the farm scale. Animal 4: 351–365.
34. Dawson LER (2010) Comparison of the performance and carbon footprint of dairy-origin beef steers. In 'Advances in Animal Biosciences': Proceedings of the British Society of Animal Science and the Agricultural Research Forum, British Society of Animal Science, Edimburgh, UK: 42.
35. Fraser MD, Theobald VJ, Dhanoa MS, Davies OD (2011) Impact on sward composition and stock performance of grazing *Molinia*-dominant grassland. Agriculture, Ecosystems and Environment 144: 102–106.
36. Richmond AS, Wylie ARG, Laidlaw AS, Lively FO, O'Connell N (2013) Methane emissions from growing beef cattle grazing semi-natural upland and improved lowland pastures. In 'Advances in Animal Agriculture': Proceedings of the 5th Greenhouse Gases and Animal Agriculture Conference (GGAA 2013), Dublin, Ireland Vol 4, Cambridge University Press: 550.
37. Fothergill M, Davies DA, Morgan CT (2001) Extensification of grassland use in the Welsh uplands: sheep performance in years 1–6. Grass and Forage Science 56: 105–117.
38. NRC (1981) Effect of Environment on Nutrient Requirements of Domestic Animals. Washington DC: The National Academies Press.
39. Fox DG, Sniffen CJ, O'Connor JD, Russell JB, Van Soest PJ (1992) A net carbohydrate and protein system for evaluating cattle diets: III. Cattle requirements and diet adequacy. Journal of Animal Science 70: 3578–3596.
40. Degen AA, Young BA (1983) Rate of metabolic heat production and rectal temperature of steers exposed to stimulated mud and rain conditions. Canadian Journal of Animal Science 73: 207–210.
41. Kitessa S, Flinn PC, Irish GG (1999) Comparison of methods used to predict the *in vivo* digestibility of feeds in ruminants. Australian Journal of Agricultural Research 50: 825–841.
42. Harper LA, Denmead OT, Freney JR, Byers FM (1999) Direct measurements of methane emissions from grazing and feedlot cattle. Journal of Animal Science 77: 1392–1401.
43. Pinares-Patiño CS, D'Hour P, Jouany JP, Martin C (2007) Effects of stocking rate on methane and carbon dioxide emissions from grazing cattle. Agriculture, Ecosystems & Environment 121: 30–46.
44. Pinares-Patiño CS, Baumont R, Martin C (2003) Methane emissions by Charolais cows grazing a monospecific pasture of timothy at four stages of maturity. Canadian Journal of Animal Science 83: 769–777.
45. Dove H, Mayes RW (1996) Plant wax components: A new approach to estimating intake and diet composition in herbivores. Journal of Nutrition 126: 13–26.
46. Waghorn GC, Clark DA (2006) Greenhouse gas mitigation opportunities with immediate application to pastoral grazing for ruminants. International Congress Series 1293: 107–110.
47. Fraser MD, Theobald VJ, Griffiths JB, Morris SM, Moorby JM (2009) Comparative diet selection by cattle and sheep grazing two contrasting heathland communities. Agriculture, Ecosystems and Environment 129: 182–192.
48. Fraser MD, Moorby JM, Vale JE, Evans DM (2014) Mixed grazing systems benefit both upland biodiversity and livestock production. PLos ONE 9: e89054.
49. Dawson LER, O'Kiely P, Moloney AP, Vipond JE, Wylie ARG, et al. (2011) Grassland systems of red meat production: integration between biodiversity, plant nutrient utilisation, greenhouse gas emissions and meat nutritional quality. Animal 5: 1432–1441.
50. Grainger C, Beauchemin KA (2011) Can enteric methane emissions from ruminants be lowered without lowering their production? Animal Feed Science and Technology 166–67: 308–320.

Label-Free and Sensitive Fluorescent Detection of Sequence-Specific Single-Strand DNA Based on S1 Nuclease Cleavage Effects

Zheng Guan[1,2], Jinchuan Liu[1], Wenhui Bai[1], Zhenzhen Lv[1], Xiaoling Jiang[1], Shuming Yang[1], Ailiang Chen[1]*, Guiyuan Lv[2]*

1 Institute of Quality Standards and Testing Technology for Agro-products, Key Laboratory of Agro-product Quality and Safety, Chinese Academy of Agricultural Sciences; Key Laboratory of Agro-food Quality and Safety, Ministry of Agriculture, Beijing, China, **2** Institute of Materia Medica, Zhejiang Chinese Medical University, Hangzhou, China

Abstract

The ability to detect sequence-specific single-strand DNA (ssDNA) in complex, contaminant-ridden samples, using a fluorescent method directly without a DNA extraction and PCR step could simplify the detection of pathogens in the field and in the clinic. Here, we have demonstrated a simple label-free sensing strategy to detect ssDNA by employing its complementary ssDNA, S1 nuclease and nucleic acid fluorescent dyes. Upon clearing away redundant complementary ssDNA and possibly mismatched double strand DNA by using S1 nuclease, the fluorescent signal-to-noise ratio could be increased dramatically. It enabled the method to be adaptable to three different types of DNA fluorescent dyes and the ability to detect target ssDNA in complex, multicomponent samples, like tissue homogenate. The method can distinguish a two-base mismatch from avian influenza A (H1N1) virus. Also, it can detect the appearance of 50 pM target ssDNA in 0.5 $\mu g\cdot mL^{-1}$ Lambda DNA, and 50 nM target ssDNA in 5 $\mu g\cdot mL^{-1}$ Lambda DNA or in tissue homogenate. It is facile and cost-effective, and could be easily extended to detect other ssDNA with many common nucleic acid fluorescent dyes.

Editor: Albert Jeltsch, Universität Stuttgart, Germany

Funding: Funding provided by The Special Fund for Agro scientific Research in the Public Interest (201203046) (http://119.253.58.231/hykj). The funders had no role in study design, data collection and analysis, decision to publish, or preparation of the manuscript.

Competing Interests: The authors have declared that no competing interests exist.

* Email: ailiang.chen@gmail.com (AC); guiyuan_lv@yeah.net (GL)

Introduction

Single strand DNA or RNA analysis plays an important role in the molecular biology, medicine and diagnosis. This has driven the development of various methods to detect sequence-specific DNA or RNA with high sensitivity and specificity. Most traditional methods for ssDNA and RNA detection employed PCR and agarose electrophoresis, or probe hybridization and fluorescent detection. Although these methods have been used successfully to detect ssDNA sensitively, many of them are often subjected to non-specific amplification or hybridization as well as complicated and tedious work. Recently, some nanomaterials including gold nanoparticles, quantum dots, carbon nanotubes and graphene were used for fluorescence assays of ssDNA and RNA [1–8]. However, these methods have also some limitations such as base selectivity, insufficient sensitivity and high-cost, especially for sequence-specific ssDNA and RNA.

To address these limitations, in this study, a highly sensitive and cost-effective approach for sequence-specific ssDNA detection was developed by using complementary single-strand DNA, S1 nuclease and nucleic acid fluorescent dyes. In the proposed method, an S1 nuclease-mediated ssDNA cleavage mechanism [9–11] was introduced to increase the assay sensitivity by eliminating nonspecific fluorescence effect of redundant complementary ssDNA sequences and mismatches. Furthermore, the fluorescence intensity with different sequence, different lengths of oligonucleotides, and their hybrid products after S1 nuclease-mediated cleavage were also studied. To test the universality and sensitivity of the method, three different types of DNA fluorescent dyes and three specific virus ssDNA sequences were investigated and the linear ranges were compared. Moreover, in order to illustrate its practical use, 4% pork muscle tissue homogenate was used to simulate the reality, and the targets in the tissue homogenate have been directly detected without a DNA extraction and PCR step. Given its universality, easy operation, cost-effectivity, high sensitivity and specificity, this strategy provides a new alternative for the detection of ssDNA in the field and in the clinic.

Materials and Methods

Ethics Statement

The tissue homogenate is made from pork, which was purchased from Beijing Chaoshifa Chain Store Co., Ltd. No live animal was used in this study.

Materials and reagents

Oligonucleotides was synthesized and purified through HPLC by Sangon Biotechnology Co., Ltd. (Shanghai, China). The sequences are listed in Table 1. The fluorescent dyes SYBR Green II (10,000× concentrated), SYBR Gold (10,000× concentrated), and PicoGreen dsDNA Reagent and Kits (200× concentrated, including 100 μg·mL^{-1} Lambda DNA standard) were purchased from Invitrogen (CA, USA). S1 nuclease was obtained from Fermentas (Beijing, China) and Takara Biotechnology Co., Ltd (Dalian, China). 96 well black polystyrene microplate (12 strips of 8 wells), MaxiSorp, were purchased from NUNC (Roskilde, Denmark). DNA hybridization buffer (HB) was prepared using Milli-Q water: 50 mM Tris-HCl buffer (pH 8.0), 0.9% (W/V) NaCl. Synthesized ssDNA dry powder samples were dissolved in Milli-Q water to obtain 10 μM stock solutions. Then it was diluted gradually from 64 nM to 50 pM ssDNA standard solutions. All other reagents were of analytical grade.

Parallel analysis of different oligonucleotides lengths and sequences

Oligonucleotides (T5, T10, T15, T20, T25, T30, A5, A10, A15, A20, A25, A30, C10, G10) were used for this analysis. Samples were hybridized in 100 μL HB (containing 20 μL 0.5 μM target ssDNA HB solution and its complementary ssDNA HB solution twice as much) by incubating at room temperature for 5 min [12]. Then 90 μL S1 nuclease solution (30 U, prepared according to the instruction: 0.1 μL S1 nuclease per 30 μL 1× reaction buffer, purchased from Fermentas, Beijing, China) was added and incubated at room temperature for 30 min. After that, 10 μL 20× PicoGreen was added and incubated for another 5 min. Then the fluorescent intensities were recorded using an Infinite F200 multifunction microplate reader (TECAN Austria GmbH, Grödig, Austria). The excitation (Ex) and emission (Em) wavelengths were 480 nm and 520 nm, respectively, and the slit width of filters both were 10 nm. All experiments were repeated three times.

Adaptability study by using three different types of DNA fluorescent dyes

To observe the universality and sensitivity of our approach, we used three different types of fluorescent DNA-dyes to react with three different virus ssDNA: avian influenza H1N1 virus (H1N1-ssDNA), cauliflower mosaic virus (CaM-ssDNA) and hepatitis C virus (HCV-ssDNA) (Table 1). Besides that, the fluorescence intensity with different lengths, different A/T number in oligonucleotides (hepatitis C virus, cauliflower mosaic virus, and H1N1 virus), and their hybrid products were also studied. The reaction system is the same as described above. One group was hybridized with complementary ssDNA solution, and the other group was hybridized without complementary ssDNA, the same volume HB was used to replace the complementary ssDNA solution. Moreover, a system blank (without DNA) has also been detected as a background fluorescent intensity control. After staining with the DNA-dye, the fluorescent spectra and intensities were obtained by an LS-55 Fluorescence Spectrometer (Perkin-Elmer, Connecticut, USA). The slit width of filters both were 10 nm. The Ex and Em wavelengths were as follows:

SYBR Green II, Ex 497 nm, Em 520 nm;
SYBR Gold, Ex 495 nm, Em 537 nm;
PicoGreen, Ex 480 nm, Em 520 nm.

Target sequence-specificity measurements

All assay conditions were the same as described in "parallel analysis" section, except the concentrations of targets: H1N1, CaM, HCV virus ssDNA (Table 1) standard solutions (0, 0.05, 0.5, 1, 2, 4, 8, 16, 32, 64 nM) and additional 5 ng·mL^{-1} Lambda DNA standard in every well as external dsDNA contamination, for their linear ranges in potential interference surroundings. The fluorescent intensities were recorded using an Infinite F200 multifunction microplate reader. Their linear ranges were

Table 1. Synthesized oligonucleotide sequences used in the experiments.

DNA	DNA base sequence	Total bases	A/T number	C/G number
H1N1-ssDNA	5′-CTACCATGCGAACAATTCAACCGACACTGTT-3′	31	17	14
C-H1N1-ssDNA	5′-AACAGTGTCGGTTGAATTGTTCGCATGGTAG-3′	31	17	14
CaM-ssDNA	5′-CATCGTTGAAGATGCCTCTGCCG-3′	23	10	13
C-CaM-ssDNA	5′-CGGCAGAGGCATCTTCAACGATG-3′	23	10	13
HCV-ssDNA	5′-TAATGAGGGCTGCGGGTGGG-3′	20	7	13
C-HCV-ssDNA	5′-CCCACCCGCAGCCCTCATTA-3′	20	7	13
H1N1-1-G	5′-AACAGTGTCGGTTGAATTGTTCG**G**ATGGTAG-3′	31	17	14
H1N1-1-A	5′-AACAGTG**A**CGGTTGAATTGTTCGCATGGTAG-3′	31	17	14
H1N1-2-CG	5′-AACAGT**C**TCGGTTGAATTGTTCG**G**ATGGTAG-3′	31	17	14
H1N1-2-AT	5′-AACAGTG**A**CGGTTGA**T**TTGTTCGCATGGTAG-3′	31	17	14
H1N1-3-CCG	5′-AACAGT**C**TCGGTT**C**AATTGTTCG**G**ATGGTAG-3′	31	17	14
H1N1-3-ATT	5′-AACAGTG**A**CGGTTGA**T**TTGTTCGC**T**TGGTAG-3′	31	17	14
A5, A10, A15, A20, A25, A30	All of the bases are adenine and the number is adenine number.			
T5, T10, T15, T20, T25, T30	All of the bases are thymine and the number is thymine number.			
G10	All of the bases are guanosine and the number is guanosine number.			
C10	All of the bases are cytosine and the number is cytosine number.			

C-H1N1-ssDNA, C-CaM-ssDNA, C-HCV-ssDNA: complementary DNA of H1N1, CaM, HCV, respectively. H1N1-1-G, H1N1-1-A, H1N1-2-CG, H1N1-2-AT, H1N1-3-CCG, H1N1-3-ATT; complementary DNA of H1N1 with one to three base mismatches, "-G, -A, -CG, -AT, -CCG, -ATT" are the variations.

acquired by deducting Lambda DNA standard background fluorescence first.

In addition, HCV (50 pM and 50 nM) was selected as an example to record the detection limit of this method, while a concentration range of dsDNA contaminations (Lambda DNA) were present. The conditions of this test were as follows: apparatus, Infinite F200 multifunction microplate reader; dye, SYBR Gold; Ex 492 nm, Em 550 nm; slit width of filters, both were 10 nm.

Method selectivity for mismatches

Method selectivity was assessed by using one to three base mutations of H1N1 complementary ssDNA (Table 1). All assay conditions were the same as described in "parallel analysis" section. The instrument parameters of this test were as follows: Ex 492 nm, Em 550 nm (dye, SYBR Gold); slit width of filters, both were 10 nm.

Evaluation of the strategy using 4% tissue homogenate samples

In order to illustrate the practical use of this method, 4% pork muscle tissue homogenate (final concentration) was used to simulate the reality, and 50 pM H1N1, CaM, and HCV virus ssDNAs in the tissue homogenate have been directly detected. The procedures are as follows:

10% pork muscle tissue homogenate (prepared by HB) were denatured for 10 min at 95°C. Then, it was centrifuged for 5 min at 5000 rpm, and the supernatant was transferred to a clean test tube. 20 μL 0.5 μM target ssDNA HB solution and 40 μL 0.5 μM complementary ssDNA HB solution were pipetted into a well and hybridized in 80 μL 10% pork muscle tissue homogenate. For control groups, 40 μL 0.5 μM complementary ssDNA HB solutions were replaced by HB; for blank control, we used 60 μL HB instead of all DNA solutions in the experiment. After incubating for 5 min at room temperature, 40 μL S1 nuclease solution (36 U, prepared according to the instruction: 0.1 μL S1 nuclease per 20 μL 1× reaction buffer, purchased from Takara, Dalian, China) was added and incubated at room temperature for 30 min. Finally, 20 μL 10× SYBR Gold was added and incubated for another 5 min, and then the fluorescent intensities were recorded (final concentration of tissue homogenate is 4%). The excitation (Ex) and emission (Em) wavelengths settings of Infinite F200 multifunction microplate reader were 492 nm and 550 nm, respectively, and the slit width of filters both were 10 nm. Experiments were repeated three times.

Statistical Analysis

All statistical analyses were performed using IBM SPSS Statistics (Version 19) software. Data are expressed as the mean ± standard deviation. Group comparisons were carried out by using standard t-test, and the significance level was measured at less than 0.05.

Results and Discussion

The simple detection strategy is presented in Fig. 1. In this strategy, S1 nuclease plays an important role which degrades single-stranded nucleic acid or cleaves dsDNA at the single-stranded region caused by a nick, gap, mismatch or loop. This ability makes it feasible to cleavage the possible small ssDNA 'bubbles' surrounding the mismatch site induced by the complementary ssDNA [10,11], which gives the strategy a discrimination capability of sequence mismatches. Additionally, S1 nuclease could also eliminate excessive complementary ssDNA or other

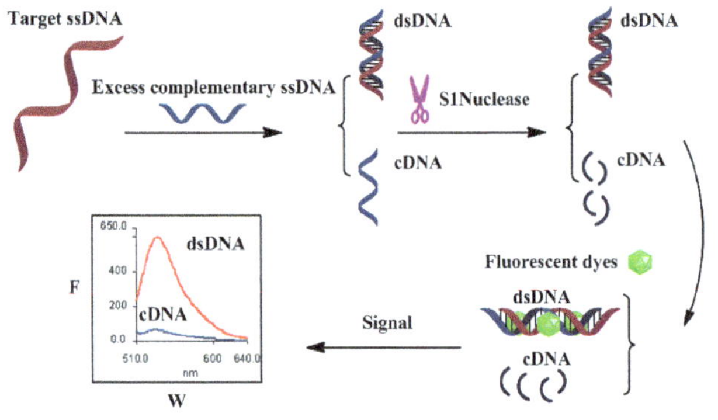

Figure 1. Illustration of the label-free ssDNA detection strategy for detecting sequence-specific ssDNA target with its complementary ssDNA, S1 nuclease and DNA fluorescent dyes.

single-stranded nucleic acid contaminations to decrease non-specific fluorescent background, therefore enhance the sensitivity and practicability of the proposed method.

As can be seen from Fig. 2A, the hybridization of virus ssDNA with the complementary ssDNA shows significantly increasing of fluorescent intensity and gives a high F/F0 value (F0 represents the fluorescent intensity of solution blank containing S1 nuclease, HB solution and DNA dyes, and F represents the fluorescent intensity of the solution as described above upon addition of target ssDNA, or target ssDNA and its complementary sequence). Since SYBR Gold exhibits >1000-fold fluorescence enhancement after binding to double- or single- stranded DNA or RNA [13], it still has excellent discrimination ability whatever there was 50 nM excessive complementary ssDNA with the S1 nuclease addition. This discrimination ability also enabled it to detect the samples in complex conditions directly. Fig. 2B is the corresponding results of the practical use. In 4% pork tissue homogenate, samples (50 nM) were determined in order to show in parallel the anti-interference capacity of the method, and the test reproduced the result of Fig. 2A. Besides that, a concentration range of lambda dsDNA was used as external contamination to investigate its discrimination ability. HCV as the lowest fluorescence efficiency sample in this test (Fig. 2A, Fig. 2B), was employed as the target to find this limit. Fig. 2C and Fig. 2D are the results of this test. 50 pM HCV-ssDNA (containing 0.5 $\mu g{\cdot}mL^{-1}$ Lambda DNA as external dsDNA contamination) induced the fluorescence increase were shown in Fig. 2C, and result was significant ($P<0.01$); also, 50 nM HCV-ssDNA can be detected in 5 $\mu g{\cdot}mL^{-1}$ Lambda DNA standard solution, $P<0.01$. Since most of the currently used methods for ssDNA detection (PCR, probe hybridization, etc.) need an extraction and purification step, this strategy would be a good alternative choice to simplify the detection of pathogens in the field and in the clinic.

Moreover, two other different fluorescent DNA-dyes SYBR Green II and PicoGreen were tested the universality of this approach. PicoGreen represents dsDNA specific dye and SYBR Green II represents ssDNA dye [14] while the above mentioned SYBR Gold is a universal nucleic acid fluorescence dye for double- or single-stranded DNA or RNA. As shown in Fig. 3, it is interesting to find that all of three DNA dyes can detect target viruses ssDNA efficiently at the presence of S1 nuclease while PicoGreen gives the highest quantum yield upon binding to dsDNA or ssDNA [15].

Compared with Zeng's ssDNA detection method using complementary ssDNA without S1 nuclease [12], the proposed

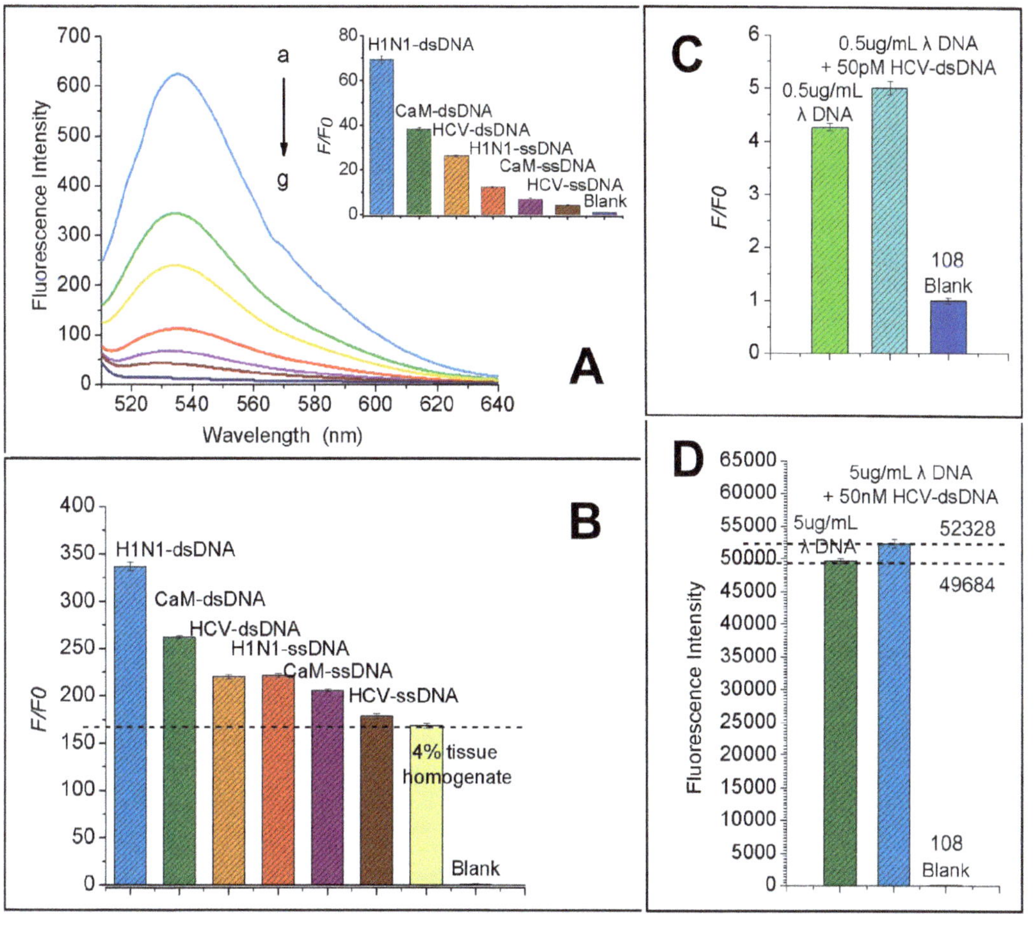

Figure 2. Detection results of Sequence-specificity ssDNA in different surroundings. (A). Fluorescence intensities of three viruses ssDNA and their hybridized products after S1 nuclease-mediated cleavage using SYBR Gold (1×). The concentration of target ssDNAs are 50 nM, and their complementary ssDNAs are 100 nM. a, H1N1-dsDNA; b, CaM-dsDNA; c, HCV-dsDNA; d, H1N1-ssDNA; e, CaM-ssDNA; f, HCV-ssDNA; g, blank. (B). Fluorescence intensities of three viruses ssDNA and their hybridized products in 4% pork muscle tissue homogenate after S1 nuclease-mediated cleavage using SYBR Gold (1×). The concentration of target ssDNAs are 50 nM, and their complementary ssDNAs are 100 nM. (C). Fluorescence intensities of 50 pM HCV-ssDNA and its hybridized products in 0.5 $\mu g \cdot mL^{-1}$ Lambda DNA standard solution after S1 nuclease-mediated cleavage using SYBR Gold (1×). (D). Fluorescence intensities of 50 nM HCV-ssDNA and its hybridized products in 5 $\mu g \cdot mL^{-1}$ Lambda DNA standard solution after S1 nuclease-mediated cleavage using SYBR Gold (1×).

method in this study shows high sensitivity, specificity and universality. It could not only detect H1N1 virus sequence but also CaM and HCV. The F/F0 value of HCV, which was reported that could not be detected by using ordinary nucleic acid fluorescent gel stains in Zeng's articles [12,16], could be detected in our research by all of the three dyes, and their F/F0 values are 17.05 (SYBR Green II), 26.43 (SYBR Gold), and 63.60 (PicoGreen). From the data, we could find that even for HCV detection, all of the F/F0 values of three dyes are higher than H1N1 in previous report [12]. We considered it as a result of S1 nuclease-mediated cleavage of redundant complementary ssDNA and nonspecific hybridization.

The effects of nucleotide composition and lengths of target ssDNA on the fluorescence intensity were investigated using different lengths oligonucleotides (5, 10, 15, 20, 25, and 30 bases) with different bases (A/T and G/C). From Fig. 4B, we could find that, compared to A/T, the G/C oligonucleotides only produced a low fluorescence signal that means PicoGreen has the nucleotide selectivity and A/T base pair playing a dominant role in the fluorescence intensity increasing. In addition (Fig. 4B), the fluorescence intensity increased significantly with increasing target ssDNA lengths. As a result of S1 nuclease-mediated cleavage, the fluorescence intensities of single-strand oligonucleotides were almost been eliminated while the fluorescence signals of their hybrid products were very strong.

Poly (T) and poly (A) with different lengths was used to further study the effect of ssDNA length on the fluorescence intensity. As shown in Fig. 4B, When different lengths of oligonucleotides were hybridized (A30 hybrid with T5, T10, T15, T20, T25 and T30 respectively or T5 hybrid with A5, A10, A15, A20, A25 and A30 respectively), the increasing fluorescence intensity has positive correlation with the lengths of hybridized dsDNA as a result of S1 nuclease-mediated cleavage of redundant ssDNA, like "A30+T5" and "A5+T5". That means the complementary sequence should have at least the same length as the target ssDNA to obtain high sensitivity by using the proposed method. The results further confirmed the S1 nuclease role in sensitivity and specificity of the proposed method as assumed above.

From Fig. 4A and 4B, it was shown that even A5/T5 hybrid products produced a fluorescence intensity of about 1000; the A10/T10 gave nearly 5000 fluorescence intensity. In Fig. 4A, the fluorescence intensity was increased by 8.27 folds from five A/T

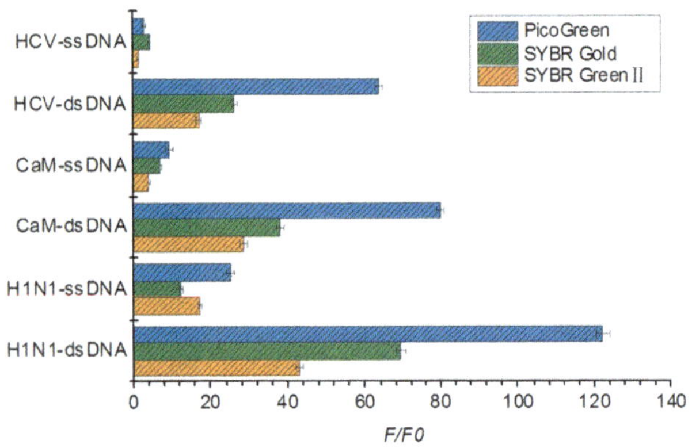

Figure 3. F/F0 values of three viruses and three types of dyes obtained from the proposed strategy. The concentrations of target ssDNA and their complementary ssDNAs are 50 nM and 100 nM respectively, and the concentration of dyes is 1×. F0 represents the fluorescent intensity of solution blank containing S1 nuclease, HB solution and DNA dyes, and F represents the fluorescent intensity of the solution as described above upon addition of target ssDNA, or target ssDNA and its complementary sequence.

base pairs to ten A/T base pairs (A5/T5 to A30/T10, Fig. 4A, green bar). Back to the HCV ssDNA we detected above, though there are only seven A/T, HCV ssDNA still gave high fluorescence intensity and could be easily detected. The results suggested that the A/T number in target ssDNAs is the key of the sensitivity of the strategy and more than five A/T is needed to use the proposed method.

To further demonstrate the proposed method sensitivity and specificity, a series of concentrations of three virus ssDNA were mixed with 5 ng·mL^{-1} Lambda DNA which was used as external

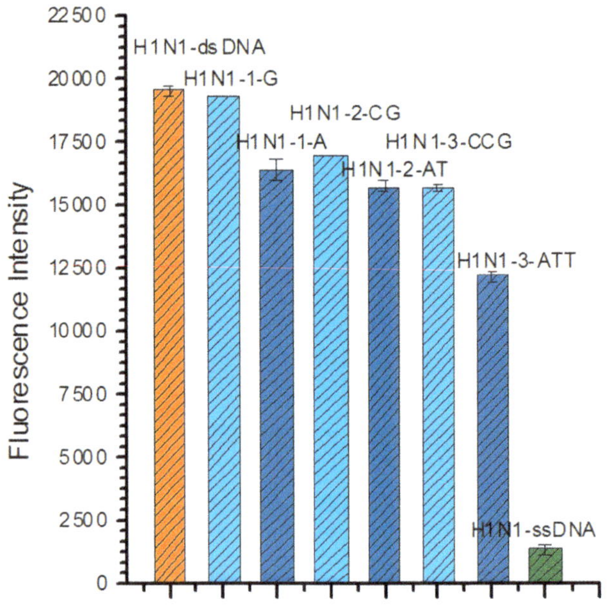

Figure 5. Method selectivity for mismatches (H1N1, 1×SYBR Gold). H1N1-1-G, H1N1-1-A: one base mismatch and the mismatched base is "G", "A", respectively. H1N1-2-CG, H1N1-2-AT: two bases mismatches and the mismatched bases are "CG", "AT", respectively. H1N1-3-CCG, H1N1-3-ATT: three bases mismatches and the mismatched bases are "CCG", "ATT", respectively. The concentration of all target ssDNAs is 50 nM, and their complementary ssDNAs is 100 nM.

dsDNA contamination. The fluorescent intensities were recorded by subtracting the background fluorescence of Lambda DNA. The linear range and sensitivity for three virus ssDNA were obtained as shown in Fig. 4C. The S1 nuclease-mediated cleavage can

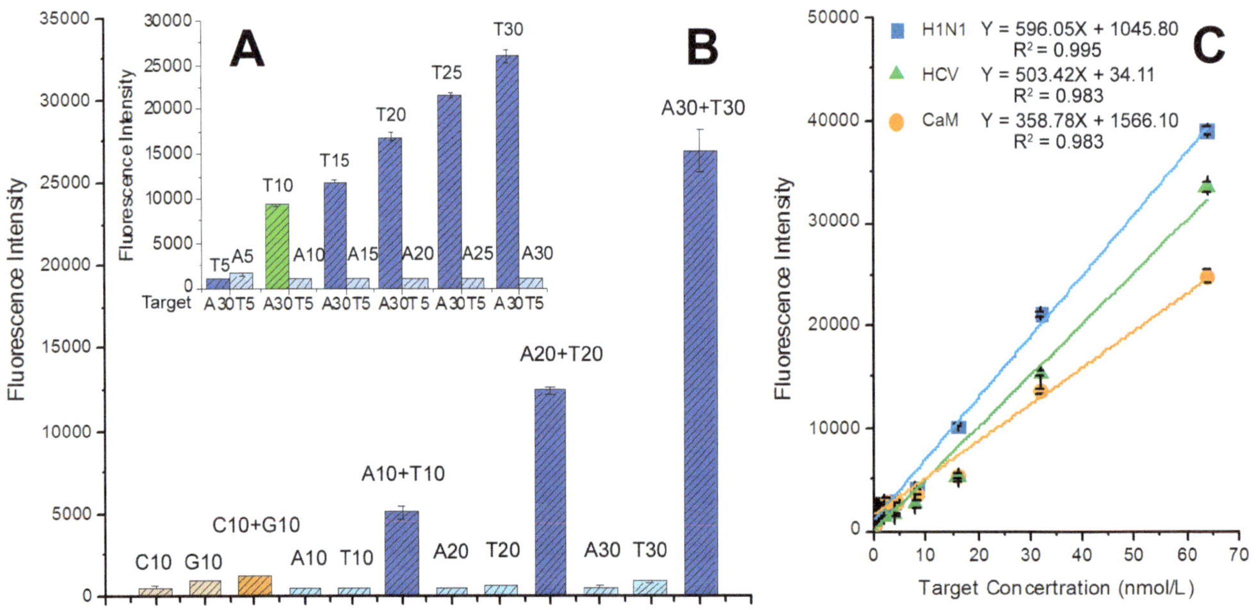

Figure 4. Fluorescence intensity of oligonucleotides hybridized products with 1× PicoGreen after S1 nuclease-mediated cleavage. The concentration of oligonucleotides and their complementary oligonucleotides is 50 nM and 100 nM respectively. (A) The effects of lengths of target ssDNA on fluorescence intensity. (B) The effects of nucleotide composition of target ssDNA on fluorescence intensity. (C) Linearity of the proposed method (three virus ssDNA). Plots of fluorescence intensity versus different concentrations of target ssDNA hybridized products (linear range, 50 pM–64 nM).

increase the fluorescent signal-to-noise ratio by reducing nonspecific background fluorescence and the measured fluorescence intensities are linearly proportional to the concentrations of the target ssDNA. As showed in Fig. 4C, for H1N1, a linear relationship of Y = 596.05X+1045.80 was found in the range of 50 pM–64 nM with $R^2 = 0.995$ and a detection limit (defined as mean of blank control +3 times the standard deviation) of 17.91 pM (n = 3); for CaM, Y = 358.78X+1566.10 with a liner range from 50 pM to 64 nM, $R^2 = 0.983$ and a detection limit of 45.23 pM; and for HCV, Y = 503.42X+34.11 with a liner range from 50 pM to 64 nM, $R^2 = 0.983$ and a detection limit of 40.51 pM. The results were also further evidences that the proposed method could specifically detect the target ssDNA even in contaminant-ridden samples. The present detection limits were much lower than that of the reported one (H1N1, 480 pM, and the other two viruses could not be quantitatively detected by common DNA dyes) [12].Thus, the high sensitivity and specificity of the strategy may fulfill the requirement for the sensitive and quantitative evaluation of most of ssDNAs.

Additionally, the method selectivity for mismatches was assessed too. By using one to three base mutations of H1N1 complementary ssDNA (Table 1), it exhibited a good selectivity for mismatches. From Fig. 5, we could find a downtrend from perfect matched H1N1-dsDNA to three base pairs mismatches, though, compare to H1N1-dsDNA a "G" variation in the sequence could not give out a significant difference (P = 0.132). However, the difference of H1N1-dsDNA and an "A" variation (or two base pairs mismatches) were significant (P<0.01). In reality, SNP-s or other variations could potentially affect the detection of the target DNA and might lead to underestimation. Alternatively, incorrect pairing to non-specific contaminating DNA (that might occur in PCR too) might also lead to overestimation of the target DNA. This experiment presented the signal changes when there are one to three mismatches between target and probe DNA. It provided a good proof for the possible use of this method in related fields in the future.

Conclusions

In this paper, we have presented a simple, sensitive, and specific label-free strategy for ssDNA detection by using its complementary ssDNA, S1 nuclease and nucleic acid fluorescent dyes. The introduction of S1 nuclease enhanced the fluorescent signal-to-noise ratio by clearing away other single-stranded nucleic acid contaminations, redundant complementary ssDNA, and possibly mismatched double strand DNAs. By taking advantage of the super fluorescence efficiency and well sequence specificity of this method, it can detect target ssDNA in complex samples directly and exhibits a high sensitivity and specificity towards target ssDNA (e.g. H1N1, with a detection limit of 17.91 pM and two base pairs mismatches). Moreover, the strategy is facile and cost-effective, and can provide a universal platform for sensitive detection of various ssDNA and RNA in the field and in the clinic.

Author Contributions

Conceived and designed the experiments: AC ZG. Performed the experiments: ZG JL WB ZL XJ. Analyzed the data: AL GL SY. Contributed reagents/materials/analysis tools: AL SY GL. Wrote the paper: AL ZG.

References

1. Zhang Y, Liu S, Wang L, Luo Y, Tian J, et al. (2012) Novel Use of Poly(3,4-ethylenedioxythiophene) Nanoparticles for Fluorescent Nucleic Acid Detection. Acs Combinatorial Science 14: 191–196.
2. Tian J, Zhao H, Liu M, Chen Y, Quan X (2012) Detection of influenza A virus based on fluorescence resonance energy transfer from quantum dots to carbon nanotubes. Analytica Chimica Acta 723: 83–87.
3. Sun W, Zhang Y, Ju X, Li G, Gao H, et al. (2012) Electrochemical deoxyribonucleic acid biosensor based on carboxyl functionalized graphene oxide and poly-L-lysine modified electrode for the detection of tlh gene sequence related to vibrio parahaemolyticus. Analytica Chimica Acta 752: 39–44.
4. Papadopoulou E, Bell SEJ (2012) Label-Free Detection of Nanomolar Unmodified Single- and Double-Stranded DNA by Using Surface-Enhanced Raman Spectroscopy on Ag and Au Colloids. Chemistry-a European Journal 18: 5394–5400.
5. Hu Y, Li F, Han D, Wu T, Zhang Q, et al. (2012) Simple and label-free electrochemical assay for signal-on DNA hybridization directly at undecorated graphene oxide. Analytica Chimica Acta 753: 82–89.
6. Du M, Yang T, Li X, Jiao K (2012) Fabrication of DNA/graphene/polyaniline nanocomplex for label-free voltammetric detection of DNA hybridization. Talanta 88: 439–444.
7. Dong H, Zhang J, Ju H, Lu H, Wang S, et al. (2012) Highly Sensitive Multiple microRNA Detection Based on Fluorescence Quenching of Graphene Oxide and Isothermal Strand-Displacement Polymerase Reaction. Analytical Chemistry 84: 4587–4593.
8. Zhou W-J, Chen Y, Corn RM (2011) Silica nanoparticles as collectors and detectors for nucleic acids detection and enhanced SPR imaging measurements. Abstracts of Papers of the American Chemical Society 241.
9. Liu M, Yuan M, Lou X, Mao H, Zheng D, et al. (2011) Label-free optical detection of single-base mismatches by the combination of nuclease and gold nanoparticles. Biosensors & Bioelectronics 26: 4294–4300.
10. Demidov V, Frank-Kamenetskii MD, Egholm M, Buchardt O, Nielsen PE (1993) Sequence selective double strand DNA cleavage by peptide nucleic acid (PNA) targeting using nuclease S1. Nucleic Acids Research 21: 2103–2107.
11. Doyle SR, Chan CK, Grant WN (2011) Enhanced annealing of mismatched oligonucleotides using a novel melting curve assay allows efficient in vitro discrimination and restriction of a single nucleotide polymorphism. BMC biotechnology 11: 83.
12. Zeng G-P, Xiang D-S, Cai J-Z (2012) A new trace analytic method for the determination of sequence-specific DNA with fluorescent probes. Analytical Letters 45: 2334–2343.
13. Tuma RS, Beaudet MP, Jin X, Jones LJ, Cheung C-Y, et al. (1999) Characterization of SYBR Gold Nucleic Acid Gel Stain: A Dye Optimized for Use with 300-nm Ultraviolet Transilluminators. Analytical Biochemistry 268: 278–288.
14. Battaglia C, Salani G, Consolandi C, Bernardi LR, De Bellis G (2000) Analysis of DNA microarrays by non-destructive fluorescent staining using SYBR green II. Biotechniques, 29: 78–81
15. Cosa G, Focsaneanu KS, McLean JRN, McNamee JP, Scaiano JC (2001) Photophysical Properties of Fluorescent DNA-dyes Bound to Single- and Double-stranded DNA in Aqueous Buffered Solution. Photochemistry and Photobiology 73: 585–599.
16. Zeng G-P, Xiang D-S, He-ZK (2011) Fluorimetric Method for the Determination of Sequence- Specific DNA with the Fluorescent Dye Hoechst 33258. Acta Chimica Sinica 69: 1450–1456.

Errors Affect Hypothetical Intertemporal Food Choice in Women

Manuela Sellitto[1,2], Giuseppe di Pellegrino[1,2]*

1 Dipartimento di Psicologia, Università di Bologna, Bologna, Italy, 2 Centro studi e ricerche in Neuroscienze Cognitive, Polo Scientifico-Didattico di Cesena, Cesena, Italy

Abstract

Growing evidence suggests that the ability to control behavior is enhanced in contexts in which errors are more frequent. Here we investigated whether pairing desirable food with errors could decrease impulsive choice during hypothetical temporal decisions about food. To this end, healthy women performed a Stop-signal task in which one food cue predicted high-error rate, and another food cue predicted low-error rate. Afterwards, we measured participants' intertemporal preferences during decisions between smaller-immediate and larger-delayed amounts of food. We expected reduced sensitivity to smaller-immediate amounts of food associated with high-error rate. Moreover, taking into account that deprivational states affect sensitivity for food, we controlled for participants' hunger. Results showed that pairing food with high-error likelihood decreased temporal discounting. This effect was modulated by hunger, indicating that, the lower the hunger level, the more participants showed reduced impulsive preference for the food previously associated with a high number of errors as compared with the other food. These findings reveal that errors, which are motivationally salient events that recruit cognitive control and drive avoidance learning against error-prone behavior, are effective in reducing impulsive choice for edible outcomes.

Editor: Luigi Cattaneo, Università di Trento, Italy

Funding: This work was supported by a Programmi di Ricerca Scientifica di Rilevante Interesse Nazionale (PRIN) grant from Ministero Istruzione Università e Ricerca (PRIN 2010, protocol number: 2010XPMFW4_009) awarded to GdP. The funders had no role in study design, data collection and analysis, decision to publish, or preparation of the manuscript.

* Email: g.dipellegrino@unibo.it

Introduction

There is increasing incidence of eating disorders, frequently resulting in obesity or other chronic weight problems (e.g., [1–4]). These abnormal behaviors reflect exceeding appetitive motivation to obtain and consume palatable edible reinforcers immediately (frequently sweet high-fat foods, e.g., [5,6]), over long-term benefits of following a healthy diet, which requires capacity for eating control [7,8]. The ability to forgo sooner gratification in favor of delayed reward is crisply captured by intertemporal choice paradigms (e.g., [9]), in which decisions involve smaller-immediate rewards vs. larger-later rewards (e.g., [10,11]). Usually, the subjective value (i.e., the utility depending on specific characteristics of a subject) of potential reward is weakened (discounted), as a function of the time until its delivery (the so-called delay or temporal discounting phenomenon; e.g., [12–17]). Suboptimal intertemporal choice (i.e., increased sensitivity to immediate temptations and increased temporal discounting) is a core feature of impulsivity (e.g., [18]) and it has been related to several pathological conditions, including drug addiction and obesity (e.g., [18–27]). Individuals suffering from eating disorders have enhanced attentional bias toward food cues [28,29], as well as increased reinforcing value placed on food [30]. However, the simple visual exposure to tempting food is a powerful trigger for immediate consumption even in healthy population [31,32].

In order to resist successfully to immediate gratification in the service of a long-term good, one must be able to control the self and refrain one's natural impulse to consume now. Self-control is clearly related to cognitive control, and involves the capacity individuals have to override or alter their predominant response tendencies, thereby allowing other more appropriate responses [33]. But how a person knows when to recruit self-control strategies? Both theoretical perspectives and empirical findings suggest that the ability to control behavior is enhanced in contexts in which errors are more frequent [34]. Errors are typically highly arousing, aversive events that elicit compensatory responses [35]. Importantly, errors represent lapses in performance (and utility) and signal the need to augment on-line the top-down control for the current and future behaviour [36]. Indeed, they drive avoidance learning against error-prone, maladaptive responses and thereby they contribute to the optimization of decision-making performance [37–40]. As aversive events, errors produce a negative neural wave (error-related negativity, ERN; [41,42]), generated in the anterior cingulate cortex (ACC) (e.g., [43]), both when subjects become aware of having committed a mistake and when they are not explicitly aware of making the error [43–44]. It has been suggested that the ERN may signify affective processing in response to errors [45], and individuals with larger ERNs showed enhanced avoidance learning for events associated with negative outcomes ([39–40,46]; see also [47]).

Here we investigated whether pairing desirable foods with errors could signal a performance-related cost (i.e., a loss in reward) and drive increased compensatory self-control strategies, thereby reducing impatient food choices [39,47]. To this aim, participants performed a Stop-signal task (adapted from [48]) in which two different foods served as cues predicting different error likelihoods in performance, high and low, respectively. Following the Stop-signal task, we measured participants' intertemporal preference for the two food items using separate Temporal Discounting tasks (adapted from [49]). More specifically, participants decided between smaller amounts of one food available immediately and larger amounts of the same food delivered after a variable delay. We expected reduced impulsive preferences for the food associated with the high-error rate as compared to the food associated with the low-error rate. Furthermore, we controlled for participants' hunger since it is known to influence the immediate evaluation of food items (e.g., [50–53]) by increasing food reinforcing value and, consequently, the discounting of future amounts of rewards [7,54–56].

Finally, since recent findings highlighted that women and men have different behavioral (e.g., [57–58]) and neural (e.g., [59–61]) responses to food cues, hunger, and satiation, we tested female participants only, to control for sources of variability.

In line with our prediction, results showed that pairing food with errors reduced impulsive choices for the food associated with the high-error rate compared with the food associated with the low-error rate, by controlling for hunger level. This result indicates that the aversive nature of errors, by signalling increased need of adaptive strategies, can be transferred on food when it has to be chosen, and that this effect is modulated by the food-related motivational state of participants. That is, participants with low level of hunger showed reduced impulsive preference for the food previously associated with a high number of errors as compared with the other food, whereas participants with higher level of hunger failed to reveal difference in the TD rates for the two foods.

Materials and Methods

Ethics statement

The study involved healthy young adult females. All subjects gave written informed consent according to the ethical guidelines of the Declaration of Helsinki [62]. The institutional Ethical Committee of the Department of Psychology of the University of Bologna specifically approved this work.

Participants

Forty young adult females took part in the study (see Table 1 for demographic information). All participants were not taking psychoactive drugs, they were not on a diet, and they were free of current or past psychiatric or neurological illness as determined by history. Subjects remained naïve as to the purpose of the study until debriefing, at the end of the experimental session.

Procedure

After collecting participants' demographics (Table 1), including height and weight in order to calculate their body mass index (BMI; [63–64]), subjects first rated their hunger level and their willingness to eat at the time of the experiment six foods depicted in picture. Following the rating session, participants performed a Stop-signal task and, afterwards, two Temporal Discounting tasks. At the end, participants filled out the External Eating Behavior subscale of the Dutch Eating Behavior Questionnaire ($DEBQ_{EEB}$; [65]).

Ratings

Hunger. Participants rated on 11-points scale their hunger level at the time of the experiment (*baseline hunger*, from −5, "not hungry at all", to 5, "extremely hungry").

Food. Following the hunger rating, participants rated on 11-points scale the willingness to eat at the moment each of six sweet food items, one at a time (*wanting*, from −5, "not at all", to 5, "extremely"). Foods were presented in high-resolution color pictures (150 dpi), matched for dimension, luminance, and contrast, on a 15-inch computer screen located approximately 40 cm away from the participants. There were no discrepancies between the size of objects depicted on the screen and their real size in the world. All pictures were presented in a random order across participants.

Stimuli selection

Following the rating session, the experimenter chose, individually for each participant, the two foods that obtained the higher score. These two foods were used as stimuli in the following Stop-signal task and in the two Temporal Discounting tasks. Since these two foods obtained often a different evaluation, they were assigned in a counterbalanced order to the two different error conditions of the Stop-signal task (see below for details). We compared stimuli ratings using nonparametric statistics since they were not normally distributed.

Stop-signal task

Based on [48]'s paradigm, a Stop-signal task was adjusted using as cues the two foods previously selected after the rating session. Two types of conditions were included. One condition had a low-error likelihood (Low-Error condition), and the other condition had a high-error likelihood (High-Error condition). One food (Low-Error Food, LEF) was used as cue for the Low-Error condition; the other food (High-Error Food, HEF) was used as cue for the High-Error condition. Hence, for a given trial, food type predicted low- versus high-error likelihood in performance, respectively.

Figure 1 illustrates the experimental paradigm. Each trial began with a black and white picture of one of the two foods appearing for 1000 ms. Later on, the black and white picture became coloured, thus prompting the Go signal. The Go signal required participants to press the down arrow button on the keyboard as

Table 1. Participants' demographic data.

N	Age	Education	BMI	Hunger	Fasting	$DEBQ_{EEB}$
40	25 (0.6)	16 (0.3)	21 (0.5)	1.7 (0.5)	4 (0.5)	3 (0.1)

BMI = Body Mass Index; $DEBQ_{EEB}$ = External Eating Behavior subscale of the Dutch Eating Behavior Questionnaire. Age and education are expressed in years. BMI is expressed in kg/m^2. Fasting is expressed in hours. Numbers in parenthesis are standard errors.

quickly as possible. However, on 33% of the trials, a Stop signal was postponed to the Go signal after a variable Stop-Signal Delay (SSD) relative to the Go signal onset. This Stop signal, a red circle appearing around the coloured picture, indicated that the response to the Go signal was no longer required. Both Go and Stop signals remained visible until a response deadline of 1000 ms after Go signal onset, which indicated a time limit of 1000 ms to produce or not a response. After each trial, a blank screen appeared for a variable intertrial interval (500, 1000, 1500, 2000 ms). Error rates (low vs. high) were explicitly set and controlled by dynamically adjusting the SSDs for each error likelihood condition independently with the use of a staircase algorithm. The Low-Error condition had shorter SSDs, whereas the High-Error condition had longer SSDs [48]. The SSD started at 200 ms (after Go signal onset) for both Low- and High-Error conditions. During the Low-Error condition, if the participant succeeded in withholding the response after the Stop signal, the SSD increased by only 5 ms; conversely, if the subject failed, the SSD decreased by 50 ms on the next trial. During the High-Error condition, if the participant succeeded in withholding the response after the Stop signal, the SSD increased by 50 ms; conversely, if the subject failed, the SSD was decreased by 50 ms on the next trial [66].

After a correct response to the Go signal or a non-response to the Stop signal, the message "Correct!" (in Italian) appeared on the screen. If participant did not respond in time to the Go signal, or if she responded to the Stop signal, a message "Error!" appeared on the screen. If participant responded to the black and white picture, a message "Too early!" appeared on the screen. Trials pertaining to the Low-Error condition and the High-Error condition were released in a random order. All cues and stimuli were presented centrally on a black background.

Participants performed 240 trials in total: 160 Go trials (80 for the Low-Error condition and 80 for the High-Error condition) and 80 Stop trials (40 for the Low-Error condition and 40 for the High-Error condition). The task lasted approximately 16 minutes.

Stop-signal task data analysis. We performed data analysis on the accuracy (number of errors) and the RTs of correct responses vs. errors (no-response trials ignored), for the Low- vs. High-Error condition, and for Go vs. Stop trials [48].

Temporal discounting task

After the Stop-signal task completion, participants underwent to two Temporal Discounting (TD) tasks, administered separately in a counterbalanced order across participants. In each of the two computerized TD tasks, participants performed a series of intertemporal choices. In each trial, they chose between a smaller amount of bites (units) of a hypothetical food [49,67–68] that could be received immediately and a larger amount of bites of the same food that could be received after some specific delay (e.g., [69–70]). One task assessed subjective preferences in time for LEF, and one task assessed subjective preferences in time for HEF. Both LEF and HEF were preselected during the rating session and were the same as in the Stop-signal task.

In each task, participants made five choices at each of six delays: 2 days, 2 weeks, 1 month, 3 months, 6 months, and 1 year. The order of blocks of choices pertaining to different delays was randomly determined across participants. Within each block of five choices, the delayed amount was always 40 units [49]. The amount of the immediate reward, on the other hand, was adjusted based on the participant's choices, using a staircase procedure that converged on the amount of the immediate reward that was equal, in subjective value, to the delayed reward [49]. The first choice was between a delayed amount of 40 units (e.g., 40 bites or tastes of muffin) and an immediate amount of 20 units (e.g., 20 bites of muffin). If the participant chose the immediate reward, then the amount of the immediate reward was decreased on the next trial; if

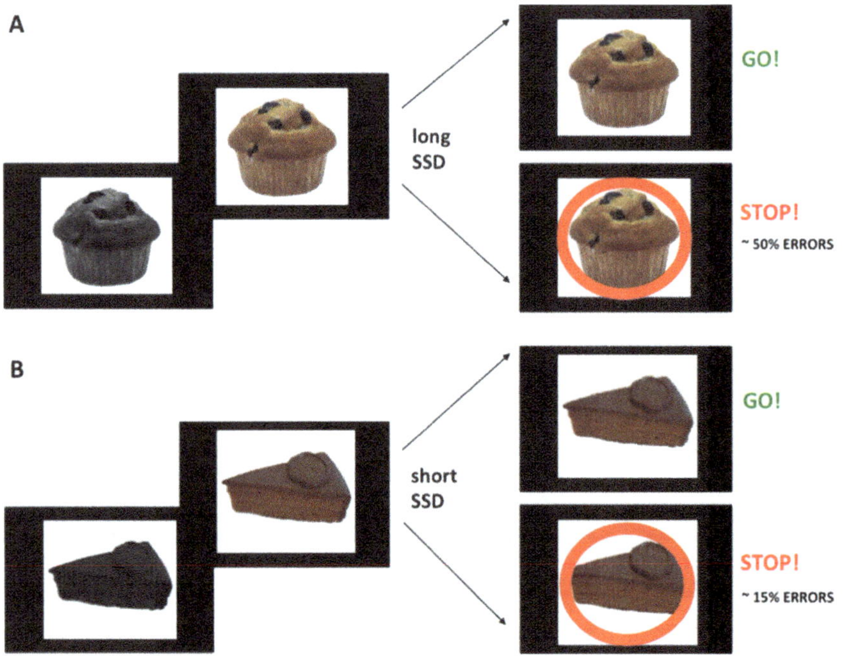

Figure 1. Stop-signal task experimental paradigm. In this trial example, the muffin (A) is assigned to the High-Error condition, whereas the chocolate cake (B) is used as cue for the Low-Error condition. Each trial began with a black and white picture displayed for 1000 ms. Then, the black and white picture became coloured: This represented the Go signal. On 33% of the trials, a Stop signal (a red circle) was postponed to the Go signal after a variable SSD relative to the Go signal onset. The High-Error condition (A) had longer SSDs. The Low-Error condition (B) had shorter SSDs. Both Go and Stop signals remained visible until a response deadline of 1000 ms after Go signal onset in both error conditions.

the subject chose the delayed reward, then the amount of the immediate reward was increased on the next trial. The size of the adjustment in the immediate reward decreased with successive choices: the first adjustment was half of the difference between the immediate and the delayed reward, whereas for subsequent choices it was half of the previous adjustment [70]. This procedure was repeated until the subject had made five choices at one specific delay, after which the subject began a new series of choices at another delay. For each trial in a block, the immediate amount represents the best guess as to the subjective value of the delayed reward. Therefore, the immediate amount that would have been presented on the sixth trial of a delay block was taken as the estimate of the subjective value of the delayed reward at that delay (see also [49]).

Participants were told that, on each trial, two amounts of hypothetical reward would appear on the screen. One could be received right now, and one could be received after a delay. They were explicitly asked to imagine receiving the two amounts of reward, and they were required to indicate the option they preferred by pressing one of two buttons [49,71]. They were informed that there were no correct or incorrect choices. Figure 2 illustrates the experimental paradigm. Each trial began with a 1 s fixation screen, followed by a screen depicting the two available options. The two options appeared on the left and right side of the screen, and clearly indicated the food type, the amount of reward, and the delay of delivery of the reward. After the participants made their choices, the non-preferred option disappeared, whereas the preferred option remained on the screen for 1 s, with a triangle underneath it. The intertrial interval was 1.5 s.

TD data analysis. For each task, the rate at which the subjective value of a reward decays with delay (TD rate) was assessed through the TD parameter (*k*) [72–74]. The hyperbolic function $SV = 1/(1+kD)$, where SV = subjective value (expressed as a fraction of the delayed amount), and D = delay (in days), was fit to the data to determine the *k* constant of the best fitting TD function, using a nonlinear, least-squares algorithm (as implemented in Statistica; Statsoft). The larger the value of *k*, the steeper the discounting function, the more participants were inclined to choose small-immediate amounts over larger-delayed amounts.

Moreover, for comparison purposes, we also assessed the fits to the data of an exponential discounting model. For each TD task, the exponential function $SV = e^{-kD}$ was fit to the data to determine the *k* constant of the best fitting TD function, using the same procedure as for the hyperbolic function.

$DEBQ_{EEB}$

This subscale ([65]; Italian version, [75]) measures the sensitivity to external edible cues, such as during food exposure, as component of eating behaviour [65]. Participants reported for each item the frequency of engagement to the described behaviors on 5-points scale. Higher scores correspond to higher sensitivity to external cues, such as sight and smell of food [65] (see Table 1).

Results

Stimuli selection

The two food cues selected after the rating session had equivalent *wanting* ratings across participants (Wilcoxon signed-rank test, T = 186, p = 0.94).

Stop-signal task

Accuracy. An ANOVA on percentage of errors with condition (Low-Error, High-Error) and trial type (Go, Stop) as within subject factors yielded a significant effect of condition ($F(1, 39) = 1537.53$, $p = 0.000001$), a significant effect of trial type ($F(1, 39) = 844.54$, $p = 0.000001$), and a significant interaction condition×trial type ($F(1, 39) = 1122.91$, $p = 0.000001$). Post hoc comparisons, performed with the Newman-Keuls test, showed that the percentage of errors was significantly higher during the High-Error condition than the Low-Error condition (28% vs. 11%; $p = 0.0001$), and that the number of errors committed during No-go trials was significantly higher than the number of errors committed during Go trials (32% vs. 7%; $p = 0.0001$). Moreover, while the percentage of errors committed during Go trials was the same for both High and Low conditions (7.07% vs. 7.09%; $p = 0.98$), the percentage of errors during No-go trials was significantly higher for the High-Error condition than the Low-Error condition (50% vs. 15%; $p = 0.0001$).

RTs. An ANOVA on RTs for correct trials with condition (Low-Error, High-Error) and trial type (Go, Stop) as within subject factors evidenced a significant effect of condition ($F(1, 39) = 40$, $p = 0.000001$), a significant effect of trial type ($F(1, 39) = 420$, $p = 0.000001$), and a significant interaction condition×trial type ($F(1, 39) = 45.5$, $p = 0.000001$). Post hoc comparisons, performed with the Newman-Keuls test, showed that RTs were significantly higher (i.e., responses were slower) during the High-Error condition than the Low-Error condition (430 ms vs. 405 ms; $p = 0.0001$), and that RTs during Go trials were significantly higher than RTs during No-go trials (454 ms vs. 381 ms; $p = 0.0001$). Moreover, while RTs for correct responses during Go trials were the same for both High and Low conditions (455 ms vs. 453 ms; $p = 0.99$), RTs for correct responses during No-go trials were significantly higher for the High-Error condition than the Low-Error condition (404 ms vs. 357 ms; $p = 0.0001$).

The above results, in line with previous findings (e.g., [48]), support the validity of the Stop-signal paradigm in producing

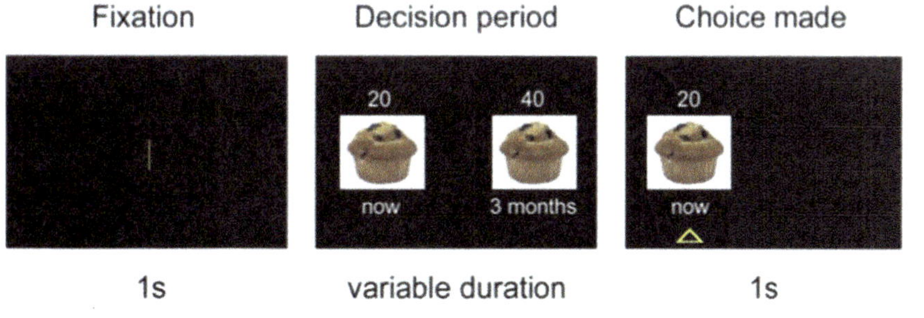

Figure 2. Temporal discounting task experimental paradigm. In each trial, after a 1000 ms fixation period, subjects chose between a small amount of reward delivered immediately and a larger amount of reward delivered after a delay. The preferred option remained highlighted for 1000 ms. Food offered was hypothetical.

different patterns of errors, and are indicative of the higher conflict experienced during the High-Error than in the Low-Error condition. Indeed, participants made clearly a significantly higher number of errors during the High-Error condition when performing Stop trials. These effects were apparently implicit: at debriefing, subjects were mostly unaware of the error manipulation even when directly prompted. This might be explained by the presentation of trials and error-conditions, which were all interspersed randomly, and by the highly demanding nature of the task, thereby requiring participants to stay focused in order to perform the task as much accurately as possible.

TD task

Figure 3 shows TD rate by food type (LEF and HEF). Bars reflect the geometric mean of the TD rate for each food cue – which corresponds to mean of the log-transformed values – and thus provides a better measure of central tendency for positively skewed metrics, such as TD rates, than does the arithmetic mean [49]. We chose bars rather than curves to represent TD rates since *k* values were quite small (e.g., [71,76–77]), in order to visually reveal better the difference between the TD rates for the two foods. The smaller the bar, the smaller the TD rate (less steep discounting), the smaller the number of impulsive choices.

First, subjective preferences were well characterized by hyperbolic functions, with no significant differences in R^2 between LEF and HEF (LEF: 0.68 vs. HEF: 0.65; $F(1, 39) = 0.26$, $p = 0.61$). The absence of differences in R^2 in describing discounting behavior applied to foods associated differently to error likelihoods indicates that error rates did not alter TD in its shape. Moreover, although both the hyperbolic and the exponential functions fit the data well, the hyperbolic function fit better than the exponential across foods. Indeed, when we entered hyperbolic and exponential R^2 scores as the dependent variables in an ANOVA for each food separately, the hyperbolic model fit better than the exponential model for both the LEF (0.68 vs. 0.58; $F(1, 39) = 31.55$, $p = 0.000002$), and the HEF (0.65 vs. 0.59; $F(1, 39) = 18.89$, $p = 0.0001$). Given the superiority of the hyperbolic over the exponential model in describing discounting behavior, hyperbolic *k* values were adopted as measures of TD [49].

Second, the hyperbolic k constants were normally distributed after log-transformation (Kolmogorov–Smirnov $d<0.14$, $p>0.2$ in all cases), and therefore, comparisons were performed using parametric statistical tests.

Thus, hyperbolic *k* values were entered in an ANOVA, with food type (LEF, HEF) as within subject factor, and *baseline* hunger as covariate to control for hunger state. We found a significant effect of food type ($F(1, 38) = 7.65$, $p = 0.01$), a significant effect of *baseline* hunger ($F(1, 38) = 6.53$, $p = 0.01$), and a significant food type×*baseline* hunger interaction ($F(1, 38) = 7.73$, $p = 0.01$). Post-hoc comparisons, performed with the Newman-Keuls test, indicated that HEF was discounted significantly less than LEF (−0.81 vs. −0.61), as determined by hunger level. Please, note that the results of this analysis on TD rates for LEF and HEF remained unaffected by including as covariates BMI and $DEBQ_{EEB}$ scores as well. No significant interaction between these two covariates and the main effect emerged ($F(1, 39)<1.5$, $p>0.23$ in all cases).

To clarify the effect of hunger on TD, we performed a regression analysis to determine the relation between the *baseline* hunger score as continuous dependent variable and the discount rates (*k*) for LEF and HEF as independent variables. We found that hunger was significantly associated with the HEF but not with the LEF (HEF: $\beta = 0.68$ vs. LEF: $\beta = -0.27$; $p = 0.002$) (Figure 4).

To better qualify this effect, we thereby applied a median split (e.g., [77]) on participants' self-reported hunger rates (median = 2.5) to create groups of 20 low- (Low-hunger) and 20 high-hunger (High-hunger) participants thus comparing their TD rates for LEF and HEF. Hyperbolic *k* values were entered in an ANOVA, with group (Low-hunger, High-hunger) as between subject factor and food type (LEF, HEF) as within subjects factor. The analysis yielded no significant effect of group ($F(1, 38) = 1.13$, $p = 0.29$), no significant effect of food type ($F(1, 38) = 2.44$, $p = 0.12$), but a significant group×food type interaction ($F(1, 38) = 7.91$, $p = 0.007$). Post-hoc comparisons, performed with the Newman-Keuls test, indicated that, while Low-hunger participants discounted significantly less the HEF than the LEF (−1.165 vs. −0.6083, $p = 0.01$), the High-hunger participants did not differ between the HEF and the LEF (−0.4581 vs. −0.6169, $p = 0.65$). Note also that the difference between groups was limited to the HEF (Low-hunger: −1.165; High-hunger: −0.4581), whereas this was not the case of the LEF (Low-hunger: −0.6083; High-hunger: −0.6169).

In line with our hypothesis, participants showed reduced sensitivity for immediate amounts of reward (i.e., reduced TD

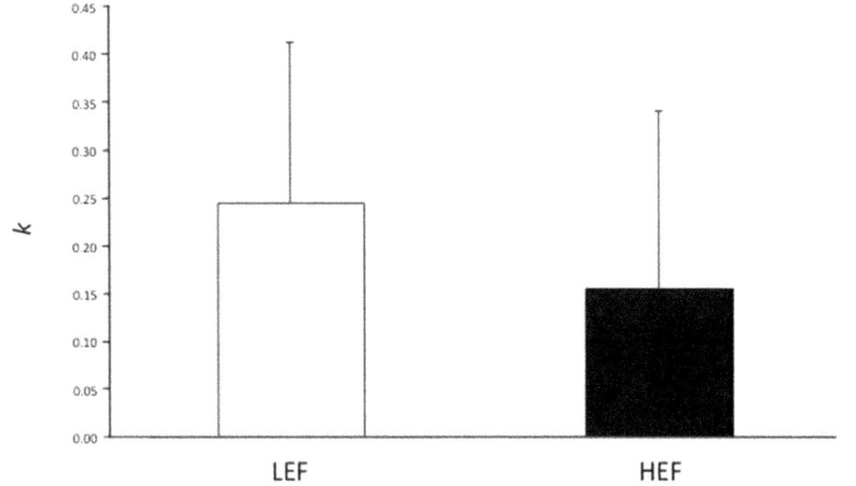

Figure 3. TD rates by food type. Bars reflect the geometric mean of TD rate *k* for LEF and HEF respectively. The smaller the bar, the smaller the TD rate, the smaller the number of impulsive choices. The error bars indicate the SEM.

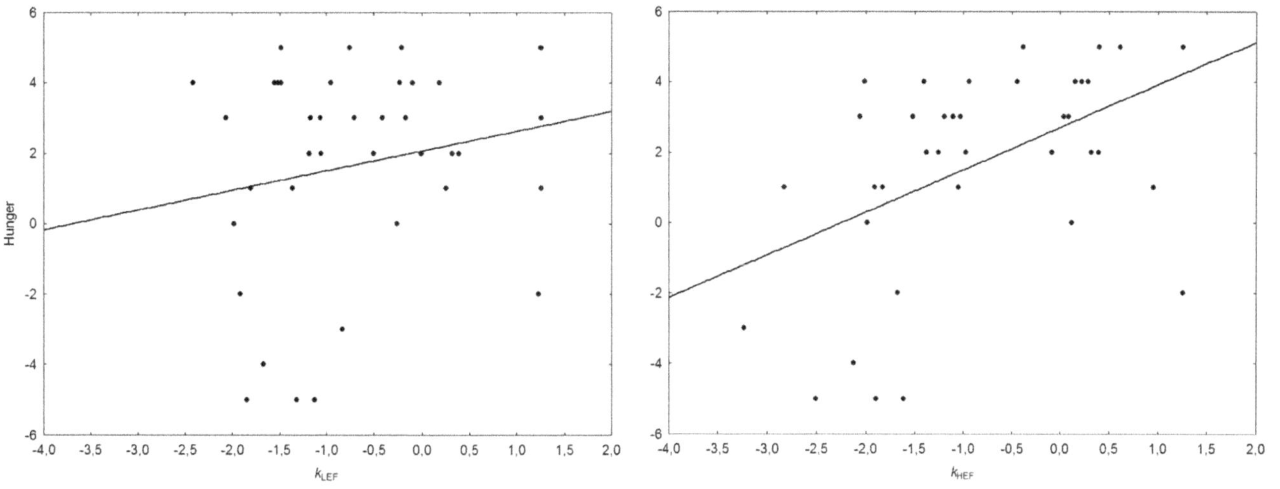

Figure 4. Regression between hunger and TD rates for LEF and HEF, separately. Scatter plot of the correlation between the hunger score and the degree of discounting (Log-*k* scores) for LEF (left panel) and HEF (right panel).

rate) when faced with the food previously associated with a high number of errors compared with the food previously associated with a low number of errors. This effect was modulated by hunger. Specifically, the lower the hunger level, the less participants made impulsive choices when faced with the food paired with high-error rate, whereas, the higher the hunger state, the more participants showed the same degree of discounting for the two foods, suggesting that the two items were comparable in terms of motivational salience.

Discussion

The present study investigated whether pairing food with errors would reduce impulsivity during food intertemporal choice, by enhancing the implementation of adaptive control strategies to promote more appropriate course of action. First, through a Stop-signal task, participants associated a different number of errors (low and high) with two different foods equally rated in the willingness to eat at the beginning of the experiment. Afterwards, they made choices between smaller-immediate and larger-later amounts of the two foods in two TD tasks, separately. Consistent with our hypothesis, foresighted food decisions were enhanced for the food previously associated with a high number of errors as compared with the food previously paired with a low number of errors. Moreover, the effect of reduced sensitivity for immediate amounts of food paired with high-error rate compared with the other food depended upon the hunger level of participants. Indeed, while less hungry individuals showed the expected reduced impatience when faced with the high-error food compared with the other food, hungrier individuals' willingness to wait for future amounts of reward was comparable across the two foods after error manipulation. These findings suggest that, during decision-making for edible rewards, when experiencing high hunger, the error manipulation is not powerful enough in reducing the degree of discounting of future reward previously paired with high-error rate. Indeed, hunger increases the reinforcing value placed on food (e.g., [7,50–56,59–60,79–82]), thereby increasing sensitivity for immediate amounts of reward (i.e., impulsivity). Thus, it might be that participants with high hunger were not able to make long-sighted choice toward the high-error food simply because this food and the low-error food were equally relevant for reducing their current state of need.

Why such errors-food pairing reduced impulsive food choice during intertemporal decisions? One possibility if that the present findings directly reflect inhibition rather than errors during the Stop-signal task, since the low-error condition is associated with successful inhibition, whereas the high-error condition is associated with unsuccessful inhibition. However, if successful inhibition can carry over from the Stop-signal task to intertemporal preference, there would have been decreased impulsive choice for the low-error food as compared with the high-error food. Conversely, our data indicate reduced discounting rate for the high-error food selectively (see also [48]). Moreover, the selective effect on high-error food rules out also the possibility that ego-depletion (e.g., [83]), negative mood [84], or induced stress or frustration [85] throughout the Stop-signal task explained our data, since we would have expected no difference in discount rate between the two foods.

Rather, we submit that errors serve as motivationally salient, warning signals that recruit cognitive control to match its anticipated demand [86]. During intertemporal choice, more visceral and automatic processes interact with more reasoned and rational mechanisms of future planning (e.g., [87]). The desire for sooner gratification competes with long-term gains maximization [9–11,87–88], and increased sensitivity to immediate temptation is a core feature of impulsivity (e.g., [18]), landmark of several pathological conditions, including drug addiction and obesity (e.g., [18–27]). In order to obtain the larger outcome, it is necessary to carefully take into account the tradeoff between costs and benefits associated with options. In this context, errors might act in two ways (e.g., [89]). One possibility is that errors, as lapses in performance, represent warning signals that adaptively increase cognitive control in order to avoid further lapses in utility [36,48]. Thus, in the present study, the high-error food cue, by enhancing the attention toward the increased likelihood of committing an error, would boost self-control over the decision [48,89–90], thereby generating more long-sighted intertemporal choice for that food selectively.

A close related possibility is that, due to their aversive nature, errors [35] would act as teaching signals of avoidance learning against events associated with negative outcomes (i.e., loss in reward) [45–47,91], which occurs through the generation of the ERN (e.g., [35–42,91–92]) in the ACC (e.g., [43]). Thus, errors would activate adaptive adjustments in control processes that minimize costs in performance toward more efficient and controlled strategies and away from error-prone behavior [37–39,91]. On this latter view, errors would act as somatic-markers guiding choice, namely, as anticipatory signals of negative outcome [93–96]. In the present study, errors committed during the Stop-signal task might have marked the high-error food so that this, in future encounters (i.e., during subsequent intertemporal choice), would have triggered adaptive self-control thus suppressing prepotent response (the choice of the tempting immediate reward) in favour of more advantageous course of actions (e.g., [97]). As such, in the present study, errors acted similarly as affective priming, which has the power of shaping even higher cognition as moral judgement (e.g., [98–99]). By inducing long-lasting carryover effect on the subsequent intertemporal choice task, errors induced more self-controlled decisions by warning against error-prone responses, thereby optimizing behavior. We thereby propose that the negative valence of errors alerts organisms toward performance monitoring and, thus, to when self-control is needed, as an *affect alarm model of control* [35,39].

More broadly, it has been suggested that a prerequisite to exercise self-control when facing a temptation is to identify the conflict correctly [100]. For example, a dieter facing a delicious dessert in an isolated occasion is less likely to identify the conflict between her ultimate goal (i.e., losing weight) and the tempting high-caloric food, than when considering dessert for multiple similar future consumptions [100]. Thus, our modified version of the Stop-signal task might have induced subjects to face, in a brief lapse of time, multiple error signals and conflict concerning a specific food, thereby priming avoidance motivation for events associated with negative outcomes and more self-controlled decisions [39–40,46–47].

Finally, since disordered eating behaviors have been recently linked consistently to drug addiction (e.g., [101]), sharing not only behavioral features like impulsivity and executive dysfunction, but also a documented dysregulation of the reward circuit (e.g., [3,102–104]), we suggest to use the method tested here as a clinical training for people suffering from obesity and binge eating disorders. Similarly to a previous study in which alcohol-related stimuli were paired to stop trials in a Go-no-go task [105], thus increasing negative attitudes toward alcohol and reducing alcohol weekly consumption, here the effect of our error manipulation lasted for enough time to influence following intertemporal food decisions through indirect error-food pairing.

Limitations

First, since recent findings highlighted that women and men have different behavioral (e.g., [57–58]) and neural (e.g., [59–61]) responses to food cues, hunger, and satiation, we tested female participants only, in order to control for sources of variability. Thus, we cannot generalize our findings to the population of healthy male young adults, and further research is needed to explore this issue. Moreover, although humans have been found to respond, both behaviorally and neurally, in a similar way to hypothetical and real rewards (e.g., [49,67–68]), further investigation on the effect of error-food pairing should involve choices among real edible outcomes. This will help in avoiding the underestimation of several factors like visceral feelings of nausea and disgust (e.g., [106]), which may influence food decisions.

Second, we chose a Stop-signal task since it is a suitable paradigm to control for participants' error rate. Indeed, we were allowed to induce all subjects making approximately the same number of errors in the low-error condition and in the high-error condition, respectively. Moreover, the low-error food served as control condition, since the adjustment we made after subject's mistakes during the low-error condition (i.e., 5 ms) was negligible, and, as said before, this task is effective in augment cognitive control in the high-error condition, selectively [48]. However, the Stop-signal task used in the present study does not help to unravelling completely between error and inhibition effects on discounting rate, thus further studies involving error task which does not imply the implementation of inhibition is needed to state that one interpretation is more likely than the other (e.g., based on [107–109]).

Acknowledgments

We thank Diego Giusti and Laura Mollica for helping during data collection. We also thank Sara Garofalo, Elena Bertossi, Martin Meier, Caterina Bertini, John Monterosso, and an anonymous reviewer for helpful comments and insightful critiques on this manuscript.

Author Contributions

Conceived and designed the experiments: MS GDP. Performed the experiments: MS. Analyzed the data: MS GDP. Wrote the paper: MS GDP. Read, corrected and approved the final manuscript: MS GDP.

References

1. Haslam DW, James WP (2005) Obesity. Lancet 366: 1197–1209.
2. Knight JA (2011) Diseases and disorders associated with excess body weight. Ann Clin Lab Sci 41: 107–121.
3. Fortuna JL (2012) The obesity epidemic and food addiction: clinical similarities to drug dependence. J Psychoactive Drugs 44: 56–63.
4. Bowden DJ, Kilburn-Toppin F, Scoffings DJ (2013) Radiology of eating disorders: a pictorial review. Radiographics 33: 1171–1193.
5. Davis C, Patte K, Levitan R, Reid C, Tweed S, et al. (2007) From motivation to behaviour: a model of reward sensitivity, overeating, and food preferences in the risk profile for obesity. Appetite 48: 12–19.
6. Dalton M, Blundell J, Finlayson G (2013) Effect of BMI and binge eating on food reward and energy intake: Further evidence for a binge eating subtype of obesity. Obes Facts 6: 348–359.
7. Epstein LH, Salvy SJ, Carr KA, Dearing KK, Bickel WK (2010) Food reinforcement, delay discounting and obesity. Physiol Behav 100: 438–445.
8. Appelhans BM, Woolf K, Pagoto SL, Kristin L, Whited MC, et al. (2011) Inhibiting food reward: delay discounting, food reward sensitivity, and palatable food intake in overweight and obese women. Obesity 19: 2175–2182.
9. Takahashi T, Ikeda K, Hasegawa T (2007) A hyperbolic decay of subjective probability of obtaining delayed rewards. Behav Brain Funct 3: 52.
10. Frederick S, Loewenstein G, O'Donoghue T (2002) Time discounting and time preference: a critical review. J Econ Lit 40: 351–401.
11. Sellitto M, Ciaramelli E, di Pellegrino G (2011) The neurobiology of intertemporal choice: insight from imaging and lesion studies. Rev Neurosci 22: 565–574.
12. Samuelson PA (1937) A note on measurement of utility. Rev Econ Stud 4: 155–161.
13. Ainslie GW (1975) Specious reward: a behavioral theory of impulsiveness and impulse control. Psychol Bull 82: 463–496.
14. Myerson J, Green L (1995) Discounting of delayed rewards: models of individual choice. J Exp Anal Behav 64: 263–276.
15. Cardinal RN, Pennicott DR, Sugathapala CL, Robbins TW, Everitt BJ (2001) Impulsive choice induced in rats by lesions of the nucleus accumbens core. Science 292: 2499–2501.
16. Kalenscher T, Windmann S, Diekamp B, Rose J, Güntürkün O, et al. (2005) Single units in the pigeon brain integrate reward amount and time-to-reward in an impulsive choice task. Curr Biol 15: 594–602.
17. Peters J, Büchel C (2010) Neural representations of subjective reward value. Behav Brain Res 213: 135–141.
18. Takahashi T (2005) Loss of self-control in intertemporal choice may be attributable to logarithmic time-perception. Med Hypotheses 65: 691–693.
19. Mischel W, Shoda Y, Peake PK (1988) The nature of adolescent competencies predicted by preschool delay of gratification. J Pers Soc Psychol 54: 687–699.

20. Davis C, Levitan RD, Muglia P, Bewell C, Kennedy JL (2004) Decision-making deficits and overeating: A Risk model for obesity. Obes Res 12: 929–935.
21. Davis C, Patte K, Curtis C, Reid C (2010) Immediate pleasures and future consequences. A neuropsychological study of binge eating and obesity. Appetite 54: 208–213.
22. Bickel WK, Miller ML, Yi R, Kowal BP, Lindquist DM, et al. (2007) Behavioral and neuroeconomics of drug addiction: competing neural systems and temporal discounting processes. Drug Alcohol Depend 90: 85–91.
23. Weller RE, Cook III E, Avsar K, Cox J (2008) Obese women show greater delay discounting than healthy-weight women. Appetite 51: 563–556.
24. Manwaring JL, Green L, Myerson J, Strube MJ, Wilfley DE (2011) Discounting of various types of rewards by women with and without binge eating disorder: Evidence for general rather than specific differences. Psychol Rec 61: 561–582.
25. Appelhans BM, Waring ME, Schneider KL, Pagoto SL, DeBiasse MA, et al. (2012) Delay discounting and intake of ready-to-eat and away-from-home foods in overweight and obese women. Appetite 59: 576–584.
26. Kishinevsky FI, Cox JE, Murdaugh DL, Stoeckel LE, Cook EW, et al. (2012) fMRI reactivity on a delay discounting task predicts weight gain in obese women. Appetite 58: 582–592.
27. Bickel WK, Wilson GA, Franck CT, Terry Mueller E, Jarmolowicz DP, et al. (2013) Using crowdsourcing to compare temporal, social temporal, and probability discounting among obese and non-obese individuals. Appetite.
28. Svaldi J, Tuschen-Caffier B, Peyk P, Blechert J (2010) Information processing of food pictures in binge eating disorder. Appetite 55: 685–694.
29. Brooks S, Prince A, Stahl D, Campbell IC, Treasure J (2011) A systematic review and meta-analysis of cognitive bias to food stimuli in people with disordered eating behaviour. Clin Psychol Rev 31: 37–51.
30. Schebendach J, Broft A, Foltin RW, Walsh BT (2013) Can the reinforcing value of food be measured in bulimia nervosa? Appetite 62: 70–75.
31. Hawk LW Jr., Baschnagel JS, Ashare RL, Epstein LH (2004) Craving and startle modification during in vivo exposure to food cues. Appetite 43: 285–294.
32. di Pellegrino G, Magarelli S, Mengarelli F (2011) Food pleasantness affects visual selective attention. Q J Exo Psychol 64: 560–571.
33. Miller EK, Cohen JD (2001) An integrative theory of prefrontal cortex function. Annu Rev Neurosci 24: 167–202.
34. Botvinick MM, Braver TS, Barch DM, Carter CS, Cohen JD (2001) Conflict monitoring and cognitive control. Psychol Rev 108: 624–652.
35. Hajcak G, Foti D (2008) Errors are aversive: defensive motivation and the error-related negativity. Psychol Sci 19: 103–108.
36. Ridderinkhof KR, van den Wildenberg WPM, Segalowitz SJ, Carter CS (2004) Neurocognitive mechanisms of cognitive control: the role of prefrontal cortex in action selection, response inhibition, performance monitoring, and reward-based learning. Brain Cogn 56: 129–140.
37. Holroyd CB, Coles MGH (2002) The neural basis of human error processing: Reinforcement learning, dopamine, and the error-related negativity. Psychol Rev 109: 679–709.
38. Yeung N, Botvinick MM, Cohen JD (2004) The neural basis of error detection: conflict monitoring and the error-related negativity. Psychol Rev 111: 931–959.
39. Shackman AJ, Salomons TV, Slagter HA, Fox AS, Winter JJ, et al. (2011) The integration of negative affect, pain and cognitive control in the cingulate cortex. Nat Rev Neurosci 12: 154–67.
40. Frank MJ, Woroch BS, Curran T (2005) Error-related negativity predicts reinforcement learning and conflict biases. Neuron 47: 495–501.
41. Falkenstein M, Hohnsbein J, Hoormann J (1991) Effects of crossmodal divided attention on late ERP components. II. Error processing in choice reaction tasks. Electroen Clin Neuro 78: 447–455.
42. Gehring WJ, Coles MGH, Meyer DE, Donchin E (1995) A brain potential manifestation of error-related processing. In Karmos G, Molnar M, Csepe V, Czigler I, Desmedt JE (Eds) Perspectives on Event-Related Potential Research. Electroen Clin Neuro 44.
43. Miltner WH, Lemke U, Weiss T, Holroyd C, Scheffers MK, et al. (2003) Implementation of error-processing in the human anterior cingulate cortex: a source analysis of the magnetic equivalent of the error-related negativity. Biol Psychol 64: 157–166.
44. Nieuwenhuis S, Ridderinkhof KR, Blom J, Band GPH, Kok A (2001) Error-related brain potentials are differentially related to awareness of response errors: evidence from an antisaccade task. Psychophysiol 38: 752–760.
45. Luu P, Collins P, Tucker DM (2000) Mood, personality, and self-monitoring: negative affect and emotionality in relation to frontal lobe mechanisms of error monitoring. J Exp Psychol Gen 129: 43–60.
46. van der Helden J, Boksem MA, Blom JH (2010) The importance of failure: feedback-related negativity predicts motor learning efficiency. Cereb Cortex 20: 1596–1603.
47. Fujita K, Han HA (2009) Moving beyond deliberative control of impulses: the effect of construal levels on evaluative associations in self-control conflicts. Psychol Sci 20: 799–804.
48. Brown JW, Braver TS (2005) Learned predictions of error likelihood in the anterior cingulate cortex. Science 307: 1118–1121.
49. Sellitto M, Ciaramelli E, di Pellegrino G (2010) Myopic discounting of future rewards after medial orbitofrontal damage in humans. J Neurosci 30: 16429–16436.
50. Kringelbach ML (2004) Food for thought: hedonic experience beyond homeostasis in the human brain. Neuroscience 126: 807–819.
51. Seibt B, Hafner M, Deutsch R (2007) Prepared to eat: How immediate affective and motivational responses to food cues are influenced by food deprivation. Eur J Soc Psychol 37: 359–379.
52. Stafford LD, Scheffler G (2008) Hunger inhibits negative associations to food but not auditory biases in attention. Appetite 1–15.
53. Piech RM, Lewis J, Parkinson CH, Owen AM, Roberts AC, et al. (2009) Neural correlates of appetite and hunger-related evaluative judgments. PLOS One 4: e6581.
54. Lappalainen R, Epstein LH (1990) A behavioral economics analysis of food choice in humans. Appetite 14: 81–93.
55. Epstein LH, Paluch R, Coleman KJ (1996) Differences in salivation to repeated food cues in obese and nonobese women. Psychosom Med 58: 160–164.
56. Epstein LH, Truesdale R, Wojcik A, Paluch RA, Raynor HA (2003) Effects of deprivation on hedonics and reinforcing value of food. Physiol Behav 78: 221–7.
57. Beer-Borst S, Hercberg S, Morabia A, Bernstein MS, Galan P, et al. (2000) Dietary patterns in six European populations: results from EURALIM, a collaborative European data harmonization and information campaign. Eur J Clin Nutr 54: 253–262.
58. Bates K, Burton S, Howlett E, Huggins K (2009) The roles of gender and motivation as moderators of the effects of calorie and nutrient information provision on away-from-home foods. J Consum Aff 43: 249–273.
59. DelParigi A, Chen K, Gautier J, Salbe AD, Pratley RE, et al. (2002) Sex differences in the human brain' s response to hunger and satiation. Am J Clin Nutr 75: 1017–22.
60. Smeets PAM, De Graaf C, Stafleu A, Van Osch MJP, Nievelstein RAJ, et al. (2006) Effect of satiety on brain activation during chocolate tasting in men and women. Am J Clin Nutr 83: 1297–1305.
61. Michalska KJ, Kinzler KD, Decety J (2013) Age-related sex differences in explicit measures of empathy do not predict brain responses across childhood and adolescence. Dev Cogn Neurosci 3: 22–32.
62. International Committee of Medical Journal Editors (1991) Statements from the Vancouver group. Brit Med J 302: 1194.
63. Smalley KJ, Knerr AN, Kendrick ZV, Colliver JA, Owen OE (1990) Reassessment of body mass indices. Am J Clin Nutr 52: 405–408.
64. Borghans L, Golsteyn BHH (2006) Time discounting and the body mass index: Evidence from the Netherlands. Econ Hum Biol 4: 39–61.
65. Van Strien T, Bergers GPA, Defares PB (1986) The Dutch Eating Behavior Questionnaire (DEBQ) for assessment of restrained, emotional, and external eating behavior. Int J Eat Disorder 5: 295–315.
66. Logan GD, Cowan WB (1984) On the ability to inhibit thought and action: a theory of an act of control. Psychol Rev 91: 295–327.
67. Bickel WK, Pitcock JA, Yi R, Angtuaco EJ (2009) Congruence of BOLD response across intertemporal choice conditions: fictive and real money gains and losses. J Neurosci 29: 8839–8846.
68. Johnson MW, Bickel WK (2002) Within-subject comparison of real and hypothetical money rewards in delay discounting. J Exp Anal Behav 77: 129–146.
69. Kirby KN, Herrnstein RJ (1995) Preference reversals due to myopic discounting of delayed reward. Psychol Sci 6: 83–89.
70. Myerson J, Green L, Hanson JS, Holt DD, Estle SJ (2003) Discounting delayed and probabilistic rewards: Processes and traits. J Econ Psychol 24: 619–635.
71. Estle SJ, Green L, Myerson J, Holt DD (2007) Discounting of monetary and directly consumable rewards. Psychol Sci 18: 58–63.
72. Mazur JE (1987) An adjusting procedure for studying delayed reinforcement. In: Quantitative analyses of behavior: The effect of delay and of intervening events on reinforcement value (Eds), 55–73. Hillsdale, NJ: Erlbaum.
73. Rachlin H, Raineri A, Cross D (1991) Subjective probability and delay. J Exp Anal Behav 55: 233–244.
74. Green L, Myerson J (2004) A discounting framework for choice with delayed and probabilistic rewards. Psychol Bull 130: 769–792.
75. Caccialanza R, Nicholls D, Cena H, Maccarini L, Rezzani C, et al. (2004) Validation of the Dutch Eating Behaviour Questionnaire parent version (DEBQ-P) in the Italian population: a screening tool to detect differences in eating behaviour among obese, overweight and normal-weight preadolescents. Eur J Clin Nutr 58: 1217–1222.
76. Odum AL, Rainaud CP (2003) Discounting of delayed hypothetical money, alcohol, and food. Behav Processes 64: 305–313.
77. Charlton SR, Fantino E (2008) Commodity specific rates of temporal discounting: does metabolic function underlie differences in rates of discounting? Behav Processes 77: 334–342.
78. Bos PA, Terburg D, Van Honk J (2010) Testosterone decreases trust in socially naïve humans Proc Nat Acad Sci U S A 1–5.
79. Channon S, Hayward A (1990) The effect of short-term fasting on processing of food cues in normal subjects. Int J Eat Disorder 9: 447–452.
80. Mogg K, Bradley BP, Hyare H, Lee S (1998) Selective attention to food-related stimuli in hunger: Are attentional biases specific to emotional and psycho-pathological states, or are they also found in normal drive states? Behav Res Ther 36: 227–237.
81. Seibt B, Häfner M, Deutsch R (2007) Prepared to eat: how immediate affective and motivational responses to food cues are influenced by food deprivation. Eur J Soc Psychol 37: 359–379.

82. Wang XT, Dvorak RD (2010) Sweet future: fluctuating blood glucose levels affect future discounting. Psychol Sci 21: 183–188.
83. Wagner DD, Altman M, Boswell RG, Kelley WM, Heatherton TF (2013) Self-regulatory depletion enhances neural responses to rewards and impairs top-down control. Psychol Sci 24: 2262–2271.
84. Wagner DD, Boswell RG, Kelley WM, Heatherton TF (2012) Inducing negative affect increases the reward value of appetizing foods in dieters. J Cogn Neurosci 24: 1625–1633.
85. Heatherton TF, Wagner DD (2011) Cognitive neuroscience of self-regulation failure. Trends Cogn Sci 15: 132–139.
86. Botvinick MM (2007) Conflict monitoring and decision making: reconciling two perspectives on anterior cingulate function. Cogn Affect Behav Neurosci 7: 356–366.
87. McClure SM, Ericson KM, Laibson DI, Loewenstein G, Cohen JD (2007) Time discounting for primary rewards. J Neurosci 27: 5796–5804.
88. Bickel WK, Yi R (2008) Temporal discounting as a measure of executive function: Insights from the competing neurobehavioral decision system hypothesis of addiction. In: Houser D, McCabe K, editors. Neuroeconomics: Advances in health economics and health services research. Bingley, UK: Emerald; 289–310.
89. Cook EW III, Turpin G (1997) Differentiating orienting, startle, and defense responses: The role of affect and its implications for psychopathology. In Lang PJ, Simons RF, Balaban MT (Eds.), Attention and orienting: Sensory and motivational processes (137–164). Hillsdale, NJ: Erlbaum.
90. Notebaert W, Houtman F, Van Opstal F, Gevers W, Fias W, et al. (2009) Post-error slowing: an orienting account. Cognition 111: 275–279.
91. Schultz W (1998) Predictive reward signal of dopamine neurons predictive reward signal of dopamine neurons. J Neurophysiol 80: 1–27.
92. Inzlicht M, Al-Khindi T (2012) ERN and the placebo: a misattribution approach to studying the arousal properties of the error-related negativity. J Exp Psychol 141: 799–807.
93. Bechara A, Damasio H, Tranel D, Damasio AR (1997) Deciding advantageously before knowing the advantageous strategy. Science 275: 1293–1295.
94. Bechara A, Damasio H, Damasio AR, Lee GP (1999) Different contributions of the human amygdala and ventromedial prefrontal cortex to decision-making. J Neurosci 19: 5473–5481.
95. Bechara A (2005) Decision making, impulse control and loss of willpower to resist drugs: a neurocognitive perspective. Nat Neurosci 8: 1458–1463.
96. Bechara A, Damasio AR (2005) The somatic marker hypothesis: a neural theory of economic decision. Games Econ Behav 52: 336–372.
97. Figner B, Knoch D, Johnson EJ, Krosch AR, Lisanby SH, et al. (2010) Lateral prefrontal cortex and self-control in intertemporal choice. Nat Neurosci 13: 538–539.
98. Valdesolo P, DeSteno D (2006) Manipulations of emotional context shape moral judgment. Psychol Sci 17: 476–477.
99. Luo S, Ainslie G, Monterosso J (2012) The behavioral and neural effect of emotional primes on intertemporal decisions. Soc Cogn Affect Neurosci 9: 283–291.
100. Myrseth KOR, Fishbach A (2009) Self-control: A function of knowing when and how to exercise restraint. Curr Dir Psychol Sci 18: 247–252.
101. Volkow ND, Wang GJ, Fowler JS, Tomasi D, Baler R (2011) Food and drug reward: Overlapping circuits in human obesity and addiction. Curr Top Behav Neurosci.
102. Avena NM, Rada P, Hoebel BG (2008) Underweight rats have enhanced dopamine release and blunted acetylcholine response in the nucleus accumbens while bingeing on sucrose. Neuroscience 156: 865–871.
103. Gearhardt AN, Yokum S, Orr PT, Stice E, Corbin WR, et al. (2011) Neural correlates of food addiction. Arch Gen Psychiatry 68: 808–816.
104. Umberg EN, Shader RI, Hsu LK, Greenblatt DJ (2012) From disordered eating to addiction: the "food drug" in bulimia nervosa. J Clin Psychopharmacol 32: 376–89.
105. Houben K, Nederkoorn C, Wiers RW, Jansen A (2011) Resisting temptation: decreasing alcohol-related affect and drinking behavior by training response inhibition. Drug Alcohol Depend 116: 132–136.
106. Kang MJ, Camerer CF (2013) fMRI evidence of a hot-cold empathy gap in hypothetical and real aversive choices. Front Neurosci 7: 104.
107. Fenske MJ, Raymond JE (2006) Affective influences of selective attention. Curr Dir Psychol Sci 15: 312–316.
108. Ferrey AE, Frischen A, Fenske MJ (2012) Hot or not: response inhibition reduces the hedonic value and motivational incentive of sexual stimuli. Front Psychol 3: 575.
109. Frischen A, Ferrey AE, Burt D, Pistchick M, Fenske MJ (2012) The affective consequences of inhibition: devaluation or neutralization? J Exp Psychol Hum Percept Perform 38: 169–179.

PERMISSIONS

All chapters in this book were first published in PLOS ONE, by The Public Library of Science; hereby published with permission under the Creative Commons Attribution License or equivalent. Every chapter published in this book has been scrutinized by our experts. Their significance has been extensively debated. The topics covered herein carry significant findings which will fuel the growth of the discipline. They may even be implemented as practical applications or may be referred to as a beginning point for another development.

The contributors of this book come from diverse backgrounds, making this book a truly international effort. This book will bring forth new frontiers with its revolutionizing research information and detailed analysis of the nascent developments around the world.

We would like to thank all the contributing authors for lending their expertise to make the book truly unique. They have played a crucial role in the development of this book. Without their invaluable contributions this book wouldn't have been possible. They have made vital efforts to compile up to date information on the varied aspects of this subject to make this book a valuable addition to the collection of many professionals and students.

This book was conceptualized with the vision of imparting up-to-date information and advanced data in this field. To ensure the same, a matchless editorial board was set up. Every individual on the board went through rigorous rounds of assessment to prove their worth. After which they invested a large part of their time researching and compiling the most relevant data for our readers.

The editorial board has been involved in producing this book since its inception. They have spent rigorous hours researching and exploring the diverse topics which have resulted in the successful publishing of this book. They have passed on their knowledge of decades through this book. To expedite this challenging task, the publisher supported the team at every step. A small team of assistant editors was also appointed to further simplify the editing procedure and attain best results for the readers.

Apart from the editorial board, the designing team has also invested a significant amount of their time in understanding the subject and creating the most relevant covers. They scrutinized every image to scout for the most suitable representation of the subject and create an appropriate cover for the book.

The publishing team has been an ardent support to the editorial, designing and production team. Their endless efforts to recruit the best for this project, has resulted in the accomplishment of this book. They are a veteran in the field of academics and their pool of knowledge is as vast as their experience in printing. Their expertise and guidance has proved useful at every step. Their uncompromising quality standards have made this book an exceptional effort. Their encouragement from time to time has been an inspiration for everyone.

The publisher and the editorial board hope that this book will prove to be a valuable piece of knowledge for researchers, students, practitioners and scholars across the globe.

LIST OF CONTRIBUTORS

Tongjit Thanchomnang
Research and Diagnostic Center for Emerging Infectious Diseases, Khon Kaen University, Khon Kaen, Thailand
Faculty of Medicine, Mahasarakham University, Mahasarakham, Thailand

Somjintana Tourtip
Faculty of Medicine, Mahasarakham University, Mahasarakham, Thailand

Chairat Tantrawatpan
Research and Diagnostic Center for Emerging Infectious Diseases, Khon Kaen University, Khon Kaen, Thailand
Division of Cell Biology, Department of Preclinical Sciences, Faculty of Medicine, Thammasat University, Rangsit Campus, Pathum Thani, Thailand

Pewpan M. Intapan, Oranuch Sanpool and Wanchai Maleewong
Research and Diagnostic Center for Emerging Infectious Diseases, Khon Kaen University, Khon Kaen, Thailand
Department of Parasitology, Faculty of Medicine, Khon Kaen University, Khon Kaen, Thailand

Penchom Janwan
Research and Diagnostic Center for Emerging Infectious Diseases, Khon Kaen University, Khon Kaen, Thailand
Department of Medical Technology, School of Allied Health Sciences and Public Health, Walailak University, Thasala, Nakhon Si Thammarat, Thailand

Viraphong Lulitanond
Research and Diagnostic Center for Emerging Infectious Diseases, Khon Kaen University, Khon Kaen, Thailand
Department of Microbiology, Faculty of Medicine, Khon Kaen University, Khon Kaen, Thailand

Hiroshi Yamasaki
Department of Parasitology, National Institute of Infectious Diseases, Tokyo, Japan

Renee M. Petr and Tim A. McAllister
Lethbridge Research Centre, Agriculture and Agri-Food Canada, Lethbridge, Alberta, Canada

Mike E. R. Dugan
Lacombe Research Centre, Agriculture and Agri-Food Canada, Lacombe, Alberta, Canada

Cletos Mapiye
Lacombe Research Centre, Agriculture and Agri-Food Canada, Lacombe, Alberta, Canada
Department of Animal Sciences, Faculty of AgriSciences, Stellenbosch University, Matieland, Western Cape, South Africa

Jan Klecka
Departmemt of Fish Ecology and Evolution, Eawag: Swiss Federal Institute of Aquatic Science and Technology, Kastanienbaum, Switzerland
Laboratory of Theoretical Ecology, Institute of Entomology, Biology Centre of the Academy of Sciences of the Czech Republic, České Budějovice, Czech Republic
Department of Ecosystems Biology, Faculty of Science, University of South Bohemia, České Budějovice, Czech Republic

Corina J. Logan
SAGE Center for the Study of the Mind, Department of Psychological and Brain Sciences, University of California Santa Barbara, Santa Barbara, California, United States of America

Sarah A. Jelbert, Russell D. Gray and Alex H. Taylor
School of Psychology, University of Auckland, Auckland, New Zealand

Alexis J. Breen
School of Psychology and Neuroscience, University of St Andrews, St Andrews, United Kingdom

Colin D. Rehm
Center for Public Health Nutrition, University of Washington, Seattle, Washington, United States of America

Adam Drewnowski
Center for Public Health Nutrition, University of Washington, Seattle, Washington, United States of America
Institute for Cardiometabolism and Nutrition, Groupe Hospitalier Pitié-Salpêtrière, Paris, France

Xueshu Xie and Roman A. Zubarev
Division of Physiological Chemistry I, Department of Medical Biochemistry and Biophysics, Karolinska Institutet, Stockholm, Sweden

Roger Schürch
Laboratory of Apiculture and Social Insects, School of Life Sciences, University of Sussex, Falmer, United Kingdom

Christoph Grüter
Departamento de Biologia da Faculdade de Filosofia, Ciências e Letras de Ribeirão Preto, Universidade de São Paulo, Ribeirão Preto, São Paulo, Brazil

Jan-Hendrik Hehemann, Adrienne Law and Alisdair B. Boraston
Department of Biochemistry & Microbiology, University of Victoria, Victoria, British Columbia, Canada

Lars Redecke
Joint Laboratory for Structural Biology of Infection and Inflammation of the Universities of Hamburg and Lübeck, c/o DESY, Hamburg, Germany

Matthew A. Davis
Children's Environmental Health and Disease Prevention Research Center at Dartmouth, Hanover, New Hampshire, United States of America
Institute for Quantitative Biomedical Sciences, Dartmouth College, Hanover, New Hampshire, United States of America
University of Michigan School of Nursing, Ann Arbor, Michigan, United States of America
Section of Biostatistics and Epidemiology, Department of Community and Family Medicine, Geisel School of Medicine at Dartmouth, Hanover, New Hampshire, United States of America

Jason H. Moore
Children's Environmental Health and Disease Prevention Research Center at Dartmouth, Hanover, New Hampshire, United States of America
Institute for Quantitative Biomedical Sciences, Dartmouth College, Hanover, New Hampshire, United States of America
Section of Biostatistics and Epidemiology, Department of Community and Family Medicine, Geisel School of Medicine at Dartmouth, Hanover, New Hampshire, United States of America
Department of Genetics, Geisel School of Medicine at Dartmouth, Hanover, New Hampshire, United States of America

H. Robert Frost
Institute for Quantitative Biomedical Sciences, Dartmouth College, Hanover, New Hampshire, United States of America
Section of Biostatistics and Epidemiology, Department of Community and Family Medicine, Geisel School of Medicine at Dartmouth, Hanover, New Hampshire, United States of America
Department of Genetics, Geisel School of Medicine at Dartmouth, Hanover, New

Scott M. Williams
Institute for Quantitative Biomedical Sciences, Dartmouth College, Hanover, New Hampshire, United States of America
Department of Genetics, Geisel School of Medicine at Dartmouth, Hanover, New

Diane Gilbert-Diamond, Margaret R. Karagas and Zhigang Li
Children's Environmental Health and Disease Prevention Research Center at Dartmouth, Hanover, New Hampshire, United States of America
Institute for Quantitative Biomedical Sciences, Dartmouth College, Hanover, New Hampshire, United States of America
Section of Biostatistics and Epidemiology, Department of Community and Family Medicine, Geisel School of Medicine at Dartmouth, Hanover, New Hampshire, United States of America

Anna Puig-Oliveras, Jordi Corominas, Josep M. Folch and Maria Ballester
Departament de Genètica Animal, Centre de Recerca en Agrigenòmica (CRAG), Bellaterra, Spain
Departament de Ciència Animal i dels Aliments, Universitat Autònoma de Barcelona (UAB), Bellaterra, Spain

Yuliaxis Ramayo-Caldas
Génétique Animale et Biologie Intégrative UMR1313 (GABI), Institut National de la Recherche Agronomique (INRA), Jouy-en-Josas, France

Jordi Estellé
Génétique Animale et Biologie Intégrative UMR1313 (GABI), Institut National de la Recherche Agronomique (INRA), Jouy-en-Josas, France
Géné tique Animale et Biologie Intégrative UMR1313 (GABI), AgroParisTech, Jouy-en-Josas, France
Laboratoire de Radiobiologie et Etude du Génome (LREG), Commissariat à l'énergie atomique et aux énergies alternatives (CEA), Jouy-en-Josas, France

Dafne Pérez-Montarelo
Departamento de Genética Animal, Instituto Nacional de Investigación y Tecnología Agraria y Alimentaria (INIA), Madrid, Spain

Nicholas J. Hudson
Computational and Systems Biology, Commonwealth Scientific and Industrial Research Organisation (CSIRO) Animal, Food and Health SciencesQLD, Brisbane, Australia

Joaquim Casellas
Departament de Ciència Animal i dels Aliments, Universitat Autònoma de Barcelona (UAB), Bellaterra, Spain
Departament de Genética i Millora Animal, Institut de Recerca i Tecnologies Agroalimentàries (IRTA), Lleida, Spain

Wei Zhao, Weizhe Zhang, Aiqin Liu and Fengkun Yang
Department of Parasitology, Harbin Medical University, Harbin, Heilongjiang, China

Longxian Zhang and Rongjun Wang
College of Animal Science and Veterinary Medicine, Henan Agricultural University Zhengzhou, Henan, China

Jianping Cao and Yujuan Shen
National Institute of Parasitic Diseases, Chinese Center for Disease Control and Prevention, Key Laboratory of Parasite and Vector Biology, Ministry of Health, WHO Collaborating Centre for Malaria, Schistosomiasis and Filariasis, Shanghai, China

Ruth Chan and Jean Woo
Department of Medicine and Therapeutics, The Chinese University of Hong Kong, Shatin, Hong Kong

Dicken Chan
The Jockey Club School of Public Health and Primary Care, The Chinese University of Hong Kong, Shatin, Hong Kong

Kim R. Hill, Jacopo Baggio, A. Magdalena Hurtado and Robert T. Boyd
School of Human Evolution and Social Change, Arizona State University, Tempe, Arizona, United States of America

Brian M. Wood
Department of Anthropology, Yale University, New Haven, Connecticut, United States of America

Stephanie M. Greer, William J. Jagust, Mark D9Esposito and Deanna L. Wallace
Helen Wills Neuroscience Institute, University of California, Berkeley, California, United States of America
Center for Cognitive Neuroimaging, Donders Institute for Brain, Cognition and Behaviour, Radboud University, Nijmegen, The Netherlands

Linh C. Dang
Helen Wills Neuroscience Institute, University of California, Berkeley, California, United States of America
Department of Psychology, Vanderbilt University, Nashville, Tennessee, United States of America

Esther Aarts
Helen Wills Neuroscience Institute, University of California, Berkeley, California, United States of America
Center for Cognitive Neuroimaging, Donders Institute for Brain, Cognition and Behaviour, Radboud University, Nijmegen, The Netherlands

Zhao-min Liu, Nelson Tang, Ruth Chan and Jean Woo
Department of Medicine &Therapeutics, the Chinese University of Hong Kong, Hong Kong Special Administrative Region, PR, China

Suzanne C. Ho
Division of Epidemiology, The Jockey Club School of Public Health and Primary Care, the Chinese University of Hong Kong, Hong Kong Special Administrative Region, PR, China

Yu-ming Chen
Department of Medical Statistics and Epidemiology, School of Public Health, Sun Yat-sen University, Guangzhou, PR, China

Daniel R. Taber and Jamie F. Chriqui
Institute for Health Research and Policy, University of Illinois at Chicago, Chicago, Illinois, United States of America

Renee Vuillaume
John F. Kennedy School of Government, HarvardUniversity, Cambridge, Massachusetts, United States of America

Frank J. Chaloupka
Institute for Health Research and Policy, University of Illinois at Chicago, Chicago, Illinois, United States of America
Department of Economics, University of Illinois at Chicago, Chicago, Illinois, United States of America

Lai Kuan Tan and Kwai Lin Thong
Microbiology Division, Institute of Biological Sciences, Faculty of Science, University of Malaya, Kuala Lumpur, Malaysia

Peck Toung Ooi
Department of Clinical Veterinary Studies, Faculty of Veterinary Medicine, University Putra Malaysia, Serdang, Malaysia

Elisabeth Carniel
Yersinia Research Unit, National Reference Laboratory and WHO Collaborating Centre for Yersinia, Institut Pasteur, Paris, France

Toshihiro Imada, Shigeru Nakamura and Kazuo Tsubota
Department of Ophthalmology, Keio University School of Medicine, Tokyo, Japan

Naoki Kitamura and Izumi Shibuya
Department of Veterinary Physiology, Faculty of Agriculture, Tottori University, Tottori, Japan

Katrina Brudzynski and Calvin Sjaarda
Bee-Biomedicals Inc., Drug Discovery and Development Department, St. Catharines, Ontario, Canada

Wei Zhang, Jing Wang and Peilong Wang
Key Laboratory of Agrifood Safety and Quality, Ministry of Agriculture, Beijing, P.R. China
Institute of Quality Standards and Testing Technology for Agriculture Products, China Agricultural Academy of Science, Beijing, P.R. China

Ruohua Zhu and Jing Jia
Department of Chemistry, Capital Normal University, Beijing, China Erik J. Tillman, Donald

Steven J. Swoap
Department of Biology, Williams College, Williamstown, Massachusetts, United States of America

A. Morgan and Kamal Rahmouni
Department of Pharmacology, University of Iowa Carver College of Medicine, Iowa City, Iowa, United States of America

Hana Kahleova, Hana Malinska, Olena Oliyarnyk, Ludmila Kazdova and Terezie Pelikanova
Institute for Clinical and Experimental Medicine, Prague, Czech Republic

Lenka Belinova
Institute for Clinical and Experimental Medicine, Prague, Czech Republic
First Faculty of Medicine, Charles University, Prague, Czech Republic

Ondrej Topolcan and Jindra Vrzalova
University Hospital in Pilsen, Pilsen, Czech Republic

Martin Hill
Institute of Endocrinology, Prague, Czech Republic

Mariecia D. Fraser, Hannah R. Fleming and Jon M. Moorby
Institute of Biological, Environmental and Rural Sciences, AberyWstwyth University, Aberystwyth, Ceredigion, United Kingdom

Jinchuan Liu, Wenhui Bai, Zhenzhen Lv, Xiaoling Jiang, Shuming Yang and Ailiang Chen
Institute of Quality Standards and Testing Technology for Agro-products, Key Laboratory of Agro-product Quality and Safety, Chinese Academy of Agricultural Sciences; Key Laboratory of Agro-food Quality and Safety, Ministry of Agriculture, Beijing, China

Zheng Guan
Institute of Quality Standards and Testing Technology for Agro-products, Key Laboratory of Agro-product Quality and Safety, Chinese Academy of Agricultural Sciences; Key Laboratory of Agro-food Quality and Safety, Ministry of Agriculture, Beijing, China
Institute of Materia Medica, Zhejiang Chinese Medical University, Hangzhou, China

Guiyuan Lv
Institute of Materia Medica, Zhejiang Chinese Medical University, Hangzhou, China

Manuela Sellitto and Giuseppe di Pellegrino
Dipartimento di Psicologia, Università di Bologna, Bologna, Italy
Centro studi e ricerche in Neuroscienze Cognitive, Polo Scientifico-Didattico di Cesena, Cesena, Italy

Index